MOVEMENT DISORDERS: TREMOR

MOVEMENT DISORDERS: TREMOR

Edited by

Leslie J. Findley

Consultant Neurologist, Regional Centre for Neurology and Neurosurgery,
Oldchurch Hospital, Romford, and Harold Wood Hospital, Romford, Essex;
Visiting Consultant Neurologist, Queen Elizabeth Military Hospital,
Woolwich, London; and Research Neurologist, MRC Neuro-Otology Unit,
Institute of Neurology, The National Hospital, Queen Square, London

and

Rudy Capildeo

Consultant Neurologist, Regional Centre for Neurology and Neurosurgery,
Oldchurch Hospital, Romford; and
Consultant Neurologist, Basildon and Orsett Hospitals, Essex

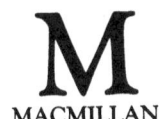

MACMILLAN

First published 1984 by
The Scientific and Medical Division
THE MACMILLAN PRESS LTD
London and Basingstoke
Associated companies in Auckland, Delhi, Dublin, Gaborone, Hamburg, Harare, Hong Kong, Johannesburg, Kuala Lumpur, Lagos, Manzini, Melbourne, Mexico City, Nairobi, New York, Singapore and Tokyo

ISBN 978-1-349-06759-6   ISBN 978-1-349-06757-2 (eBook)
DOI 10.1007/978-1-349-06757-2

Contents

Contributors   ix

Preface   xv

SECTION 1   GENERAL ASPECTS   1
1   Classification of tremor   3
    R. Capildeo and L. J. Findley
2   Definition, analysis and genesis of tremor   15
    M. A. Gresty and L. J. Findley
3   Differential diagnosis of motor disorders by tremor analysis   27
    H.-J. Freund, H. Hefter, V. Hömberg and K. Reiners
4   Origins of normal and pathological tremor   37
    C. D. Marsden
5   Pharmacological differentiation of tremor   85
    S. Fahn
6   Pathology of tremor   95
    A. Marshall

SECTION 2   NEUROPHYSIOLOGY OF TREMOR   125
7   Physiological and enhanced physiological tremor   127
    R. R. Young
8   Segmental reflex, muscle mechanical and central mechanisms
    underlying human physiological tremor   135
    J. H. J. Allum
9   Muscle spindle discharge patterns in tremor and clonus   157
    K.-E. Hagbarth
10   Rebound excitation as the physiological basis for tremor: a
    biophysical study of the oscillatory properties of mammalian
    central neurones *in vitro*   165
    R. R. Llinás
11   Animals models of physiological, essential and parkinsonian-like
    tremors   183
    Y. Lamarre
12   Determinants of tremor rate   195
    H.-J. Freund, H. Hefter, V. Hömberg and K. Reiners

SECTION 3   ESSENTIAL TREMOR   205

13   Essential tremor: introductory remarks   207
          L. J. Findley
14   Epidemiology of essential tremor   211
          I. Rautakorpi, R. J. Marttila and U. K. Rinne
15   Problems in the differential diagnosis of essential tremor   219
          P. Salisachs and L. J. Findley
16   Beta-adrenoceptor involvement in tremor production: possible
          defects in essential tremor   225
          S. Kilfeather, A. Massarella, P. Turner and L. J. Findley
17   Essential tremor: treatment with beta-adrenoceptor blocking drugs   245
          J. F. Wilson, R. W. Marshall and A. Richens
18   D,L-Propranolol and D-propranolol in essential tremor   261
          S. Calzetti and L. J. Findley
19   Primidone in essential tremor   271
          L. J. Findley, S. Calzetti and L. Cleeves

SECTION 4   THE TREMORS OF PARKINSON'S DISEASE   283

20   Parkinson's disease complex—restyling an old overcoat!   285
          R. Capildeo
21   Tremor and rhythmical involuntary movements in Parkinson's disease   295
          L. J. Findley and M. A. Gresty
22   Neurochemical basis of parkinsonian tremor   305
          P. Jenner and C. D. Marsden
23   Assessment of resting tremor in Parkinson's disease   321
          M. A. Gresty, R. McCarthy and L. J. Findley
24   Medical treatment of tremor in Parkinson's disease   331
          J. A. Obeso and J. M. Martinez Lage
25   Surgical treatment of tremor   339
          J. Andrew

SECTION 5   CEREBELLAR TREMOR   353

26   Cerebellar tremor: clinical aspects   355
          S. Fahn
27   Motor control in cerebellar tremor   365
          P. Rondot and N. Bathien
28   Treatment of cerebellar tremor   377
          N. J. Legg

SECTION 6   TREMORS IN PERIPHERAL NEUROPATHY   387

29   Tremor associated with peripheral neuropathy   389
          B. T. Shahani

30 Tremor in peripheral neuropathy   399
        I. S. Smith, P. Furness and P. K. Thomas

SECTION 7   TREMULOUS AND TREMOR-LIKE MOVEMENTS
                       OF THE EYES   407
31 Mechanisms of ocular oscillations   409
        D. S. Zee and L. M. Optican
32 Pendular nystagmus (ocular myoclonus) and related somatic tremors:
        their pharmacological modification and treatment   421
        J. J. Ell, L. J. Findley and M. A. Gresty

SECTION 8   DIVERSE TREMULOUS STATES   429
33 Atypical tremors, rare tremors and unclassified tremors   431
        S. Fahn
34 Drug-induced tremor   445
        R. M. Pinder
35 Tremor in relation to certain other movement disorders   463
        R. R. Young

SECTION 9   SIGNIFICANCE OF TREMOR IN THE ONTOGENY
                       OF THE NERVOUS SYSTEM   473
36 Possible role of tremor in the organisation of the nervous system   475
        R. R. Llinás

Glossary of terms   479

Index   487

Contributors

J. H. J. Allum
Brain Research Institute,
University of Zürich; and
HNO Klinik,
Kantonsspital,
CH-4031 Basel,
Switzerland

J. Andrew
Department of Neurosurgery,
The Middlesex Hospital,
Mortimer Street,
London W1; and
Regional Centre for Neurology and Neurosurgery,
Oldchurch Hospital,
Romford,
Essex

N. Bathien
Centre Hospitalier Sainte-Anne,
Faculté de Médecine Cochin Port-Royal,
Service de Neurologie,
1 Rue Cabanis,
75674 Paris,
France

S. Calzetti
Istituto di Clinica Neurologica,
Via del Quartiere 4,
I-43100 Parma,
Italy; and
MRC Neuro-Otology Unit,
Institute of Neurology,
The National Hospital,
Queen Square,
London WC1N 3BG

R. Capildeo
Regional Centre for Neurology and Neurosurgery,
Oldchurch Hospital,
Romford,
Essex

Lynn Cleeves
Regional Centre for Neurology and Neurosurgery,
Oldchurch Hospital,
Romford,
Essex

J. J. Ell
    MRC Neuro-Otology Unit,
    Institute of Neurology,
    The National Hospital,
    Queen Square,
    London WC1N 3BG

S. Fahn
    Department of Neurology,
    College of Physicians and Surgeons,
    Columbia University,
    New York; and
    The Neurological Institute,
    710 West 168th Street,
    New York,
    NY 10032,
    USA

L. J. Findley
    Regional Centre for Neurology and Neurosurgery,
    Oldchurch Hospital,
    Romford,
    Essex; and
    MRC Neuro-Otology Unit,
    Institute of Neurology,
    The National Hospital,
    Queen Square,
    London WC1N 3BG

H.-J. Freund,
    Medizinische Einrichtungen der Universitat Düsseldorf,
    Neurologische Klinik,
    Morrenstrasse 5,
    4000 Düsseldorf 1,
    West Germany

P. Furness
    Institute of Neurology,
    The National Hospital,
    Queen Square,
    London WC1N 3BG

M. A. Gresty
    MRC Neuro-Otology Unit,
    Institute of Neurology,
    The National Hospital,
    Queen Square,
    London WC1N 3BG

K.-E. Hagbarth
    Department of Clinical Neurophysiology,
    University Hospital,
    S-751 85 Uppsala,
    Sweden

H. Hefter
     Medizinische Einrichtungen der Universitat Düsseldorf,
     Neurologische Klinik,
     Morrenstrasse 5,
     4000 Düsseldorf 1,
     West Germany

V. Hömberg
     Medizinische Einrichtungen der Universitat Düsseldorf,
     Neurologische Klinik,
     Morrenstrasse 5,
     4000 Düsseldorf 1,
     West Germany

P. Jenner
     University Department of Neurology,
     Institute of Psychiatry and King's College Hospital Medical School,
     De Crespigny Park,
     Denmark Hill,
     London SE5 8AF

S. Kilfeather
     Department of Clinical Pharmacology,
     St Bartholomew's Hospital Medical College,
     London EC1A 7BE

Y. Lamarre
     Centre de Recherche en Sciences Neurologiques,
     Faculté de Médecine,
     Université de Montréal,
     CP 6128 A, Montréal,
     Québec,
     H3C 3J7,
     Canada

N. J. Legg
     Royal Postgraduate Medical School,
     Hammersmith Hospital,
     Ducane Road,
     London W12 0HS

R. R. Llinás
     Department of Physiology and Biophysics,
     New York University Medical Center,
     School of Medicine,
     550 First Avenue,
     New York,
     NY 10016,
     USA

Rosaleen McCarthy
     Department of Psychology,
     The National Hospital,
     Queen Square,
     London WC1N 3BG

C. D. Marsden
University Department of Neurology,
Institute of Psychiatry and King's College Hospital Medical School,
De Crespigny Park,
Denmark Hill,
London SE5 8AF

Ann Marshall
Department of Neuropathology,
Regional Centre for Neurology and Neurosurgery,
Oldchurch Hospital,
Romford,
Essex

R. W. Marshall
Department of Pharmacology and Therapeutics,
Welsh National School of Medicine,
Heath Park,
Cardiff CF4 4XN

J. M. Martínez Lage
Department de Neurologia,
Clinica Universitaria,
Facultad de Medicina,
Universidad de Navarra,
Pamplona,
Spain

R. J. Marttila
Department of Neurology,
University of Turku,
SF-20520 Turku 52,
Finland

A. Massarella
Department of Clinical Pharmacology,
St Bartholomew's Hospital,
London EC1A 7BE

J. A. Obeso
Department de Neurologia,
Clinica Universitaria,
Facultad de Medicina,
Universidad de Navarra,
Pamplona,
Spain

L. M. Optican
Clinical Branch and Laboratory of Sensorimotor Research,
National Institutes of Health,
Bethesda, MD; and
Departments of Neurology and Ophthalmology,
Johns Hopkins Hospital,
600 North Wolfe Street,
Baltimore,
MD 21205,
USA

R. Pinder
    Scientific Development Group,
    Organon,
    Oss,
    The Netherlands

I. Rautakorpi
    Department of Neurology,
    University of Turku,
    SF-20520 Turku 52; and
    Department of Neurology,
    Lappi Central Hospital,
    SF-97145 Totonvaara,
    Finland

K. Reiners
    Medizinische Einrichtungen der Universitat Düsseldorf,
    Neurologische Klinik,
    Morrenstrasse 5,
    4000 Düsseldorf 1,
    West Germany

A. Richens
    Department of Pharmacology and Therapeutics,
    Welsh National School of Medicine,
    Heath Park,
    Cardiff CF4 4XN

U. K. Rinne
    Department of Neurology,
    University of Turku,
    SF-20520 Turku 52,
    Finland

P. Rondot
    Centre Hospitalier Sainte-Anne,
    Faculté de Médecine Cochin Port-Royal,
    Service de Neurologie,
    1 Rue Cabanis,
    75674 Paris,
    France

P. Salisachs
    MRC Neuro-Otology Unit,
    The National Hospital,
    Queen Square,
    London WC1N 3BG; and
    Servicio de Neurologia,
    Residencia Sanitaria de la Seguridad Social,
    Badalona,
    Barcelona,
    Spain

B. T. Shahani
Clinical Neurophysiology Laboratory,
Department of Neurology,
Massachusetts General Hospital and Harvard Medical School,
Fruit Street,
Boston,
MA 02114,
USA

I. S. Smith
Department of Clinical Neurophysiology,
The National Hospital,
Queen Square,
London WC1N 3BG

P. K. Thomas
Institute of Neurology,
The National Hospital,
Queen Square,
London WC1N 3BG

P. Turner
Department of Clinical Pharmacology,
St Bartholomew's Hospital,
London EC1A 7BE

J. F. Wilson
Department of Pharmacology and Therapeutics,
Welsh National School of Medicine,
Heath Park,
Cardiff CF4 4XN

R. R. Young
Movement Disorder Clinic and Clinical Neurophysiology Laboratory,
Department of Neurology,
Massachusetts General Hospital and Harvard Medical School,
Fruit Street,
Boston,
MA 02114,
USA

D. S. Zee
Clinical Branch and Laboratory of Sensorimotor Research,
National Institutes of Health,
Bethesda, MD; and
Departments of Neurology and Ophthalmology,
Johns Hopkins Hospital,
600 North Wolfe Street,
Baltimore,
MD 21205,
USA

Preface

Tremor is a manifestation of normal or abnormal functioning of the nervous system. Although our knowledge of the causes of tremor is incomplete, it is apparent that all tremors involve a combination of peripheral and central mechanisms. These mechanisms are diverse in nature, including the passive mechanical properties of body appendages, oscillatory instabilities in both short and long 'reflex' loops and intrinsic electrochemical instabilities in individual neurones and neuronal assemblages. Thus the study of tremors is of necessity a multidisciplinary undertaking.

This book presents the views of specialists from various disciplines who share a common interest in tremor phenomena. The participants joined in a 'workshop' whose aim was to forge an integrative approach to tremor research. The contributions represent individual approaches to the subject, written retrospectively and tempered by the discussions that took place.

The purpose of the book is to give a comprehensive, current account of the 'state of the art' in tremor research. Sections are included dealing with techniques of tremor analysis, normal and abnormal physiology, epidemiology, anatomical and chemical pathology, behavioural neurology, pharmacology, and medical and surgical treatment.

It was apparent to all participants that the initial and considerable difficulty confronting discussion of tremor was semasiological. For this reason, a glossary of definitions has been appended. The definitions in this glossary are not those necessarily adopted throughout the book but are based on a consensus view of the editors, and of Professor David Marsden FRS and Dr Michael Gresty. The intention of the glossary is to provoke comment, criticism and further clarification of terms so that, eventually, we may arrive at a universally acceptable terminology.

The editors would like to acknowledge the help of Dr Michael Gresty in advising on the scientific contributions to this volume and Professor David Marsden FRS for his support and encouragement. The workshop was supported financially by a charitable grant from Sandoz Products Limited.

Spring 1984   Leslie J. Findley and Rudy Capildeo

SECTION 1
GENERAL ASPECTS

1
Classification of tremor

RUDY CAPILDEO and LESLIE J. FINDLEY

INTRODUCTION

The classification most widely used throughout the world is that published by the World Health Organisation and revised every 10 years. The Ninth International Statistical Classification of Diseases, Injuries and Causes of Death (ICD 9) was revised in 1974 and volume 1 published in 1977 and volume 2 in 1978. In the United Kingdom all hospital discharge summaries have up to five diagnoses listed and each diagnosis is coded using the WHO classification. This information is collected regionally and forms the basis for the Hospital Inpatient Activities Analysis. It has not yet been extended to outpatient clinics or general practitioner surgeries. The WHO classification is based on a four-digit code. The Ninth Revision has been strongly criticised by Kurtzke (1979) who has demonstrated that ICD 9 is 'a regression toward a less specific and more symptom-orientated code than its predecessors. It is particularly poor in the category of neurologic disorders with admixtures of disparate entities even at the fourth-digit level. This holds also for neurologic states coded under circulatory, musculo-skeletal and congenital anomalies sections.'

There is no universally accepted definition or classification of tremor. In ICD 9 tremor is classified in both section VI 'Diseases of the nervous system and sense organs' and also in section XVI 'Symptoms, signs and ill-defined conditions'. In section VI, tremor is classified after Parkinson's disease (see table). It will be noted that the remaining digits, 332.2 to 332.9, have not been used to specify which type of parkinsonism. If the terms were more accurately defined and anachronisms removed (viz. paralysis agitans) then parkinsonism 'not otherwise specified' could have been separated from 'idiopathic' parkinsonism. With tremor only a single digit is available, viz. '333.1 Essential and other specified forms of tremor' namely 'Benign essential tremor and familial tremor'. There is no room for expansion since 333.2 is 'Myoclonus' followed by a diverse group of disorders from 'Tics' to 'Huntington's chorea'. In section XVI, 'Tremor, not otherwise specified' is classified with 'Abnormal head movements, fasciculation and spasm' under 781.0 (see table).

With the strict adherence to a four-digit code there is little room for adaptation. Yet, within the WHO classification, the section on 'Morphology of neo-

WHO classification (ICD 9)
Section VI   Diseases of the nervous system and sense organs

332	Parkinson's disease

332.0	Paralysis agitans
	Parkinsonism or Parkinson's disease
	    NOS*
	    idiopathic
	    primary

332.1	Secondary parkinsonism
	Parkinsonism
	    due to drugs
	    syphilitic (094.8)
	Use additional E code † if desired to identify drug, if drug-induced

333	Other extrapyramidal disease and abnormal movement disorders
	    Includes: other forms of extrapyramidal basal ganglia or striato-pallidal disease
	    Excludes: abnormal movements of head NOS* (781.0)

333.1	Essential and other specified forms of tremor
	    Benign essential tremor Familial tremor
	    Use additional E code
	    Excludes: tremor NOS* (781.0)

(See text for reference)
*NOS = not otherwise specified
†E code = external causes

WHO classification (ICD 9)
Section XVI   Symptoms, signs and ill-defined conditions (symptoms 780–789)

781	Symptoms involving nervous and musculoskeletal systems

781.0	Abnormal involuntary movements
	    Abnormal head movements Spasm NOS
	    Fasciculation Tremor NOS
	    Excludes: Chorea NOS (333.5)
	                  Infantile spasms (345.6)
	                  Spastic paralysis (342–344)
	                  Specified movement disorders classifiable to 333
	                  When of non-organic origin (307.2, 307.3)

plasms' is identified by a letter, M. and five digits, e.g. 'M9530/0 Meningioma not otherwise specified' to 'M9539/3 Meningeal sarcomatosis'. If this system was adopted for central nervous diseases, more clinical categories could be usefully classified since the object here is to 'define a homogeneous patient group as accurately as possible' (Capildeo et al., 1980).

The single most important reason to suggest a new classification is that existing classifications do not satisfy the needs of clinicians or scientists working in a particular disease category. Tremor presents a special challenge since it is both a symptom and a sign; it can be a normal or an abnormal phenomenon (both of which are worthy of study); it may be the 'only' feature of disease of the central nervous system as in 'benign essential heredofamilial tremor' when the failure to develop further neurological signs distinguishes it from other more progressive diseases of the central nervous system; it is an interdisciplinary phenomenon of interest to physiologists, clinicians, pharmacologists, epidemiologists and pathologists—as demonstrated in this volume. Tremor can be measured objectively. The scientist can therefore help the clinician. However, can the clinician define a clinically homogeneous patient group for the scientist? Certainly not by any of the existing classifications.

The ideas put forward in this chapter will, it is hoped, form a basis for future discussion and thus enable clinicians, using such a classification, to make direct comparisons between patients seen in different centres by different physicians and at different times.

TERMINOLOGY

Tremor is an involuntary periodic oscillation of a body member (Findley and Gresty, 1981). The movement is continuous and rhythmical in appearance and these properties jointly distinguish tremor from other involuntary movements. Other tremor-like involuntary movements, clonus and myoclonus should probably be classified with tremor (Findley *et al.*, 1981).

Clonus is defined as a rhythmical involuntary movement that is evoked by passive stretch of a muscle or muscle group and may be transient or sustained for many hours (Findley and Gresty, 1981).

CLASSIFICATION

Tremors have been classified according to the behavioural circumstances in which they are evoked, as in resting tremor (the part of the body supported), postural tremor (with the part of the body maintaining a posture), action tremor (when the part of the body is actively moving) and intention tremor (a refinement of action tremor, when the execution of the task is goal-directed, as in the finger-to-nose test).

Tremor can also be classified according to the body part affected, duration of the tremor, the presence or absence of other neurological signs, the frequency of the tremor, response to drug treatment, the presence of associated conditions, a family history of tremor or other neurological disease. These nine features form the basis of the proposed classification, which when added to the basic demographic data of any patient will form that patient's clinical profile, indicating not only the essential clinical features but also *the basis on which the diagnosis was made* (see appendix). Another clinician reviewing these data independently, without recourse to the patient, will be readily able to see whether he agrees with the diagnosis or not. On a different scale, data collected in this way, say, for epidemiological studies, could be reviewed by a computer programmed to select out certain features in the patient's profile as 'compatible with the diagnosis, not compatible, or possible'.

TABLES

The tables 1.1–1.9 will be discussed in more detail.

Clinical I (table 1.1)

Table 1.1   Clinical I: upper limbs.

		Left arm		Right arm
	0	Unknown		
At rest	1	Present	16	Present
Posture	2	Present	32	Present
Intention	4	Present	64	Present
Clonus	8	Present	128	Present
			......	(Total)

Tremor most commonly presents in the upper limbs. This table is used to indicate which arm is affected or whether both arms are affected and the characteristics of the tremor according to the behavioural characteristics. A cumulative numbering system (see below) has been used so that more than one item can be indicated. The total number is unique since it indicates the components on which it is based. A 'score of 3' would indicate the presence of a resting and postural tremor in the left arm.

Clinical II (table 1.2)

Table 1.2   Clinical II: duration of tremor.

0	Unknown
1	Less than 1 year
2	More than 1 year less than 2, etc.
....	Code according to number of years

Tremor present for many years without much change and in the absence of other neurological symptoms or signs would suggest benign essential tremor. If the tremor was present for only a short time then the specificity and sensitivity of this table would be low. Taken in conjunction with table 1.1 increases its usefulness.

Clinical III (table 1.3)

Tremor may affect many different parts of the body. The frequencies of the tremors may be similar or several different tremors may be identified.

Table 1.3   Clinical III: other somatic tremors.

0	Unknown	32	Trunk
1	Tremor of voice	64	Left leg
2	Head (pathological)	128	Right leg
4	Eyes–congenital nystagmus	888	Other
8	Eyes–acquired pendular nystagmus	999	None
16	Buccolingual, chin	......	(Total)

Clinical IV (table 1.4)

Table 1.4   Clinical IV: other neurological signs.

0	Unknown	128	Dissociation of eye movements
1	Parkinsonian facies	256	Rigidity
2	Spasmodic torticollis	512	Spasticity
4	Dysarthria	1024	Dystonia
8	Dysphasia	2048	Peripheral neuropathy
16	Optic atrophy	8888	Other
32	Disorder of pursuit eye movement	9999	None
64	Nystagmus	....	(Total)

The presence (or absence) of other neurological signs further defines the basis for the clinical diagnosis (see appendix).

Quantification of tremor: frequency (table 1.5)

Table 1.5   Quantification of tremor: frequency.

0	Unknown	
	Dominant frequency	....
	Secondary frequency	....

The frequency of a tremor is the number of times the limb oscillates backwards and forwards in one second and is expressed in hertz. In general, tremors fall into four frequency bands which are of diagnostic significance. These frequency bands are 2–3 Hz, 4–5 Hz, around 6 Hz and 6.5–11 Hz. The wild tremulous 'waving' of the whole arm during action seen in some patients with multiple sclerosis is at 2–3 Hz. The classical resting tremor of Parkinson's disease lies between 4 and 5 Hz. 'Around 6 Hz' is the frequency at which the leg trembles when muscles are tired and contracting. It can be the frequency for the postural tremor of Parkinson's disease. Upper and lower motor neurone lesions affecting the arms, tremor associated with peripheral neuropathy, drug intoxications and even a low-frequency form of essential tremor may be seen around 6 Hz. Normal physiological tremor is seen between 6.5 and 11 Hz. Anxiety states, thyrotoxicosis and stress situations may cause postural tremors in the highest frequency band of 7 to 11 Hz.

The amplitude of tremor is not a reliable diagnostic criterion since it can fluctuate not only from examination to examination but within a single examination session. Too many extraneous factors may also affect amplitude, such as anxiety, level of arousal of the patient and previous activity.

Although more than one type of tremor may be measured, it is suggested that the predominant frequency is recorded. Other peaks could be recorded if felt useful.

Response to drug treatment (table 1.6)

Table 1.6   Response to drug treatment (greater than 50% response to objective measurements).

0	Unknown	16	Primidone
1	Propranolol	32	Bromocriptine
2	Levodopa	88	Other
4	Anticholinergic drug	99	None
8	Amantidine	......	(Total)

This can be defined as a '50% response to objective measurements'. Response to drug treatment can be of diagnostic importance. Essential tremor may respond to propranolol or primidone but not to levodopa or Bromocriptine. Parkinsonian tremor should respond to dopaminergic drugs providing the patient has 'idiopathic parkinsonism'. Response to alcohol could be included but it is unlikely that patients would consider it seriously as a regular treatment regime in the same way as propranolol or levodopa.

Associated conditions (table 1.7)

Table 1.7   Associated conditions.

0	Unknown	
1	Drug ingestion (specify)	....
2	Heavy-metal poisoning (specify)	....
4	Other neurotoxins	
8	Head injury	
16	Alcohol abuse	
32	Thyrotoxicosis	
64	Systemic/metabolic disease (code separately)	
128	Hysteria	
888	Other	
999	None	
......	(Total)	

This provides information on possible underlying causes. It is not possible to predict all possible associations but any coexisting symptoms, signs or diseases could be classified separately using the WHO classification. This table relates directly to tremor and does not include the equivalent of the E code (external cause) in the WHO classification where it is possible to define the drug (or type of drug) and whether 'accident, suicide or undetermined'.

Family history: tremor (table 1.8)

Table 1.8 Family history: tremor (similar clinical picture).

0	Unknown
1	Father
2	Mother
4	Other siblings
8	Grandparents
99	None
......	(Total)

This with the clinical details in table 1.1–1.4 would establish that if there is a family history then, for example, the label 'familial' can be justifiably added to the clinical diagnosis of essential tremor.

Family history: other neurological disease (table 1.9)

Table 1.9 Family history: other neurological disease.

0	Unknown	
1	Father	(specify)
2	Mother	....
4	Other siblings	....
8	Grandparents	....
99	None	
......	(Total)	

Involuntary movements, including tremor, may be a feature in a variety of inherited diseases. The neurological disease must be specified and coded as appropriate.

Cumulative numbering system

This shorthand system was devised whilst preparing a new classification of stroke (Capildeo *et al.*, 1977). In each section '0' is used for unknown information and

'9' or serial '9s' used to indicate 'none'. The cumulative number obtained in tables 1.1, 1.3, 1.4, 1.6, 1.7, 1.8 and 1.9 is in each case unique since only one possible combination of numbers will arrive at this total. In table 1.1, '48' is made up of '16 + 32', i.e. tremor in the right arm, present at rest and posture. The 'uniqueness' of each cumulative number is the principle of the cumulative numbering system.

DISCUSSION

This method of classification has been used to classify stroke, multiple sclerosis, Parkinson's disease (Capildeo *et al.*, 1978, 1980, 1981) and migraine (Capildeo and Rose, 1982). It has not been used to classify a 'symptom or sign'. The tables provide a collective database. From this database, the different types of tremor can be classified in a way that most clinicians understand, namely, using clinical description augmented where possible by simple scientific measurement. This method of classification can, for example, easily separate the tremors seen in 'benign familial essential tremor', 'idiopathic Parkinson's disease' and 'multiple sclerosis' (see appendix).

The database can be used to monitor change over time (both through clinical reassessments and through quantification of the frequency of the tremor), response to therapy, the development of other neurological symptoms and signs, and allow new features to be described and easily recognised through the use of '8' or serial '8s' in the clinical tables. When information is recorded as 'unknown' this will, according to the sensitivity and specificity of the individual tables, bring the clinical diagnosis into doubt. It also puts a strong emphasis on collecting and recording all known information. In those rare instances when a 'clinical label' is not possible, then straightforward description is the only alternative. Yet out of this type of description, new diseases or symptom complexes may be recognised which might open up new therapeutic possibilities and afford neurochemical and pathological correlation.

CONCLUSIONS

The next version of the International Statistical Classification of Diseases, Injuries and Causes of Death should allow more space for the classification of diseases of the nervous system. This could be done simply by using a fifth digit and possibly by a letter prefix, e.g. 'N'.

Even if this was carried out it still would not completely satisfy the needs of clinicians and research workers. For this reason we recommend that an additional classification be used to fulfil this purpose. The classification suggested in this chapter will, it is hoped, be used as a basis for future discussion.

APPENDIX

Example 1

A 60-year-old male with 'tremor'
Clinical diagnosis: 'Benign familial essential tremor'

Table	1.1	Clinical I	'2 + 32' = tremor on posture, left and right arms
	1.2	Clinical II (duration)	15 years
	1.3	Clinical III (other somatic tremors)	'2' = tremor of head
	1.4	Clinical IV (other neurological features)	None
	1.5	Quantification of tremor	7–11 Hz
	1.6	Response to drug treatment	'1 + 16' = propranolol and primidone
	1.7	Associated conditions	None
	1.8	Family history (tremor)	'1' = father
	1.9	Family history (other neurological disease)	None

Comment

The presence of *postural tremor in both hands*, for *15 years*, with *tremor of the head*, with a tremor *frequency* of *7–11 Hz*, responding to *propranolol* and *primidone*, with a *family history* (father) would support the clinical diagnosis of 'benign familial essential tremor'.

Example 2

A 70-year-old male with 'tremor'
Clinical diagnosis: 'Idiopathic Parkinson's disease'

Table	1.1	Clinical I	'1 + 16' = tremor at rest, left and right arms
	1.2	Clinical II (duration)	3 years
	1.3	Clinical III (other somatic tremors)	None
	1.4	Clinical IV (other neurological features)	'1 + 256' = parkinsonian facies and rigidity
	1.5	Quantification of tremor	4–5 Hz .
	1.6	Response to drug treatment	'2 + 4 + 32' = levodopa, anticholinergic and Bromocriptine
	1.7	Associated conditions	None
	1.8	Family history (tremor)	None
	1.9	Family history (other neurological disease)	None

Comment

The presence of *tremor at rest in both hands*, for *3 years*, with *other neurological features*, including *parkinsonian facies* and *rigidity*, with a tremor *frequency* of *4–5 Hz*, responding to *levodopa, an anticholinergic drug and Bromocriptine*, with no known associated conditions or family history would support the clinical diagnosis of 'idiopathic Parkinson's disease'.

Example 3

A 42-year-old female with 'tremor'
Clinical diagnosis: 'Multiple sclerosis'

Table	1.1	Clinical I	'2 + 4 + 32 + 64' = tremor on posture and with intention in both arms
	1.2	Clinical II (duration)	12 years
	1.3	Clinical III (other somatic tremors)	'1 + 2 + 32' = voice, head, trunk
	1.4	Clinical IV (other neurological features)	'4 + 16 + 64 + 128 + 512' = dysarthria, optic atrophy, nystagmus, dissociation of eye movements and spasticity
	1.5	Quantification of tremor	2–3 Hz
	1.6	Response to drug treatment	None
	1.7	Associated conditions	None
	1.8	Family history (tremor)	None
	1.9	Family history (other neurological disease)	None

Comment

The presence of *tremor on posture and with intention in both arms*, for *12 years*, with *voice, head and trunk* also affected by tremor, with *other neurological features*, including *dysarthria, optic atrophy, dissociation of eye movements* and *spasticity* with a tremor *frequency* of *2–3 Hz*, *no response* to therapy, and without a family history of tremor or other neurological disease would support the clinical diagnosis of 'multiple sclerosis'.

REFERENCES

Capildeo, R., Haberman, S. and Rose, F. C. (1977). New classification of stroke: preliminary communication. *Br. Med. J.*, 2, 1578–80.
Capildeo, R., Haberman, S. and Rose, F. C. (1978). A new classification of stroke. *Q. J. Med.*, 47, 177–96.

Capildeo, R., Haberman, S. and Rose, F. C. (1980). The classification and coding of neurological disease. In Rose, F. C. (ed.), *Clinical Neuroepidemiology*, Pitman Medical, Tunbridge Wells, pp. 28–36.

Capildeo, R., Haberman, S. and Rose, F. C. (1981). A new classification of parkinsonism. In Rose, F. C. and Capildeo, R. (eds), *Research Progress in Parkinson's Disease*, Pitman Medical, Tunbridge Wells, pp. 17–24.

Capildeo, R. and Rose, F. C. (1982). Towards a new classification of migraine. In Rose, F. C. (ed), *Advances in Migraine Research and Therapy*, Raven Press, New York, pp. 1–7.

Findley, L. J. and Gresty, M. A. (1981). Tremor. *Br. J. Hosp. Med.*, **26**, 16–32.

Findley, L. J., Gresty, M. A. and Halmagyi, G. M. (1981) Tremor, the cogwheel phenomenon and clonus in Parkinson's disease. *J. Neurol. Neurosurg. Psychiatr.*, **44**, 534–46.

Kurtzke, J. F. (1979). ICD 9: A regression. *Am. J. Epidemiol.*, **109**, 383–93.

WHO (1974). *Manual of the International Statistical Classification of Diseases, Injuries and Causes of Death*, Ninth Revision, 1974, vol. 1, 1977, and vol. 2, 1978, World Health Organisation, Geneva.

2
Definition, analysis and genesis of tremor

M. A. GRESTY and L. J. FINDLEY

DEFINITION: THE CHARACTERISTICS OF TREMOR

A definition of tremor is of importance because good definitions aid our approach to measurement. An exhaustive review of definitions of tremor is given by Brumlik and Yap (1970). Since there is considerable agreement, it would be pointless here to recapitulate the various viewpoints so the following is a distillation. The appearance of tremor is that of a rhythmical movement of a part of the body. This appearance implies that the movement has a relatively fixed periodicity and possesses an amplitude and waveform which are to some extent invariable over reasonable amounts of time. If these characteristics do not hold then movements have an irregular appearance and historically have been classified as different phenomena.

The inherent rhythmicity of tremor allows its characterisation in terms of certain parameters. These are frequency (and its converse, periodicity), waveform and amplitude. It is implicitly understood that the periodicity of tremor bears an important relationship to the nature of the underlying mechanism and some schools of thought take the view that frequency can be of value in the diagnosis of specific pathophysiology (Holmes, 1904). Waveform is a less valuable parameter of tremor and reflects the specific distribution and timing sequence of muscular activity involved. Amplitude determines symptomaticity but is arguably the least valuable aspect of tremor from the point of view of understanding mechanism, for it is well established that amplitude varies with both internal and external psychological and physiological factors. Because of its inherent variability, the measurement of amplitude is the major problem in the assessment of potential drugs for the treatment of tremor.

Certain rare involuntary movements in nervous diseases have the appearance of crescendo–decrescendo oscillations of a body member. An example of this is the transient oscillation of the head occurring occasionally in children in response to novel stimuli which is termed 'startle myoclonus' (Gresty and Halmagyi, 1979). Such movements are commonly called 'myoclonic' and yet, regardless of specific pathophysiology, it is appropriate to analyse them in terms of frequency and waveform, modulated by time course, in the same fashion as continuous tremor.

15

The origin of these involuntary movements remains obscure, yet the likelihood that they lie on some continuum with tremor renders the use of the term myoclonus misleading (Gresty *et al.*, 1982). On occasion, in earlier texts, they have been termed 'shuddering' tremors.

STANDARDISATION OF TREMOR OBSERVATIONS

The point of the following observations is that they appeal for standardisation of the behavioural characteristics of tremor and the situations within which tremor is assessed.

By the turn of the century it was well established in neurological practice that tremor varied with the behavioural situation. Clear distinctions were made between resting and postural tremor, between tremors which developed through or at the termination of movement and by intentional or passive movements. Clinicians were aware that tremor could be brought out by specific attitudes of flexion or extension and could involve isolated, reciprocal or co-contractive muscle activity. Unfortunately few studies in the physiological or biophysical literature which have dealt with pathological tremor have taken the varied behavioural characteristics into account.

Two areas in this respect are worthy of particular mention, the first relating to animal models of parkinsonian tremor. An experimental model of parkinsonian tremor can be produced in monkeys by lesions of the ventromedial tegmentum of the brainstem (e.g. Poirier *et al.*, 1975). Unfortunately the physiological studies tend not to report the behavioural characteristics of the experimental tremor in sufficient detail which would allow comparison with tremor in patients. For example, one would like to know the typical amplitudes and frequencies of the induced tremor and whether the character of the tremor changes with movement and posture. The second major criticism concerns experiments such as weighting or passively perturbing or vibrating a limb in order to observe the effects on tremor. There may be radical consequences of these procedures on different types of pathological tremor. Tremor amplitude reflects the depths of modulation of motor neurone activity, upon which activity the neural input due to passive stretch of the muscle is imposed. In order to appreciate the subtleties of interaction between these two events the energy inputs delivered by the perturbations have to be scaled carefully. A small stretch reflex input to a big tremor has little opportunity of affecting the activity of the neurone pool; conversely a strong input to a weak tremor could well swamp tremogenic activity. These relationships are described in more detail in a later section of this paper and are illustrated in figure 2.2. There is a further problem with this type of experiment which arises from the characteristics of some pathological tremors and, in particular, parkinsonian tremors. This is that the tremor may change frequency, amplitude and waveform characteristics when the limb is moved either passively or actively or when it is loaded. These fundamental changes in the characteristics of the tremor make interpretation of behavioural experiments difficult and are frequently overlooked in the experimental literature. In summary, future experimental or clinical investigations of tremor have the onus to define the phenomenon carefully, having regard for frequency and waveform characteristics, typical amplitude and their fluctuations and behavioural characteristics. These observations are of particular relevance to the crucially important area of animal studies which attempt to construct experimental paradigms of pathological processes.

TRANSDUCTION OF TREMOR AND UNITS OF MEASUREMENT

The skeleton is a system of jointed rods and the appropriate way of describing body movement is with reference to rotations about the joints. This requires goniometric transducers such as angular accelerometers. Angular transducers tend to be bulky and expensive but fortunately we can approximate most tremulous movements of the body by reference to the linear displacement of a suitable site on the limb in the line of trajectory of the centroid of mass. For small movements the record produced by a linear accelerometer can readily be transformed to an angular acceleration which is relatively uncontaminated by artefactual signals arising from the deviation of the sensitive axis of the device from the line of the gravity vector. Linear accelerometers have the advantages that they may be of minute size and are relatively inexpensive.

There are several overriding reasons why acceleration should be the dimension of choice in transducing tremor. First, accelerometers are much more sensitive to higher-frequency vibrations than are velocity or displacement devices; secondly, the acceleration of a limb most directly reflects the underlying muscular contraction; and thirdly, the signals derived from an accelerometer may be integrated digitally to produce viable velocity and displacement records. In contrast, displacement and tachometric transducer signals are not so easily differentiated to produce acceleration records because of the amplification of high-frequency noise inherent in the differentiation process.

Under some circumstances it is useful to have an immediate record of the displacement of a limb because the actual visible appearance of movement is that of change of position. One does not 'see' velocity or acceleration, for these entities are abstractions from the phenomenological world. Perhaps the simplest and cheapest device available for the transduction of displacement in two dimensions is the Schottky barrier photodetector which may be set up to 'view' a source of light mounted on a limb (Findley *et al.*, 1980). The detector gives continuous electrical signals corresponding to the *x* and *y* coordinates in cartesian geometry of the trajectory of movement of the light. Disadvantages of the method are that ambient and source illumination must stay constant and the optics must be appropriate to the field of view, so that the setting-up procedure may be troublesome. An extensive review of methods of transducing tremor is given by Brumlik and Yap (1970).

APPLICATIONS OF SPECTRAL ANALYSIS TO TREMOR

The purpose of this section is to illustrate the applications of spectral analysis to the investigation of tremor. The advent of cheap spectral analysers has enabled many laboratories to deal with tremor in the frequency domain. This form of representation may deter many with little mathematical background; however all should take heart. The method of representing signals in the frequency domain has many intuitive aspects. Detailed technical discussions of applications of spectral analysis are available in numerous texts. Some of note are Jenkins and Watts (1968); Glaser and Rutchkin (1976), for particular applications to neurobiological signals; approachable short texts for use alongside a signal analyser are published by Solartron (1981) and Hewlett-Packard (1978) and are of value in the initial intuitive approach to spectral analysis.

The rationale for the spectral analysis of tremor derives from the fact that tremor is a periodic phenomenon. According to Fourier's theorem a periodic waveform may be represented by a series of sinusoidal components, each of which has an amplitude and is fixed in phase with respect to the others. The first component of lowest frequency is called the fundamental, whilst the rest are the harmonics. The fundamental component is at a frequency corresponding to the overall 'cycle time' or period of the waveform. A waveform that is a pure sine wave in shape has only one component, which is the fundamental. Waveforms that have more complex shapes have components at 'harmonic frequencies', which means whole-number multiples of the fundamental frequency. The amplitudes of the components indicate the shape of the waveform. The Fourier transform of a signal is represented in a spectrum. Along the abscissa of a spectrum is plotted frequency. The ordinate scales magnitude of the frequency components. These relationships are illustrated in figure 2.1. The applications of spectral analysis to tremor studies that will be illustrated here have been performed on either a Hewlett-Packard 5000 series computer or on a Solartron 1200.

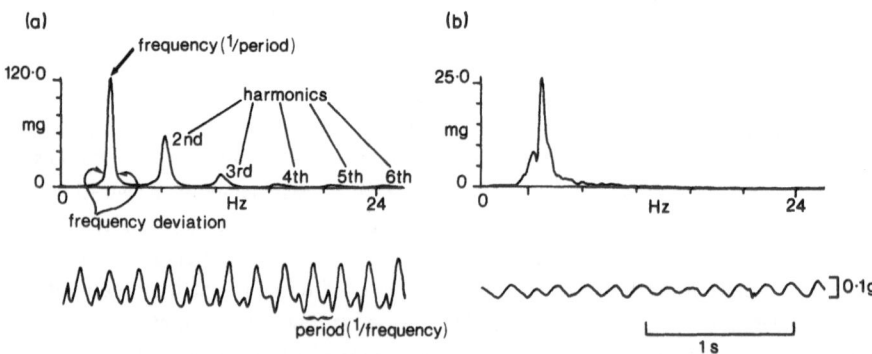

Figure 2.1 Raw records and derived spectra from a tremor with extensive harmonic distortion (a) and one with a more or less pure sinusoidal waveform (b) illustrating the spectral appearance of the different waveforms and exemplifying the terminology used in waveform analysis. (Note that in figures illustrating spectra, g and mg refer to acceleration due to gravity; mg = milli-g = 9.81×10^{-3} m s^{-2}.)

Use of spectra in the assessment of the tremolytic and tremogenic effects of drugs

Averaged spectra are useful in the assessment of the efficacy of tremolytic agents. A time sample of tremor activity may be divided into suitable epochs for frequency analysis. Spectra are calculated for each of the epochs and averaged. Suitable measurements to be taken from the averaged spectra are the frequency of the dominant component of the tremor, which usually corresponds to the cycle time of the tremor waveform, and the amplitude of this component. If the tremor has a fairly simple waveform then these values correspond to the dominant events. In the case of complex waveforms it is necessary to have an estimate of all frequency components. The most useful measurement of these is the total power content of the spectrum, which is calculated as the sum of the squares of the individual frequency components. If the tremor was measured using an accelerometer then the spectrum may be transformed to a velocity spectrum whose total power content is proportional to the kinetic energy dissipated by the tremor, $\frac{1}{2} \times$ (mass of limb) $\times$ (velocity squared). This produces a powerful measurement which has a physical basis and compensates for changes in waveform.

Use of spectral analysis in intervention experiments

In the introductory section of this chapter, which was concerned with standardisation of tremor observations and experiments, a critique was made of intervention experiments in which perturbations are applied to the limb. An example of such, aimed at determining the stretch reflex contribution to tremor, is to vibrate a tremulous limb and observe whether the vibration entrains or beats with the tremor. The problem here is to balance energy input/output relationships and for this spectral analysers are indispensable. A modern instrument has of the order of 110 dB range of resolution, which is capable of detecting a minute tremor in the presence of one of large amplitude. This permits one to detect the concurrence of two vibration frequencies at levels below visible signs of 'beating' of the two frequencies. Furthermore, the accurate measurement of the vibratory input to the limb in relationship to the tremor amplitude allows one to balance the energy relationship with care. Some of the relationships discussed in this section are illustrated in figure 2.2.

Applications of the coherence function

Associated with the spectral analysis of signals is an important function termed coherence. Coherence is somewhat similar to a correlation coefficient and indicates the degree of causal relationship between two signals scaled from 0 indicating complete independence to 1 indicating a completely deterministic relationship. Coherence is a function in the frequency domain, and a level of coherence is calculated for each frequency present in the two signals under consideration.

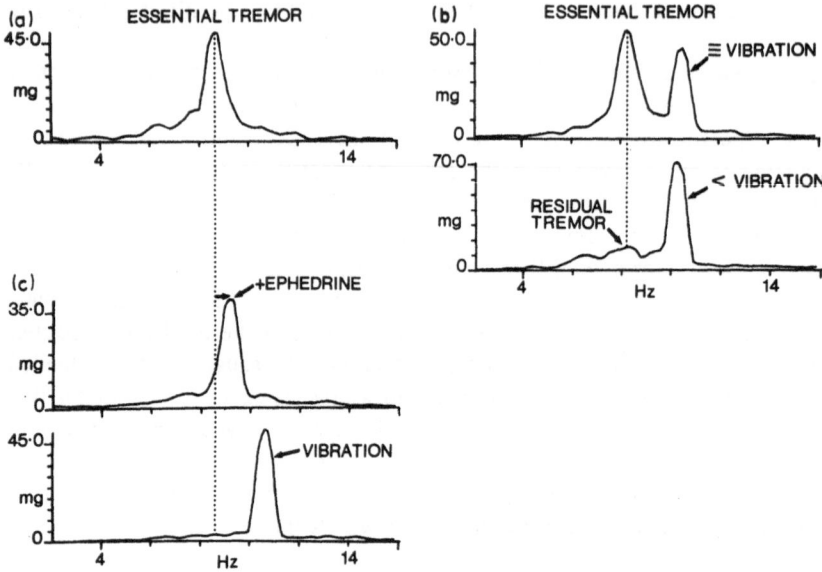

Figure 2.2 Spectra illustrating the effect of various intensities of vibration of the hand using a torque motor on small-amplitude/high-frequency essential tremor and upon an ephedrine-induced tremor. (a) Averaged spectrum of an essential tremor calculated from four 10.24 s samples of tremor recording. (b) Vibratory input at equivalent energy levels to those dissipated by the tremor do not modify the tremor in amplitude or frequency. Vibratory input with an energy level greater than that dissipated by the tremor reduces the tremor greatly in amplitude; however, the high-resolution spectrum shows that the tremor is still present. The tremor would be almost undetectable in the appearance of the raw movement and it could be taken that the vibration had entrained the tremor. (c) Tremor in the same subject half an hour after oral administration of 50 mg ephedrine. The tremor is of similar amplitude but has increased by almost 1 Hz in frequency. Vibration now does completely entrain the tremor, demonstrating that it is an enhanced physiological tremor. The vertical dotted lines indicate synchronisation.

The coherence function involves averaging cross-spectra with respect to individual autospectra and is associated with levels of statistical significance which become more reliable with increased numbers of averages:

$$\text{Coherence} = \frac{\text{Average (squared cross-spectrum)}}{\text{Average (one signal power spectrum)} * \text{Average (second signal power spectrum)}}$$

There are two important applications of the coherence calculation. One is in the estimation of the amount of passive transmission from the movement of one limb to another part of the body. Typical examples of this application are estimating the amount of head shaking induced by truncal tremor or the extent of transmission of tremor from left to right hand (illustrated in figure 2.3). A further

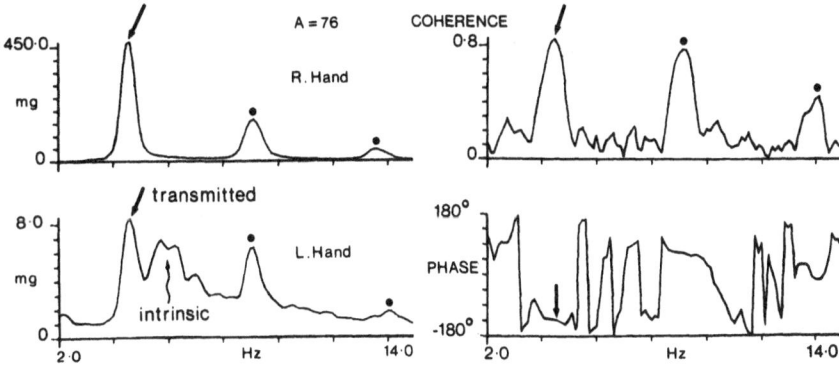

Figure 2.3 Use of the coherence function in determining the proportion of passive transmission of a resting tremor from the right hand to the left hand. The level of the coherence function indicates that 90% of the energy in the left hand at the frequency of the tremor of the right hand is passively transmitted. The phase delay of 170° indicates a time lag of about 120 ms between events in the right and left hands. Straight arrows indicate the tremor of the right hand with harmonics marked with dots. The wavy, upwards pointing arrow on the spectrum of the left hand indicates the intrinsic tremor.

application of coherence is in determining whether tremors in two separate parts of the body have a common rhythm generator (e.g. Marsden *et al.*, 1969; Ell *et al.*, 1982). Thus, in chapter 32 in this volume, Ell *et al.* have shown that, in some cases of multiple tremors, tremor in very different parts of the body such as eyes and hand can be perfectly synchronised and covary in amplitude. The coherence calculation for the movements in these cases gives values close to unity. The conclusion derived from this analysis is that a common rhythm generator must have access to discharge to both body parts.

Coherence may be used to assess more than the relationship between two movements. With suitable demodulation of the frequency coding of the signals, coherence may be applied to the relationship between muscle spike activity (electromyogram, EMG) or neuronal action potentials and overall movement (e.g. Elble and Randall, 1976). An application of coherence would be in estimating the relationship between neuronal activity in the thalamus and tremor during stereotaxis. It would be quite possible to give an estimate of the degree of relationship between the activity of thalamic structures being probed and ongoing tremor which may help to improve the accuracy of tremolytic lesions.

AN OVERVIEW OF TREMOR: CLASSIFICATION AND INTERPRETATION BASED ON FREQUENCY

The following classification which we have made is based on our own experience with a wide variety of nervous diseases. There are many ways of classifying tremor including behavioural characteristics and pharmacological response. Because the general clinical appearance of tremor relates to the period of the movement with amplitude and behaviour as close secondary characteristics, we have chosen frequency as the primary criterion of classification. In practice, with the notable exceptions of the 'essential tremors' and ocular 'myoclonus', a combination of frequency and behavioural characteristics are the most useful attributes for diagnostically useful classification.

1.5 to 3 Hz band

Tremors in this frequency band are usually called the 'ataxic' or 'coarse' tremors and typically occur in the head, trunk and upper limbs. They are most frequently seen in demyelinating disease with multiple lesions. Historically this type of tremor has been ascribed to a predominantly cerebellar pathology (Schuster, 1924). However, we have observed similar tremor in one patient with a large infiltrating thalamic tumour. There is a specific form of tremor at about 3 Hz which has been shown to arise from delayed and enhanced long-latency reflexes resulting from atrophy of the anterior lobe of the cerebellum (Mauritz *et al.*, 1981). This tremor has the characteristic that its rhythm may be 'reset' by an external activation of the reflex and is thus not a true tremor and should be classified as a dysmetria (see Llinás, chapter 10, this volume). The ataxic tremors can be violent with acceleration amplitudes that can be in excess of 1 g, which renders them self-injuring. The frequency of these tremors is not finely tuned and the amplitudes vary greatly. They are typically brought out in posture and intention but may also occur when the patient is lying supported on the bed, most notably in cases of alcoholic degeneration. Ataxic tremor may be temporarily suppressed with hyoscine and intravenous lignocaine, and some respond to oral lignocaine (Ell *et al.*, chapter 32, this volume). The tremulous movements of the body (but not those of the eyes) in 'oculo-palatal-diaphragmatic-etc. myoclonus' are also in this frequency band, whilst others are in the 4 to 5 Hz band (see below).

4 to 5 Hz band

Tremor in this frequency band is characteristically the most identifiable and has known pathophysiology which has features in common with tremor in the low-frequency band. The most useful subdivision is with respect to behavioural characteristics. These tremors are generally found in the upper trunk, head and limbs. 4 Hz tremor present on posture and during intentional movement is termed 'cerebellar tremor', when present at rest and in posture it is called 'rubral' and when present largely at rest is identifiable as parkinsonian resting tremor. All these forms of tremor are thought to arise from lesions of the cerebello-mesencephalic-thalamic projection pathways (Struppler *et al.*, 1978). At the level of the cerebellar nuclei and peduncles, postural tremor is provoked. Rubral tremor is associated with intrinsic mesencephalic lesions, whilst at the higher levels the resting tremor is produced which is attributed to functional deafferentation of the thalamus. Postural and resting tremor are both very variable in amplitude. Whenever we have encountered a case of rubral tremor with established pathology the movement has tended to be violent to the point of self-injury. Resting and rubral tremor can be responsive to levodopa therapy, and all three tremors may be temporarily suppressed with hyoscine. Postural tremor is suppressed with intravenous lignocaine.

6 Hz band

A variety of tremulous movements have a fixed frequency within 0.2 Hz of 6 Hz. Generally speaking these tremors are found in the limbs. Several are associated with Parkinson's disease and include the postural tremor, the rhythmicity of the cogwheel phenomenon and action tremors, and a clonus-like response to passive or active stretch (Findley and Gresty, chapter 21, this volume). Clonus typically found in pyramidal tract lesions has a frequency of 6 Hz. We have observed postural tremor at 6 Hz with focal infarcts of the basal ganglia. Occasionally patients with peripheral neuropathy have a well organised tremor at this frequency. Most 6 Hz tremor is of relatively small amplitude; typical postural tremors will be less than 0.1 g although the clonuses and clonus-like movements may be much larger. On the basis that all these forms of tremor involve abnormal patterns of activity at the level of the spinal neurone pool, it has been postulated that they share a common tremogenic mechanism (Jung, 1941) which derives its rhythmicity from structures at a spinal cord level (Findley *et al.*, 1981).

8 to 12 Hz band

Symptomatic tremors in the highest-frequency band are frequently termed 'exaggerated physiological tremor'. Although this term is misleading it does usefully imply that their origins may be diverse (Marsden, 1978). The many possible mechanisms for tremor at high frequencies include hyperdynamic circulation, potentiation of reflexes and unusual synchronisation in the recruitment of motor units. Visible tremor may represent an unusual amplitude of passive mechanical resonance in the limb or muscle activity. Tremors in this frequency band are most commonly associated with anxiety. Alternatively high-frequency tremor is seen in some cortical infarcts and degenerations, in some cases of peripheral neuropathy in which there are individual violent muscle twitches and in many states of drug intoxication. In some patients with high cord lesions clonus at high frequency may be evoked by passive stretch. Similarly in Parkinson's disease, the cogwheel phenomenon, action tremor and clonus-like tremor in response to passive stretch may be evoked at these frequencies.

The rhythmical myoclonuses

Rhythmical crescendo–decrescendo movements in 'startle myoclonus' have frequencies and amplitudes similar to cerebellar tremor and may be related in pathophysiology (Gresty and Halmagyi, 1979).

Ocular myoclonus and pendular nystagmus, which may be related in aetiology, are the only rhythmical involuntary eye movements with a sinusoidal motion and therefore should be classified as tremors. They have a frequency from 2.5 to 6 Hz with a modal frequency of 4 Hz. Associated somatic tremor may be in any part of the body (larynx, pharynx, diaphragm, limbs) and tends to be in the frequency range of 3 to 5 Hz, thus identifiable with the ataxic and the cerebello-thalamic tremors (Gresty *et al.*, 1982; Ell *et al.*, 1982). The relationships between 'oculo-palatal myoclonus' and other forms of tremor are discussed at greater length by Ell *et al.* in chapter 32 in this volume.

Essential tremor

Essential tremor most frequently affects the upper limbs and may involve the head and other body parts. The tremor develops most frequently on posture and through guided or ballistic movement. Frequencies of essential tremor of the upper limbs range from 4 Hz to about 9 Hz with amplitudes up to 1 g (1 cm) displacement of the middle dorsum). There is an approximately inverse linear relationship between amplitude and frequency. Essential tremor of the head, as with other body parts, is usually at about 4 Hz. The pathophysiology of essential tremor is unknown and it is possible that the term covers a heterogeneous group of disorders. Some types of essential tremor are attenuated by beta-adrenoceptor blockade (Wilson *et al.*, chapter 17, this volume). Recently it has been shown that some cases of essential tremor can be controlled with primidone (Findley *et al.*, chapter 19, this volume).

CONCLUSIONS

Jung (1941), considering the relationship between tremor and normal physiological processes, proposed that tremor represents phylogenetically primitive mechanisms concerned with locomotion which are 'released' by insults to the nervous system which cause disintegration of higher-order control mechanisms. We would like to propose an extension of this hypothesis which emphasises the point that tremor mechanisms may not necessarily be phylogenetically vestigial but are of current importance to the motor coordination of the organism.

There are two prime considerations relating to body movement. The first, which is common to all engineering problems, is the overriding necessity to prevent structures from going into oscillation and to contain and dampen out unwanted oscillation where necessary. The second consideration derives from the unique structure of the body, which consists of a jointed rod framework supporting inertial loads with viscoelastic properties and is controlled by a muscular system which works at a mechanical disadvantage! The problem of working with mechanical disadvantage can be offset to some extent by operating at close to the natural resonant frequency of the structure. Thus the control of the nervous system is faced with the dilemma of wishing to avoid resonance in the body and yet make use of the natural tendencies to resonance in order to conserve energy.

We propose that tremor arises in structures normally responsible for coordinating movement and is the risk that the nervous system takes to conserve energy. Tremors occur at similar frequencies because of the necessity to coordinate movement in several body parts, each of considerable mass. There is ample evidence that frequency and time synchronisation occurs at the level of neuronal membranes as exemplified by the coupling of cells in the inferior olive (Llinás and Yarom, 1980; Llinás and Volkind, 1973). This is precisely what one would expect for strict timing, queuing and frequency regulation of movement control signals. In addition one could expect that long and short loop reflexes could share similar cycle times with each other and with tremogenic processes. These considerations may explain much of the conflicting opinions on the nature of motor organisation. The conflict arises because experimental results are frequently equivocal and may reflect the workings of any of several parallel and synchronised systems.

REFERENCES

Brumlik, J. and Yap, C.-B. (1970). *Normal Tremor: A Comparative Study*, Charles C. Thomas, Springfield, Illinois.

Elble, R. J. and Randall, J. E. (1976). Motor unit activity responsible for 8 to 12 Hz component of finger tremor. *J. Neurophysiol.*, **39**, 370–83.

Ell, J. J., Gresty, M. A., Chambers, B. R. and Findley, L. J. (1982). Acquired pendular nystagmus: characteristics, pathophysiology and pharmacological modification. In Rocoux, A. (ed.), *Physiological and Pathological Aspects of Eye Movements*, Proceedings of the European Communities Workshop, Chateau Pont d'Oye, Belgium, Pergamon Press, Oxford and New York (to appear).

Findley, L. J., Gresty, M. A. and Halmagyi, G. M. (1980). A novel method of recording arm movements: a survey of common abnormalities. *Arch. Neurol.*, **38**, 38–42.

Findley, L. J., Gresty, M. A. and Halmagyi, G. M. (1981). Tremor, the cogwheel phenomenon and clonus in Parkinson's disease. *J. Neurol. Neurosurg. Psychiatr.*, **44**, 534–46.

Glaser, E. M. and Rutchkin, D. S. (1976). *Principles of Neurobiological Signal Analysis*, Academic Press, New York.

Gresty, M. A., Ell, J. J. and Findley, L. J. (1982). Acquired pendular nystagmus: its characteristics, localising value and pathophysiology. *J. Neurol. Neurosurg. Psychiatr.*, **45**, 431–9.

Gresty, M. A. and Halmagyi, G. M. (1979). Abnormal head movements. *J. Neurol. Neurosurg. Psychiatr.*, **42**, 705–14.

Hewlett-Packard (1978). *5420 A Digital Signal Analyzer User's Guide*, Part no. 05420-90033.

Holmes, G. (1904). On certain tremors in organic cerebral lesions. *Brain*, 27, 360-75.

Jenkins, G. M. and Watts, D. G. (1968). *Spectral Analysis and its Applications*, Holden Day, San Francisco.

Jung, R. (1941). Physiologische untersuchungen uber den Parkinsontremor und andere zitterformen beim menschen. *Z. Ges. Neurol. Psychiatr.*, 173, 263-330.

Llinás, R. and Volkind, R. A. (1973). The olivo-cerebellar system: functional properties as revealed by harmaline induced tremor. *Exp. Brain Res.*, 18, 69-87.

Llinás, R. and Yarom, Y. (1980). Electrophysiological properties of mammalian inferior olivary cells *in vitro*. In de Montigny, C. (ed.), *Anatomy and Physiology of the Inferior Olive*, Raven Press, New York.

Marsden, C. D. (1978). The mechanisms of physiological tremor and their significance for pathological tremor. In Desmedt, J. E. (ed.), *Physiological Tremor, Pathological Tremor and Clonus, Progress in Clinical Neurophysiology*, vol. 5, Karger, Basel, pp. 1-16.

Marsden, C. D., Meadows, J. C., Lange, G. W. and Watson, R. S. (1969). The relation between physiological tremor of the two hands in healthy subjects. *EEG Clin. Neurophysiol.*, 27, 179-85.

Mauritz, K. H., Schmitt, C. and Dichgans, J. (1981). Delayed and enhanced long latency reflexes as the possible cause of postural tremor in late cerebellar atrophy. *Brain*, 104, 97-116.

Poirier, L. J., Filion, M., Larochelle, L. and Pechadre, J.-C. (1975). Physiopathology of experimental Parkinsonism in the monkey. *J. Can. Sci. Neurol.*, 2, 256-63.

Schuster, P. (1924). Die im hoheren lebensalter vorkommenden kleinhirnerkrankungen nebst bemerkungen uber den cerebellaren wackeltremor. *Z. Ges. Neurol. Psychiatr.*, 91, 521-50.

Solartron–Schlumberger (1981). *Using Digital Spectral Techniques*, Welstead, P. E., 1200 Signal processor operating manual, Part no. 12000006.

Struppler, A., Erbel, F. and Velho, F. (1978). An overview of the pathophysiology of Parkinsonian and other pathological tremors. In Desmedt, J. E. (ed.), *Physiological Tremor, Pathological Tremor and Clonus, Progress in Clinical Neurophysiology*, vol. 5, Karger, Basel, pp. 114-28.

3
Differential diagnosis of motor disorders by tremor analysis

H.-J. FREUND, H. HEFTER, V. HÖMBERG and K. REINERS

INTRODUCTION

Tremor is regarded as something pathological when it becomes so strong that it disturbs the patient and is evident to the clinician. Thus it is the increase in the 'strength' of tremor which underlies its classification as pathological tremor. Additional information can be obtained from observation of the conditions under which tremor is stronger. Tremor at rest, action and intention tremor are useful and traditional categories of tremor, providing diagnostic clues about the clinical syndrome. In terms of the underlying mechanisms, closer synchronisation between motor units represents the neuronal mechanism underlying the development of augmented physiological tremor and pathological tremor. In the power spectrum, such tremors are characterised by a sharp peak at motor unit onset firing rates. The high amplitude of this peak and low peak frequency are typical features of pathological tremor (see Freund *et al.*, chapter 12, this volume).

Tremor is also and always present under physiological conditions. It is an inevitable side-product of muscle activity and of movement. It is known from studies on spectral analysis of physiological tremor that the power spectra are characterised by a relatively broad frequency distribution between 0 and 30 Hz Allum *et al.*, 1978; Halliday and Redfearn, 1956; Sutton and Sykes, 1967). In the normal situation the power spectrum does not show a prominent peak.

This raises the question: what then are the tremor-generating mechanisms in the absence of synchronisation between the motor units? A two-component model of physiological tremor has recently been proposed by Allum *et al.* (1978). According to this model the power spectrum of physiological tremor originates from two different sources (cf. figure 3.1):

(a) The *low-frequency* part (<6 Hz) is produced by slow force variations due to changes in the net output of the motoneurone pool.
(b) The *high-frequency* part (>6 Hz) reflects unfused parts of the twitch contractions produced by motor units discharging at the corresponding rates. This part of the spectrum corresponds to the range of firing rates between recruitment and obvious fusion (6–20/30 Hz). The steep decay of this part

27

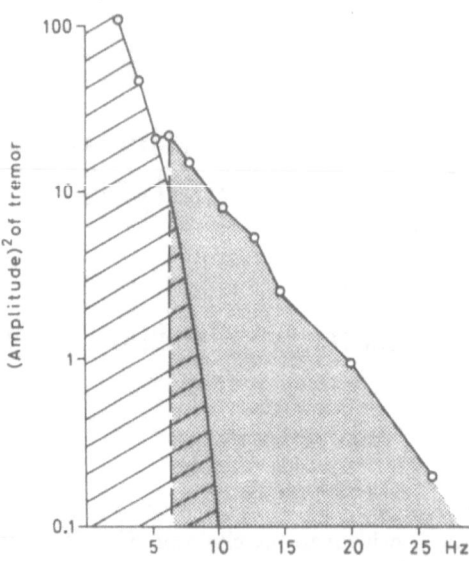

Figure 3.1 Schematic illustration of the tremor-generating mechanisms. The hatched area represents the part of the power spectrum which is produced by the force variations due to changes of the net activity of the whole motoneurone pool. The dotted area is produced by the unfused parts of the twitch contractions of single motor units. (From Allum *et al.*, 1978.)

of the tremor spectrum (−43 dB/decade) is the consequence of the reduction in amplitude of the unfused parts of the muscle fibre contractions with increasing rates (−38 dB/decade). It reflects the mechanical properties of the muscle resembling a second-order damped system (Bawa and Stein, 1976). This hypothesis is in agreement with the old concept of Marshall and Walsh (1956) that physiological tremor is generated by the asynchronous discharges of motor nerve fibres 'converted to mechanical ripples by the muscles'. This assumption was corroborated by asynchronous stimulation of ventral root fibres (Allum *et al.*, 1978) and by the frequency characteristics of ocular tremor (Alpern, 1972). The motor unit discharge and tremor rates of the eye muscles are both much higher than those of skeletal muscles.

In the context of this chapter, the use of power spectra of force recordings for diagnostic purposes and for the study of pathophysiological mechanisms was not examined for such tremors which can already be sufficiently recognised and categorised by clinical analysis. The investigations concentrated on testing the hypothesis proposed in an earlier study (Allum *et al.*, 1978) that the power spectrum of tremor force recordings provides information on the activity of motor units in the tremor-producing muscle, and whether or not they are synchronised. In that case, the majority of motor disorders should lead to changes in the power spectrum of the force record. When the higher-frequency part of the spectrum is generated by unfused parts of motor units twitch contractions, the frequency distribution should reveal the range of firing rates of the motor units of the muscle. Alterations of the range of firing rates in pathological conditions could then be recognised by changes in the spectrum. We have therefore examined various motor disorders that are not associated with pathological tremor.

METHODOLOGY

High-gain, AC-coupled force recordings were obtained via a strain gauge during extension of the forefinger. We have restricted the analysis to force recordings because they are unbiased by the various mechanical factors influencing the recording of movement. Low-gain, DC-coupled force was also monitored. Both were fed into a small computer for display and spectral analysis. The smallest force increment that can be recorded from the force transducer was $50\,\mu g$. The filters were arranged in such a way that both slow force deviations and all frequencies up to 30 Hz were properly displayed: corner frequencies were 0.5 and 30 Hz. The 40 dB decay of the spectrum due to mechanical damping with increasing fusion of motor unit contractions at increasing firing rates was compensated by the program in order to get a better display of the higher frequencies. The degree of compensation of mechanical damping was tested by microstimulation of the muscle. When a tiny contraction (0.5 g) is produced by electrical microstimulation of one or a few motor units, the amplitude in the resulting peak in the power spectrum remains approximately constant at all stimulus frequencies throughout the spectrum.

A further change from the conventional display of power spectra of tremor was made by displaying consecutive spectra three-dimensionally as a function of time. In this way spectral analysis of high-gain force records is not restricted to stationary conditions but can be expanded for dynamic studies. Rapid contractions cannot be recorded because of the sampling time necessary for each force segment. For the same reason consecutive spectra are derived from partially overlapping force segments so that rapid force changes are not properly reflected by this method.

The muscle activity spectrum

Figures 3.2 and 3.3 show the difference between a conventional spectrum of tremor force (figure 3.2) and the new method (figure 3.3). Usually, the spectra are displayed on a semilogarithmic plot. In figure 3.2 the low frequencies show high amplitudes with a steep decay towards higher frequencies. The effect of different filters is illustrated by the two curves as explained in the legend. Figure 3.3 shows consecutive force spectra during a similar stationary contraction. The higher frequencies can be recognised better on a linear abscissa and with correc-

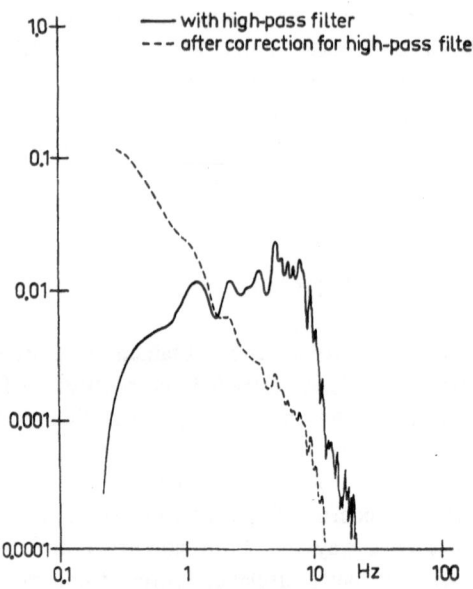

Figure 3.2   Power spectra of physiological force tremor (10 N) before (broken line) and after (full line) high-pass filtering. The abscissa is in logarithmic units. Note increased resolution of frequencies above 6 Hz in the high-pass-filtered spectrum. Owing to mechanical damping, frequencies above 10 Hz show steep decrease in amplitude. (From Allum *et al.*, 1978.)

tion for damping. This spectrum is typical for such a weak isometric contraction and shows frequencies between 8 and 25 Hz. They indicate motor unit firing at corresponding rates. Most power is spread to frequencies between 8 and 14 Hz. Frequencies below 6 Hz are of much lower amplitude as compared to figure 3.2 as a consequence of different filters. The scale is, however, selected to allow a proper display of stronger force fluctuations as they occur at non-stationary contractions or in patients with ataxia. The main purpose of the muscle activity spectrum (MAS) is, however, to provide a proper display of the range of motor unit firing rates. The stronger the force exerted, the more are higher frequencies found in the spectrum.

The assumption that small contractions like partially fused twitch contractions of synchronously discharging motor units are really reflected in these spectra has been proven by microstimulation. Unfused twitch contractions with amplitudes of 200 µg at a stimulus rate of 4 Hz still appear in the spectrum up to stimulus rates of 24 Hz. Further evidence for detection precision of motor unit activity in the muscle comes from the systematic examination of force levels and of ramp contractions. The changes in the spectrum always occur according to the changes in the number of active units and in firing rate modulation. That the frequencies in the 6–10 Hz range reflect the activity of those motor units discharging at their slowest maintained firing rates could be proven by simultaneous recordings of

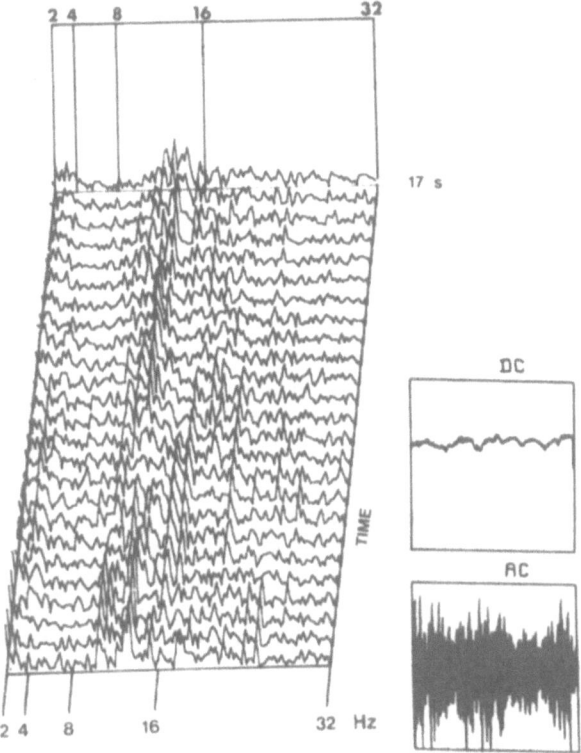

Figure 3.3 Series of partly overlapping force tremor spectra recorded during a steady isometric contraction (6 N) of the index finger extensor maintained by a normal individual for 17 s. Each single spectrum was computed over a period of 4.25 s. To correct for effects of mechanical damping, higher-frequency parts (above 8 Hz) are enhanced following a slope of 40 dB/decade. As typical for such weak steady contractions, spectra show predominantly frequencies between 8 and 20 Hz corresponding to the range of motor unit firing rates.

single motor units, and by the fact that the increase in amplitude of the frequencies as occurs in activated physiological or pathological tremor is invariably the result of motor unit firing or bursting synchronously at these rates. The prominent peak resulting from this synchronisation demarcates the left end of the range of motor unit firing rates, as reflected in such spectra much clearer than in the normal case (see Freund *et al.*, chapter 12, this volume). In most pathological tremors, the peak is not only larger but also shifted to the left as compared with physiological tremor. This corresponds to the slower onset firing rates of the motor units in such cases.

Since the method seems to be suitable to assess the activity of the motoneurone pool innervating the force-producing muscle, we have chosen the term 'muscle activity spectrum' (MAS) for this type of spectrum. This takes into account that these spectra reflect changes in the force output of the muscle as well as the force produced by the motor units: the MAS can be used for the display of tremor, but its potential reaches beyond that scale. It holds a promise to provide information about the activity of motor units that cannot be obtained by other methods.

Motor unit activity as revealed by muscle activity spectra

The need for this sort of information is shown by our lack of knowledge of essential properties of motor units in various motor disorders. Any disturbance of muscle innervation is associated with alterations of motor unit activity. Paresis, no matter whether central or peripheral in nature, can only be the consequence of a reduction in the number of units recruited or of an impairment of firing rate modulation. Almost nothing is known about the differential involvement of these two force-generating mechanisms of the final common path. This is due to the difficulty in assessing firing rate modulation of enough motor units throughout the working range of the muscle by single unit recording, as it is impossible to measure the number of units recruited.

The difficulty in obtaining information about the two force-generating mechanisms has led to various approaches to obtain this information by other methods. Frequency analysis of surface or needle EMG (Verroust et al., 1981) and the relationship between force and surface EMG (Tang and Rymer, 1981) have been developed to fill this gap. These methods provide, however, only limited information. What can we expect from the MAS?

As shown by Freund et al. (chapter 12, this volume), pathological tremor can be nicely displayed. Changes in onset firing rates as they occur in Parkinson's disease or lesions of cerebellar or other subcortical motor nuclei can be easily recognised. It is then possible to determine the characteristic peak frequencies of individual patients or of groups of patients with different tremor forms.

Whenever synchronisation between motor units is increased in extra-pyramidal motor disorders, there are fewer frequency components at higher frequencies since motor unit firing rates seem to be 'clamped' to low frequencies. This is indicative of an impairment of firing rate modulation. This impairment could be responsible for the slight weakness in such disorders. It has already been recognised by Parkinson (1817) that patients with the shaking palsy show an apparent weakness. Holmes (1917) has described a weakness in patients with cerebellar lesions. The impairment of firing rate modulation would be able to explain such a weakness as well as a slowing of rapid movements in these disorders. The generation of strong or fast contractions both depend on the capacity of the motoneurones to produce high-frequency discharges.

In contrast to the impairment of firing rate modulation in some extrapyramidal motor disorders the situation is inverse in cases with *myopathies*. It has already been observed in single unit recordings that the firing rates of the motor units are higher than normal in some patients with a myopathy (Dietz et al., 1975). The MAS of a patient suffering from a muscular dystrophy was characterised by a shift in the range of firing rates towards the higher frequencies. This is shown in figure 3.4 for one of these patients. There is not much activity at the lower frequencies,

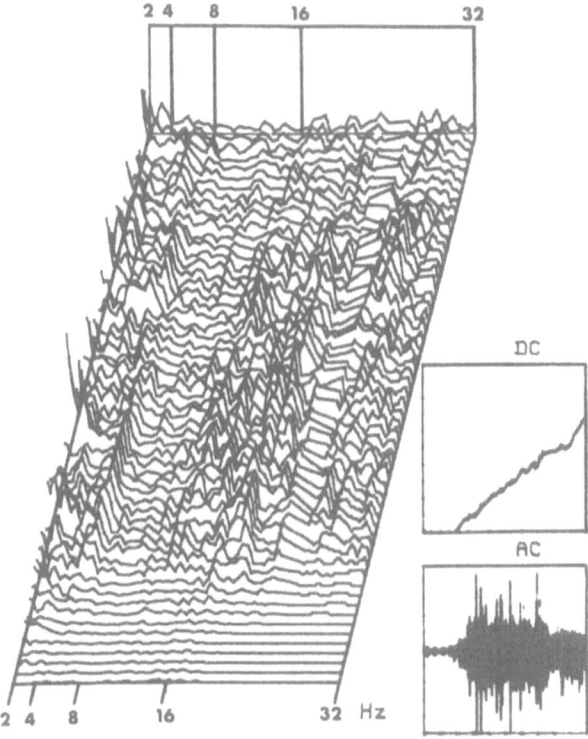

Figure 3.4 Muscle activity spectra of a patient with a myopathy during slowly increasing isometric force of the right extensor indicis muscle. In contrast to spectra of a normal person (figure 3.3) there is almost no activity in the range between 4 and 14 Hz but very much spectral power at higher frequencies. This corresponds well to increased onset firing rates in the motor units of patients with muscular dystrophy. In addition, more power is seen at low frequencies (0–5 Hz). This is due to the force change during the ramp contraction (non-stationary contraction).

but there is also almost no activity between 6 and 14 Hz where most of the power is distributed in normal subjects. In the myopathic patients the power is spread to frequencies higher than 14 Hz already at weak muscular efforts. According to our assumptions on the generation of the MAS, this is regarded as evidence that the firing range is shifted to higher frequencies. The onset firing rates are as high as 15–16 Hz. This raises the question why motor units should fire at higher rates in a pathological condition where the contractile mechanism is primarily damaged. We conjecture that motor units increase their firing rates as compensation for the diminution of the amplitudes of the twitch contractions. The motoneurone pool would then use increasing fusion to compensate for the decreased amplitudes. Similar MAS were observed in a patient with a peripheral neuropathy. Although the weakness of the hands and forearms was only mild, the frequency distribution was similar to that shown in figure 3.4. The increase in the firing rates could indicate a substantial reduction in the number of motor units that can be recruited. The increase in firing rate would again represent a compensatory mechanism for a decreased capability of the motor units to produce the required force.

A different pathological configuration was seen in patients with a moderate hemiparesis of the arm. The MAS showed less power than usual and the distribution was limited to a narrow range. But this range corresponds to the normal range, as it is seen at very weak efforts. It is therefore likely that the paresis is the consequence of an impairment of both the number of units that can be recruited and the firing rate modulation.

DISCUSSION

On the basis of such examples it seems possible that the MAS can serve as a semiquantitative method for the assessment of the activity of a motoneurone pool. It can provide information about the activity of ensembles of motor units that cannot be obtained by any other method. The distribution of frequencies in the range above 6 Hz (or in pathological cases even above 3–4 Hz) indicates that the range of firing rates and the power at different frequencies give an estimate of the number of motor units producing it. The latter is shown by cases with synchronisation of motor units at their onset firing rates. The more units that are synchronised, the stronger is the force at this frequency so that this small part of the power spectrum causes a force oscillation or movement. Since the force contribution of a single motor unit is unknown, it is impossible to draw any inferences about the number of motor units active at each frequency. The MAS can therefore only be regarded as a semiquantitative method: the frequencies can be determined quantitatively as well as the power, but one cannot determine how many motor units produce this power. Furthermore, the power can be falsified by a number of factors. Changes in the net force output of the muscles are the generators of the low-frequency part of the spectrum. There is a certain amount of overlap with the part of the spectrum generated by the twitch contractions in cases where the force fluctuations are large. In cases with stronger tremors and a corresponding high peak in the power spectrum, peaks at the harmonic frequencies are added to the 'true' power generated at that frequency. Another source of error comes from the fact that almost any muscle action is the result of synergistic innervation. For our recording situation with extension of the forefinger (to which is fixed a ring) wrist extension can support finger extension considerably via the friction of the finger joint. It is therefore essential for the method that the subject really activates the extensor indicis muscle. If this is not the case, it can readily be recognised because almost no power appears in the spectrum. For practical purposes the shortcomings of the method with respect to an accurate measurement of the spectral power does not hamper the application of the method significantly. It clearly seems possible to obtain a rough estimate of the proportion of units firing at different rates. For more accurate assessment of motor unit activity, the increase in the contractile amplitude of higher threshold motor units was also taken into account.

CONCLUSIONS

These kinds of tremor analyses open new possibilities for the exploration of the activity of motor units in various motor disorders. The examples shown in this chapter have only illustrated a few pathological cases indicating diagnostic possibilities. Further systematic studies have to expand these observations and test how certain changes in the muscle activity spectrum reflect motor unit dysfunction typical for lesions of different parts of the motor system. At this stage it is only possible to say that a method derived from tremor analysis offers considerably more information in addition to that concerning the tremor itself. This is the consequence of better insights into the tremor-generating mechanisms. Tremor is only one aspect of the force output of a muscle. Spectral analysis of muscle force has shown that the analysis of mechanical events may be worth while. The results reveal that it offers information which is complementary to that obtained by EMG analysis.

REFERENCES

Allum, J. H. J., Dietz, V. and Freund, H.-J. (1978). Neuronal mechanisms underlying physiological tremor. *J. Neurophysiol.*, **41**, 557–71.

Alpern, J. (1972). Eye movements. In Jameson, D. and Hurvich, L. M. (eds), *Handbook of Sensory Physiology*, vol. 7, Springer, Berlin, pp. 303–30.

Bawa, C. C. and Stein, R. B. (1976). Frequency responses of human soleus muscle. *J. Neurophysiol.*, **39**, 788–93.

Dietz, V., Büdingen, H. J., Hillesheimer, W. and Freund, H.-J. (1975). Discharge characteristics of single motor fibres of hand muscles in lower motoneurone diseases and myopathies. In Kunze and Desmedt (eds), *Studies on Neuromuscular Diseases*, Karger, Basel, pp. 122–7.

Halliday, A. M. and Redfearn, J. W. T. (1956). An analysis of finger tremor in healthy subjects. *J. Physiol. (Lond.)*, **134**, 600–11.

Holmes, G. (1917). The symptoms of acute cerebellar injuries due to gunshot wounds. *Brain*, **40**, 461–535.

Marshall, J. and Walsh, E. G. (1956). Physiological tremor. *J. Neurol. Neurosurg. Psychiatr.*, **19**, 260–7.

Parkinson, J. (1817). *An Essay on the Shaking Palsy*, Sherwood, Neely and Jones, London. (Reprinted, 1922, in *Arch. Neurol. Psychiatr.*, **7**, 682–710.)

Sutton, G. G. and Sykes, K. (1967). The variation in hand tremor with force in healthy subjects. *J. Physiol. (Lond.)*, **191**, 699–711.

Tang, H. and Rymer, W. Z. (1981). Abnormal force–EMG relations in paretic limbs of hemiparetic human subjects. *J. Neurol. Neurosurg. Psychiatr.*, **44**, 690–8.

Verroust, J., Blinowska, A. and Cannet, G. (1981). Functioning of the ensemble of motor units of the muscle determined from global EMG-signal. *EMG Clin. Neurophysiol.*, **21**, 21–4.

4
Origins of normal and pathological tremor

C. D. MARSDEN

INTRODUCTION

Tremors, perhaps because they are so obvious, have always fascinated neuro-physiologists and neurologists, even though their causes are often uncertain and their origins disputed.

There is no satisfactory classification of tremor, and many different terms are used ambiguously. That presented in tables 4.1 and 4.2 represents this author's prejudices.

The simple classification of tremor by appearance (table 4.1) is practical. The clinical significance of a rest tremor is different from that of an action tremor,

Table 4.1 Classification of tremor by appearance.

(1) Rest
(2) Action
    (a) Postural
    (b) Movement (kinetic or intention)
        (i) Initial
        (ii) Transition
        (iii) Terminal

Table 4.2 Classification of tremor by cause.

	Rest	Postural	Movement
Physiological	−	+	+/−
Enhanced physiological	−	++	+
Benign essential	−	+++	+
Severe essential	++	++++	++
Parkinsonian – Rest	++++	++	+
Postural	+	+++	+
Rubral	++	+++	++++
Cerebellar	−	+	+++

and a postural tremor may have a different origin to a kinetic or movement tremor. The common causes of tremor are shown in table 4.2, in relation to the clinical picture of the tremor.

In this chapter I will review the pathophysiology of the common types of tremor encountered in clinical practice, with particular emphasis upon the physiological mechanisms involved. The chapter builds upon and develops the themes presented in an earlier review (Marsden, 1978).

PHYSIOLOGICAL TREMOR

We are all aware that our hands shake from time to time, particularly under conditions of fright. Such a physiological action tremor causes no disability, but has fascinated physiologists who see it as a clue to the operation of the motor nervous system.

Unfortunately, the literature on physiological tremor abounds with confusion arising from dogmatic belief that there is but one cause of the phenomenon. In fact, physiological tremor represents the sum of a large number of different interacting mechanisms (table 4.3). All contribute to produce the oscillation of the outstretched hands at a frequency of 8–12 Hz that can be recorded by many different techniques. This is not surprising. Oscillation of a mechanical system,

Table 4.3 Causes of physiological tremor.

(1) Ballistocardiogram – heart-beat vs mechanical resonance
(2) Muscle properties – low-pass filter
(3) Motoneurone firing – size principle
(4) Spindle feedback – synchronisation of discharges
(5) Supraspinal influences – visual
(6) Pharmacological influences – beta-receptors

such as a human limb, is a function of both the inherent mechanical properties of the system, and of the input into the system. The final output, in this case a tremor oscillation, is influenced by both, and can be changed in amplitude or frequency by alteration of either the mechanical properties or the input. In fact, any tremor comprises a number of oscillations at different frequencies, some dependent on passive mechanical properties, others on the form of the input.

The frequency components of a tremor are conveniently separated by the technique of spectral analysis. This reveals the presence of an unexpected peak at around 8–10 Hz in the oscillations of the outstretched fingers (figure 4.1). (It should be noted that the size of this peak is larger in records of acceleration or velocity, as shown in figure 4.1, where the size of the tremor is expressed as power spectral density. In raw records of displacement alone, this 9 Hz peak is much smaller.) It will be noted that the size and frequency of the tremor peak illustrated in figure 4.1 is remarkably stable. What is responsible for this phenomenon?

Mechanical factors in physiological tremor

The human limb possesses inertia and stiffness, so that it acts as a passive mass-spring system, which has a natural frequency at which it oscillates freely. The greater the mass of such a system, the lower will be its natural resonant frequency and the more damped will be its oscillations. The natural frequency of the finger (about 25 Hz) is higher than that of the wrist (about 9 Hz), which is higher than that of the elbow (about 2 Hz). These natural mechanical resonances can be identified in tremor spectra from finger, wrist and elbow by adding mass, which increases inertia and causes resonant frequencies to decrease. However, both in the case of finger and elbow, another component exists at around 9 Hz, whose frequency is unaffected by added mass. This component, illustrated in figure 4.1, must be generated by the nature of the input into the system.

The mechanical properties of the limb, however, do confer certain filtering characteristics on the effect of any input into the system. For example (figure 4.2), increasing the speed of muscle contraction dramatically increases the amplitude of oscillation provoked by a fixed input. Conversely, if the central nervous system (CNS) generates an input into the limb at a frequency well above or well below the natural frequency of oscillation of the limb, the amplitude of the resulting tremor is likely to be small. In particular, if the frequency of activation exceeds the tetanic fusion frequency of the muscle, the resulting oscillation will be negligible. Voluntary movements of limbs can be made at various frequencies, up to a limit of about 6 Hz. Tetanic fusion frequency for human muscle is around 15-20 Hz.

Two mechanical factors, therefore, will determine the amplitude of any tremor generated by central input into the passive limb system:

(1) the natural resonant frequency, which is a function of load and therefore changes with the task undertaken;
(2) the tetanic fusion frequency of muscle, which confers the properties of a low-pass filter on input into the system.

These passive mechanical properties determine the impact of any input into the limb, whether that input is the result of added external force, or due to forces generated by the body itself, either from the heart or from muscle contraction. (For a review of the influence of muscle mechanics on motor performance, see Rack (1978, 1981).)

The role of heart-beat

The mechanical thrust of the heart generates small oscillations which can be recorded throughout the body. This ballistocardiac impulse is responsible for 'tremor' of the relaxed limb and contributes a little (perhaps less than 10%) to the tremor of the outstretched hands (Marsden *et al.*, 1969b). The fundamental frequency of oscillation produced by heart-beat is around 1 Hz although harmonics at higher frequencies are evident.

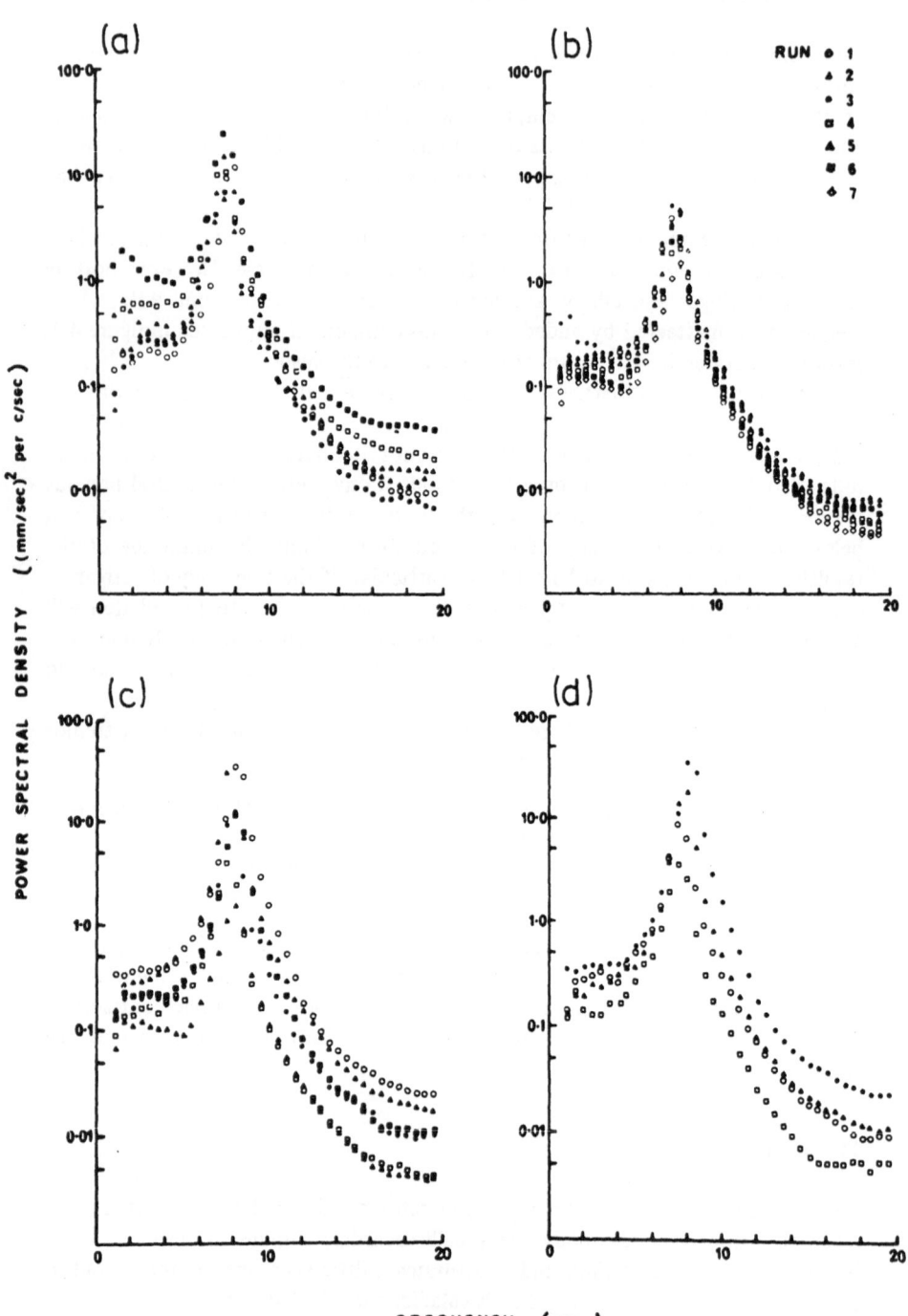

FREQUENCY   (c/sec)

Figure 4.1 (*opposite*) Tremor of the right index finger recorded with an accelero-meter from a single subject on repeated occasions. Each period of recording lasted 1 to 2 min and was repeated up to seven times: (a) at 3 min intervals over 15 min; (b) at 10 min intervals over 1 h; (c) at 1 h intervals over 6 h; and (d) daily for 4 days. Each tremor recording was subjected to spectral analysis at 0.5 Hz intervals up to 20 Hz. Note the consistent size and frequency of the tremor peak at around 9 Hz in this subject. (Reproduced from Marsden *et al.* (1969a), *EEG Clin. Neurophysiol.*, 27, 169–78, with permission.)

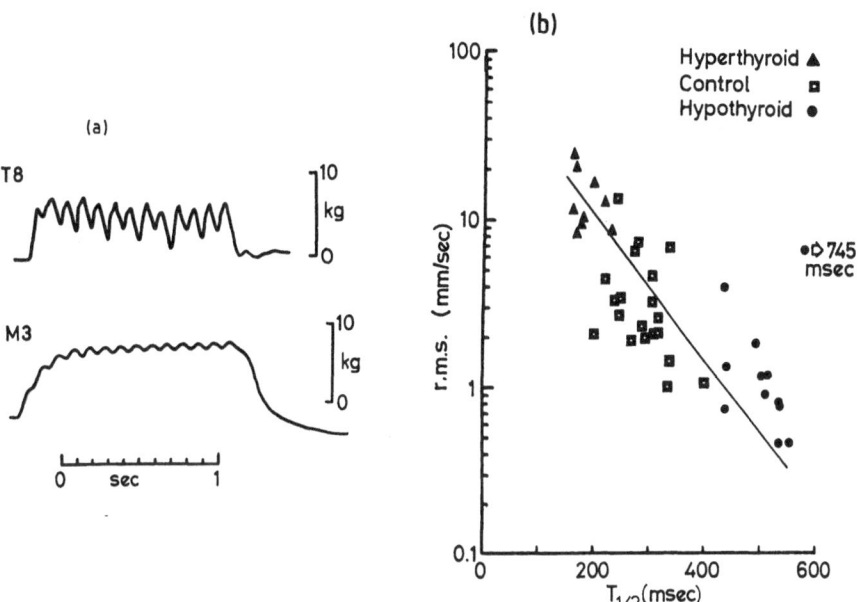

Figure 4.2 Effect of speed of muscle contraction on physiological tremor. (a) Effect of difference in speed of calf muscle contraction of a patient with thyro-toxicosis (case T8, with $T_{1/2}$ = 173 ms) compared to one with myxoedema (case M3, with $T_{1/2}$ = 491 ms) in response to a brief tetanus at 10 Hz delivered to the medial popliteal nerve at the knee, recording isometric force of plantar flexion. The faster muscle twitch in the thyrotoxic patient allows an unfused tetanus of around 5 kg, while the slow twitch in myxoedema produces a nearly fused tetanus approaching 10 kg to the same neural stimulus. (b) The amplitude of finger tremor (as r.m.s. velocity in millimetres per second between 0.5 and 20 Hz) in groups of thyrotoxic, normal and myxoedematous subjects, plotted against their speed of calf muscle contraction (shown as half-relaxation time or $T_{1/2}$). The faster the muscles contract, the greater the amplitude of the tremor ($r = 0.83$, $p < 0.001$), and vice versa, although the peak frequency of the tremor scarcely alters. (Reproduced from Marsden *et al.* (1970), *J. Neurol. Neurosurg. Psychiatr.*, 33, 776–82, with permission.)

The contribution of motor neurone firing characteristics

Two features of motor neurone firing contribute to physiological tremor. The first is that most motor neurones commence firing at a frequency of around 8 Hz (Milner-Brown *et al.*, 1973a,b,c; Freund *et al.*, 1975) (which is below tetanic fusion frequency for human muscle, so causes oscillation) (figure 4.3). As the force of contraction increases, the frequency of recruited motor units also increases above that required to produce fusion of contraction, so faster firing units make less and less mechanical contribution to tremor (Marshall and Walsh, 1956; Allum *et al.*, 1978).

The second factor is related to the size principle of Henneman (Henneman *et al.*, 1965, 1974). This states, in general, that recruitment of motor units is an orderly process with smaller units firing at lower forces than larger units. It turns out that the size of the unit recruited is more or less proportional to the mean force level over a wide range (figure 4.4). As a result, the fractional increment of force generated by each newly recruited unit remains more or less constant. However, as each unit that is brought in fires at around 8 Hz, there will be a constant ripple of unfused tension on top of the existing fused contraction produced by the earlier and faster firing units. This superimposed ripple will remain a more or less constant fraction of the force exerted, because of the size principle. This

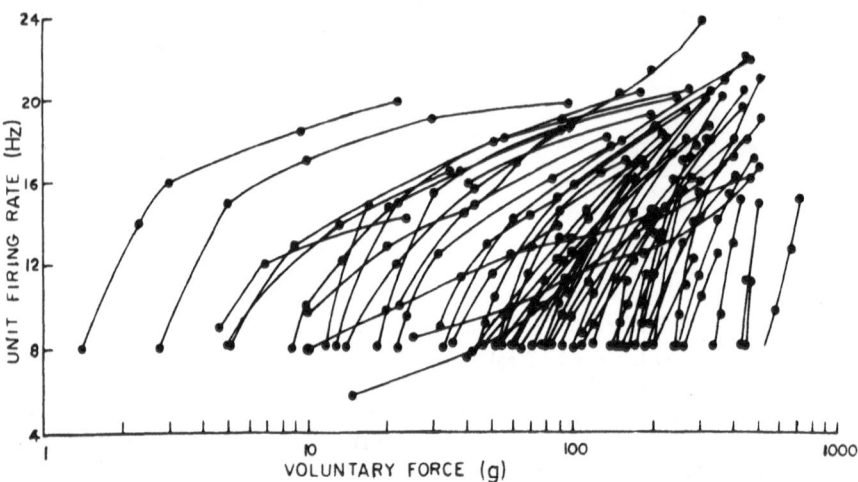

Figure 4.3 Steady firing frequencies (ordinate) of single motor units in human extensor digitorum communis, recorded during voluntary contractions over a range of forces. Note that all units start firing at about 8 Hz. As force increases, their firing rates are raised progressively to 16–24 Hz (frequency modulation). Those units brought in at higher forces show a tendency to increase their firing frequency more rapidly for smaller force increments. (Reproduced from Burke (1981), in Brooks (ed.), *Handbook of Physiology. The Nervous System, Motor Control*, part 1, pp. 345–422, with permission.)

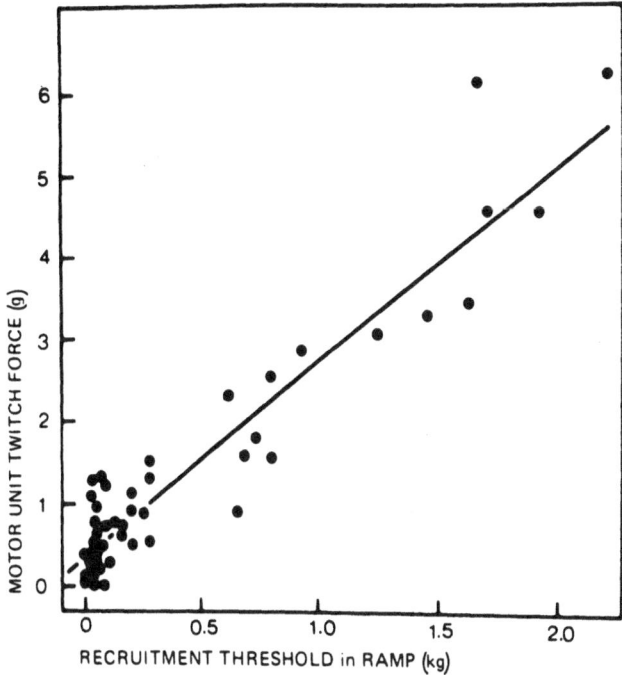

Figure 4.4 Behaviour of single motor units from human first dorsal interosseous during slow voluntary abduction of the index finger. The threshold tension at which each of the 50 units was recruited is shown on the abscissa. The twitch force generated by each unit, extracted by spike-triggered averaging, is shown on the ordinate. Note the linear relation between the size of the motor unit and the threshold force at which it is recruited. (Reproduced from Desmedt (1981), *Progress in Clinical Neurophysiology*, vol. 9, pp. 97–136, with permission.)

concept receives support from the observation that the amplitude of hand tremor increases linearly with the force exerted (until one approaches maximal forces) (Sutton and Sykes, 1967a) (figure 4.5).

This idea that motor neurone firing characteristics combined with the size principle is responsible for physiological tremor does not require any degree of synchronisation of motor neurone firing. However, any synchronisation that does occur inevitably will increase the amplitude of tremor. The extent to which such synchronisation takes place, and the mechanisms responsible, are subjects of controversy.

Examination of simple EMG records of the muscles involved in physiological tremor usually does not reveal evidence of synchronisation. Surface EMG recordings of a pair of antagonistic muscles usually show a continuous voluntary 'interference pattern'. Furthermore, most authors agree that impulses from different motor units in a single muscle often are remarkably independent of each other. Indeed, such synchronisation that does occur during normal human

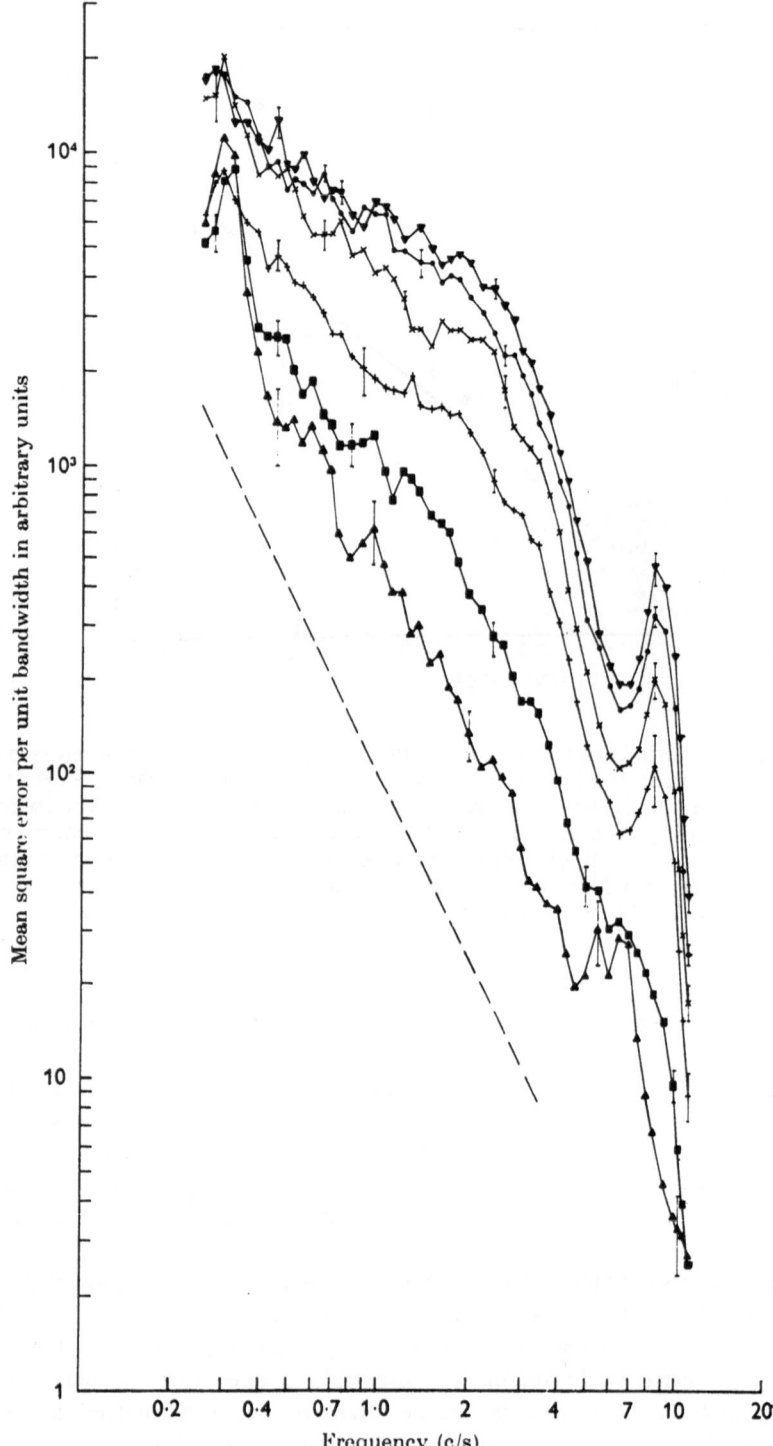

muscle contraction may be weak (Milner-Brown *et al*., 1975), and some have claimed that even this is the result of chance occurrence (Taylor, 1962). Dietz *et al*. (1976), however, by simultaneous recording from pairs of motor units in the first dorsal interosseous muscle, or in soleus and gastrocnemius, were able to demonstrate a tendency to synchronisation greater than could be explained by chance. Indeed, the greater the degree of synchronisation, the greater the tremor in their studies. However, tremor could still be present even in the absence of synchronisation.

The conclusion that synchronisation of motor unit discharge is not essential for the generation of normal physiological tremor certainly appears justified. However, obviously the greater the tendency for synchronisation of motor unit discharge at frequencies below tetanic fusion frequency, the greater will be the physiological tremor. There are occasions when great synchronisation can be provoked, for example, when the subject is anxious or subjected to adrenaline infusion (see later), or when the limb is suddenly disturbed (Lippold, 1970) (figure 4.6). In these situations, grouping of motor unit action potentials around 9 Hz is obvious, even in the surface electromyogram, and is associated with marked tremor oscillations. Such grouping of motor unit discharge often seems to be the result of activation of stretch reflex mechanisms, which tend to pull motor neurone discharges together (Hagbarth and Young, 1979). In addition, recurrent Renshaw cell inhibition may contribute.

The stretch reflex and physiological tremor

The majority of motor neurones innervating a muscle receive excitation from each muscle spindle afferent, so muscle stretch synchronises motor neurone discharge. Many investigators have been attracted to the similarity between the spinal stretch reflex and mechanical linear servo-systems. The latter may exhibit instability and oscillate at a particular frequency related to the delay around the servo-loop. The delay in operation of the monosynaptic spinal stretch reflex arc has been considered by some authors to be such as to generate a tremor at about 9 Hz (Halliday and Redfearn, 1956; Lippold *et al*., 1957). A linear servo-

---

Figure 4.5 (*opposite*) Effect of force of contraction on hand tremor in one normal subject. The subject held a stiff joystick as if it were a pen, and was asked to press it medially with a fixed force of 0.45 kg (▲), 0.91 kg (■), 1.36 kg (+), 1.81 kg (×), 2.27 kg (●) and 2.72 kg (▼). The means of eight recordings of tremor amplitude (as mean square error per unit bandwidth), each lasting 1 min, are shown (± 1 SEM) at 52 frequencies between 0.256 and 12.5 Hz. Note that in general the amplitude of tremor decreased with increasing frequency with a slope of about 6 dB/octave, but that there also is a 9 Hz peak of tremor. The amplitude of the tremor increases at all frequencies with increasing force, but the frequency of the tremor peak remains more or less the same. (Reproduced from Sutton and Sykes (1967a), *J. Physiol*., **191**, 699–711, with permission.)

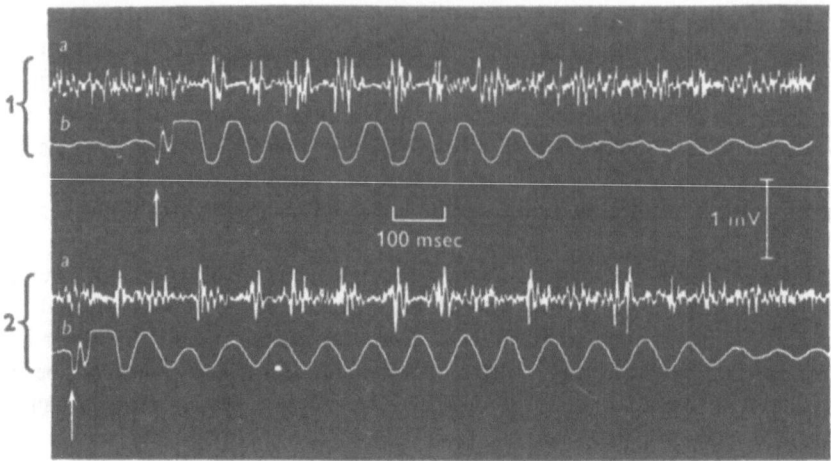

Figure 4.6 Oscillations produced by prodding the nail of the outstretched middle finger downwards at the times indicated by the arrows. In both records 1 and 2, the upper trace (a) is the EMG recorded from surface electrodes over the extensor digitorum communis, while the lower trace (b) is of finger position recorded photometrically. (Reproduced from Lippold (1970), *J. Physiol.*, **206**, 359–82, with permission.)

system tends to oscillate at a period equal to twice the delay around the loop, when negative feedback becomes positive. A loop delay of around 50 ms could easily generate an oscillation at the requisite frequency. But the delay from the response of muscle spindles to muscle activation in, for example, the human forearm is only about 20 ms, which clearly is too short a time to generate a finger tremor with a peak frequency of 9 Hz. There is also the additional and greater delay required to generate muscle contraction. In physiological tremor, each spindle burst occurs only once in each cycle (Hagbarth and Young, 1979), during muscle lengthening, so that loop delay must include not only neuronal conduction time, but also the time required to generate force. In addition, account must be taken of antagonistic muscles. Some tremors could be generated by alternating contraction of agonist and antagonist, in which case the delay introduced by muscle contraction becomes minimal—the spindles in the antagonist are immediately activated by the beginnings of contraction of the agonist.

Whatever the theoretical arguments about stretch reflex involvement in physiological tremor, the true contribution it makes must be made evident by the effects of deafferentation. Our own data on a single patient with surgical section of the posterior roots of C5–T2 (Marsden *et al.*, 1967b), and on nine patients with tabes dorsalis and seven patients with a severe polyneuropathy with slowed maximal motor conduction velocities (Marsden, 1978), suggest that afferent feedback is not critical to physiological tremor. Thus, a 9 Hz peak was evident in the deafferented patient's hand tremor (figure 4.7), a 9 Hz peak was present in the

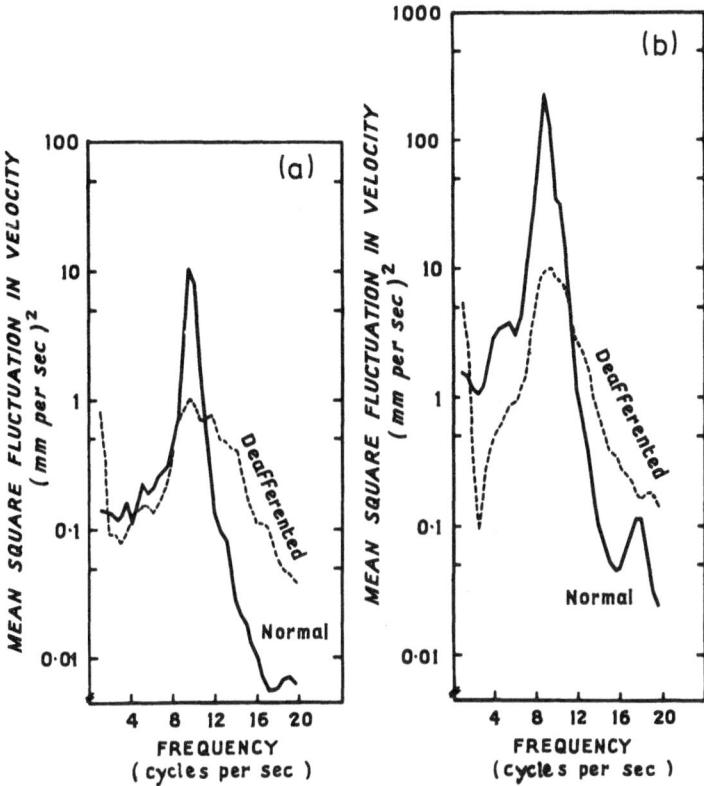

Figure 4.7 Effect of deafferentation on physiological tremor. Spectral analysis of tremor of the outstretched index fingers of both hands of a 51-year-old woman whose posterior roots from C5 to T2 inclusive on the right-hand side had been divided at open operation: (a) before infusion and (b) during the third to fifth minutes of infusion of adrenaline (10 μg/min i.v.). Note the presence of a 9 Hz tremor peak in the deafferented arm, and the greater effect of adrenaline upon the normal arm's tremor peak. (Reproduced from Marsden *et al.* (1967b), *Lancet*, 2, 700–2, with permission.)

patients affected by tabes dorsalis, and finger tremor frequency was not markedly different from normal in the patients with polyneuropathy; three of the latter recovered, but merely showed a shift in tremor peak from about 7 Hz to 8.7 Hz, despite recovery of conduction velocity from a mean of 27 to 45 m s^{-1}.

While the effect of deafferentation upon tremor frequency seems slight, its effect upon tremor amplitude is more obvious. The size of the 9 Hz tremor peak was smaller in the patient with the deafferented arm, and in many of those with tabes or a peripheral neuropathy, while the width of the peak was broader.

The general conclusion from observations such as these is that physiological tremor can occur in the absence of afferent feedback, but its amplitude probably is modulated by the effects of spindle input synchronising motor neurone discharge. Indeed, there are circumstances when such a mechanism may become of crucial importance to the genesis of a tremor, as for example in the die-away oscillations provoked by prodding a finger, as illustrated in figure 4.6. Indeed, it was analysis of this phenomenon that confirmed Lippold's belief in the role of the stretch reflex arc in physiological tremor—'physiological tremor will also involve stretch receptor activation in phase with it' (Lippold, 1970).

Another situation in which stretch reflex mechanisms become of considerable importance is when the subject exerts a muscular force against a suitably tuned mechanical load. Joyce and Rack (1974), for example, showed that a compliant system opposing human elbow flexion encourages tremor, in which the stretch reflex participates (see Joyce *et al.*, 1974). Subsequently, Matthews and Muir (1980) confirmed that when a subject exerted a high force of elbow flexion against a compliant spring, a vigorous 10 Hz tremor developed. This disappeared when the subject exerted the same force against a rigid restraint. Smaller forces exerted against the compliant spring caused smaller 10 Hz tremors. Matthews and Muir (1980) also concluded that tremor generated by strong contractions against compliant loads 'resulted from the central action of a similar rhythmicity of afferent input from the moving limb'.

It remained for Hagbarth and Young (1979) and Young and Hagbarth (1980) to demonstrate such rhythmicity of spindle input by direct recording of afferent activity in man during physiological tremor. They found that human muscle spindles in nerves supplying mainly the wrist and finger flexors, and identified as primary endings on the basis of their response to an electrically induced muscle twitch, were exquisitely sensitive to the minute movements of physiological tremor. In fact, the spindles discharged rhythmically, silencing during muscle shortening and firing when the muscle lengthened. Thus, the spindles discharged only once during each tremor cycle, and there was no evidence of alpha-gamma coactivation during the unloading phase. However, despite this rhythmic spindle activity, there was no evidence of synchronisation of motor unit discharge in the active muscle's electromyogram during low-amplitude physiological tremor.

When, however, physiological tremor was enhanced by fatigue or other means, such rhythmic bursts of spindle discharge then begin to synchronise motor unit firing after a delay appropriate to operation of the spinal stretch reflex. So, in enhanced physiological tremor the electromyogram reveals rhythmic bursts of activity, whose timing is such as to produce force pulses which increase tremor amplitude (a positive feedback effect of stretch reflex action). However, Hagbarth and Young (1979) also noted that the same spinal stretch reflex could act as a negative feedback system in response to large perturbations, such as those produced by prodding the finger. In these circumstances, the high dynamic sensitivity of primary spindles caused them still to fire early in the stretch, so that the resulting monosynaptic motoneurone discharge now generated force at a time when stretch might still be continuing. In these circumstances the stretch reflex tended to damp rather than reinforce oscillation.

Supraspinal influences on physiological tremor

There have been many suggestions concerning the possible influence of the brain upon physiological tremor. Perhaps the most striking was that of Gordon Holmes, who observed that normal postural tremor of the outstretched hand disappeared after unilateral damage to the cerebellum (an observation that we can confirm from personal observation). However, most of the studies investigating central contributions to physiological tremor have been dismissed or ignored.

Certainly there seems no relation between the alpha rhythm and physiological tremor (Lindqvist, 1941). There is, however, an intriguing and unexplained influence of vision. In certain circumstances, the 9 Hz tremor of the hand disappears when vision is abolished (Sutton and Sykes, 1967b) (figure 4.8). This is particularly and dramatically evident when tremor is recorded in a tracking or holding task employing visual feedback. Indeed, the introduction of time delays in the visual feedback may actually shift the 9 Hz physiological tremor; the longer the delay the lower the frequency (Merton *et al.*, 1967) (figure 4.9). These observations remain unexplained and unexplored.

Lamarre (1975), however, has drawn attention to the presence of rhythmic activity at 7-12 Hz in the olivo-cerebello-bulbar system of the awake and decerebrate monkey, particularly when given the drug harmaline. Harmaline generates a muscular tremor at 7-12 Hz in the monkey. Lamarre and his colleagues showed that harmaline caused the inferior olives to behave as a 10 Hz generator, perhaps by altering calcium conductances. He put forward the hypothesis that some physiological tremors, such as those dependent upon visual feedback (as described by Sutton and Sykes, 1967b, and by Merton *et al.*, 1967), might be due to synchronised rhythmic activity of this olivary generator.

Pharmacological influences on physiological tremor

'We shake with fright' is a commonplace, but it has a pharmacological basis. Intravenous infusions of adrenaline or isoprenaline considerably increase the amplitude of physiological finger tremor, an effect mediated by peripheral beta-adrenergic receptors (Marsden *et al.*, 1967a) (figure 4.10). The responsible receptors lie in the forearm, for the effect of intravenous adrenaline can be abolished by intra-arterial propranolol, and can be reproduced by intra-arterial adrenaline. At least a part of this pharmacological effect is due to alterations of muscle contractile properties. Thus, beta-agonists increase the speed of contraction of human muscle, thereby raising tetanic fusion frequency (Marsden and Meadows, 1970) (figure 4.11). As a result, input at around 9 Hz causes greater oscillations. However, this is not the only explanation for the tremogenic effects of peripheral beta-receptor activation, for adrenaline has less effect on finger tremor of the deafferented arm (see figure 4.7). There is some evidence that beta-agonists actually increase spindle feedback, perhaps by an action upon intrafusal muscle fibres (Hodgson *et al.*, 1969).

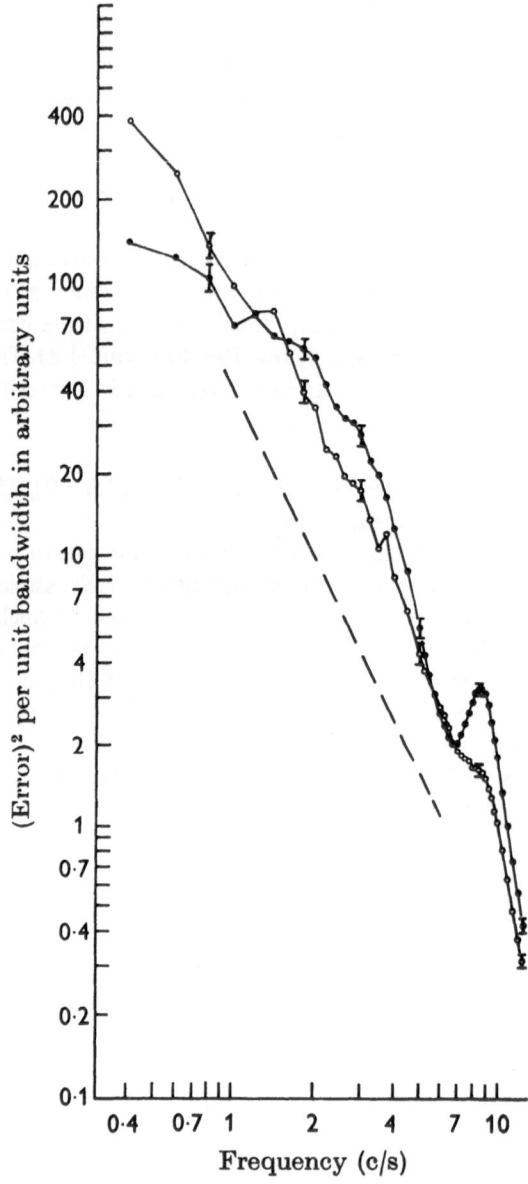

Figure 4.8 Effect of withdrawal of vision on hand tremor. Tremor of the hand was recorded as described in the legend to figure 4.5. The subject tried to maintain a constant force of 2.3 kg by pushing the joystick medially, with reference to a display of the position of the joystick provided on a cathode ray tube. Mean error per unit bandwidth is shown for 16 runs with the eyes open (solid circles) and for 16 runs with the eyes shut (open circles). Note that the tremor peak at about 9 Hz in this normal subject disappears when the eyes are shut. (Reproduced from Sutton and Sykes (1967b), *J. Physiol.*, **190**, 281–93, with permission.)

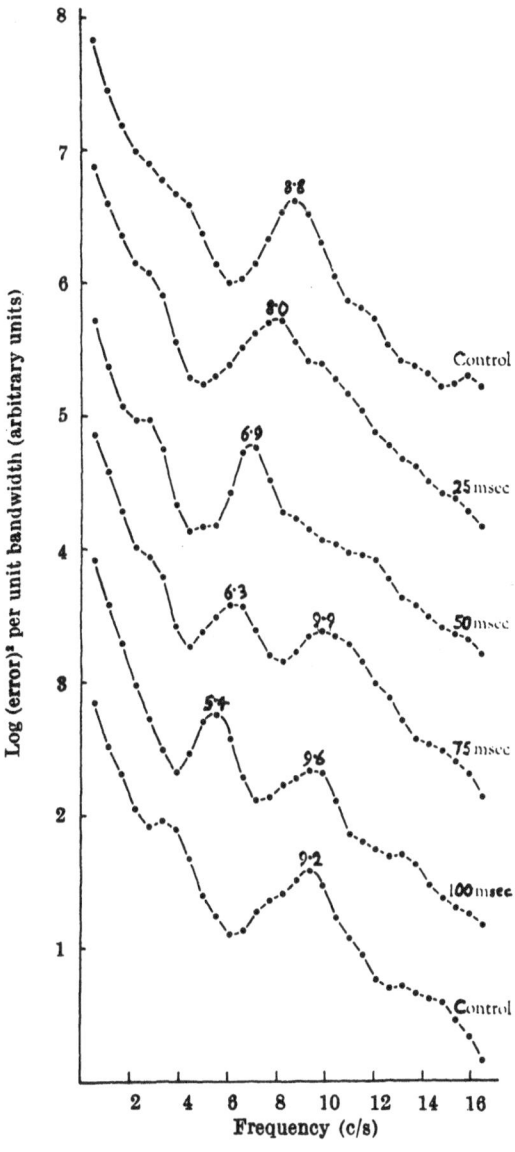

Figure 4.9 Effect of added visual delay on the frequency of the 9 Hz tremor peak. Tremor was recorded as described in the legends to figures 4.5 and 4.8. Time delays were added between the joystick and the cathode ray tube. The power spectra of successive 30 s runs of hand tremor are shown, beginning and ending with control runs, and with delays of 25, 50, 75 and 100 ms. To avoid overlap, consecutive spectra are displaced down by one log unit. The frequencies of the main peaks are given above them in Hz. Note that added delay increasingly slows the peak of tremor from around 9 Hz down to 5.4 Hz, while another higher-frequency peak also appears. (Reproduced from Merton *et al.* (1967), *Nature*, 216, 583-4, with permission.)

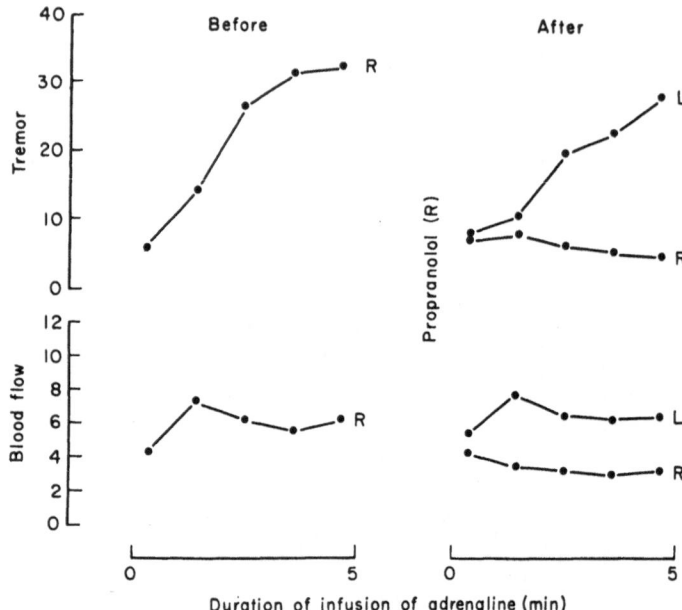

Figure 4.10 Effect of adrenaline (10 μg/min i.v.) on finger tremor and forearm blood flow in a single subject whose right arm was beta-blocked by direct intra-arterial injection of propranolol (0.5 mg) into the right brachial artery at the elbow. Note that both adrenaline and isoprenaline increased tremor and forearm blood flow in the left normal arm, but not in the beta-blocked right arm. (Reproduced from Marsden *et al.* (1967a), *Clin. Sci.*, **33**, 53–65, with permission.)

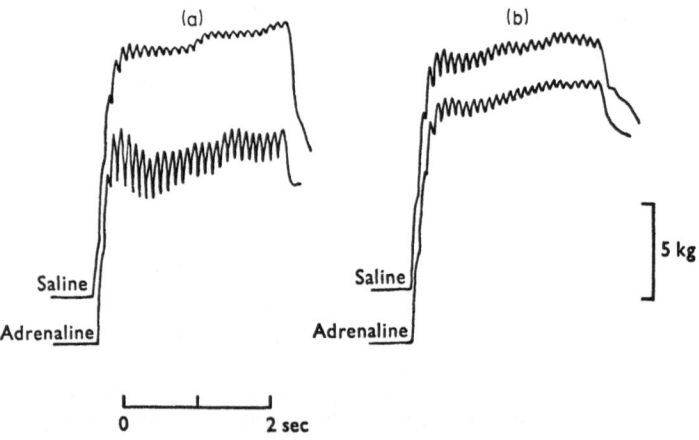

Figure 4.11 The effect of adrenaline (10 μg/min i.v.) on human calf muscle tension evoked by a 10 Hz tetanus for 2 s: (a) before and (b) after propranolol (5 mg i.v.). Note that adrenaline infusion reduces the degree of fusion of the 10 Hz tetanus, an effect abolished by prior beta-blockade. (Reproduced from Marsden and Meadows (1970), *J. Physiol.*, **207**, 429–48, with permission.)

Summary

Physiological tremor thus appears to be the result of a complex interaction of a number of factors including:

(1) The natural resonance of the limb, which is dependent upon the inertia and stiffness of the system.

(2) An interaction between the initial firing rates of motor neurones and the low-pass filter properties of the muscle system. The latter cuts out any tendency to oscillate when motor neurones fire at frequencies above about 15 Hz.

(3) The size principle of motor unit activation. As force is increased, those units already engaged increase their firing rate, so contribute less and less to tremor as a result of the filtering properties of muscle. However, newer and larger motor units are recruited at the lower frequency, so superimposing an oscillation roughly proportional to the force of contraction.

(4) The effect of spindle input which, via spinal pathways, tends to synchronise motor neurone discharge at around 9 Hz, particularly in enhanced physiological tremor.

(5) Supraspinal influences which, in the case of visually determined tasks, maybe dictate the presence and frequency of tremor.

(6) The ballistocardiogram (and any other form of mechanical disturbance such as a passing train!) which will add to the overall tremor.

(7) Circulating catecholamines and the general sympathomimetic tone, which also modulates tremor intensity.

A mechanical recording of tremor consists of the sum of all these various factors, in varying proportions depending upon the amplitude and nature of the tremor.

ENHANCED PHYSIOLOGICAL TREMOR

Knowledge of the many mechanisms that combine to create physiological tremor has helped to explain the variety of enhanced physiological tremors that are encountered in clinical practice (table 4.4). Such tremors have the frequency of physiological tremor (around 8–12 Hz), and have the same characteristics (they are absent at rest, appear on posture, and are present but not intensified on movement). However, they are characterised by a much greater tendency for synchronisation of single motor unit discharges, and surface recordings of the EMG from the active muscle show discrete bursts (Young *et al.*, 1975; Hagbarth and Young, 1979; Young and Hagbarth, 1980).

One of the commonest general mechanisms of enhanced or exaggerated physiological tremor is increased beta-adrenergic stimulation. As discussed above, stimulation of peripheral beta-adrenoceptors causes muscle to contract and relax more rapidly, and may even alter the output of muscle spindles. Both effects

Table 4.4   Enhanced physiological tremor.

	Beta-adrenergic overactivity
(1) Anxiety	+
(2) Thyrotoxicosis	+
(3) Phaeochromocytoma	+
(4) Hypoglycaemia	+
(5) Bronchodilators	+
(6) Alcohol	+ (−)
(7) Lithium	?
(8) Other drugs	?
(9) Exercise	−
(10) Fatigue	−

increase the size of the bursts of group 1a muscle spindle impulses that occur during the lengthening phases of the small ripples of contraction of human fore-arm muscles (Hagbarth and Young, 1979). Indeed, the synchronisation of motor unit discharge provoked by these exaggerated 1a spindle bursts appears to be responsible for these forms of enhanced physiological tremor.

The commonest enhanced physiological tremor is seen during fright. Those who have experienced the problem of the tapping toe and shaking hands while kneeling in church will have no hesitation in accepting the biblical phrase of shaking with fright! Such tremor is reduced by beta-adrenergic blockade (Marsden *et al.*, 1968), as is the tremor encountered in patients with phaeochromocytoma or hypoglycaemia. The tremor of thyrotoxicosis also is reduced by beta-blockade (Marsden *et al.*, 1968), so this also probably is the result of beta-adrenergic stimulation. The tremor produced as an unwanted effect of treatment of asthma with bronchodilators (designed to stimulate selectively $beta_2$-adrenoceptors) now is common. The tremor of alcoholics also has a beta-adrenergic component. Alcohol-withdrawal tremor may be improved by beta-adrenergic antagonists, but whether this is the complete explanation for all alcoholic tremor is not yet certain. Likewise, the cause of tremor induced by drugs such as lithium may involve beta-adrenergic mechanisms, but proof is lacking.

Another type of enhanced physiological tremor occurs during exercise and fatigue. Even a brief but strong muscle contraction has been found to produce long-lasting increases in hand tremor (Furness *et al.*, 1977). This exercise-induced tremor occurred only in the muscles previously contracted, so was unlikely to be due to circulating catecholamine action. Nor could it be mimicked by replacing the prior period of voluntary contraction with a similar period of electrically induced tetanus. In fact, it occurred even if the subject only attempted to undertake the prior contraction, but could not because the muscle had been subjected to ischaemic paralysis. This led the authors to conclude that such exercise-induced tremor must have been due to changes in synchronisation of motor unit firing (see Lippold, 1981). Another sort of tremor develops during prolonged muscle contraction. After 15 min or so of continued contraction, finger or hand tremor gradually begins to increase in amplitude, not only at the usual peak frequency around 9 Hz, but also at lower frequencies particularly around 4-6 Hz (Stiles, 1976; Lippold, 1981). This is not due to any significant change in muscle mechanics, but must represent an alteration in motor unit firing frequency. What is responsible for such a change is unknown.

ESSENTIAL TREMOR

The clinical diagnosis of essential tremor is crude. A tremor conforming to the characteristics of (1) absent at rest, (2) present on maintaining a posture particularly of the outstretched arms, (3) not made strikingly worse by movement, and (4) the absence of signs of parkinsonism or cerebellar disease, will usually mean that essential tremor can be diagnosed. A number of entities conform to this description (table 4.5).

Table 4.5 'Essential tremor'.

A postural tremor, absent at rest and not made strikingly worse on movement, without signs of parkinsonism or cerebellar deficit.
(1) Enhanced physiological tremor
(2) Classical benign essential tremor
(a) Sensitive to beta-antagonists
(b) Insensitive to beta-antagonists
(c) Sensitive to primidone
(d) Sensitive to alcohol
(3) Severe essential tremor
(4) Symptomatic essential tremor

Enhanced physiological tremor

This has been discussed in detail earlier. The mechanisms responsible for enhanced physiological tremor probably are quite distinct from those causing classical essential tremor. Unfortunately, however, many patients complaining only of a postural tremor of the hands are diagnosed as cases of 'essential tremor' when the correct description is one of enhanced physiological tremor (Marsden, 1978; Shahani and Young, 1978). This occurs when the response of primary muscle spindles to the minute fluctuations of force or position inherent in any muscle contraction is increased so as to cause synchronisation of motor unit discharge at physiological tremor frequencies around 8-10 Hz (Hagbarth and Young, 1979; Young and Hagbarth, 1980). Enhanced physiological tremor thus presents as a fast fine postural tremor.

Classical essential tremor

In contrast to enhanced physiological tremor, classical essential tremor is of larger amplitude and slower frequency. It is characterised by a postural tremor of the arms, occasionally of the head, and rarely of the legs (Critchley, 1972). No tremor is evident at rest. The tremor disappears during movement, although it may reappear as the finger hits the point of aim and adopts a posture. This distinction from kinetic or movement tremor sometimes can be exceedingly difficult. True kinetic or movement tremor gets increasingly worse during movement, while essential tremor only appears when the movement is completed. Another crucial diagnostic distinction is that there are no signs of parkinsonism (no akinesia or rigidity, although cogwheeling may be present due to tremor interrupting passive movement), and there are no signs of cerebellar deficit. The latter may be difficult to establish if the tremor is particularly severe. However, the crucial feature is that a patient with cerebellar disease of sufficient severity to cause a postural tremor will be grossly disabled by kinetic tremor and ataxia such that they will be unable to use the arms to dress or feed. In striking contrast, the patient with essential tremor who exhibits moderate to severe postural tremor of the outstretched arms is not so severely disabled. Handwriting may be clumsy, and it may be difficult to manipulate a cup or buttons, but such individuals are independent. They do not exhibit the disastrous motor incapacity of someone with cerebellar disease sufficient to produce the same intensity of postural tremor.

Classical essential tremor may appear in childhood, adolescence (juvenile tremor), early adult life or old age (senile tremor). Its cause is unknown. A positive family history is claimed on over half of such patients, and the pattern of inheritance indicates an autosomal dominant trait. No pathological or biochemical abnormality has been identified, but few cases have come to necropsy.

The pharmacology of essential tremor

There are distinctive pharmacological characteristics of classical essential tremor.

Most patients become aware that alcohol, even in small doses, dramatically decreases the amplitude of the tremor (Growdon et al., 1975). The mechanism responsible for alcohol's effect, however, has not been established.

Some patients can be successfully treated with beta-adrenergic antagonists (Winkler and Young, 1974; Young et al., 1975; Jefferson et al., 1979). The mechanism of action of beta-adrenoceptor antagonists in essential tremor is disputed. Some workers, struck by the fact that so-called cardioselective beta-blockers such as metoprolol and atenolol may ameliorate this tremor, have claimed that blockade of $beta_1$-receptors is necessary for tremor control. Others have suggested that the effects of a drug such as propranolol may be due to its central actions in the brain, rather than to any peripheral effect. These questions now are being resolved by the use of the present generation of selective beta-adrenoceptor antagonists (table 4.6). For example, Jefferson *et al.* (1979), in a double-blind placebo-controlled trial of doses of drugs having equipotent effects on the heart, were able to show that:

(1) A drug that has difficulty entering the brain (sotalol) was as effective in controlling essential tremor as a standard drug that enters the brain with ease (propranolol), indicating that it is the peripheral actions of these compounds that are important in reducing tremor.

(2) The cardioselective drug atenolol was less potent than either propranolol or sotalol, suggesting that blockade of beta$_2$-receptors is the crucial anti-tremor action.

Table 4.6 Beta-adrenoceptor antagonists in benign essential tremor.*

| | *Membrane stabilising action* | *Antagonist at* | | *Central action in brain* | *Effect on benign essential tremor* |
		Beta$_1$- receptors	*Beta$_2$- receptors*		
Propranolol	+	+	+	+	+++
Sotalol	0	+	+	+/−	+++
Atenolol	+	+	+/−	+/−	++
Metoprolol	+	+	+/−	+	+

*Based upon data in Jefferson *et al.* (1979) and Leigh *et al.* (1983).

Despite contrary claims, these conclusions have received further support from a more recent study (Leigh *et al.*, 1983) in which atenolol (which has difficulty entering the brain) was more effective than metoprolol (which enters the nervous system with relative ease), but neither of these cardioselective beta-blockers was as effective as propranolol, all being administered in equipotent doses. All this evidence suggests that blockade of peripheral beta$_2$-adrenoceptors is the critical action responsible for the anti-tremor effect of these drugs. However, there are other conflicting reports, so the matter is not settled finally. In any case, only a proportion of patients with benign essential tremor are helped by such beta-blocking drugs. Why they are of no value in many others (perhaps 50% or more of patients) has not been established. The degree of response does not appear to be related to plasma propranolol levels (Jefferson *et al.*, 1979).

Another drug that has been found to be of benefit in benign essential tremor recently is the anticonvulsant primidone (O'Brien *et al.*, 1981; Findley and Calzetti, 1982), but the exact mechanism of this action also is in dispute. O'Brien and his colleagues originally suggested that primidone's anti-tremor action was mediated by its metabolite phenylethylmalonamide, but administration of the compound by itself had no effect on essential tremor (Calzetti *et al.*, 1981). Indeed, Procaccianti *et al.* (1981) recently have confirmed the traditional value of phenobarbitone in essential tremor.

Variants of classical essential tremor

There are a number of variants of essential tremor, affecting other parts of the body. For instance, about 50% of patients with essential tremor of the hands also have a tremor of the head (titubation). Occasionally, one encounters families with inherited head tremor without hand tremor; the tremor may be 'yes-yes', or 'no-no'. Another variant is isolated writing tremor. Such patients develop a typical essential tremor only while writing, but exhibit no postural tremor of the out-stretched arms. Isolated writing tremor, which is a fragment of essential tremor, must be distinguished from the rarer primary writing tremor described by Rothwell *et al.* (1979). Occasionally one encounters patients who develop a typical essential tremor only on other particular acts. Musicians may find it interfering with particular actions while playing the piano or bowing strings, and even wind instrumentalists occasionally experience an action tremor of the lips and mouth. Sportsmen may present with an isolated specific tremor for one particular phase of their own game. Thus, golfers may present with tremor during the backswing (easily distinguished from the 'yips'); darts throwers may develop a shake of the arm when drawn back to throw the quiver. Such individuals have no other signs of essential tremor.

Mechanisms of essential tremor

Some authors have suggested that essential tremor is merely exaggerated physio-logical tremor (Marshall, 1962). This seems unlikely. In the forms of enhanced physiological tremor described above, the frequency remains the same as that of physiological tremor. Classical essential tremor, however, usually is of a somewhat lower frequency, 5-8 Hz, which is faster than that of classical parkinsonian rest tremor (4-5 Hz), but slower than that of typical physiological tremor (8-12 Hz).

Simultaneous surface EMG records of antagonistic muscles of the arm in essential tremor usually show discrete bursts of EMG activity often occurring synchronously (Shahani and Young, 1976). However, such co-contraction is not found in all patients with essential tremor. Many exhibit typical alternating contractions in agonist and antagonist (figure 4.12). The significance of this finding at present is not known. The similarity to the tremor of Parkinson's disease is apparent, but whether such patients go on to develop parkinsonism has not been established. However, it is believed that there may be an association between essential tremor and Parkinson's disease (Critchley, 1949; Schwab and Young, 1971). Some patients with the latter illness give a long history of essential tremor prior to the appearance of signs of parkinsonism. In addition, the incidence of essential tremor may be higher in the families of patients with Parkinson's disease than it is in the normal population.

The exaggerated oscillations responsible for essential tremor could be due to one or all of a number of abnormal mechanisms (table 4.7).

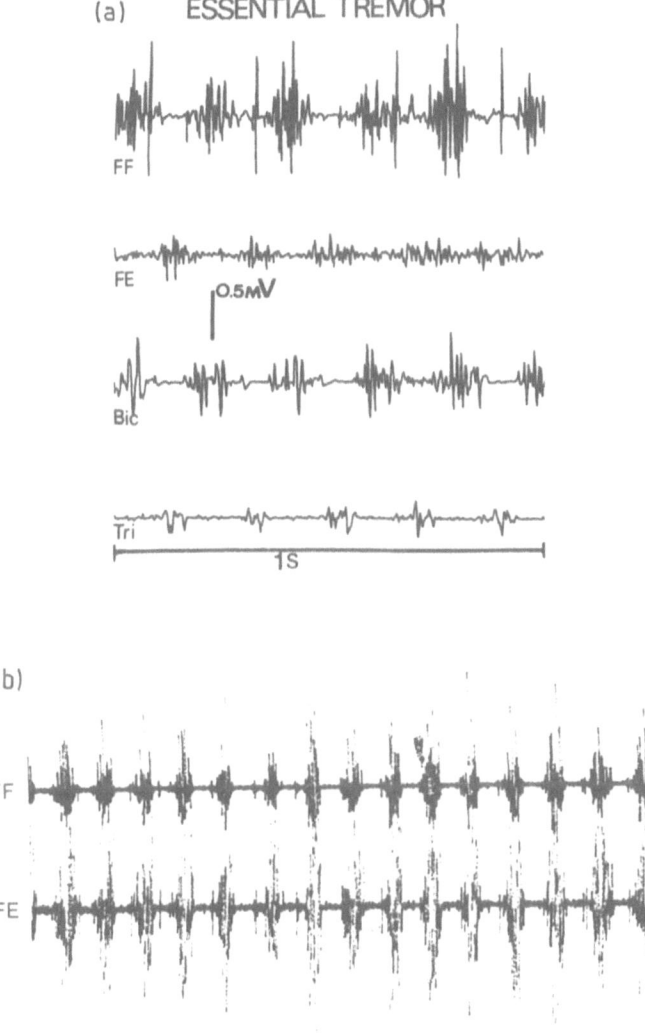

Figure 4.12 Electromyogram recordings from two patients with typical benign essential tremor, holding the arms outstretched (FF = finger flexors, FE = finger extensors, Bic = biceps, and Tri = triceps). In (a) note the obvious alternating contraction in biceps and triceps and, to a lesser extent, in the long finger muscles. In (b) note the co-contraction of finger flexors and extensors. (Reproduced from Marsden *et al.* (1983), in Yahr (ed.), *Current Concepts in Parkinson's Disease*, pp. 31–46, with permission.)

Table 4.7 Exaggerated tremor.

---

(1) Altered mechanical properties
(2) Altered motoneurone firing
(3) Altered spindle feedback
(4) Central pacemaker

There is no evidence of altered mechanical properties of the limbs in essential tremor.

Shahani and Young (1978) and Young and Shahani (1979) have described abnormalities of the behaviour of single motor units in patients with essential tremor, quite different from those found in physiological tremor or in Parkinson's disease. Within each tremor burst, single motor units do not follow the usual order of recruitment seen in normal subjects. Individual single motor units may have instantaneous firing frequencies of 20–50 Hz. Similar bursts of fast firing units, with instantaneous firing frequencies of 20–50 Hz are seen in the tremor of Parkinson's disease, although normal recruitment order is preserved. In addition, there is a tendency in the latter disease for single units to fire in doublets or triplets at about 50 Hz in each tremor burst. What is responsible for these abnormalities of motoneurone firing in different forms of tremor is not known.

There is no evidence for abnormality of muscle spindle feedback in essential tremor. Monosynaptic spinal reflexes appear normal, and we have found the size and latency of long-latency stretch reflexes to be normal (Marsden *et al.*, 1983) (table 4.8). However, stretch may cause repetitive muscle contractions and a tendency to oscillate at the usual tremor frequency, a tendency that can be diminished by administration of propranolol (Marsden *et al.*, 1983) (figure 4.13). Indeed, peripheral input can reset essential tremor (Lee and Stein, 1981; Marsden *et al.*, 1983) (figures 4.14 and 4.15).

Table 4.8 Size of long-latency stretch reflexes.*

		Speed of stretch†	
	n	*Medium (56°/s)*	*Fast (135°/s)*
Control subjects	10	163 ± 25	193 ± 18
Essential tremor	11	200 ± 31	237 ± 28
Parkinson's disease	8	295 ± 17‡	416 ± 26‡

The size of the long-latency stretch reflex (as a percentage of control) was measured from the integrated EMG record from flexor pollicis longus after steady ramp displacement of the top joint of the thumb at the speeds shown. The patients with essential tremor and Parkinson's disease (all of whom were rigid) were matched for age and sex with the control subjects.

---

*From Marsden *et al.* (1983).
† Mean ± SEM shown.
‡ $p < 0.01$ (Student's *t*-test).

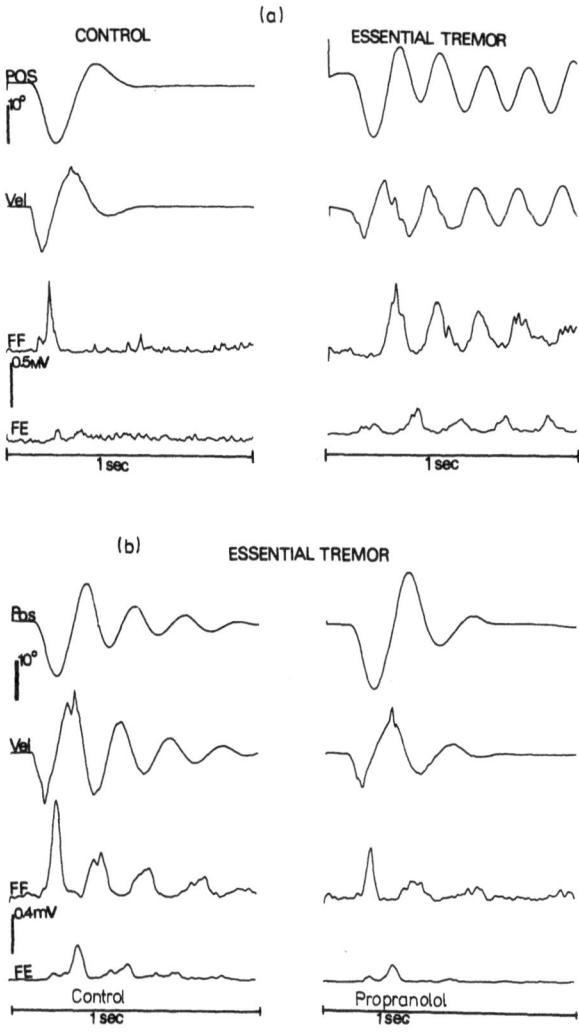

Figure 4.13 Long-latency stretch reflexes in (a) a normal subject (left) and a patient with typical benign essential tremor (right), and (b) a patient with typical benign essential tremor before (left) and after (right) administration of propranolol (1.5 mg i.v.). The subject exerted a small force of index finger flexion against the resistance offered by a torque motor. A short pulse stretch was applied, 100 ms after the start of the sweep, when the torque of the motor was suddenly increased so as to extend the finger through about 15°. The traces are (from top down) finger position and velocity, and rectified EMG recorded from finger flexors (FF) and finger extensors (FE). Note (1) that the pulse stretch does not generate an abnormally large initial stretch reflex in the patient with benign essential tremor, but that the response subsequently oscillates, and (2) that propranolol considerably reduces such oscillations. (Reproduced from Marsden *et al.* (1983), in Yahr (ed.), *Current Concepts in Parkinson's Disease*, pp. 31–46, with permission.)

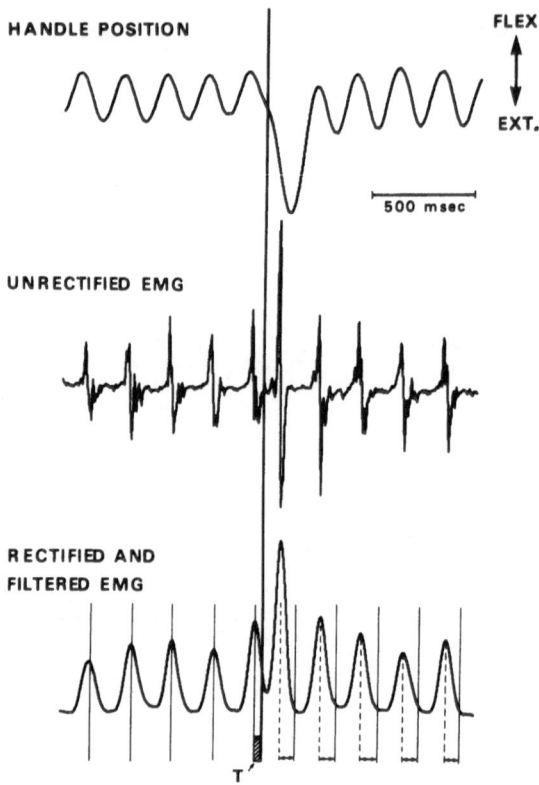

HANDLE POSITION

FLEX

EXT.

500 msec

UNRECTIFIED EMG

RECTIFIED AND
FILTERED EMG

T

Figure 4.14 Effect of a sudden perturbation on essential tremor. The patient grasped a handle linked to a torque motor, which recorded the ongoing tremor and delivered an abrupt wrist extension movement at the time indicated by the vertical bar. The EMG of the wrist flexors was recorded by surface electrodes. The small vertical bars on the rectified EMG recording coincide with the peaks of tremor before the perturbation, and with the predicted time of tremor peaks afterwards. (Reproduced from Lee and Stein (1981), *Ann. Neurol.*, **10**, 523–31, with permission.)

The extent to which a tremor may be reset by peripheral input depends upon the size of the perturbation and the time in the tremor cycle that it is given. Even a tremor due primarily to a rhythmically discharging autonomous central pacemaker may be reset if a large enough peripheral input is introduced. Conclusions as to whether a tremor is of central or peripheral origin, depending upon the degree of resetting introduced by external input, can only be based on data obtained with inputs appropriate to the size of the tremor.

Assuming an appropriate input, the time at which that is introduced in the tremor cycle may influence the extent to which it is capable of resetting the tremor. If a tremor can be completely reset by appropriate external input, then this will occur irrespective of the time of the input in the tremor cycle. In other words, wherever the external perturbation is applied, the next tremor beat will

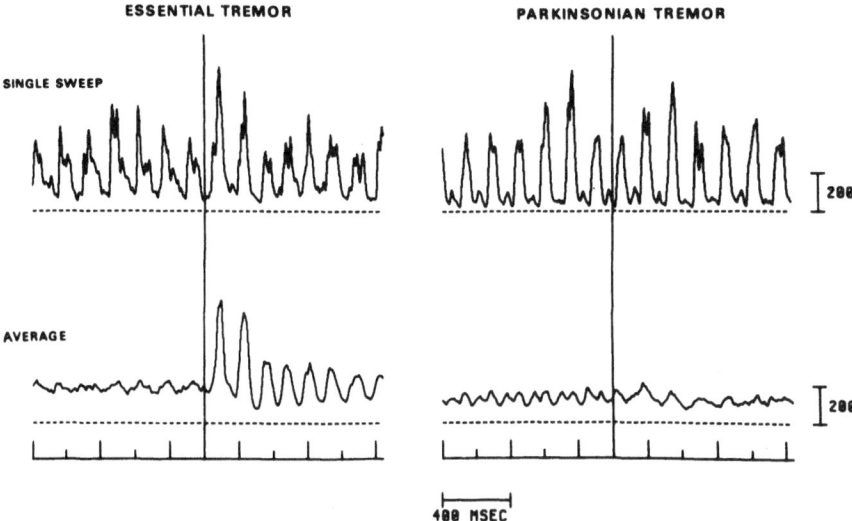

Figure 4.15 Resetting of essential tremor but not of parkinsonian tremor by a sudden perturbation, introduced as illustrated in figure 4.14 at the time of the vertical bar. The upper traces show single 2 s recordings of tremor. The lower traces are the average of 50 such recordings. Note that averaging cancels out the tremor bursts in both patients prior to the perturbations, but that in the case of essential tremor, the wrist extension resets the tremor which becomes time-locked to the stimulus. (Reproduced from Lee and Stein (1981), *Ann. Neurol.*, **10**, 523–31, with permission.)

occur at a fixed latency thereafter. Plotting the time of the stimulus after the preceding tremor peak against the deviation of the next peak will produce, in those circumstances, a linear relationship with a slope of 1, indicating complete resetting. In contrast, if there is a purely central origin for a tremor, then the slope of the relationship between time of input to deviation of next peak will be 0, i.e. no resetting occurs. Intermediate examples can be imagined where tremor involves both interaction between reflex mechanisms and central oscillators.

Applying this reasoning to essential tremor, Lee and Stein (1981) found that the resetting index for patients with essential tremor was relatively high, indicating a strong involvement of sensory feedback (figure 4.16). However, their experiments may be criticised on the grounds that the step input used to reset the tremor was considerably greater than the on-going tremor itself (see figure 4.14).

Other experiments have given different answers. Walsh (1976) utilised the technique of application of an external rhythmic displacement to decide whether clonus of the ankle in patients with spasticity was due to reflex re-excitation or to some central generator triggered by stretch. If clonus were dependent on such a self re-exciting peripheral reflex, it would be expected that the application of a rhythmic external force to the foot should entrain the rhythm to that of the applied frequency. However, Walsh found that clonus in spasticity could not be

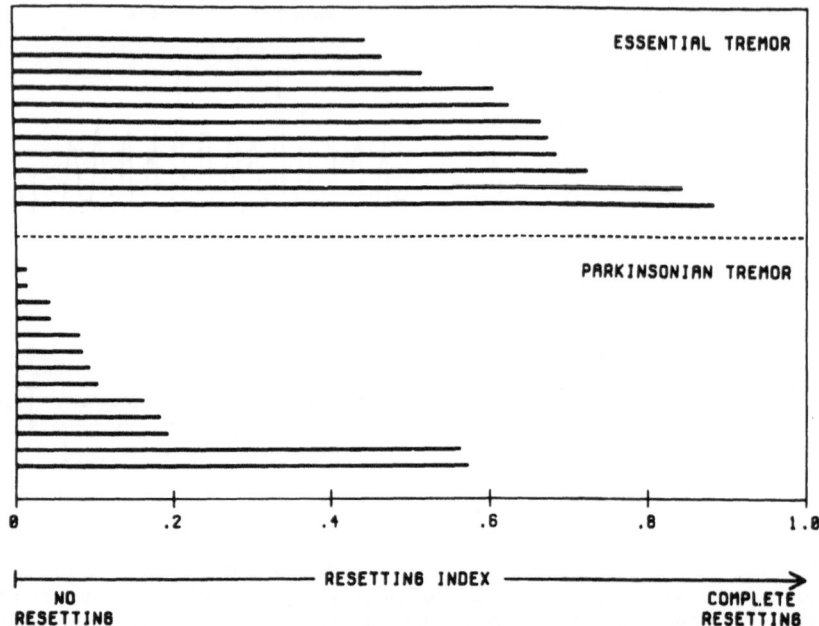

Figure 4.16 Resetting indices for 13 patients with essential tremor and 11 patients with Parkinson's disease. For details of the calculation of the resetting index, see text. An index of 0 indicates that the perturbation had no effect on the tremor. An index of 1 indicates that the tremor was completely reset. (Reproduced from Lee and Stein (1981), *Ann. Neurol.*, **10**, 523-31, with permission.)

entrained. What happened was that beats were set up, with waxing and waning of the amplitude of the oscillation, in response to the applied rhythmic force. This strongly suggested that the oscillation of clonus was the result of the activity of an autonomous central pacemaker. Obviously, the oscillations were set off by sudden stretch input, but thereafter the generator appeared to run free, providing that proprioceptive input continued.

Application of a similar technique to patients with essential tremor also has suggested the presence of an autonomous central generator (Marsden *et al.*, 1983). Rhythmic oscillations of the outstretched fingers at frequencies other than that of the spontaneous tremor caused marked beating in many patients with essential tremor, even when the applied force was relatively small (figure 4.17). The presence of such beating does not disprove the existence of peripheral feedback contributing to tremor, but it does suggest that there is, in addition, some central pacemaker that is involved.

Of course, the matter could be resolved by deafferentation, but no example of loss of proprioceptive and other sensation in a patient with essential tremor has been reported. It is, however, known that essential tremor disappears on the side of a hemiplegia (Mylle and van Bogaert, 1940), and that it can be abolished by a suitably placed lesion in the thalamus (Ohye *et al.*, 1982a,b) (figure 4.18). Ohye

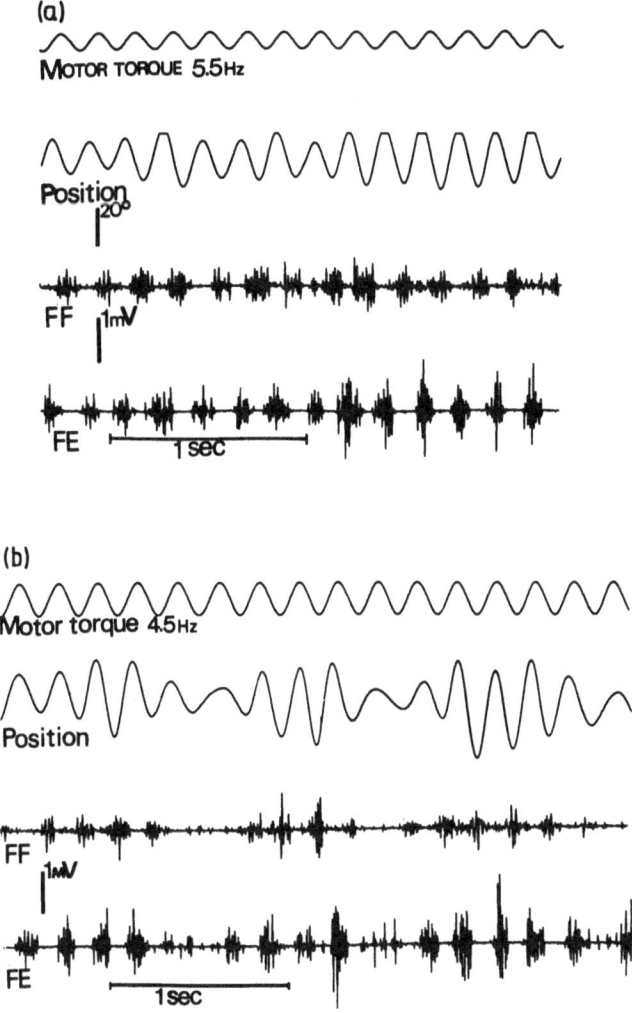

(a)

MOTOR TORQUE 5.5Hz

Position
|20°

FF |1mV

FE ├─────1sec─────┤

(b)

Motor torque 4.5Hz

Position

FF |1mV

FE ├─────1sec─────┤

Figure 4.17 Effect of application of a rhythmic sinusoidal torque to the fingers in a patient with typical benign essential tremor. The experimental arrangements were as described in the legend to figure 4.13. The traces are (from top down) motor torque, finger position, and EMG recorded from the finger flexors (FF) and finger extensors (FE). The sinusoidal oscillation was delivered to the finger by the torque motor, in (a) at 5.5 Hz, which was the frequency of the patient's spontaneous tremor, and in (b) at 4.5 Hz. When the finger was driven at the frequency of spontaneous tremor, the oscillation produced remained more or less sinusoidal, as judged from the position trace. However, when the finger was driven below its normal tremor frequency, obvious 'beating' occurred in the position record, suggesting the existence of some central tremor generator. (Reproduced from Marsden *et al.* (1983), in Yahr (ed.), *Current Concepts in Parkinson's Disease*, pp. 31–46, with permission.)

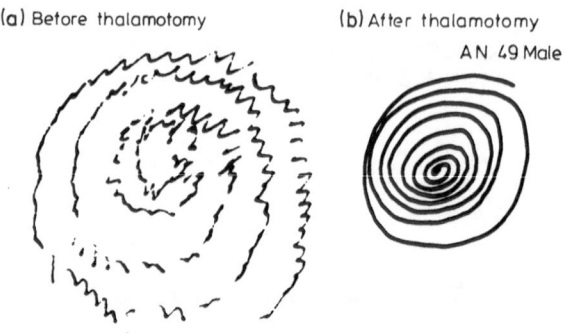

Figure 4.18 Stereotactic Vim thalamotomy abolishes essential tremor of writing. (Reproduced from Ohye *et al.* (1982b), *J. Neurol. Neurosurg. Psychiatr.*, **45**, 988–97, with permission.)

and his colleagues have recorded rhythmic bursting neuronal discharges in the thalamic nucleus ventralis intermedius (Vim) in patients with essential tremor. This nucleus Vim, which receives proprioceptive input, is the standard target for stereotactic surgery for tremor. The rhythmic discharges recorded in this nucleus in patients with essential tremor appear linked to the tremor beats, and are similar to those found in Parkinson's disease at the same operation (see later).

In summary, the origins of essential tremor remain debated. On the one hand there is the evidence that tremor can be reset with a fair degree of ease by peripheral input. On the other hand there is the evidence from lack of entrainment by rhythmic inputs for the existence of a central oscillator. On balance, it seems likely that both may be involved but to what degree is uncertain.

Severe essential tremor

The majority of patients with classical essential tremor are not grossly disabled by their disorder. The tremor may interfere with writing, and make holding a cup or glass difficult, but the disability usually is not severe. A minority of patients, however, experience considerable problems with increasingly severe essential tremor which eventually becomes so bad that they can be rendered helpless. The shaking on attempting to hold an object is so gross that they have to drink through a straw and be fed. They become quite incapable of dressing. Since the legs usually are not as badly affected, such patients often can walk, although often unsteadily. Tremor of the jaw and mouth leads to severe dysarthria.

Whether this picture of severe essential tremor is merely an extreme of a spectrum of the disorder or whether it is a separate illness with different pathophysiology is not established. Most such patients are elderly and give a long history of tremor, initially much less disabling. The supposition, therefore, is that these patients represent a final outcome of progressive but severe essential tremor.

Symptomatic essential tremor

A tremor with all the characteristics of essential tremor, being absent at rest, present on maintaining a posture, but not made strikingly worse on action, may be seen in a variety of established neurological diseases.

Such a tremor may occur in association with several different types of peripheral neuropathy. It may occur in some patients with inherited neuropathies such as those of Charcot–Marie–Tooth (HMSN I) (Salisachs, 1976) or of Dejerine and Sottas (HMSN III) (Salisachs and Lapresle, 1973). A similar tremor may be observed in some patients recovering from the Guillain-Barré-Strohl syndrome (acute post-infective polyneuropathy) (Shahani *et al.*, 1973). It has also been described in patients with IgM neuropathies (Smith *et al.*, 1983). Indeed, it is now evident that a neuropathic tremor of this nature may be seen in a wide variety of different conditions affecting the peripheral nerves.

The pathophysiology of such neuropathic tremor is uncertain. Not every patient with peripheral neuropathy develops the condition, so simple concepts of deafferentation do not seem adequate. Although many of the patients exhibiting the phenomenon have profoundly slowed nerve conduction, this is not universal. Furthermore, other patients with a similar degree of nerve conduction slowing do not exhibit such tremor. Some subtlety of selective deafferentation, perhaps involving proprioceptive feedback of one sort or another, may be responsible, but remains to be proven. Two other possibilities require consideration. Many of these patients are profoundly weak, so that in some cases the reported tremor may be simply that of fatigue. In other situations of inherited neuropathy, the tremor may be a coexisting inherited abnormality. In other words, such patients may have inherited benign essential tremor as well as their neuropathy.

An action tremor identical to that of essential tremor also is seen in at least 10% of patients with the syndrome of idiopathic torsion dystonia (Marsden, 1976). Whether this means that the abnormality of torsion dystonia predisposes such patients to develop this sort of tremor, or whether such patients have inherited two separate genes, one for dystonia and the other for essential tremor, is unknown.

The same considerations apply to the problem of essential tremor in Parkinson's disease. As noted earlier, it sometimes happens that both conditions occur in the same family or even in the same patient. The significance of these observations remains unknown.

PARKINSON'S DISEASE

There is more than one sort of tremor in Parkinson's disease (figure 4.19). Findley *et al.* (1981) have put forward strong arguments that the classical parkinsonian rest tremor has an origin different from that of other sorts of tremor in this condition. They suggest that postural tremor, kinetic tremor, intention tremor, the

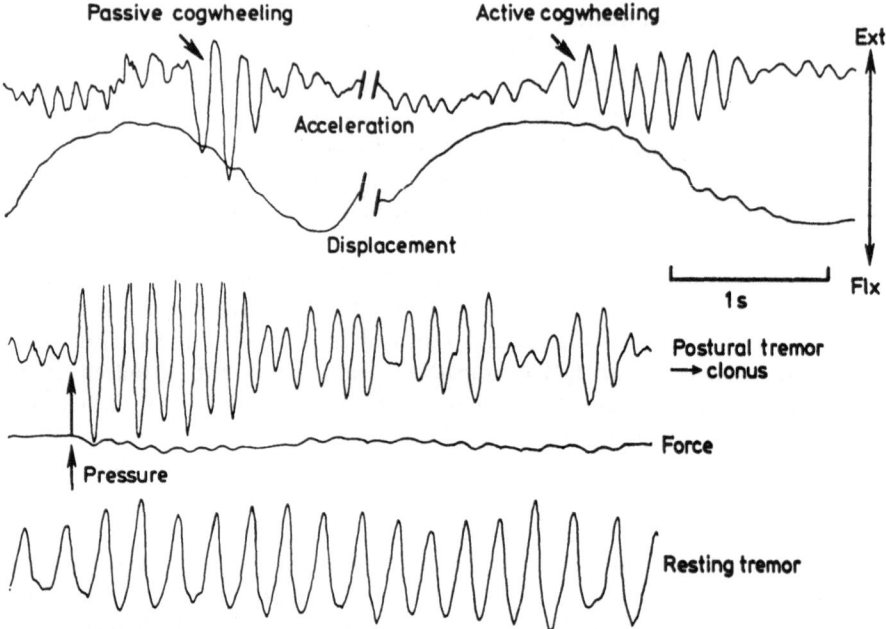

Figure 4.19 Different types of tremor in Parkinson's disease. The records are all from one patient, taken within a few minutes of each other at the same recording session. The accelerometer recording gain was the same in all records. The upper pair of traces show hand acceleration and position. To the left, the wrist was passively flexed, evoking passive cogwheeling at 6 Hz. A few seconds later the patient moved his own hand from extension into flexion, evoking active cogwheeling tremor at 6 Hz. The middle pair of traces are of hand acceleration (upper record), initially with the hand in posture. The patient then pressed down on a force transducer (lower record), causing the hand to go into clonus at 6 Hz. In the lowest trace of hand acceleration, the hand is at rest, and develops a typical tremor at 4.3 Hz. (Reproduced from Findley *et al.* (1981), *J. Neurol. Neurosurg. Psychiatr.*, **44**, 534–46, with permission.)

cogwheel phenomenon and clonus in Parkinson's disease all have a common spinal origin. They base this conclusion on a careful analysis of the frequency spectra characteristics of the various types of tremor encountered (table 4.9). Classical rest tremor has a remarkably stable and reproducible frequency of around 4–5 Hz. Postural tremor, kinetic tremor, cogwheeling and clonus are of higher frequency at around 6 Hz. This is lower than the frequency of physiological tremor (8–9 Hz), so they believe that postural and kinetic tremor, as well as cogwheeling and clonus, are not related to the mechanisms responsible for physiological tremor. This contrasts with the views of Lance *et al.* (1963), who felt that the action tremor seen in Parkinson's disease might be an exaggeration of physiological tremor. In addition, Stiles and Pozos (1976) found a continuous range of frequencies in parkinsonian tremor between 4 and 9 Hz, the frequency varying inversely with tremor amplitude. Teravainen and Calne (1980) were of the opinion that action tremor (the

Table 4.9 Tremors in Parkinson's disease.*

Rest tremor	4–5 Hz
Postural tremor ⎫ Movement tremor ⎬ 6 Hz Cogwheeling Clonus ⎭	6 Hz
Physiological tremor	8–9 Hz

*After Findley *et al.* (1981).

term they used to describe tremor during movement) was similar in its pathophysiology to that occurring at rest. They based this conclusion on the finding that voluntary movement of pronation or supination of the wrist often could provoke action tremor with alternating contraction of agonists and antagonists, similar to the pattern seen in parkinsonian rest tremor. However, the frequency of such action tremor usually was between 6 and 9 Hz, similar to the cogwheel phenomenon and intention tremor described by Findley *et al.* (1981), but quite different from the frequency of parkinsonian rest tremor. Teravainen and Calne (1980) argue that rest and action tremor in Parkinson's disease are of similar origin, perhaps due to oscillation within an 'internal feedback loop between motor cortex and spinal cord'. Findley *et al.* (1981), on the other hand, argue that the difference in frequency between rest and action tremor indicates that they are of different origin. This also was the conclusion of Lance *et al.* (1963), not only on the basis of the difference in frequency between rest and action tremor, but also because rest tremor was characterised by reciprocal activity in agonist and antagonist muscles, while action tremor often occurred with synchronous contraction of opposing muscle groups.

This discussion will concentrate on the rest tremor of Parkinson's disease which is the major distinctive tremor of the illness.

Pathophysiology of rest tremor

It is fortunate that it is possible to create a tremor more or less identical to that seen in Parkinson's disease in experimental primates (Ward *et al.*, 1948). This has allowed a careful analysis of the factors responsible for experimental rest tremor. These will be considered first, and then observations in patients with Parkinson's disease will be discussed in relation to the experimental work.

Experimental rest tremor

Lesions involving the midbrain ventromedial tegmental area in monkeys (figure 4.20) produce a spontaneous sustained tremor similar to that of Parkinson's disease (Poirier *et al.*, 1966). Only a proportion of animals lesioned at this site exhibit

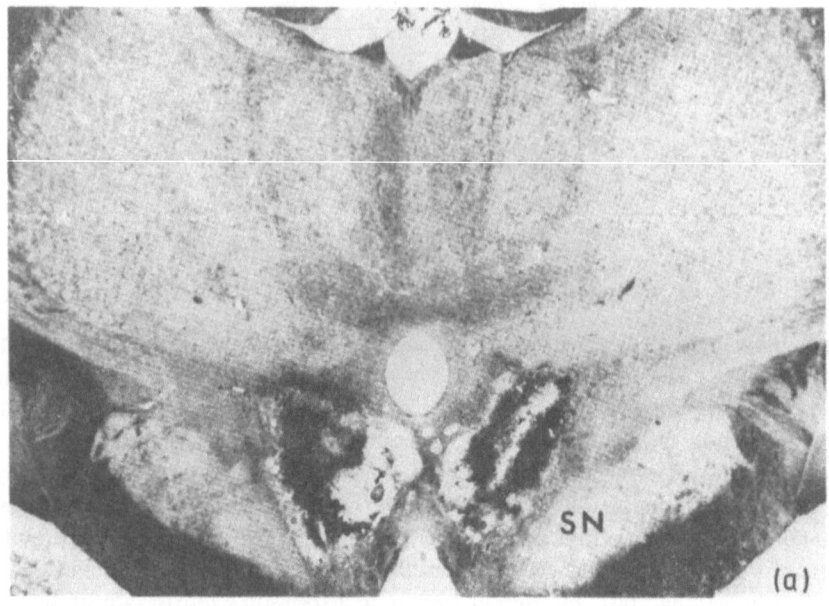

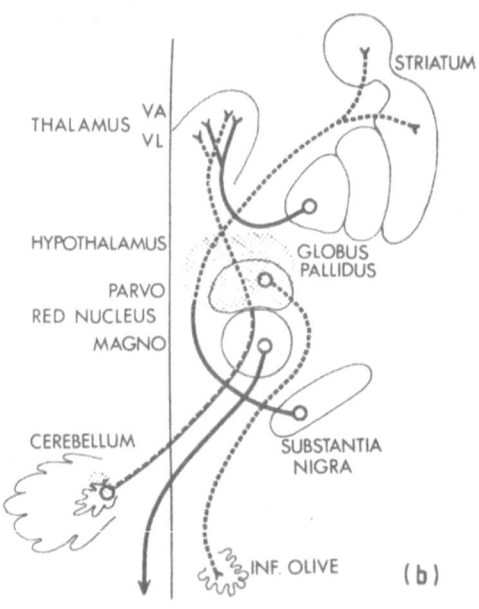

Figure 4.20 Ventromedial tegmental lesion in the midbrain of the monkey which can cause a rest tremor similar to that seen in Parkinson's disease. (a) Transverse section through the midbrain of a monkey which had received bilateral incomplete lesions of the dentate nuclei nine months prior to the bilateral

ventromedial tegmental lesions illustrated (×4; basic fuchsin and fast blue; SN = substantia nigra). The cerebellar lesions produced no motor impairment. Following the bilateral midbrain lesions the animal became aphagic, profoundly akinetic and displayed tremor and rigidity of all four limbs. Intramuscular apomorphine (0.125–0.2 mg/kg i.m.) overcame these motor disturbances. The tegmental lesions caused almost complete degeneration of the substantia nigra and adjacent pigmented nuclei, destroyed the parvocellular portion of the red nucleus and interrupted the ascending cerebellothalamic pathways. (b) Schematic drawing to illustrate the main nervous pathways involved bilaterally in this monkey. Note loss of the ascending nigrostriatal, cerebellorubral and cerebellothalamic projections, and of the descending rubro-olivary pathway. (Reproduced from Pechadre *et al.* (1976), *J. Neurol. Sci.*, **28**, 147–57, with permission.)

---

tremor. The administration of harmaline to lesioned animals may induce tremor when it was not present beforehand, or may greatly enhance existing tremor (Poirier *et al.*, 1966). Such lesions damage several structures and pathways, including portions of the ventral component of the brachium conjunctivum, the descending rubral systems and the substantia nigra and its efferents. Lesions confined to the brachium conjunctivum cause ataxia. Lesions confined to the substantia nigra cause neither ataxia nor tremor. Lesions involving the cerebellar output to red nucleus and thalamus, and the descending rubral pathways, do not cause tremor alone, but if such animals are then treated with drugs inhibiting the actions of dopamine (α-methyl-*p*-tyrosine to prevent synthesis, reserpine to prevent storage, or phenothiazines to block receptors), then typical rest tremor develops (Bedard *et al.*, 1970; Larochelle *et al.*, 1970, 1971). Such experimental rest tremor can be abolished by administration of dopamine agonists.

The conclusion is that rest tremor is the result of damage to the nigrostriatal dopaminergic pathway in combination with damage to the cerebellorubral and cerebellothalamic pathways. Either alone is insufficient. Additional damage to descending rubral pathways often coexists but does not seem essential.

Further study of such animals has shown that the motor cortex (Poirier *et al.*, 1969) and ventrolateral thalamus must be intact for such experimental tremor to be present. However, sectioning the corticospinal tract did not prevent appearance of the tremor (Poirier *et al.*, 1966, 1969; Ohye *et al.*, 1970), indicating that non-pyramidal efferents from the motor cortex must play a major role in its transmission to the spinal cord. (This is in contrast to hemiballism due to subthalamic lesions, which is abolished by damage to the corticospinal tract.)

Electrophysiological investigation of such experimental animals, by recording of single-unit activity, has shown neurones firing in phase with the tremor bursts in the contralateral sensorimotor cortex (Cordeau *et al.*, 1960; Lamarre and Joffroy, 1979) and in ventrolateral thalamus (in the specific relay nuclei VPlo and posterior VLo and VLc) (Lamarre and Joffroy, 1970, 1971, 1979; Lamarre *et al.*, 1971). The area in the thalamus where such tremor bursts were found corresponds to nucleus ventralis intermedius (Vim) in man. It contains those neurones known to project to the arm area of the motor cortex (Strick, 1976). However, such spontaneous discharges in thalamus and motor cortex might be the cause or the consequence of the tremor.

Two approaches to this problem have been made, first by paralysing such animals, and secondly by deafferentation of the trembling limb by section of dorsal roots. Deafferentation does not prevent the occurrence of experimental parkinsonian tremor (Ohye et al., 1970), nor does it abolish rhythmic discharges in the motor cortex or thalamus time-locked to tremor bursts (Joffroy and Lamarre, 1971; Lamarre and Joffroy, 1979). Paralysis of such animals with curare or gallamine also does not abolish rhythmic bursting of neuronal activity at 3–6 Hz in that area of the primate thalamus corresponding to the human Vim (Lamarre and Joffroy, 1970, 1979). Nor does it abolish similar rhythmic unit activity at tremor frequency in the motor cortex (Cordeau and Lamarre, 1966; Lamarre and Joffroy, 1979).

These results, as well as the relationship between the timing of the motor cortex neuronal activity and the muscle tremor bursts, support the notion that it is a spontaneous rhythmic discharge of neurones in the motor cortex that is responsible for experimental parkinsonian tremor.

It is impossible to be certain whether the motor cortex is driven by a thalamic generator or whether bursting activity at both sites merely represents their inter-connections. Thalamic neurones are known to show a propensity to rhythmic firing at a frequency of about 5 Hz in normal circumstances (Lamarre and Joffroy, 1971). This activity is greatest at rest, and tends to disappear on arousal. Deaffer-entation of the thalamus as a result of the ventral tegmental lesion might lead to permanent rhythmic bursting at 3–6 Hz which then could drive the motor cortex (Lamarre, 1975) (see below).

Rest tremor in patients with Parkinson's disease

Many of the observations in experimental animals have also been made in patients with Parkinson's disease. Thus, parkinsonian rest tremor is not abolished by dorsal root section, although rigidity disappears (Leriche, 1914; Pollock and Davis, 1930; Foerster, 1936). Damage to the motor cortex also abolishes parkinsonian tremor (Klemme, 1940; Bucy and Case, 1949). Selective lesions to that part of the human thalamus corresponding to the area of the primate thalamus from which tremor bursts can be recorded is now the standard operation for relief of parkinsonian tremor (Narabayashi, 1982). Such stereotactic surgery is centred on the nucleus Vim (figure 4.21), which is that part of the thalamic relay nuclei that receives proprioceptive information from limbs (Ohye et al., 1974; Ohye and Narabayashi, 1979). A small lesion at this site will abolish tremor although a larger lesion intruding into more anterior portions of ventralis lateralis (VL), to include the nuclei Voa and Vop of Hassler, are required for relief of rigidity.

Microelectrode recordings (about 10 μm in tip size) of neuronal activity in the thalamus at the time of stereotaxis have revealed the presence of burst discharges synchronous with tremor in nucleus Vim (Albe-Fessard et al., 1963, 1966; Jasper and Bertrand, 1966; Ohye et al., 1974). Stimulation through the same micro-electrode at high frequency stops or suppresses parkinsonian rest tremor immedi-ately, and electrocoagulation within that area stops tremor permanently.

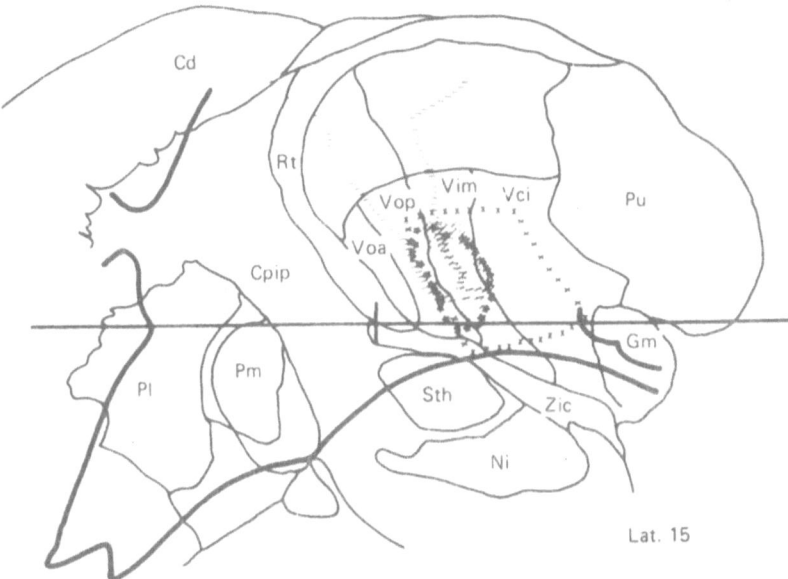

Figure 4.21 Diagram of saggital section, 15 mm lateral to the midline, through thalamus according to the atlas of Bailey and Schaltenbrand, to show the position of the nucleus ventralis intermedius (Vim). This is the target for stereotactic lesions designed to relieve tremor. Note the relation of Vim to other thalamic sensory relay nuclei (Vop and Vci), to the subthalamus (Sth), substantia nigra (Ni), zona incerta (Zic), caudate nucleus (Cd) and pulvinar (Pu). (Reproduced from Narabayashi (1982), in Marsden and Fahn (eds), *Movement Disorders*, pp. 292–9, with permission.)

The general similarity of these findings in man to those in the experimental animal is remarkable. The overall conclusion must be that parkinsonian rest tremor is the consequence of spontaneous bursting discharge in the thalamus, and perhaps the motor cortex. This arises as a result of loss of inputs due to damage in the region of the ventral tegmental area but must involve the nigrostriatal dopaminergic pathway. The latter is made evident by the finding that parkinsonian rest tremor often is abolished by treatment with levodopa or other dopamine agonists.

There are, however, some findings which, at first sight, seem incompatible with this notion of a central generator for parkinsonian tremor. Thus, Teravainen *et al.* (1979) were able to reset the phase of rest tremor (and of postural tremor) by short external perturbations flexing or extending the wrist. Displacements delivered in the absence of tremor could trigger tremor in phase with the input (see also Teravainen, 1980). These observations could be taken to suggest the influence of peripheral factors in generating parkinsonian tremor. However, they illustrate the difficulties of interpreting such results. Resetting of the phase of rest tremor occurred only with strong, large perturbations and lasted for only a few cycles. Such behaviour is typical of the effects of peripheral inputs on a central generator, whose activity may be temporarily disturbed if that input is large enough. Lee and Stein (1981), examining their resetting index, were able to show that this is low in Parkinson's disease, much lower than that found in essential tremor (figure 4.16). These results do not, therefore, disturb the overall conclusion that parkinsonian tremor is driven by a central oscillator, although this obviously is influenced by peripheral input.

The nature of any central oscillator generating parkinsonian tremor is controversial. Teravainen and colleagues favoured the notion that it was a consequence of oscillation within the supraspinal neuronal loop from motor cortex to spinal cord and back via the ventral spinocerebellar pathway to the cerebellum, thence via nucleus ventralis lateralis of the thalamus to the motor cortex. They interpreted their findings that peripheral perturbations could reset or trigger parkinsonian tremor to indicate that such inputs could modify or trigger oscillatory activity in this hypothetical loop. In contrast, Lamarre (1975), from his extensive studies of experimental tremor in the monkey, has concluded that the likeliest mechanism for parkinsonian tremor rests in the ability of thalamic neurones in the monkey to fire rhythmically at about 5 Hz (Lamarre and Joffroy, 1971). Such synchronised bursting activity is evident at rest and relaxation, but is replaced by desynchronised continuous firing when the animal is aroused. Lamarre suggests that the lesion responsible for parkinsonian tremor may effectively deafferent the thalamus, causing a state of more or less permanent rhythmic synchronised bursting activity at about 5 Hz. If sufficient thalamic neurones behaved in this fashion, they could drive the motor cortex to generate typical parkinsonian rest tremor.

CEREBELLAR TREMOR

There is more than one type of tremor in cerebellar disease ('all tremors occurring in cerebellar disease are not of the same nature' (Holmes, 1922)), and cerebellar tremor often is confused with ataxia. The disturbance of the trajectory of movement that characterises the dysmetria of cerebellar disease is not a rhythmical oscillation, so is not a tremor. True cerebellar tremor is of three types.

Tremor that occurs during movement, increasing in amplitude as the point of aim is reached, is conventionally designated 'intention tremor'. However, this term has been criticised as ambiguous, for 'it can be used in reference to tremors on contemplating, initiating, performing, or completing a movement' (Gilman et al., 1981). For this reason the term 'cerebellar kinetic tremor' is preferred. In its mildest form, cerebellar kinetic tremor only appears at the end of movement, just as the target is reached. The frequency of such oscillations is around 3-4 Hz. The more severe the tremor, the earlier in the movement does it appear, but still it increases as the target is approached. In severe cases, such tremor may be apparent on attempting to hold a posture. In the most dramatic cases, as for example occur in multiple sclerosis, there even may be tremor at apparent rest, which then gets much worse on adopting a posture, and becomes uncontrollable on attempted movement. For reasons to be discussed below, such tremor sometimes is referred to as 'midbrain' or 'rubral' tremor.

A second form of cerebellar tremor is that occurring mainly in posture. The outstretched arms, after a few seconds, develop a rhythmic oscillation at the shoulder; if the leg is held extended, a rhythmic oscillation develops at the hip. Holmes (1922) considered this to be a consequence of fatigue and weakness: ... 'But as the muscles holding the limb up begin to tire an irregular tremor develops. Its oscillations are mostly in the line of gravity, and can be seen on careful inspection to be due to a failure in the tonic contractions of the muscles that maintain the attitude, with the result that the limb falls with gravity and is replaced by voluntary efforts.' Such patients may or may not also exhibit kinetic tremor.

The third type of tremor that occurs in cerebellar disease is titubation, which consists of a rhythmic oscillation of the head, and sometimes of the trunk. At its mildest, there may be only a barely perceptible to-and-fro oscillation of the head. When severe, the whole body may shake. Titubation may occur in those with severe kinetic tremor. It also sometimes appears in isolation. The mechanisms of titubation may be similar to those of kinetic tremor, but there is insufficient information to be sure of this point.

Cerebellar kinetic (intention) tremor

Such a tremor is characteristic of injury or disease of the cerebellar outflow, as when the dentate nucleus or its projections to the red nucleus and thalamus, via the brachium conjunctivum, are damaged. Thus it may appear with lesions of the cerebellum itself, or of the midbrain ('rubral tremor'). The greater the damage to the cerebellar outflow, the worse is the kinetic tremor.

In their extensive experimental studies in primates, Carrea and Mettler (1947, 1955) established that cerebellar tremor is not just the consequence of severe ataxia. They were able to show that interrupting different parts of the superior cerebellar peduncle differentially affected ataxia and tremor. Lesions of the ventral segment of the ascending limb of the brachium conjunctivum produced a tremor, while lesions interrupting the descending limb caused ataxia.

Typical cerebellar kinetic tremor has been produced by cerebellectomy (Gilman *et al.*, 1976), by selective stereotactic lesions involving the dentate nucleus (Growdon *et al.*, 1967), by reversible cooling of the deep cerebellar nuclei (Brooks *et al.*, 1973; Cooke and Thomas, 1976; Villis and Hore, 1977), by lesions of the red nucleus (Ranish and Soechting, 1976), or by damage to the superior cerebellar peduncle.

Recent experiments utilising cooling of the dentate nucleus have given further insight into the mechanisms responsible for cerebellar tremor. Dentate nucleus cooling leads to oscillations in the course of self-paced goal-directed movement (Cooke and Thomas, 1976). The frequency of such oscillations, at about 3-5 Hz, is similar to typical intention tremor seen in such animals. Experimental cerebellar intention tremor survives deafferentation, so cannot be due to any oscillation in stretch reflex machinery (Gilman *et al.*, 1976). However, as is the case with Parkinson's disease, the tremor generated by abnormal function resulting from lesions of dentate nucleus and cerebellar output pathways can be modified by peripheral input (Villis and Hore, 1977).

There is a major problem in interpreting the differences between cerebellar intention tremor and parkinsonian rest tremor. There is a striking similarity in the site of lesions that may produce such tremors in the experimental animal. Indeed, it appears necessary to damage those cerebellar pathways responsible for intention tremor to produce experimental parkinsonian rest tremor. Observations such as these have led to the proposition that there is no real fundamental difference between the two (Narabayashi, 1973). Whether the tremor appears at rest or not merely depends on whether or not there is muscle contraction at 'apparent rest'. Thus, the addition of rigidity caused by nigrostriatal dopaminergic deficiency represents a background muscle contraction which, by its presence, ensures the appearance of tremor at rest as a result of the additional damage to the cerebello-rubro-thalamic system.

Such an interpretation has the merit of simplicity, but comes up against one major problem. It is difficult to see why parkinsonian rest tremor should not then convert into a typical cerebellar intention tremor on movement. There may be some simple explanation for this discrepancy but none is immediately apparent.

'Rubral tremor'

This has the characteristics of a parkinsonian tremor at rest, which becomes worse on maintaining a posture, and even worse on carrying out a movement. Thus it has the characteristics of rest, postural and intention tremor combined. It is seen in circumstances associated with midbrain damage, due to stroke, head trauma and occasionally tumour or demyelination. The tremor appears in the limbs opposite to the side of midbrain damage. All such lesions focused on the midbrain may involve the red nucleus, but there is no evidence to show that this is the crucial site of damage responsible for the problem. Indeed, it seems more likely that this form of tremor represents massive damage to cerebello-rubro-thalamic pathways in combination with nigral deficit. In the light of the earlier discussion, this seems to be the sort of tremor to be expected when cerebellar intention tremor is combined with dopamine deficiency. Indeed, there is a single case report indicating that levodopa may abolish this type of rubral tremor (Findley and Gresty, 1980).

CONCLUSIONS

This chapter has reviewed the pathophysiology of physiological tremor and of various pathological tremors, including enhanced physiological tremor, essential tremor, parkinsonian tremor and cerebellar tremor. I will conclude by listing some areas of uncertainty and debate that remain.

Physiological tremor

(1) To what extent, if at all, is spindle feedback and the stretch reflex involved in normal physiological tremor?

(2) In what circumstances does the stretch reflex enhance physiological tremor, and when does it damp it?

(3) How do monosynaptic spinal stretch reflexes and long-latency, perhaps transcortical, stretch reflexes interact in enhanced physiological tremor?

(4) Why does a cerebellar lesion decrease ipsilateral physiological tremor?

(5) Why can visual deprivation abolish, and visual delay slow, some types of physiological tremor?

(6) To what extent is the tendency for the inferior olive to exhibit rhythmic activity involved in some forms of physiological tremor?

(7) Do sympathomimetics increase physiological tremor in part by altering spindle feedback?

(8) What is the cause of the enhanced physiological tremor seen in alcoholics?

(9) How does lithium enhance physiological tremor?

(10) Why does a brief strong muscle contraction increase physiological tremor?

(11) How does prolonged muscular effort enhance and slow physiological tremor?

Essential tremor

(1) Is there more than one type of essential tremor?

(2) How does alcohol reduce essential tremor?

(3) Are mechanisms other than peripheral beta$_2$-adrenoceptor blockade involved in the beneficial effects of beta-blocking drugs in essential tremor (for example, central actions or beta$_1$-effects)?

(4) Why do only some patients with essential tremor respond to beta-blockers?

(5) How does primidone (and phenobarbitone) benefit essential tremor, and why again do only some respond?

(6) What is the relation of typical essential tremor to isolated head or voice tremors, to isolated writing tremor and to isolated 'musical' or 'sports' tremors?

(7) What is the relation of essential tremor to Parkinson's disease?

(8) What is responsible for the abnormalities in motor unit firing seen in essential tremor?

(9) Is essential tremor driven by an abnormal response to spindle feedback or by some central oscillator?

(10) If a central oscillator is involved, where is it?

(11) Is severe disabling essential tremor the end of the spectrum of one illness, or a separate disease?

(12) What is responsible for the tremor seen in some peripheral neuropathies and in torsion dystonia?

Parkinson's disease

(1) Are the postural tremor, cogwheel phenomenon and clonus of Parkinson's disease of common spinal origin and distinct from physiological tremor?

(2) Is the action tremor of Parkinson's disease distinct from rest tremor?

(3) Is the rest tremor of Parkinson's disease driven by abnormal thalamic rhythmic activity?

(4) If so, what causes the thalamus to behave in this way?

(5) What lesions, in addition to damage to the nigrostriatal system, are essential for the appearance of parkinsonian rest tremor?

(6) To what extent can parkinsonian rest tremor be reset by peripheral input?

(7) What is the relation of parkinsonian rest tremor, which may require damage to cerebellar outflow pathways in addition to the nigrostriatal lesion, to the tremors of cerebellar disease?

Cerebellar tremor

(1) What is the relation of titubation to cerebellar tremors of the limbs?

(2) Is so-called 'midbrain' or 'rubral' tremor merely the most severe degree of cerebellar kinetic (intention) tremor, due to the most massive damage to cerebellar output pathways?

(3) Alternatively, does 'midbrain' or 'rubral' tremor require damage to other structures?

(4) Since cerebellar kinetic (intention) tremor survives deafferentation, does it represent an oscillation in some internal feedback circuit?

(5) Alternatively, is cerebellar kinetic (intention) tremor driven by some internal oscillator triggered by movement, and, if so, where is such an oscillator?

These are some of the areas of dispute or ignorance in the field of tremor at the present time. They illustrate the many avenues for future research into tremor, the results of which may well justify revision of the present review.

REFERENCES

Albe-Fessard, D., Arfel, G. and Guiot, G. (1963). Activités électriques characteristiques de quelques structures cérébrales chez l'homme. *Ann. Chir.*, **17**, 1185–214.

Albe-Fessard, D., Guiot, G., Lamarre, Y. and Arfel, G. (1966). Activation of thalamo-cortical projections related to tremorogenic process. In Yahr, M. and Purpura, D. (eds), *The Thalamus*, Columbia University Press, New York, pp. 237–54.

Allum, J. H. J., Dietz, V. and Freund, H.-J. (1978). Neuronal mechanisms underlying physiological tremor. *J. Neurophysiol.*, 41, 557–71.

Bedard, P., Larochelle, L., Poirier, L. J. and Sourkes, T. L. (1970). Reversible effect of L-DOPA on tremor and catatonia induced by α-methyl-*p*-tyrosine. *Can. J. Physiol. Pharmacol.*, 48, 82–4.

Brooks, V. B., Kozlovskaya, I. B., Atkin, A., Horvath, F. E. and Uno, M. (1973). Effects of cooling dentate nucleus on tracking-task performance in monkeys. *J. Neurophysiol.*, 36, 974–95.

Bucy, P. C. and Case, T. J. (1949). Tremor: physiologic mechanism and abolition by surgical means. *Arch. Neurol. Psychiatr.*, 41, 721–46.

Burke, R. E. (1981). Motor units: anatomy, physiology, and functional organisation. In Brookes, V. B. (ed.), *Handbook of Physiology. The Nervous System, Motor Control*, part 1, Williams and Wilkins, Baltimore, pp. 345–422.

Calzetti, S., Findley, L. J., Pisani, F. and Richens, A. (1981). Phenylethylmalonamide in essential tremor. A double-blind controlled study. *J. Neurol. Neurosurg. Psychiatr.*, 44, 932–4.

Carrea, R. M. E. and Mettler, F. A. (1947). Physiologic consequences following extensive removal of cerebellar cortex and deep cerebellar nuclei and effect of secondary cerebral ablations in the primate. *J. Comp. Neurol.*, 87, 169–288.

Carrea, R. M. E. and Mettler, F. A. (1955). Function of the primate brachium conjunctivum and related structures. *J. Comp. Neurol.*, 102, 151–322.

Cooke, J. D. and Thomas, J. S. (1976). Fore-arm oscillation during cooling of the dentate nucleus in the monkey. *Can. J. Physiol. Pharmacol.*, 54, 430–6,

Cordeau, J. P., Gybels, J., Jasper, H. H. and Poirier, L. J. (1960). Micro-electrode studies of unit discharges in the sensorimotor cortex: investigations in monkeys with experimental tremors. *Neurology (Minneap.)*, 10, 591–600.

Cordeau, J. P. and Lamarre, Y. (1966). Further studies on patterns of central unit activity in relation with tremor. *J. Neurosurg.*, 24, 213–18.

Critchley, E. M. R. (1972). Clinical manifestations of essential tremor. *J. Neurol. Neurosurg. Psychiatr.*, 35, 365–72.

Critchley, M. (1949). Observations on essential (heredo-familial) tremor. *Brain*, 72, 113–39.

Desmedt, J. E. (1981). The size principle of motoneuron recruitment in ballistic or ramp voluntary contractions in man. In Desmedt, J. E. (ed.), *Motor Unit Types, Recruitment and Plasticity in Health and Disease, Progress in Clinical Neurophysiology*, vol. 9, Karger, Basel, pp. 97–136.

Dietz, V., Bischofberger, E., Wita, C. and Freund, H. J. (1976). Correlation between discharges of two simultaneously recorded motor units and physiological tremor. *EEG Clin. Neurophysiol.*, 40, 97–105.

Findley, L. J. and Calzetti, S. (1982). Double-blind controlled study of primidone in essential tremor: preliminary results. *Br. Med. J.*, 285, 608.

Findley, L. J. and Gresty, M. A. (1980). Supression of 'rubral' tremor with levodopa. *Br. Med. J.*, 281, 1043.

Findley, L. J., Gresty, M. A. and Halmagyi, G. M. (1981). Tremor, the cogwheel phenomenon and clonus in Parkinson's disease. *J. Neurol. Neurosurg. Psychiatr.*, 44, 534–46.

Foerster, O. (1936). Symptomatologie der Erkrankungen des Ruckenmarks und seiner Wurzeln. In Bumke, R. and Foerster, O. (eds), *Handbuch der Neurologie*, vol. 5, Springer-Verlag, Berlin, pp. 1–403.

Freund, H.-J., Budingen, H. J. and Dietz, V. (1975). Activity of single motor units from human fore-arm muscles during voluntary isometric contractions. *J. Neurophysiol.*, **38**, 933-46.

Furness, P., Jessop, J. and Lippold, O. C. J. (1977). Long-lasting increases in the tremor of human hand muscles following brief, strong effort. *J. Physiol. (Lond.)*, **265**, 821-31.

Gilman, S., Bloedell, J. R. and Lechtenberg, R. (1981). *Disorders of the Cerebellum, Contemporary Neurology Series*, vol. 21, Davis, Philadelphia.

Gilman, S., Carr, D. and Hollenberg, J. (1976). Kinematic effects of deafferentation and cerebellar ablation. *Brain*, **99**, 311-30.

Growdon, H., Chambers, W. W. and Liu, C. N. (1967). An experimental dyskinesia in the Rhesus monkey. *Brain*, **90**, 603-32.

Growdon, J. H., Shahani, B. T. and Young, R. R. (1975). The effect of alcohol on essential tremor. *Neurology (Minneap.)*, **25**, 259-62.

Hagbarth, K. E. and Young, R. R. (1979). Participation of the stretch reflex in human physiological tremor. *Brain*, **102**, 509-26.

Halliday, A. M. and Redfearn, J. W. T. (1956). An analysis of the frequencies of finger tremor in healthy subjects. *J. Physiol. (Lond.)*, **134**, 600-11.

Henneman, E., Clamann, H. P., Gillies, J. D. and Skinner, R. D. (1974). Rank-order of motoneurons within a pool: law of combination. *J. Neurophysiol.*, **37**, 1338-49.

Henneman, E., Somjen, G. and Carpenter, D. O. (1965). Functional significance of cell size in spinal motoneurons. *J. Neurophysiol.*, **28**, 560-80.

Hodgson, H. J. F., Marsden, C. D. and Meadows, J. C. (1969). The effect of adrenaline on the response to muscle vibration in man. *J. Physiol. (Lond.)*, **202**, 98-99p.

Holmes, G. (1922). Clinical symptoms of cerebellar diseases (The Croonian Lectures). *Lancet*, **1**, 1177-82, 1231-7, and **2**, 59-65, 111-15.

Jasper, H. H. and Bertrand, G. (1966). Recording from micro-electrode in stereotaxic surgery for Parkinson's disease. *J. Neurosurg.*, **24**, 219-21.

Jefferson, D., Jenner, P. and Marsden, C. D. (1979). β-Adrenoreceptor antagonists in essential tremor. *J. Neurol. Neurosurg. Psychiatr.*, **42**, 904-9.

Joffroy, A. J. and Lamarre, Y. (1971). Rhythmic unit firing in the precentral cortex in relation with postural tremor in a deafferented limb. *Brain Res.*, **27**, 386-9.

Joyce, G. C. and Rack, P. M. H. (1974). The effects of load and force on tremor at the normal human elbow joint. *J. Physiol. (Lond.)*, **240**, 375-96.

Joyce, G. C., Rack, P. M. H. and Ross, H. F. (1974). The forces generated at the human elbow joint in response to imposed sinusoidal movements of the forearm. *J. Physiol. (Lond.)*, **240**, 351-74.

Klemme, R. M. (1940). Surgical treatment of dystonia, paralysis agitans and athetosis. *Arch. Neurol. Psychiatr.*, **44**, 926.

Lamarre, Y. (1975). Tremorogenic mechanisms in primates. In Meldrum, B. S. and Marsden, C. D. (eds), *Primate Models of Neurological Disorders, Advances in Neurology*, vol. 10, Raven Press, New York, pp. 23-34.

Lamarre, Y. and Joffroy, A. J. (1970). Thalamic unit activity in monkey with experimental tremor. In Barbeau, A. and McDowell, S. H. (eds), *L-Dopa and Parkinsonism*, Davis, Philadelphia, pp. 163-70.

Lamarre, Y. and Joffroy, A. J. (1971). Spontaneous unit activity in the ventrolateral thalamus of the chronic monkey. *Int. J. Neurol.*, **8**, 190-7.

Lamarre, Y. and Joffroy, A. J. (1979). Experimental tremor in monkey: activity of thalamic and precentral cortical neurons in the absence of feedback. In Poirier, L. J., Sourkes, T. L. and Bedard, P. J. (eds), *Advances in Neurology*, vol. 24, Raven Press, New York, pp. 109-22.

Lamarre, Y., de Montigny, C., Dumont, M. and Weiss, M. (1971). Harmaline-induced rhythmic activity of cerebellar and lower brainstem neurons. *Brain Res.*, 32, 246–50.

Lance, J. W., Schwab, R. S. and Peterson, E. A. (1963). Action tremor and the cogwheel phenomenon in Parkinson's disease. *Brain*, 86, 95–110.

Larochelle, L., Bedard, P., Boucher, R. and Poirier, L. J. (1970). The rubro-olivo-cerebello-rubral loop and postural tremor in the monkey. *J. Neurol. Sci.*, 11, 53–64.

Larochelle, L., Bedard, P., Poirier, L. J. and Sourkes, T. L. (1971). Correlative neuroanatomical and neuropharmacological study of tremor and catatonia in the monkey. *Neuropharmacology*, 10, 273–88.

Lee, R. G. and Stein, R. B. (1981). Resetting of tremor by mechanical perturbations: a comparison of essential tremor and Parkinsonian tremor. *Ann. Neurol.*, 10, 523–31.

Leigh, P. N., Jefferson, D., Twomey, A. and Marsden, C. D. (1983). Beta-adrenoreceptor mechanisms in essential tremor; a double-blind placebo-controlled trial of metoprolol, sotalol and atenolol. *J. Neurol. Neurosurg. Psychiatr.*, 46 (8), 710–15.

Leriche, R. (1914). Radiocotomie cerricale pour un tremblement parkinsonism. *Lyon Med.*, 122, 1075–6.

Lindqvist, T. (1941). Finger tremor and the alpha waves of the electroencephalogram. *Acta Med. Scand.*, 108, 580–5.

Lippold, O. C. J. (1970). Oscillation in the stretch reflex arc and the origin of the rhythmical 8-12 c/s component of physiological tremor. *J. Physiol. (Lond.)*, 206, 359–82.

Lippold, O. C. J. (1981). The tremor in fatigue. In *Human Muscle Fatigue: Physiological Mechanisms, Ciba Foundation Symposium*, No. 82, pp. 234–48.

Lippold, O. C. J., Redfearn, J. W. T. and Vuco, J. (1957). The rhythmical activity of groups of motor units in the voluntary contraction of muscle. *J. Physiol. (Lond.)*, 137, 473–87.

Marsden, C. D. (1976). The spectrum of dystonia. In Yahr, M. D. (ed.), *The Basal Ganglia*, Association for Research in Nervous and Mental Disease, vol. 55, pp. 351–67.

Marsden, C. D. (1978). The mechanisms of physiological tremor and their significance for pathological tremors. In Desmedt, J. E. (ed.), *Physiological Tremor, Pathological Tremors and Clonus, Progress in Clinical Neurophysiology*, vol. 5, Karger, Basel, pp. 1–16.

Marsden, C. D., Foley, T. H., Owen, D. A. L. and McAllister, R. G. (1967a). Peripheral β-adrenergic receptors concerned with tremor. *Clin. Sci.*, 33, 53–65.

Marsden, C. D., Gimlette, T. M. D., McAllister, R. G., Owen, D. A. L. and Miller, T. M. (1968). Effect of β-adrenergic blockade on finger tremor and Achilles reflex time on anxious and thyrotoxic patients. *Acta Endocrinol. (Copenh.)*, 57, 353–62.

Marsden, C. D. and Meadows, J. C. (1970). The effect of adrenaline on the contraction of human muscle. *J. Physiol. (Lond.)*, 207, 429–48.

Marsden, C. D., Meadows, J. C. and Lange, G. W. (1970). Effect of speed of muscle contraction on physiological tremor in normal subjects and in patients with thyrotoxicosis and myxoedema. *J. Neurol. Neurosurg. Psychiatr.*, 33, 776–82.

Marsden, C. D., Meadows, J. C., Lange, G. W. and Watson, R. S. (1967b). Effect of deafferentation on human physiological tremor. *Lancet*, 2, 700–2.

Marsden, C. D., Meadows, J. C., Lange, G. W. and Watson, R. S. (1969a). Variations in human physiological finger tremor with particular reference to changes with age. *EEG Clin. Neurophysiol.*, 27, 169–78.

Marsden, C. D., Meadows, J. C., Lange, G. W. and Watson, R. S. (1969b). The role of the ballistocardiac impulse in the genesis of physiological tremor. *Brain*, 92, 647–62.

Marsden, C. D., Obeso, J. and Rothwell, J. C. (1983). Benign essential tremor is not a single entity. In Yahr, M. D. (ed.), *Current Concepts in Parkinson's Disease*, Excerpta Medica, Amsterdam, pp. 31–46.

Marshall, J. (1962). Observations on essential tremor. *J. Neurol. Neurosurg. Psychiatr.*, 25, 122–5.

Marshall, J. and Walsh, E. G. (1956). Physiological tremor. *J. Neurol. Neurosurg. Psychiatr.*, 19, 260–7.

Matthews, P. B. C. and Muir, R. B. (1980). Comparison of electromyogram spectra with force spectra during human elbow tremor. *J. Physiol. (Lond.)*, 302, 427–41.

Merton, P. A., Morton, H. B. and Rashbass, C. (1967). Visual feedback in hand tremor. *Nature (Lond.)*, 216, 583–4.

Milner-Brown, H. S., Stein, R. B. and Lee, R. G. (1975). Synchronization of human motor units: possible roles of exercise and supraspinal reflexes. *EEG Clin. Neurophysiol.*, 38, 245–54.

Milner-Brown, H. S., Stein, R. B. and Yemm, R. (1973a). The contractile properties of human motor units during voluntary isometric contractions. *J. Physiol. (Lond.)*, 228, 285–306.

Milner-Brown, H. S., Stein, R. B. and Yemm, R. (1973b). The orderly recruitment of human motor units during voluntary isometric contractions. *J. Physiol. (Lond.)*, 230, 359–70.

Milner-Brown, H. S., Stein, R. B. and Yemm, R. (1973c). Changes in firing rate of human motor units during linearly changing voluntary contractions. *J. Physiol. (Lond.)*, 230, 371–90.

Mylle, G. and van Bogaert, L. (1940). Etudes anatomo-cliniques de syndromes hypercinetiques complexes. I. Sur le tremblement familial. *Monatsschr. Psychiatr. Neurol.*, 103, 28–43.

Narabayashi, H. (1973). Importance of muscle tone in production or modification of tremorous movements. In Siegfried, J. (ed.), *Parkinson's Disease*, Huber, Bern, pp. 27–36.

Narabayashi, H. (1982). Surgical approach to tremor. In Marsden, C. D. and Fahn, S. (eds), *Movement Disorders*, Butterworths, London, pp. 292–9.

O'Brien, M. D., Upton, A. R. and Toseland, P. A. (1981). Benign familial tremor treated with primidone. *Br. Med. J.*, 282, 178–80.

Ohye, C., Bouchard, R., Larochelle, L., Bedard, P., Boucher, R., Raphy, B. and Poirier, L. J. (1970). Effect of dorsal rhizotomy on postural tremor in the monkey. *Exp. Brain Res.*, 10, 140–50.

Ohye, C., Hirai, T., Miyazaki, M., Shbazaki, T. and Nakajima, H. (1982a). Vim thalamotomy for the treatment of various kinds of tremor. *Appl. Neurophysiol.*, 45, 275–80.

Ohye, C., Miyazaki, M., Hirai, T., Shibazaki, T., Nakajima, H. and Nagaseki, Y. (1982b). Primary writing tremor treated by stereotactic selective thalamotomy. *J. Neurol. Neurosurg. Psychiatr.*, 45, 988–97.

Ohye, C. and Narabayashi, H. (1979). Physiological study of presumed ventralis intermedius neurons in the human thalamus. *J. Neurosurg.*, 50, 290–7.

Ohye, C., Saito, Y., Fukamachi, A. and Narabayashi, H. (1974). An analysis of the spontaneous and rhythmic and non-rhythmic burst discharges in the human thalamus. *J. Neurol. Sci.*, 22, 245–59.

Pechadre, J. C., Larochelle, L. and Poirier, L. J. (1976). Parkinsonian akinesia, rigidity and tremor in the monkey. *J. Neurol. Sci.*, 28, 147–57.

Poirier, L. J., Bouvier, G., Bedard, P., Boucher, R., Larochelle, L., Oliver, A. and

Singh, P. (1969). Essai sur les circuits neuronaux impliqués dans le tremblement postural et l'hypokinesie. *Rev. Neurol. (Paris)*, **120**, 15–40.

Poirier, L. J., Sourkes, T. L., Bouvier, G., Boucher, R. and Carabin, S. (1966). Striatal amines, experimental tremor and the effect of harmaline in the monkey. *Brain*, **89**, 37–52.

Pollock, L. J. and Davis, L. (1930). Muscle tone in Parkinsonian states. *Arch. Neurol. Psychiatr.*, **23**, 303–19.

Procaccianti, G., Martinelli, P., Baruzzi, A., Pazzaglia, P. and Lugaresi, E. (1981). Benign familial tremor treated with primidone. *Br. Med. J.*, **283**, 558.

Rack, P. M. H. (1978). Mechanical and reflex factors in human tremor. In Desmedt, J. E. (ed.), *Physiological Tremor, Pathological Tremors and Clonus, Progress in Clinical Neurophysiology*, vol. 5, Karger, Basel, pp. 17–27.

Rack, P. M. H. (1981). Limitations of somatosensory feedback in the control of posture and movement. In Brooks, V. B. (ed.), *Handbook of Physiology. The Nervous System, Motor Control*, part 1, Williams and Wilkins, Baltimore, pp. 229–56.

Ranish, N. A. and Soechting, J. F. (1976). Studies on the control of some simple motor tasks. Effects of thalamic and red nuclei lesions. *Brain Res.*, **102**, 334–45.

Rothwell, J. C., Traub, M. M. and Marsden, C. D. (1979). Primary writing tremor. *J. Neurol. Neurosurg. Psychiatr.*, **42**, 1106–14.

Salisachs, P. (1976). Charcot–Marie–Tooth disease associated with essential tremor. *J. Neurol. Sci.*, **28**, 17–40.

Salisachs, P. and Lapresle, J. (1973). Nevrite hypertrophique avec atrophie peronière associée à une dyskinesie volitionelle d'attitude. *Rev. Neurol. (Paris)*, **123**, 119–25.

Schwab, R. S. and Young, R. R. (1971). Non-resting tremor in Parkinson's disease. *Trans. Am. Neurol. Assoc.*, **96**, 305–7.

Shahani, B. T. and Young, R. R. (1976). Physiological and pharmacological aids in the differential diagnosis of tremor. *J. Neurol. Neurosurg. Psychiatr.*, **39**, 772–83.

Shahani, B. T. and Young, R. R. (1978). Action tremors: a clinical neurophysiological review. In Desmedt, J. E. (ed.), *Physiological Tremor, Pathological Tremors and Clonus, Progress in Clinical Neurophysiology*, vol. 5, Karger, Basel, pp. 129–37.

Shahani, B. T., Young, R. R. and Adams, R. D. (1973). Neuropathic tremor. *EEG Clin. Neurophysiol.*, **34**, 800.

Smith, I. S., Kahn, S. N., Lacey, B. W., King, R. H. M., Eames, R. A., Whybrew, D. J. and Thomas, P. K. (1983). Chronic demyelinating neuropathy associated with benign IgM paraproteinemia. *Brain*, **106**, 169–96.

Stiles, R. B. and Pozos, R. S. (1976). A mechanical-reflex oscillator hypothesis for Parkinsonian hand tremor. *J. Appl. Physiol.*, **40**, 990–8.

Stiles, R. N. (1976). Frequency and displacement amplitude relations for normal hand tremor. *J. Appl. Physiol.*, **40**, 44–54.

Strick, P. L. (1976). Anatomical analysis of ventrolateral thalamic input into primate motor cortex. *J. Neurophysiol.*, **39**, 1020–31.

Sutton, G. G. and Sykes, K. (1967a). The variation in hand tremor with force in healthy subjects. *J. Physiol. (Lond.)*, **191**, 699–711.

Sutton, G. G. and Sykes, K. (1967b). The effect of withdrawal of visual presentation of errors upon the frequency spectrum of tremor in a manual task. *J. Physiol. (Lond.)*, **190**, 281–93.

Taylor, A. (1962). The significance of grouping of motor unit activity. *J. Physiol. (Lond.)*, **162**, 259–69.

Teravainen, H. (1980). Oscillatory electromyographic responses to limb displacement in Parkinsonism. *J. Neurol. Neurosurg. Psychiatr.*, **43**, 419–26.

Teravainen, H. and Calne, D. B. (1980). Action tremor in Parkinson's disease. *J. Neurol. Neurosurg. Psychiatr.*, **43**, 257–63.

Teravainen, H., Evarts, E. and Calne, D. B. (1979). Effects of kinesthetic inputs on Parkinsonian tremor. In Poirier, L. J., Sourkes, T. L. and Bedard, P. J. (eds), *Advances in Neurology*, vol. 24, Raven Press, New York, pp. 161–73.

Villis, T. and Hore, J. (1977). Effects of changes in mechanical state of limb on cerebellar intention tremor. *J. Neurophysiol.*, **40**, 1214–24.

Walsh, E. G. (1976). Clonus: beats provoked by the application of a rhythmic force. *J. Neurol. Neurosurg. Psychiatr.*, **39**, 266–74.

Ward, A. A., McCulloch, W. S. and Magoun, H. W. (1948). Production of an alternating tremor at rest in monkeys. *J. Neurophysiol.*, **11**, 317–30.

Winkler, J. F. and Young, R. R. (1974). Efficacy of chronic propranolol therapy in action tremors of the familial, senile, or essential varieties. *New Engl. J. Med.*, **290**, 984–8.

Young, R. R., Growdon, J. H. and Shahani, B. T. (1975). Beta-adrenergic mechanisms in action tremor. *New Engl. J. Med.*, **293**, 950–3.

Young, R. R. and Hagbarth, K.-E. (1980). Physiological tremor enhanced by manoeuvres affecting the segmental stretch reflex. *J. Neurol. Neurosurg. Psychiatr.*, **43**, 248–56.

Young, R. R. and Shahani, B. T. (1979). Single unit behaviour in human muscle afferent and efferent systems. In Poirier, L. J., Sourkes, T. L. and Bedard, P. J. (eds), *Advances in Neurology*, vol. 24, Raven Press, New York, pp. 175–83.

5
Pharmacological differentiation of tremor

STANLEY FAHN

HISTORICAL ASPECTS

The rest tremor of Parkinson's disease probably was the first type of tremor to be successfully ameliorated by pharmacologic agents. Atropine was introduced by Charcot (1879), and scopolamine by Erb (1908). Duvoisin (1967) pointed out that a student of Charcot, Ordenstein, first suggested the use of belladonna alkaloids. The belladonna-like drugs have been used for partial symptomatic relief since that time. Because of fewer systemic side-effects, the synthetic centrally acting anticholinergic drugs, introduced in the early 1950s, have largely replaced the natural alkaloids. These agents rarely provided complete relief of the tremor, and it took the introduction of high-dosage levodopa (Cotzias *et al.*, 1967) for the elimination of the tremor by a pharmacologic approach to become a reality. By then, stereotactic surgery had already been shown by Cooper (1955) to be effective in eliminating parkinsonian tremor. In patients not responding to levodopa alone, a combination of levodopa and an anticholinergic agent may be effective. The newly introduced direct-acting dopamine receptor agonists can substitute for levodopa in some patients (Lieberman and Goldstein, 1982).

It had been known for a long time that alcohol can relieve essential tremor (Critchley, 1949), but except for a drink before dinner or on social occasions, alcohol has consistently and intentionally not been recommended as a means of chronic pharmacotherapy because of the potential for alcohol abuse and its consequence. As with parkinsonian tremor, surgical relief of essential tremor was already demonstrated by Cooper (1962) before practical pharmacologic therapy was discovered.

Although the discovery of the beneficial effects of propranolol in the treatment of essential tremor was by serendipity (Winkler and Young, 1971, 1974; Sevitt, 1971), there were strong clues already in the literature that beta-adrenergic blockers may have some usefulness. Marshall and Schnieden (1966) had reported that intravenous infusion of epinephrine enhanced essential tremor (and also anxiety tremor, parkinsonian tremor and cerebellar tremor). Marsden and his associates showed that epinephrine (Marsden *et al.*, 1967), but not norepinephrine

85

(Marsden *et al.*, 1969), increased the amplitude (but not the frequency) of physiologic tremor. They reasoned that since the former drug has a greater effect stimulating beta-adrenergic receptors, and the latter has a greater effect on the
alpha-receptors, the enhancement of physiologic tremor is due to stimulation of
beta-receptors. Previously, Owen and Marsden (1965) had shown that beta-
adrenergic blockade reduced the worsening of parkinsonian tremor induced by
infusion of epinephrine, whereas it could not be abolished by the alpha-adrenergic
blocker, phentolamine (Constas, 1962). Marsden *et al.* (1968) also showed that
intravenous propranolol, a beta-adrenergic blocker, can also reduce the accentuated
physiologic tremor of anxiety and thyrotoxicosis.

Fewer studies have been conducted on cerebellar tremors, and most of these
have not yielded newer approaches to their pharmacotherapy. Two exceptions
are the reports on 5-hydroxytryptophan by Rascol *et al.* (1981) and isoniazid by
Sabra *et al.* (1982). Both of these reports await confirmation.

DRUG EFFECTS ON TREMOR

In order to determine whether the utilisation of drugs can aid in the diagnosis of
different types and aetiologies of tremor, it is important to review briefly their
known effects, which are listed in table 5.1.

Parkinsonian tremors

Two types of tremor are found in patients with parkinsonism: the classical rest
tremor and also an action tremor (Lance *et al.*, 1963). Both types occur in a
majority of patients. The rest tremor of Parkinson's disease can usually be
ameliorated by dopaminergic agents, both levodopa and the direct-acting dopamine
receptor agonists, such as bromocriptine, lisuride and pergolide. Not uncommonly, the tremor can be completely eliminated. Anticholinergic drugs, amantadine (believed to have both dopaminergic and anticholinergic activity) and antihistaminics (probably due to their anticholinergic activity) can also reduce the
tremor. Too much has been written about these effects to go into any more detail
about them. Rajput *et al.* (1975) evaluated the effect of ethanol on parkinsonian
tremor. Ostensibly trying to determine if ethanol affects the action tremor of
parkinsonism, it was not clear from their report that they could clearly separate
out the effect on action tremor from rest tremor. In any event tremor was reduced
in 47% of parkinsonian patients.

Duvoisin (1967) demonstrated that, whereas anticholinergic drugs can ameliorate parkinsonian rest tremor, the central action of the cholinomimetic drug,
physostigmine, can increase this tremor. Similarly, antidopaminergic agents, such
as the antipsychotic drugs that act by blocking dopamine receptors, can worsen
parkinsonian rest tremor, and even antagonise the benefit obtained from levodopa
(Klawans and Weiner, 1974, Tarsy *et al.*, 1975). It had long been known that

Table 5.1 Drug effects on tremor.

Disease state	Improvement	Worsening
Parkinsonism		
Rest tremor	Levodopa	Physostigmine
	Dopamine agonists	Isoproterenol
	Anticholinergics	Epinephrine
	Amantadine	Antipsychotics
	Antihistamines	
	Alcohol	
Action tremor	Alcohol	Isoproterenol
	Beta-adrenergic blockers	Epinephrine
	Benzodiazepines	Antipsychotics
		Levodopa
Essential tremor	Alcohol	Isoproterenol
	Beta-adrenergic blockers	Epinephrine
	Primidone	Antipsychotics
	Benzodiazepines	Levodopa
	Amantadine	
Accentuated physiologic	Alcohol	Isoproterenol
tremor, examples:	Beta-adrenergic blockers	Epinephrine
Thyrotoxicosis	Benzodiazepines	Antipsychotics
Hypoglycaemia		Levodopa
Alcohol withdrawal		
Lithium		
Cerebellar disease		
Postural tremor	5-HTP (?)	Epinephrine
		Alcohol
Intention tremor	5-HTP (?)	Epinephrine
(multiple sclerosis)	Isoniazid (?)	Alcohol
Wilson's disease	D-Penicillamine	D-Penicillamine
		(transient)

See text for details.

anxiety can worsen parkinsonian rest tremor. This is probably related to beta-adrenergic receptor stimulation; drugs, such as isoproterenol and epinephrine, that stimulate these receptors also increase this tremor (Barcroft *et al.*, 1952; Constas, 1962; Owen and Marsden, 1965; Marshall and Schnieden, 1966). This increase of parkinsonian tremor can be abolished by beta-adrenergic antagonists (Owen and Marsden, 1965).

Although some patients with Parkinson's disease have an associated essential tremor, as determined by typical features of essential tremor during much of their adult life prior to the onset of symptoms of parkinsonism, many more patients have an action tremor related directly to Parkinson's disease itself. This tremor occurs in a majority of patients and may be present instead of the more classical rest tremor, but most patients have both a rest tremor and an action tremor.

Young and Shahani (1979) placed the action tremor of parkinsonism in the category of essential tremor based on the lack of response from intravenous propranolol (Shahani and Young, 1976). However, because of the long duration and positive family history in patients with rather typical essential tremor in addition to Parkinson's disease, it seems reasonable to categorise the more common action tremor of parkinsonism as being distinct from essential tremor. On this basis, Jankovic and Fahn (1980) considered the action tremor of parkinsonism as being due to enhanced physiologic tremor rather than as part of essential tremor. However, the lack of improvement with intravenous ethanol suggests that this placement is incorrect also. It may be best to create a separate category for the action tremor of parkinsonism.

Regardless of the category in which it is placed, it does respond somewhat to oral propranolol (Schwab and Young, 1971; Rajput et al., 1975; Shahani and Young, 1976). As with typical accentuated physiologic tremor or with essential tremor, the action tremor of parkinsonism also lessens with ethanol (Rajput et al., 1975) and worsens with isoproterenol, epinephrine, levodopa and anti-psychotic drugs (Shahani and Young, 1976; Young and Shahani, 1979). Since parkinsonian patients will usually require levodopa for the treatment of other symptoms of this disorder, and since the presence of any action tremor may be made worse with levodopa, the addition of propranolol may be required (Abramsky et al., 1971; Shahani and Young, 1976).

Essential tremor

Alcohol can have the most dramatic effect on essential tremor; one or two drinks can eliminate the tremor in most patients. However, some patients, with otherwise clinically typical essential tremor, fail to respond. Rajput et al. (1975) reported that 62% of 21 patients improved. They also found that a higher percentage (92%) of patients improved with propranolol than with ethanol. Nevertheless, the degree of improvement of tremor amplitude with propranolol is much less than that with ethanol in my experience. The effect of ethanol appears to be in the central nervous system, since it is not effective when infused into the brachial artery (Growdon et al., 1975).

The initial reports by Winkler and Young (1971) and Sevitt (1971) that pro-pranolol can reduce the amplitude of essential tremor have been confirmed by a large number of studies (e.g. Tolosa and Loewenson, 1975; McAllister et al., 1977; Jefferson et al., 1979; Sorensen et al., 1981). Many of these studies utilised electromyographic recordings of tremor as a means of assessing improvement. By using a clinical scoring scale, Sweet et al. (1974) found propranolol not to be very effective. From personal experience, I have noticed that tremor affecting the hands responds better than that affecting the neck or voice. Whereas I have not had any success in reducing voice tremor with propranolol, Massey and Paulson (1982) reported some benefit. Other beta-adrenergic blockers have also been found to ameliorate essential tremor (Newman and Jacobs, 1980; Calzetti et al., 1981; Larsen and Teravainen, in press).

Young *et al.* (1975) showed that intra-arterial infusion of propranolol did not relieve essential tremor in contrast to chronic oral propranolol, and suggested that the effect of propranolol is from an action on the central nervous system. Shahani and Young (1976) proposed that the effect of intravenous propranolol could differentiate essential tremor from accentuated physiologic tremor, such as that produced by isoproterenol. The former would not respond, and the latter would respond.

Benzodiazepines and sedatives are not very effective in controlling essential tremor, but benzodiazepines in combination with propranolol can sometimes be beneficial (Fahn, 1972; Shahani and Young, 1976). O'Brien *et al.* (1981) recently reported that primidone can be effective in reducing essential tremor. Amantadine has been found to be helpful in some patients (Manyam, 1981). Epinephrine (Marshall and Schnieden, 1966), isoproterenol, levodopa and antipsychotic agents (Shahani and Young, 1976) aggravate essential tremor.

Accentuated physiologic tremor

As discussed above, increased beta-adrenergic activity can produce tremor. This has been associated with an increase of physiologic tremor. Examples include tremor induced with isoproterenol and many other drugs (e.g. levodopa, tricyclic antidepressants, lithium) and tremor associated with thyrotoxicosis, hypoglycaemia and alcohol withdrawal. Beta-adrenergic blockers can suppress this type of tremor (Kirk *et al.*, 1973; Zilm *et al.*, 1975; Shahani and Young, 1976; Pickles *et al.*, 1981). Furthermore, Shahani and Young (1976) reported that intravenous propranolol is effective against this type of tremor. In fact, these authors suggest that this response can serve as a useful diagnostic test to diagnose this form of tremor. Essential tremor does not respond to intravenous propranolol.

Benzodiazepines, perhaps by reducing anxiety, have some beneficial effect on this type of tremor (Shahani and Young, 1976). Ethanol may act in a similar manner (Shahani and Young, 1976). Drugs that increase beta-adrenergic activity make the tremor more severe. These include epinephrine (Marshall and Schnieden, 1966), isoproterenol and terbutaline (Young and Shahani, 1979). Young and Shahani (1979) mention that levodopa with or without carbidopa can increase this form of tremor. In the presence of carbidopa, peripheral formation of catecholamines is prevented. Therefore, it is possible that central mechanisms as well as peripheral ones may affect accentuated physiologic tremor. These authors also mention that antipsychotic drugs aggravate this tremor, which again suggests that other mechanisms not yet understood can also be involved.

Cerebellar disease

There have been very few gains in the pharmacologic understanding of cerebellar tremors. Rascol *et al.* (1981) reported that the serotonin precursor, 5-hydroxytryptophan, can ameliorate intention and postural tremors as well as ataxia in patients with cerebellar diseases. Sabra *et al.* (1982) have recently reported that isoniazid can reduce severe intention tremor in patients with multiple sclerosis. These reports await confirmation.

Infusions of epinephrine increase cerebellar tremors, according to Marshall and Schnieden (1966). Ethanol appears to make cerebellar tremors worse (Rajput *et al.*, 1975).

Chelation of copper is specific therapy for Wilson's disease, and D-penicillamine is the most commonly utilised drug for this purpose. In the early stage of treatment, D-penicillamine can aggravate the symptoms of Wilson's disease. This paradoxical response is believed to be due to removal of copper from systemic organs, causing increased copper in the circulation and subsequent increased deposition in the brain. With continued treatment with D-penicillamine, the symptoms will gradually fade.

PHARMACOLOGICAL DIFFERENTIATION OF TREMOR

Since many drugs can alter the severity of tremors of various aetiologies, it would be ideal if they could be utilised to aid in the diagnosis of each type of tremor. Unfortunately, the lack of specificity by most drugs (false positives) and the failure of some usually responsive tremors to be affected (false negatives) limit the role of drugs in this regard. One possible exception is the rest tremor of parkinsonism which usually responds to levodopa and anticholinergic drugs. There do not appear to be any false positive responses to these drugs, although there are false negative ones. In other words, a positive response to these medications supports the diagnosis that the tremor is due to parkinsonism, but a lack of response does not exclude this diagnosis.

Although essential tremor frequently is ameliorated by beta-blockers, there are too many patients who fail to respond adequately, and these drugs also can suppress the action tremor of parkinsonism as well as accentuated physiologic tremor, for such a clinical response to be of diagnostic value. Alcohol, the most potent drug suppressing essential tremor, has also been shown not to be specific for this type of tremor. On the other hand, Young and Shahani (1979) believe that accentuated physiologic tremor can be differentiated from essential tremor because the former responds to intravenous propranolol, while the latter does not. They may be correct, but it is important that other investigators confirm their findings before this concept is accepted. If they are correct, then this approach would serve as a major criterion in the differential diagnosis of action tremors.

It has recently been reported that intention tremor can be ameliorated by isoniazid, but insufficient experience with this drug prevents us from drawing any conclusions about the specificity of this action or about the incidence of false negatives. Amelioration of tremor with D-penicillamine would reinforce a diagnosis of Wilson's disease, which can be established by the presence of a Kayser–Fleischer ring and various chemical tests.

More careful work is needed to extend our knowledge about the specificity of response of various tremors to pharmacologic agents. The rest tremor of parkinsonism appears to be the only tremor that improves from levodopa and the anticholinergic agents. Even so, there are many causes of parkinsonism, many of which can respond to these agents. The list includes Parkinson's disease, postencephalitic parkinsonism, reserpine-induced parkinsonism and others. If the specificity of intravenous propranolol to reduce only accentuated physiologic tremor is substantiated, there still remains the problem as to the exact aetiology for each patient with this type of tremor, much like the problem with parkinsonism, but even more so since there are a great many causes of accentuated physiologic tremor.

It is expected that with more careful clinical pharmacologic studies we will be able to rely more heavily on drug trials to aid us in the clinical diagnosis of tremors.

REFERENCES

Abramsky, O., Carmon, A. and Lavy, S. (1971). Combined treatment of Parkinsonian tremor with propranolol and levodopa. *J. Neurol. Sci.*, **14**, 491–4.

Barcroft, H., Peterson, E. and Schwab, R. S. (1952). Action of adrenaline and noradrenaline on the tremor in Parkinson's disease. *Neurology*, **2**, 154–60.

Calzetti, S., Findley, L. J., Gresty, M. A., Perucca, E. and Richens, A. (1981). Metoprolol and propranolol in essential tremor: a double-blind, controlled study. *J. Neurol. Neurosurg. Psychiatr.*, **44**, 814–19.

Charcot, J. M. (1879). *Clinical Lectures on Diseases of the Nervous System*, vol. I, 2nd edn, transl. Sigerson, G., Henry C. Lea, Philadelphia.

Constas, C. (1962). The effects of adrenaline, noradrenaline, and isoprenaline on Parkinsonian tremor. *J. Neurol. Neurosurg. Psychiatr.*, **25**, 116–21.

Cooper, I. S. (1955). Chemopalledectomy, an investigative technique in geriatric parkinsonians. *Science*, **121**, 217–18.

Cooper, I. S. (1962). Heredofamilial tremor abolition by chemothalamectomy. *Arch. Neurol.*, **7**, 129–31.

Cotzias, G. C., Van Woert, M. H. and Schiffer, L. M. (1967). Aromatic amino acids and modification of parkinsonism. *New Engl. J. Med.*, **276**, 374–9.

Critchley, M. (1949). Observations on essential (heredofamilial) tremor. *Brain*, **72**, 113–39.

Duvoisin, R. C. (1967). Cholinergic–anticholinergic antagonism in parkinsonism. *Arch. Neurol.*, **17**, 124–36.

Erb, W. (1908). Paralysis agitans (Parkinson's disease). In Church, A. (ed.) *Diseases, of the Nervous System*, D. Appleton, New York, pp. 801–98.

Fahn, S. (1972). Differential diagnosis of tremors. *Med. Clin. N. Am.*, **56**, 1363–75.

Growdon, J. H., Shahani, B. T. and Young, R. R. (1975). The effect of alcohol on essential tremor. *Neurology*, **25**, 259–62.

Jankovic, J. and Fahn, S. (1980). Physiologic and pathologic tremors. Diagnosis, mechanism, and management. *Ann. Intern. Med.*, **93**, 460–5.

Jefferson, D., Jenner, P. and Marsden, C. D. (1979). Relationship between plasma propranolol concentration and relief of essential tremor. *J. Neurol. Neurosurg. Psychiatr.*, **42**, 831–7.

Kirk, L., Baastrup, P. C. and Schou, M. (1973). Propranolol treatment of lithium-induced tremor. *Lancet*, **2**, 1086–7.

Klawans, H. L., Jr, and Weiner, W. J. (1974). Attempted use of haloperidol in the treatment of L-dopa induced dyskinesias. *J. Neurol. Neurosurg. Psychiatr.*, **37**, 427-30.

Lance, J. W., Schwab, R. S. and Peterson, E. A. (1963). Action tremor and the cogwheel phenomenon in Parkinson's disease. *Brain*, **86**, 95-110.

Larsen, T. A. and Teravainen, H. (in press). Beta-1 vs non-selective blockade in therapy of essential tremor. In Fahn, S., Calne, D. B. and Shoulson, I. (eds), *Experimental Therapeutics of Movement Disorders*, Raven Press, New York.

Lieberman, A. N. and Goldstein, M. (1982). Treatment of advanced Parkinson's disease with dopamine agonists. In Marsden, C. D. and Fahn, S. (eds), *Movement Disorders*, Butterworth Scientific, London, pp. 146-65.

McAllister, R. G., Jr, Markesbery, W. R., Ware, R. W. and Howell, S. M. (1977). Suppression of essential tremor by propranolol: correlation of effect with drug plasma levels and intensity of beta-adrenergic blockade. *Ann. Neurol.*, **1**, 160-6.

Manyam, B. V. (1981). Amantadine in essential tremor. *Ann. Neurol.*, **9**, 198-9.

Marsden, C. D., Foley, T. H., Owen, D. A. L. and McAllister, R. G. (1967). Peripheral beta-adrenergic receptors concerned with tremor. *Clin. Sci.*, **33**, 53-65.

Marsden, C. D., Gimlette, T. M., McAllister, R. G., Owen, D. A. L. and Miller, T. N. (1968). Effects of beta-adrenergic blockade on finger tremor and Achilles reflex time in anxious and thyrotoxic patients. *Acta Endocrinol.*, **57**, 353-62.

Marsden, C. D., Meadows, J. C. and Lowe, R. D. (1969). The influence of noradrenaline, tyramine and activation of sympathetic nerves on physiological tremor in man. *Clin. Sci.*, **37**, 243-52.

Marshall, J. and Schnieden, H. (1966). Effect of adrenaline, noradrenaline, atropine, and nicotine on some types of human tremor. *J. Neurol. Neurosurg. Psychiatr.*, **29**, 214-18.

Massey, E. W. and Paulson, G. (1982). Essential vocal tremor: response to therapy. *Neurology*, **32**, 113.

Newman, R. P. and Jacobs, L. (1980). Metoprolol in essential tremor. *Arch. Neurol.*, **37**, 596-7.

O'Brien, M. D., Upton, A. R. and Toseland, P. A. (1981). Benign familial tremor treated with primidone. *Br. Med. J.*, **282**, 178-80.

Owen, D. A. L. and Marsden, C. D. (1965). Effect of adrenergic beta-blockade on Parkinsonian tremor. *Lancet*, **2**, 1259-62.

Pickles, H., Perucca, E., Fish, A. and Richens, A. (1981). Propranolol and sotalol as antagonists of isoproterenol-enhanced physiologic tremor. *Clin. Pharmacol. Ther.*, **30**, 303-10.

Rajput, A. H., Jamieson, H., Hirsh, S. and Quraishi, A. (1975). Relative efficacy of alcohol and propranolol in action tremor. *Can. J. Neurol. Sci.*, **2**, 31-5.

Rascol, A., Clanet, M., Montastruc, J. L., Delage, W. and Guiraud-Chaumeil, B. (1981). L5H Tryptophan in the cerebellar syndrome treatment. *Biomedicine*, **35**, 112-13.

Sabra, A. F., Hallett, M., Sudarsky, L. and Mullally, W. (1982). Treatment of action tremor in multiple sclerosis with isoniazid. *Neurology*, **32**, A113.

Schwab, R. S. and Young, R. R. (1971). Non-resting tremor in Parkinson's disease. *Trans. Am. Neurol. Assoc.*, **96**, 305-6.

Sevitt, I. (1971). The effect of adrenergic beta-receptor blocking drugs on tremor. *Practitioner*, **207**, 677-8.

Shahani, B. T. and Young, R. R. (1976). Physiological and pharmacological aids in the differential diagnosis of tremor. *J. Neurol. Neurosurg. Psychiatr.*, **39**, 772-83.

Sorensen, P. S., Paulson, O. B., Steiness, E. and Jansen, E. K. (1981). Essential tremor treated with propranolol: lack of correlation between clinical effect and plasma propranolol levels. *Ann. Neurol.*, **9**, 53–7.

Sweet, R. D., Blumberg, J., Lee, J. E. and McDowell, F. H. (1974). Propranolol treatment of essential tremor. *Neurology*, **24**, 64–7.

Tarsy, D., Parkes, J. D. and Marsden, C. D. (1975). Metoclopramide and pimozide in Parkinson's disease and levodopa-induced dyskinesias. *J. Neurol. Neurosurg. Psychiatr.*, **38**, 331–5.

Tolosa, E. S. and Loewenson, R. B. (1975). Essential tremor: treatment with propranolol. *Neurology*, **25**, 1041–4.

Winkler, G. F. and Young, R. R. (1971). The control of essential tremor by propranolol. *Trans. Am. Neurol. Assoc.*, **96**, 66–8.

Winkler, G. F. and Young, R. R. (1974). Efficacy of chronic propranolol therapy in action tremors of the familial senile or essential varieties. *New Engl. J. Med.*, **290**, 984–8.

Young, R. R., Growdon, J. H. and Shahani, B. T. (1975). Beta-adrenergic mechanisms in action tremor. *New Engl. J. Med.*, **293**, 950–3.

Young, R. R. and Shahani, B. T. (1979). Pharmacology of tremor. *Clin. Neuropharmacol.*, **4**, 139–56.

Zilm, D. H., Sellers, E. M., MacLeod, S. M. and Degani, N. (1975). Propranolol effect on tremor in alcoholic withdrawal. *Ann. Intern. Med.*, **83**, 234.

6

Pathology of tremor

ANN MARSHALL

INTRODUCTION

Tremor is a dynamic state involving contraction and relaxation of muscles around a joint. It leaves no specific marker in the brain after death and there is as yet no 'pathology'. In some conditions, such as Parkinson's disease, the tremor is generated by structural alterations within the central nervous system; in others, such as enhanced physiological and essential tremors, such structural alterations have not been recognised. Since, as Oppenheimer (1976) states, in so-called extrapyramidal diseases 'it is still not possible to account for individual symptoms such as tremor, rigidity or athetosis in terms of normal or abnormal function of a particular nucleus', it is not possible to assess any particular structural lesion seen in the brain in terms of the contribution it made to the presence of the tremor.

There are several distinct types of tremor recognisable clinically and by electrophysiological methods (Findley and Gresty, 1981). From a pathological point of view, pathological tremors may be broadly divided into parkinsonian tremors, present at rest and abolished by movement, and postural and intention tremors which occur with muscular activity in a limb. Typical cerebellar intention tremor is a function of the profound hypotonia that is characteristic of cerebellar diseases (Dow, 1969). Lesions of the superior cerebellar peduncle and the dentate nucleus are particularly prone to produce intention-type tremor in animals (Brodal, 1981), and lesions of the upper midbrain produce a coarse postural, so-called 'rubral' tremor (Findley and Gresty, 1981) in man.

PARKINSONIAN (RESTING) TREMOR

The tremor of Parkinson's disease appears to result from impulses arising within the brain, possibly the result of a release of inhibition by interruption of intracerebral pathways (Selby, 1968). These pathways are very complex but there is a major relay station in the thalamus, the rostral part of the ventrolateral nucleus of which is shown to fire impulses in bursts, synchronous with frequency of the tremor (Nashold and Slaughter, 1969). These abnormal rhythmic bursts may be either produced locally in the thalamus or triggered from other structures. Fibres

95

from the dentate nucleus and the globus pallidus (the relay nucleus for fibres from other basal ganglia) relay in the anterior ventral nuclei of the thalamus. There are reciprocal connections between the cerebellar and the pallidal pathways (Snider and Snider, 1982). It is probable that all types of movement are influenced by cerebellar activity.

Parkinsonian tremors are relieved by stereotactic thalamotomy. Using the Marchi method to show degenerating projections, Marion Smith (1966) examined the brains of 46 patients who had undergone stereotactic thalamotomy during life; 33 of these patients had suffered from parkinsonism. She found that satisfactory results, i.e. relief of tremor in the contralateral limb and decrease in rigidity, were obtained from large or small lesions over a wide area within the globus pallidus, the internal capsule, the lateral ventricular nucleus of the thalamus as well as the field of Forel immediately ventral to it. That is, lesions that interrupted the pallidofugal fibres or dentato-rubro-thalamic fibres were effective in relieving tremor. Beck and Bignami (1968) studied the brains of 10 patients who had had stereotactic operations. It was found that the lesion also interrupted fibres projecting to the cortex from the centromedian thalamic nucleus and fibres from the cortex projecting to the red nucleus.

Anatomy and neurochemistry

Since the discovery by Ehringer and Hornykiewicz (1960) of low dopamine levels in the striatum and substantia nigra in the brains of patients with Parkinson's disease, and the later demonstration of the dopaminergic nigrostriatal tract (Andén et al., 1966), many discoveries about the neurochemical anatomy of the basal ganglia have been made and these have been described by Pearce (1979), together with the methods used. Details of modern and older established neuroanatomical methods are given by Brodal (1981).

Methods of examination

Histological examination; silver technique and Marchi methods

Many of the older neuroanatomical methods depend upon observing degenerative changes after experimental or pathological lesions of the brain. After such lesions, Wallerian degeneration in nerve fibre tracts can be shown by the Marchi method, in which degenerating myelin products appear black when impregnated with osmic acid, while retrograde and transneuronal changes can be seen in the perikarya.

Standard histological preparations of the brain have for many years included impregnation with silver to show nerve bodies and fibres. Despite their many limitations, silver methods are still widely used to demonstrate neural pathways— often in combination with other methods of examination such as electron microscopy and histochemistry.

Fluorescent visualisation

In the beautiful Falck and Hillarp method, cells and fibres are mapped in animal brains according to their monoamine content. These amines react with gaseous formaldehyde to form fluorescent isoquinolines, which can be seen microscopically. Pathways so visualised include the nigrostriatal tract and several adrenergic projections from the locus coeruleus.

Axonal transport

Nuclear projections can be demonstrated experimentally by using the phenomenon in which endogenous molecular substances are transported centrifugally along the axon to the terminal branches. Tritiated amino acids injected stereotactically are rapidly transported to terminals and can be seen autoradiographically. Exogenous substances such as horseradish peroxidase (HRP) are transported retrogradely to the perikaryon, along the axon. This method is used to determine the origin of a projection. After staining, the peroxidase can be observed by either light or electron microscopy.

Histochemical methods

Storage vesicles transport the enzymes concerned in neurotransmission, such as dopamine beta-hydroxylase (DBH) or gamma-aminobutyric acid (GABA), from the perikaryon to the nerve terminals. These enzymes can be labelled using specific antisera and the reaction products visualised by histological methods (for details see, e.g., Burns, 1978).

Biochemical analyses

Many chemical transmitters and related enzymes are fairly stable in the brain at post-mortem (Bird, 1978). This has enabled the chemical changes in many varieties of Parkinson's and other cerebral diseases to be analysed directly. In all types of parkinsonism there is a deficiency of striatal dopamine and its metabolite homovanillic acid (Hornykiewicz, 1982).

Connections of the basal ganglia

Greenfield and Bosanquet (1953) showed that degenerative changes in the substantia nigra and locus coeruleus are the hallmark of Parkinson's disease, which results in a profound decrease in the neurotransmitter dopamine (Marsden, 1982).

Dopaminergic fibres project from the substantia nigra to the neostriatum (caudate nucleus and putamen), which also receives glutaminergic efferents from the cortex, cholinergic fibres from the midline thalamic nuclei and serotonergic fibres from the raphe nuclei. Noradrenergic fibres from the locus coeruleus project widely to the cortex, limbic system and elsewhere. GABA-ergic, and some peptidergic, fibres from the neostriatum project to the globus pallidus whence efferents in the medial segment project to the ventral nuclei of the thalamus and efferents from the lateral segments are reciprocally connected with the subthalamic nucleus. GABA-ergic striatofugal fibres terminate in the substantia nigra. Through thalamic efferents the basal ganglia are connected to the motor cortex and the frontal lobes. The zona reticulata of the substantia nigra has a GABA-ergic efferent projection to the centromedian thalamic nucleus, to the reticular formation and to the superior colliculus. Dopaminergic fibres from the tegmental region of the midbrain project to the limbic system and the hypothalamus (taken from Brodal, 1981, and Marsden, 1982).

The normal functioning of the striatum depends on a proper balance between the incoming dopaminergic fibres and the intrinsic cholinergic neurones. Deficiency of dopamine or increase in cholinergic activity in the striatum produce hypokinesia, catalepsy, rigidity of the skeletal muscles and tremor (Hornykiewicz, 1982).

Causes of Parkinson's disease

> Idiopathic parkinsonism (paralysis agitans, Lewy body disease)
> Infections (post-encephalitic or encephalitic)
> Trauma
> Vascular diseases
> Drugs, poisons and toxic metabolites
> Unexplained system degeneration and multiple system atrophies
> Parkinsonism–dementia complex of Guam

Other infections and tumours are discussed in the section of 'Tremor of activity'.

Idiopathic parkinsonism

(Synonyms for this are paralysis agitans and Lewy body disease.) Idiopathic Parkinson's disease is a slowly progressive disabling common disorder of unknown cause which occurs predominantly in late-middle or old age. Tretiakoff (1919) identified inclusions in cytoplasm of nerve cell bodies in the substantia nigra which resembled those concentric hyaline inclusions described by Lewy (1912) in cells of the substantia innominata (nucleus basalis) of the hemisphere and also in the dorsal motor nucleus of the vagus in the medulla (Greenfield, 1963). Greenfield and Bosanquet (1953) examined the brains of 19 cases of (idiopathic) Parkinson's disease, 10 cases of post-encephalitic parkinsonism, five cases in which the diagnosis was uncertain and 22 controls. Lewy bodies were seen in the cytoplasm of the neurones in the substantia nigra and/or the locus coeruleus in all 19 cases of idiopathic parkinsonism. Neurofibrillary tangles, another type of primary intracytoplasmic degeneration, were found in nine out of 10 of the cases of post-encephalitic Parkinson's disease, in one of the idiopathic cases and in one atypical case (parkinsonism with amyotrophy). Lewy bodies were present in one patient aged 64 who was demented and had the typical changes of Alzheimer's disease elsewhere. Greenfield and Bosanquet concluded that the changes in the substantia nigra and locus coeruleus are responsible for the clinical features of Parkinson's disease, that the Lewy body is the characteristic finding and that Lewy bodies and neurofibrillary tangles rarely coexist in these sites. These are still the most important neuropathological, as opposed to neurobiochemical, observations about the disease, and they have been reinforced by findings of later workers such as Stadlan *et al.* (1966) and Forno and Alvord (1971).

At post-mortem, death in idiopathic parkinsonism is usually found to be due to intercurrent disease, often also closely associated with ageing, such as ischaemic cerebral or cardiac disease. The brain may show features of such intercurrent disease as well as changes of normal ageing, but in uncomplicated Parkinson's disease it is of normal or only slightly under normal weight for age. It shows no external abnormality and the grey and white matter in the cerebral hemispheres appear normal. Macroscopic and microscopic abnormalities are present in the mid-brain where the pigmented part of the substantia nigra, the dark line lying between the cerebral peduncles (figure 6.1), is obviously much paler than normal, although in idiopathic as opposed to post-encephalitic parkinsonism the normal brown colour is not usually totally lost. The medial part of the nucleus is often obviously less affected than the lateral. Elsewhere the brainstem appears normal. Microscopically there is obvious overall loss in the numbers of large cell bodies which normally lie irregularly clustered together, in a line about five cells deep, rostral to the cerebral peduncles, and which contain large golden brown granules of melanin pigment (figure 6.2). The loss of neurones is reflected in a concomitant gliosis and shrinkage of the nucleus. Melanin particles can be seen lying loose in the neuropil or within macrophages or in small groups around blood vessels. Variable numbers of surviving neurones are seen to contain the characteristic Lewy body. These are round or oval hyaline eosinophilic intracytoplasmic inclusion bodies. They are from 5 to 25 μm in diameter and have a pale outer zone and a strongly acidophilic core which stains a deep red with many dyes such as Masson's trichrome. These inclusions lie among the melanin granules, which tend to surround them unevenly, or in non-pigmented perikarya. The smaller forms are sometimes multiple. They are non-laminar, argyrophilic, non-birefringent, non-congophilic and do not react with stains for iron or fat. They are PAS (periodic acid Schiff reagent) negative (Greenfield and Bosanquet, 1953). Ultrastructurally a typical Lewy body has an electron-dense amorphous central core surrounded by radiating filaments, giving them sunflower-like appearance (Duffy and Tennyson, 1965).

Changes have been described in the cerebral and cerebellar cortex, the dentate nucleus and deep grey matter. They include neuronal loss, lipofuchsin accumulation and senile plaques in the cortex. They are probably non-specific and associated with ageing (Greenfield, 1963).

Lewy bodies are seen in idiopathic parkinsonism, regularly in the substantia

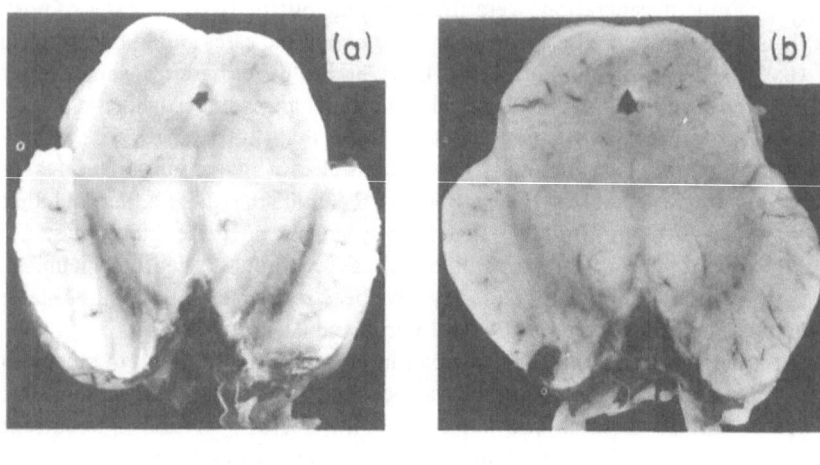

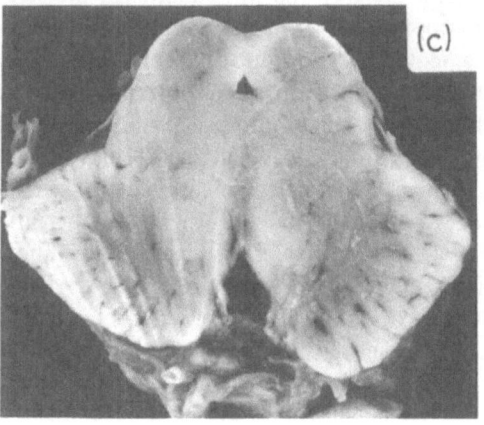

Figure 6.1 The midbrain in Parkinson's disease. (a) The normal appearance. (b) Idiopathic Parkinson's disease—the substantia nigra on both sides is paler than normal. (c) Post-encephalitic Parkinson's disease—pigment has disappeared from the substantia nigra which is grey and shrunken, due to gliosis.

nigra and locus coeruleus but also in other pigmented and some non-pigmented nuclei—commonly in the substantia innominata, the dorsal motor nucleus of the vagus, the hypothalamus, the raphe nuclei of the midbrain and the rostral pons, and the sympathetic ganglia; rarely in the cerebral cortex, the neostriatum, the globus pallidus, the pontine nuclei and the inferior olives. They are never seen in the cerebellum (Forno, 1982). According to Forno and Alvord (1971) 'the only melanin containing cells known not to contain Lewy bodies in idiopathic Parkin-

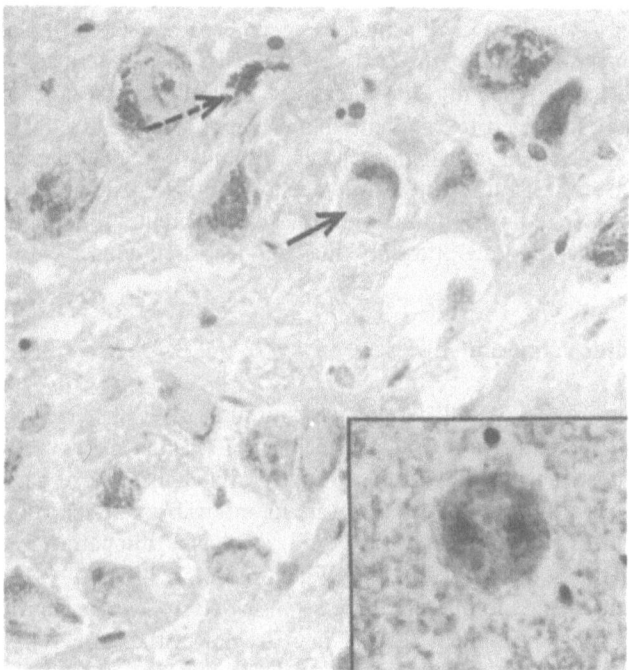

Figure 6.2 Lewy bodies. A Lewy body (arrowed) is seen lying eccentrically within a pigmented nerve cell body. Melanin granules lie to one side. Loose melanin granules (broken arrow) lie in the neuropil. *Inset*: A perikaryon containing multiple smaller Lewy bodies of varying shape. (Haematoxylin and eosin × 330.)

sonism are the primary sensory neurones of the dorsal root ganglia'. Lewy bodies are composed of cytoplasmic protein and sphingomyelin (Forno and Alvord, 1971). They may be situated in the perikarya or in the cell processes, especially the dendrites, the 'intraneuritic Lewy bodies'. They apparently reflect the actual nerve cell loss due to the disease and this loss is reflected in the loss of neurotransmitter substances in affected pathways (Forno, 1982).

The degree of dopamine depletion in the corpus striatum parallels the severity of the parkinsonism. For parkinsonism to appear 80% of the striatal dopamine must be lost—until then compensation takes place presynaptically by the dopaminergic neurones in the substantia nigra increasing their activity and postsynaptically by an increase in the number of dopamine receptors in the striatum (Marsden, 1982). The application of immunohistochemical techniques and silver impregnation methods to electron microscopy of human material has produced evidence of a compensatory increase in synaptic vesicles in the nerve terminals (Forno, 1982). Dopamine deficiency has also been demonstrated in the cortex, the limbic system and the hypothalamus. Other biochemical changes include a decrease in noradrenaline in the nucleus accumbens and in the hypothalamus, reflecting damage to part of the pathway from the locus coeruleus, a decrease in GABA-ergic activity in the substantia nigra as well as decrease in cholinergic activity in the frontal cortex and the hippocampus (Marsden, 1982). There has been some discussion about whether globus pallidus shows abnormalities in idiopathic parkinsonism, but quantitative measurements (Pakkenberg, 1963) have failed to demonstrate any abnormalities of size or content although the neuronal cytoplasm may be abnormal, possibly due to a decreased concentration of RNA.

Post-encephalitic Parkinson's disease

Although some patients still develop parkinsonism after an encephalitic illness (Rail *et al.*, 1981) and although it has been suggested that many cases of parkinsonism are post-encephalitic, most observers think that most cases of post-encephalitic parkinsonism followed at varying intervals an attack of encephalitis lethargica contracted during the 1918–28 epidemic. Idiopathic parkinsonism (Parkinson's disease) is an entirely different nosological entity (Yahr, 1981). Post-encephalitic and idiopathic parkinsonism differ clinically; rigidity, for example, is a more prominent feature than tremor in the former and there is a much greater association of other neurological damage and psychiatric disorders. Pathologically the lesions in post-encephalitic parkinsonism are much more widespread, with much more obvious shrinkage and pallor of the substantia nigra. Approximately a quarter of the infected patients died during the acute attack of encephalitis lethargica. In these cases the brainstem bore the brunt of the acute inflammatory changes. They were also seen in the deep grey matter, the cortex, the spinal cord and the white matter of the hemisphere. Microscopically there was dense perivascular lymphocytic inflammatory cuffing and focal mononuclear infiltration, leading, in longer surviving cases, to neuronal loss and gliosis that was particularly dense in the brainstem (McMenemy, 1966). The acute changes were seen in the brain for a considerable time, to be replaced, in those patients who developed post-encephalitic parkinsonism, by widespread evidence of damage in the form of glial scars and nerve cell loss, accompanied, in many surviving neurones, by a primary cytoplasmic degeneration—neurofibrillary tangles. This change is most severe in the midbrain, diffusely, but especially in the substantia nigra and in the locus coeruleus. So extensive may the damage be that sometimes no surviving neurones are seen at all. Greenfield and Bosanquet (1953) found neurofibrillary tangles in the substantia nigra and/or locus coeruleus in nine out of 10 of their cases of post-encephalitic parkinsonism, and neurofibrillary tangles have since been described in the substantia nigra, locus coeruleus, the brainstem reticular nuclei, the periaqueductal region, the dentate nucleus, the subthalamic nucleus, throughout the basal ganglia, in the hypothalamus and in the cortex (Blackwood, 1981). Rail *et al.* (1981) found tangles in the brainstem, dentate nuclei and corpus striatum in their two cases whose brains were examined, one of which also showed tangles, without senile plaques, in the cortex.

Trauma

Repeated hard blows to the head may cause the 'punch drunk syndrome' well known in boxers. This is a progressive disease in which there is dementia and other neurological disorders, frequently including parkinsonian rigidity and sometimes tremor. The neuropathology was fully investigated and described by Corsellis *et al.* (1973). They found changes suggestive of damage to midline structures in the brain throughout its extent, probably as a result of tearing and rotational forces as well as of a sudden rise in intraventricular pressure. Microscopically there was neuronal loss mainly in the midline structures, including frontal and temporal lobes, cerebellum and substantia nigra, which was pale. Many surviving neurones contained neurofibrillary tangles; neither senile plaques nor Lewy bodies were seen.

Cerebrovascular disease

The substantia nigra, red nucleus and related structures are supplied by the posterior cerebral artery. Vascular disease in this territory may produce a coarse postural tremor, 'rubral tremor'.

The term 'arteriosclerotic parkinsonism' has been applied to vascular disease affecting the corpus striatum and thalamus (Critchley, 1929). The striatum is supplied by striate branches of the anterior and middle cerebral arteries and the anterior choroidal artery. Strokes resulting from thromboembolism of diseased arteries in their territories may give rise to parkinsonian rigidity but rarely to tremor (Critchley, 1981) (figure 6.3).

Small infarcts and organising haemorrhages, visible to the naked eye as cystic softenings, are a common finding at post-mortem especially in the outer part of the putamen where they are usually symptomless. More medially they may give rise to symptoms. Microscopically there is necrosis, cavitation and reactive gliosis around or near a diseased, thickened, hyalinised, often calcified blood vessel. These lesions contain lipid-laden or iron-pigment-containing macrophages resulting from phagocytosis of dead tissue or from old organising haemorrhages.

Arteriosclerotic degeneration, often associated with hypertension, and with superimposed thromboembolism, is by far the commonest but not the only cause of this type of vascular disease (see below).

Striatonigral degeneration and multisystem atrophy

Parkinsonian syndromes can occur, alone or in combination with other neurological disturbances, in specific conditions in which there are degenerations of nuclei or groups of nerve cells and their projections. These diseases may be hereditary or isolated, and the underlying biochemical defects are unknown (Weller *et al.*, 1982).

Striatonigral degenerations may occur alone, in olivo-ponto-cerebellar atrophy or as part of a combination of lesions in the Shy–Drager syndrome, progressive

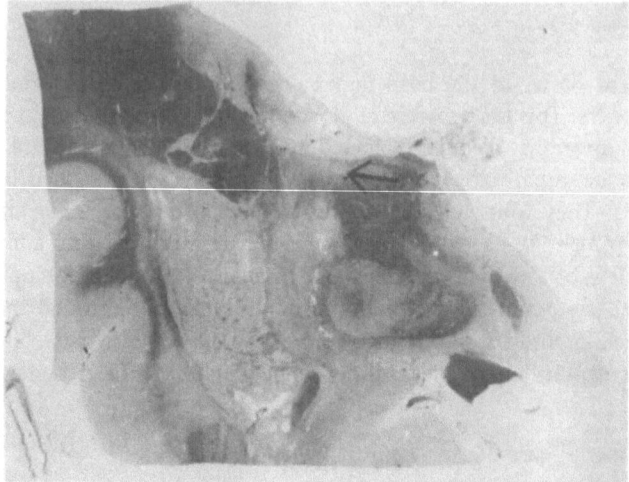

Figure 6.3 Infarcts in the basal ganglia. Multiple old infarcts, seen as irregular pale areas in the caudate nucleus, putamen and globus pallidus. The adjacent internal capsule is also involved (arrow). The patient was a 63-year-old man who had suffered from parkinsonian rigidity but no tremor. (Luxol fast blue and Nissl × 2.2.)

autonomic failure with parkinsonism. The term 'multiple system atrophy' usefully covers such combinations (see Bannister and Oppenheimer, 1982). Atrophy of the affected system is seen in the brain and shrinkage and discoloration of the area with neuronal loss and reactive gliosis (Spokes *et al.*, 1979).

Striatonigral degeneration is a true supranigral form of parkinsonism in which there is degeneration of the putamen. Rigidity predominates and tremor may not be seen. Lewy bodies are not a feature. There is a loss of nerve cells in and gliosis of the putamen, which is shrunken (Adams, 1968). Borit *et al.* (1975) found in it an accumulation of neuromelanin, among other breakdown pigments. In their three cases the substantia nigra was normal or only slightly abnormal.

Olivo-ponto-cerebellar atrophy

In olivo-ponto-cerebellar atrophy there is shrinkage of the ventral pons, of the inferior olives, usually obvious to the naked eye, and of the middle cerebellar peduncle with diffuse loss of Purkinje cells, mainly from the lateral lobes of the cerebellum with gliosis replacing neurones in the dentate nucleus (Oppenheimer, 1976). Tremor at rest is characteristic of the disease (Weller *et al.*, 1982).

Shy–Drager syndrome

In some cases of parkinsonism, tremor and rigidity are accompanied by postural hypotension and other signs of autonomic failure such as loss of sphincter tone and loss of sweating. Such patients are said to have the Shy–Drager syndrome, although, as Bannister and Oppenheimer (1982) point out, the syndrome actually consists of 'progressive autonomic failure and a variety of neurological disturbances'. Parkinsonism is by far the commonest of those. Pathologically there may be Lewy body degeneration or striatonigral degeneration, either alone or as part of a multisystem atrophy, combined with a loss of preganglionic sympathetic cells in the spinal cord.

Parkinsonism–dementia complex of Guam

One of the races which inhabit the western Pacific island of Guam, the Chamarro Indians, show a most unusual incidence both of motor neurone disease (amyotrophic lateral sclerosis, ALS) and of a fatal neurological condition in which there is severe progressive dementia and parkinsonism. In a significant number of cases ALS and parkinsonism-dementia complex coexist. The cause of both conditions is unknown. The disease, usually of the fifth and sixth decade, accounts for 7% of deaths on Guam. Two-thirds of the cases have parkinsonism and dementia only, half the rest also have signs of upper motor neurone involvement, and the other half typical amyotrophic lateral sclerosis. Akinesia is a striking feature of the parkinsonism but in 32 of the 47 cases originally reported by Hirano *et al.* (1961a), who described the clinical features, tremor was present, although sometimes not typically a resting tremor and involving only part of the limb.

The pathological features were described by Hirano *et al.* (1961b) in a companion paper. The brains of 17 patients were examined. They were small with bilateral atrophy of the globus pallidus, the frontal and temporal regions and the substantia nigra. Microscopically there was widespread neuronal loss in the affected regions with many neurofibrillary tangles in the surviving neuronal cytoplasm. Other types of degeneration typically seen in Alzheimer's disease were also present: granulovacuolar degeneration; oval intracytoplasmic granules 1-5 μm across, with a central argyrophilic core, lying in the cytoplasm of the cell bodies in the hippocampus; and Hirano bodies (rod-like hyaline cytoplasmic inclusions). There were no senile plaques. The worst affected regions were the medial temporal cortex, the substantia nigra and the hypothalamus. Severely involved also were the frontal and anterior temporal cortex, the periaqueductal and tectal regions. Changes were also seen in the amygdala, the globus pallidus, thalamus, reticular formation, cranial nerve nuclei, olfactory bulb and spinal cord grey matter. The cerebellum and visual cortex were not involved.

The diagnosis, nature and significance of cytoplasmic inclusions in parkinsonism

Lewy bodies are characteristic but not pathognomonic of idiopathic parkinsonism. They are found in about 5% of routine autopsies, usually in elderly patients, and in conditions unrelated to parkinsonism (Lipkin, 1959). Autopsies may fail to show either Lewy bodies or tangles in patients with parkinsonism (Alvord *et al.*,

1974). By light microscopy Lewy bodies somewhat resemble corpora amylacea, but these are basophilic and strongly PAS positive, and Pick's bodies which are non-laminar and found in the cortex. Ultrastructurally, Pick's bodies consist of compact aggregates of neurofibrillary and neurotubular material (Wisniewski *et al.*, 1972). Lewy bodies have a dense central core of granular material surrounded by radiating peripheral fibrils or one formed entirely of fibrils (Roy and Wolman, 1969).

Neurofibrillary tangles are a manifestation of nerve cell degeneration seen in many organic brain diseases, such as Alzheimer's disease and senile dementia, post-encephalitic parkinsonism, parkinsonism–dementia complex, boxer's brains, Down's syndrome, motor neurone disease and progressive supranuclear palsy; in the latter there is parkinsonian rigidity, but no tremor (see Behrman *et al.*, 1969). They occur to a limited extent in normal ageing. Tangles are seen by light micro-scopy as a thickening and tortuosity of fibrils within the neuronal cytoplasm, and, as they grow, they displace the nucleus to one side. They stain with silver and with congo red dye. Their shapes vary, depending on the shape of the cells in which they arise (Janota, 1981). Elongated triangular 'flame-shaped' forms are seen in cortical pyramidal cells, and oval 'globose' forms in the brainstem (figure 6.4). Ultrastructurally they are not all the same (see, for example, Iqbal *et al.*, 1977). In post-encephalitic parkinsonism tangles resembling those seen in Alzheimer's disease have been described. These are paired helical filaments, with a periodicity of about 80 nm, from 20 to 10 nm wide, which have a tubular appearance on cross-section (Wisniewski *et al.*, 1970) (figure 6.5). Wisniewski *et al.*

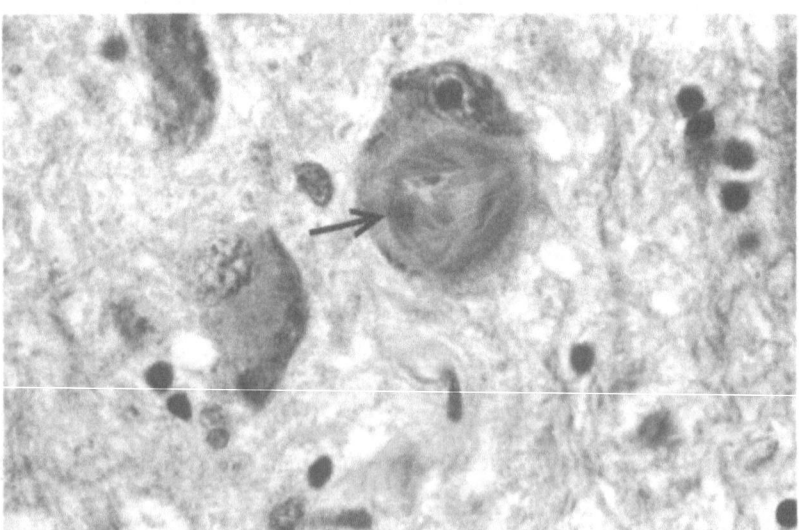

Figure 6.4 Neurofibrillary tangle in post-encephalitic Parkinson's disease. A nerve cell body in which the cytoplasm is distended with abnormal twisted filaments. (Haematoxylin and eosin × 780.)

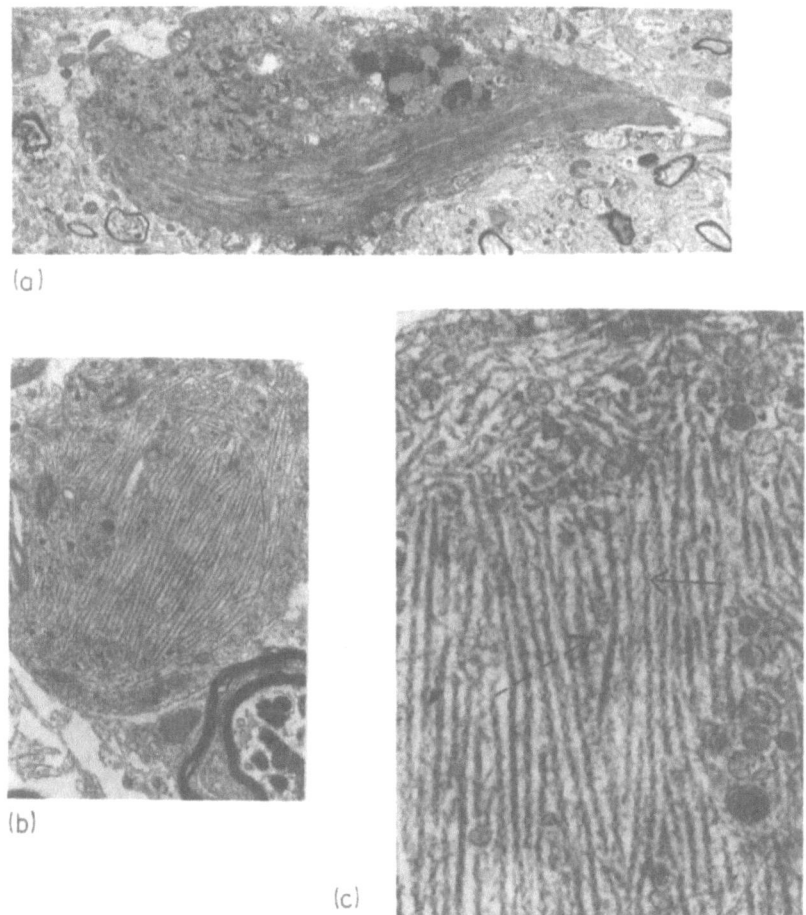

(a)

(b)

(c)

Figure 6.5 Neurofibrillary tangle—ultrastructure. (a) A neurofibrillary tangle in Alzheimer's disease showing displacement of the nucleus and intracytoplasmic organelles. (Longitudinal section × 3500.) (b) A neurofibrillary tangle showing paired helical filaments. (Transverse section × 1050.) (c) A neurofibrillary tangle: longitudinal section (arrow) showing paired helical filaments and cross-section (broken arrow) showing their tubular appearance. (× 30 420.) (By courtesy of Dr L. H. Carrasco.)

(1970) found tangles of this sort in the locus coeruleus in a brain from a patient with post-encephalitic parkinsonism, which had been preserved in formalin for five years before being processed for electron microscopy. Ishii and Nakamura (1981) examined the brains of four patients with post-encephalitic parkinsonism. Electron microscopy of the most affected regions, brainstem, hypothalamus and Ammon's horn, showed Alzheimer-like twisted tubules in all four, but, in three, straight tubules were also seen resembling those described in progressive supranuclear palsy and other conditions (Powell *et al.*, 1974).

About a third of patients with idiopathic Parkinson's disease develop dementia (Marsden, 1982). The incidence of Alzheimer-type neurofibrillary tangles, senile plaques and other cortical changes of Alzheimer's disease is increased compared to controls (Alvord *et al.*, 1974) but it is often not possible to find morphological evidence of a 'dementing' disease in such cases. There may, however, be degeneration of cholinergic pathways as shown by a decrease in choline acetyl transferase in the cortex (Rossor, 1982). In Alzheimer's disease there is degeneration of cholinergic pathways (Perry *et al.*, 1978). Tangles are not uncommonly found in the brainstem in Alzheimer's disease without parkinsonism (Corsellis, 1976). Lewy bodies are very occasionally found in the cortex. Okazaki *et al.* (1961) described two cases of dementia without parkinsonism in which, on light microscopy, Lewy bodies were identified in the cortex and in 'various levels in the nervous system'. Dementia had been present in the cases of Kosoka (1978) and in that of Yagishita *et al.* (1980) in which, in a 59-year-old woman, features of Alzheimer's disease, neurofibrillary tangles, senile plaques, granulovacuolar degeneration and Hirano bodies were also present. Ikeda *et al.* (1978) have described cortical Lewy bodies in a 35-year-old man with clinical and pathological Parkinson's disease but without dementia. There were some histochemical and ultrastructural differences between the cortical and brainstem inclusions.

Although usually, either one or the other inclusion is seen, Lewy bodies and tangles may coexist in parkinsonism, as was found in 21% of the cases studied by Alvord *et al.* (1974). According to Alvord (1968) incidence of Lewy bodies increases with increasing age in patients with post-encephalitic parkinsonism and Forno and Alvord (1971) found 'a statistically defined pattern' in which the loss of nerve cells and accumulation of Lewy bodies was directly proportional to the severity of parkinsonism.

There is therefore some histological support for the idea that Lewy bodies increase as dopamine levels decrease and that non-parkinsonian patients with Lewy bodies have a presymptomatic form of the disease (Marsden, 1982). However, it is not yet certain what Lewy bodies are nor what eventually happens to cells which contain them.

TREMOR OF ACTIVITY

Tremor may occur in lesions of the cerebellum or its projections. Such a tremor depends on the limb being held in position and is not present at rest. Cerebellar and brainstem pathways are intimately and intricately connected. Cerebellar efferents relay in the ventrolateral nucleus of the thalamus, having passed through the field of Forel to it where they lie close to the pallidal outflow. The nucleus projects to the motor cortex.

A coarse postural tremor is now considered typical of lesions in the red nucleus and superior cerebellar peduncle (Andrew *et al.*, 1982) and was first described by

Holmes (1904) particularly in lesions in the upper brainstem in the region of the red nucleus and superior cerebellar peduncle. In two cases autopsies were done and showed tumours. These had destroyed or largely destroyed the midbrain and structures extending from the rostral part of the fourth ventrical to the posterior thalamus and medial temporal region; one by direct extension, the other by compression.

In monkeys, lesions of the cerebellar hemisphere typically produce ipsilateral reflex and postural disturbances which are the result of profound hypotonia and these disturbances include an intention tremor. Ablation of the cerebellar hemispheres produces hypotonia with clumsiness and asynergia, and if the dentate nucleus or its projection in the superior cerebellar peduncles are also damaged these features are exacerbated and accompanied by intention tremor (Dow, 1969). It is said that intention tremor particularly occurs in man in disease of the cerebellum when the roof nuclei and the superior cerebellar peduncles and brainstem connections are involved (Findley and Gresty, 1981). Pathological examinations do not always support this assertion in man, but well-documented lesions in some patients have been shown to produce a 3 Hz tremor (F. Afshar, 1983, personal communication; Cooper, 1977).

Anatomy and neurochemistry

The anatomy of the cerebellum and its projections is described by Brodal (1981). Vestibular and spinal fibres project directly to the cerebellum or relay in the vestibular nuclei and inferior olive respectively; the fibres pass in the inferior cerebellar peduncle. Vestibular fibres terminate in the phylogenetically older vermis and flocculonodular lobe. Impulses from the limbs, with projections from the red nucleus, the superior colliculus, the cortex, and the contralateral cerebellum, relay in the inferior olive and to the cerebellar cortex as climbing fibres in the contralateral cerebellar peduncle. Corticopontine fibres, with tectopontine and cerebellar pontine, relay in the basal pontine nuclei and pass in the, mainly contralateral, middle cerebellar peduncle to the lateral parts of the cerebellar hemispheres (the neocerebellum). Other projections include those from the reticular nuclei which pass in the superior cerebellar peduncle as a ventral cross-descending tract. Most cerebellar fibres are GABA-ergic (Krnjevic, 1982). There is a projection of noradrenergic fibres from the locus coeruleus in the pons, which so often shows cytoplasmic degeneration in Parkinson's disease and other conditions, and serotonergic fibres from the raphe nuclei (Palay, 1982). There are reciprocal connections between the monoamine systems of the cerebellum and basal ganglia (Snider and Snider, 1982).

Cerebellar efferents are the axons of Purkinje cells which relay in the cerebellar nuclei, of which the nucleus lateralis or dentate nucleus in man is by far the largest. Efferents from the nuclei pass in the superior cerebellar peduncles, cross in the midbrain and pass through the red nucleus to the ventrolateral nucleus of the thalamus or pass to the inferior olive, the pontine or anterior nuclei, to elsewhere in the cerebellar cortex or to the oculomotor nuclei. It is apparent that lesions in man in the upper midbrain and in the region of the red nucleus will probably involve cerebellar efferent pathways as well as the nigrostriatal tract and reciprocal connections between the substantia nigra and the striatum.

Causes of tremor of activity

    Cerebellar and vascular diseases
    Hereditary system degeneration
    Trauma
    Infections
    Tumours
    Poisons and toxic metabolites
    Liver failure
    Huntington's chorea

Cerebellar diseases

Diseases of the cerebellar hemispheres, nuclei and connections may cause cerebellar signs and symptoms, including tremor, but localisation is poor and such symptoms and signs are not specific to the cerebellum and its connections for a number of well known reasons, including the fact that lesions seldom involve only one area. Other areas and connections may be affected by pressure or circulatory disturbance, factors which are of particular importance in the posterior fossa. An additional modifying feature is the degree of compensation of which the cerebellum is capable (Brodal, 1981).

Multiple sclerosis

The most important cause of typical cerebellar intention tremor is multiple sclerosis, the cause of which is still unknown. The wide variety of the clinical disease reflects the multiplicity of the lesions and their variation in size and distribution. The pathological appearance of a typical case is unmistakable, the significance of the various microscopical changes is obscure and the aetiology of the disease is uncertain; neither do we know which lesions produce the tremor. Allen (1981) has discussed the present state of pathological knowledge.

    The clinical disease is the result of focal destruction of central nervous system myelin. There is some evidence that changes such as increased lysosomal atrophy in the white matter precede the myelin breakdown (Cuzner, 1980). Established plaques are typically irregular, well demarcated grey areas with a firm texture and of irregular size and shape, and they are very widely scattered throughout the brain, although some particular sites such as the ventricular angle are much more commonly affected than others. The tendency for watershed areas to be affected has been noted (Brownell and Hughes, 1962).

Pathological interest has centred on the 'early lesions and the edges of plaques' (Oppenheimer, 1976). The changes which precede myelin breakdown are unknown. Reported changes include the presence of populations of T and B lymphocytes as well as increased concentration of IgG in the cerebrospinal fluid (Cuzner, 1980). As the breakdown progresses swelling and fragmentation appear, free stainable lipid accumulates and is taken up by macrophages. There is reactive gliosis, both in the plaques and diffusely in the white matter (Allen and McKeown, 1979) and an infiltration of microglial cells. A mononuclear inflammatory infiltrate consisting of lipid macrophages and lymphocytes, including immunologically competent cells, is present around the adjacent blood vessels. Lysosomal enzymes are increased in established plaques. In an established plaque myelin is absent (figure 6.6) and there is dense fibrous gliosis. The lesions lie around or near a blood vessel. Oligodendrocytes are not seen but there is perivascular lymphocytic cuffing around the area. The axons, though they may show abnormalities, are relatively preserved in the early stages but later disintegrate.

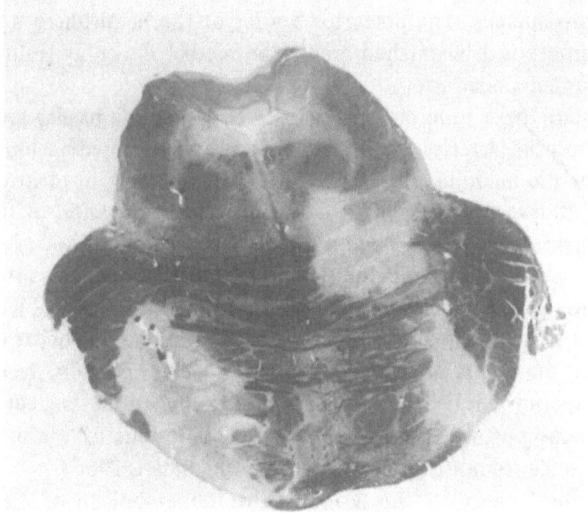

Figure 6.6 Multiple sclerosis. A long-standing case showing areas of demyelination in the pons. (Luxol fast blue and Nissl × 2.3.)

The aetiology of these changes is much debated. Possibilities include auto-immune reaction, reaction to abnormal myelin, virus infection or a combination of a viral and allergic response. There is some evidence that the function of T cells is impaired and this impairment might alter the lymphocytic response to many different agents (Cuzner, 1980).

Vascular diseases

The arterial supply to the midbrain, brainstem and cerebellum depends on the vertebrobasilar system. The vertebral arteries are very vulnerable to disease outside the brain. Occlusions and compression of the vertebral arteries in the neck, particularly within the vertebral canal, can and frequently do cause infarction in the brainstem and cerebellum at some distance from the actual obstruction (Yates, 1976).

Midbrain structures, the posterior two-thirds of the cerebral peduncles, the substantia nigra, the superior cerebellar peduncle (also supplied by the superior cerebellar artery) and the red nucleus are supplied by the posterior cerebral artery which also supplies the visual cortex and is vulnerable to compression against the edge of the tentorium as well as to atherosclerotic and thrombotic occlusion. The middle and inferior cerebellar peduncles are supplied by the anterior inferior cerebellar artery, as is the adjacent tegmentum, the more caudal parts of which are supplied by the posterior inferior cerebellar artery and the more rostral by the superior cerebellar artery. The cerebellar hemispheres are supplied by the superior cerebellar artery superiorly and the posterior inferior cerebellar artery posteriorly, as is the dentate nucleus. The posterior border of the hemisphere where the two systems anastamose is a 'watershed area'. The medial flocculus is supplied by the anterior inferior cerebellar artery.

In addition to these long circumferential branches the basilar artery supplies short circumferential arteries to the cerebellum and paramedian branches to the ventral parts of the medulla and pons. Both are vulnerable in obstructive disease of the basilar and vertebral arteries. Occlusion or compression of the supplying artery or of a vessel feeding it from a distance causes infarction of the territory of supply. These are common in the posterior inferior cerebellar artery territory in which unilateral cerebellar signs are associated with signs of involvement of the medulla (Papworth, 1971). They are also common in the cerebellar hemispheres, at the base of the pons, and in the posterior cerebral artery territory which includes the superior cerebellar peduncles, and produce ipsilateral cerebellar signs, including a coarse postural tremor. Such vascular lesions of the brainstem elsewhere may produce tremor or rigidity of both (Harriman, 1966).

The commonest cause of the lesion is thromboembolism of diseased—often atheromatous—cerebral arteries. In atheroma the diseased artery shows eccentric intimal fibrosis and subintimal lipid accumulation, with duplication of the elastic lamina and degeneration of the media. Other arterial disorders include: endarteritis obliterans, a feature of most bacterial infections, in which there is perivascular inflammation and concentric intimal thickening; other primary inflammatory conditions such as polyarteritis nodosa, in which there is medial necrosis and inflammatory infiltration; giant cell and granulomatous arteritis (Nurick et al., 1972) and disseminated lupus erythematosis, in which there is either inflammatory necrosis of the media and elastica as in polyarteritis nodosa, or a bland endarteritis with preserved elastica (Urich, 1976).

The arterial obstruction may also be embolic in the form of blood clots from the heart, fragments of fat from fractures, nitrogen (in caisson disease), air emboli and atheromatous detachments. External compression of vessels is especially common in the posterior fossa often as a result of downward herniation of supratentorial structures in the presence of space-occupying lesions of the hemispheres.

Hereditary system degeneration

Friedreich's ataxia is the commonest, autosomal dominant, form of hereditary spinocerebellar degeneration of which several types exist (Weller *et al.*, 1982). Oppenheimer (1976) has described the pathology of various primary degenerations, including 15 personally observed cases of Friedreich's ataxia. Primary cortical cerebellar degeneration (Holmes type) is very much rarer.

In Friedreich's ataxia and similar conditions there is degeneration of the peripheral and central spinal sensory pathways of the spinocerebellar tracts and their nuclei, and of corticospinal fibres—the more distal parts of the latter being more affected ('dying back' phenomenon). Other variable changes seen in the brain in Friedreich's ataxia include degeneration of (sensory) cranial nerves, and cell loss in the dentate, in the vestibular and the cochlear nuclei.

Acquired spinocerebellar degenerations

These may accompany degenerations of the posterior and lateral columns in acquired myelopathies, such as vitamin deficiency (Smith, 1976).

Trauma

Some concussive blows cause, in addition to local deformation and damage, lesions in long tracts of white matter including the superior cerebellar peduncles, due to either shearing stresses from rotation of the brain (Strich, 1961) or vascular compression (Adams, 1975). In surviving patients such damage may give rise to a coarse postural tremor, like that described by Holmes (1904). This tremor was seen clinically in three out of nine cases of midbrain injury by Kremer *et al.* (1947).

Infections

A host of pathogenic and opportunistic organisms can seriously damage the brain, which 'offers less resistance to infection than any other tissue' (Greenfield, 1963). Tremor may be produced in a variety of ways by which the relevant parts of the brain, basal ganglia, midbrain and cerebellum, may be damaged.

Infectious organisms and the inflammation they excite may directly damage and destroy relevant parts of the brain. The very marked midbrain damage in encephalitis lethargica is a well known example. Virus infections in general tend to damage certain parts of the brain preferentially (see Adams, 1976).

Space-occupying lesions such as abscesses and granulomas cause direct destruction and also swelling. The latter is due to inflammatory and vasogenic oedema, enhanced by the involvement of blood vessels in the inflammatory process (Klatzo, 1979). Infarction in the territories of large arteries may follow swelling and herniation of the cerebral hemispheres. Midbrain structures are vulnerable in the posterior cerebral artery compression that accompanies supratentorial lesions such as temporal lobe abscess.

All forms of inflammation are associated with venous thrombosis and with endarteritis obliterans. The latter is especially marked in chronic granulomatous infection such as meningovascular syphilis or tuberculous meningitis. In tuberculosis the inflammation involves the meningeal and the basal arteries characteristically producing multiple infarction. Tremor may follow involvement of the penetrating arteries at the base of the brain which supply the basal ganglia (Greenfield, 1963).

Some special types of infection of the CNS

The brain is vulnerable to opportunistic infection. Progressive multifocal leucoencephalopathy is an interesting viral example. The disease occurs in immunologically compromised patients, particularly with lymphomas, and produces mental disturbance, alteration of consciousness and focal lesions with brainstem and cerebellar disturbance. There is striking and widespread focal demyelination, and ultrastructurally, virus particles are seen in the abnormal oligodendroglial nuclei (Henson and Urich, 1982).

Neither these nor any other features of inflammation are seen in slow virus infection. Slow viruses are filterable transmissible agents which cause fatal spongiform encephalopathies including the human diseases of Kuru and Creutzfeldt-Jakob disease.

Kuru was a disease of the Fore tribe in New Guinea caused by eating infected humans (Matthews *et al.*, 1968). The disease consisted of gross progressive cerebellar tremor and ataxia. Pathologically (Beck *et al.*, 1970) there was severe loss of and degeneration in cerebellar neurones, congophilic plaque formation and dense gliosis with spongiform degeneration elsewhere in the cortical grey matter and deep grey matter.

Creutzfeldt–Jakob disease is a disease of late-middle and old age in which progressive dementia is accompanied by many other neurological disorders, including gross disturbance of movement and tone. The disease affects the cortex widely, as well as the deep grey matter, the brainstem, cerebellum and spinal cord (Daniel, 1972).

In spongiform degeneration there is loss of cortical nerve cells, intense proliferin the grey matter which contains many closely packed microcysts (Adams *et al.*, 1974). The cysts lie in the processes of astrocytes and neurones (Lampert *et al.*, 1969).

Tumours

Tumours of all types may produce tremors depending on their locality. Parkinsonian tremor may also occur in the presence of massive frontal lobe tumours which are not in contact with the basal ganglia (see Northfield, 1973). Non-metastatic neurological syndromes which occur in association with cancer, such as brainstem encephalomyelitis or cerebellar degeneration, may also be associated with tremor (see Henson and Urich, 1982).

Poisons and toxic metabolites

Drugs such as phenytoin probably damage the cerebellar cortical neurones directly (Reynolds, 1968), as do some metals and organic compounds. Alcohol may also directly and selectively damage cerebellar cortical neurones (Smith, 1976), but there is evidence that alcoholic cerebellar damage is primarily nutritional (Adams, 1968). There is atrophy particularly of the medial part of the cerebellum, and cerebellar cortical damage is seen as a loss of Purkinje rather than the granule cells. This is seen in many other cerebellar degenerations, mercury poisoning being an interesting exception.

Inorganic mercury produces in man a typical coarse tremor (hatters' shakes'), and disturbance of higher cerebral function–'erythism'–(Hunter, 1975). Mercurous chloride (a very poisonous insoluble form) causes a peripheral neuropathy in infants with 'pink disease'. Organic mercury compounds produce a sensory peripheral neuropathy, with cerebellar, basal ganglia and cortical signs. Experimentally methyl mercury poisoning causes a loss of small neurones in the cerebral and cerebellar cortex where there is atrophy of the granular layer with preservation of Purkinje cells (Cavanagh, 1979). Cavanagh and his colleagues consider that organic mercury poisoning is more rapid and more destructive but essentially the same as inorganic. Ultrastructurally both show damage to ribosomes and rough endoplasmic reticulum in cell bodies–this damage being probably proportionally greater in the small granule than the large Purkinje cells.

Other diseases of the basal ganglia

(See also Vascular disease and Infections (above).) There appears to be no absolute distinction between abnormal movements and tremor in some diseases of the basal ganglia. In Wilson's disease the one appears to merge with the other (Martin, 1968). In manganese poisoning the one is described in man, the other is apparent in monkeys (Pentschew, 1966). Chorea and a choreoathetosis are typical of Huntington's chorea, but, with advancing disability, dystonia and parkinsonism are observed more frequently (Shoulson, 1982).

Liver failure

The clinical and biochemical disorders in hepatic encephalopathy have been described by Sherlock (1977). Liver cell failure and portal systemic shunting cause retention of nitrogenous substances in the blood and abnormally high concentrations of ammonia, amines and aromatic amino acids reach the brain. Also, in acute liver cell failure, the blood–brain barrier is breached (Potvin *et al.*, 1976), and there is cerebral oedema. In addition to the classical flapping tremor, which is also seen in uraemia and hypercapnia, the neuropsychiatric disorders in chronic hepatocellular failure may include parkinsonism, cerebellar disturbance and features of Wilson's disease.

In patients with chronic hepatic failure and portal systemic encephalopathy, macroscopic cerebral damage seen as a linear, patchy, spongy degeneration of the cortex and superficial white matter, the basal ganglia, cerebellum and brainstem has been described by Adams (1968). The sponginess appears to be due to vacuolation in the astrocytic cytoplasm (Plum and Hindfelt, 1976). However, in most patients who die with hepatocerebral failure the brain is macroscopically normal and light microscopy shows little or no damage to neurones. The abnormalities are confined to the astrocytes. Their nuclei are abnormally swollen and indented, with prominent nucleoli. These are Alzheimer's type II astrocytes; they are most obvious in the basal ganglia, the dentate nucleus, the inner layers of the cortex and the anterior horn cells in the spinal cord. They are non-specific, occurring in all forms of liver disease and states of hyperammonaemia, being the result of increased metabolic activity in the presence of high circulating ammonia levels (Cavanagh and Kyu, 1971, 63–75; Cavanagh, 1972).

Unlike acquired hepatocellular failure, in Wilson's disease (hereditary hepatolenticular degeneration) there is neuronal degeneration especially of the striatum. In this disease, as well as type II, Alzheimer's type I astrocytes are seen. There are also large cells with granular, eosinophilic cytoplasm (these are Opalski cells), which are probably histiocytes (Greenfield, 1963). Type I astrocytes are large with multilobular, multinucleolate, tetraploid nuclei. Cavanagh and Kyu (1971, 241–61) produced type I astrocytes around needle wounds in rats with portal systemic shunts and showed that they were the result of a failure of spindle function in cell division. Cavanagh and colleagues (Cavanagh, 1972) showed that this failure of the spindle mechanism is directly related to the high plasma ammonia levels which cause a disturbance of microtubular function. Microtubular damage was also seen ultrastructurally in oligodendrocytes and nerve cells. It is most obvious in astroglia since this is where most glutamine synthesis upon which deamination depends, probably takes place.

Huntington's chorea

In Huntington's chorea, as in idiopathic Parkinson's disease, there is an imbalance between neurotransmitters. There is relative overactivity of dopaminergic transmission from the substantia nigra due to a loss of small striatal interneurones. GABA and its biosynthetic enzyme GAD are decreased in the striatum but not in the frontal cortex at post-mortem in the brains of patients with the disease (Bird, 1978).

Macroscopically the brain in Huntington's chorea is smaller than normal with a variable degree of atrophy but with obvious dilation of the lateral ventricles due to shrinkage of the caudate and putamen (figure 6.7). The globus pallidus is also shrunken and brownish in colour. It contains abnormal amounts of iron. The substantia nigra appears normal or darker than normal. Microscopically there is loss of neurones in the anterior basal ganglia, particularly of small nerve cells. There is prominence of fibrous glia, but probably no actual increase (Lange *et al.*, 1976).

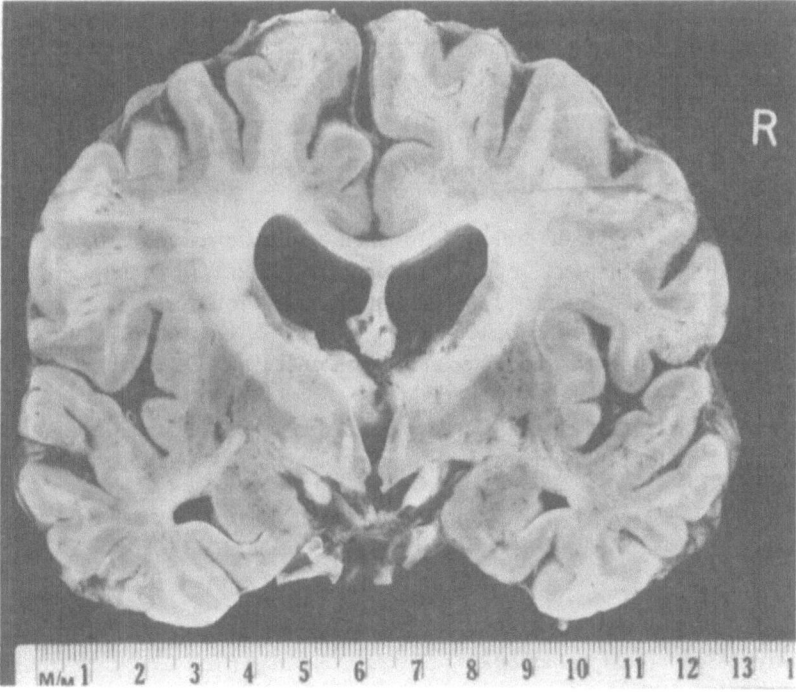

Figure 6.7 Huntington's chorea. Coronal section of the brain of a woman of 67 years with Huntington's chorea for eight years. She came from an affected family. Compared to the temporal horns, which are slightly dilated, the anterior horns of the lateral ventricles are very enlarged and their lateral angles are abnormally rounded. The head of the caudate nucleus is reduced to a narrow ribbon 3–4 mm wide. The putamen and the globus pallidus are also smaller than normal.

OTHER TYPES

Essential tremor

Benign essential tremor is a common postural tremor in which no structural abnormality has so far been identified in the brain. Standard routine examinations have shown pathological and biochemical changes attributable to ageing only (Hersovits and Blackwood, 1969). Fuller and further neuropathological examinations are necessary but may prove fruitless. Marsden (1981) has summarised what is known, and as yet it is still not clear to what extent peripheral or central mechanisms are involved.

CONCLUSIONS

In Parkinson's disease it is not possible to determine structural changes that relate solely to the specific symptoms of tremor. Essential tremor as yet has no recognised structural pathology. Patients with tremors of cerebellar or brainstem origin can show pathology in which precise anatomical localisation is possible.

ACKNOWLEDGEMENTS

It is a pleasure to thank the following for their helpful advice and criticism in the preparation of this chapter: Dr A. Taghizadeh, Dr I. Janota, Dr L. Carrasco, Dr P. Ellis, Dr C. Scholtz, Professor J. A. N. Corsellis and Professor C. D. Marsden. I should also like to thank the Histology Departments of Oldchurch, Runwell and the London Hospitals for much technical assistance, and Mrs P. Finney in the Academic Centre at Oldchurch Hospital.

I am very grateful to Dr Luis Carrasco for all his help in the preparation of the illustrations and for supplying much of the pathological material used.

REFERENCES

Adams, J. H. (1975). The neuropathology of head injury. In Vinken, P. J. and Bruyn, G. W. (eds), *Handbook of Clinical Neurology*, vol. 23, North-Holland, Amsterdam, pp. 35–65.

Adams, J. H. (1976). Virus diseases of the nervous system. In Blackwood, W. and Corsellis, J. A. N. (eds), *Greenfield's Neuropathology*, 3rd edn, Edward Arnold, London, chap. 8, pp. 292–326.

Adams, J. H., Beck, E. and Shenkin, A. M. (1974). Creutzfeld–Jakob disease. Further similarities with Kuru. *J. Neurol. Neurosurg. Psychiatr.*, **37**, 195–200.

Adams, R. D. (1968). Striato-nigral degenerations; and Acquired hepato-cellular degeneration. In Vinken, P. J. and Bruyn, G. W. (eds), *Handbook of Clinical Neurology*, vol. 6, North-Holland, Amsterdam, pp. 694–702 and 279–97.

Allen, I. V. (1981). The pathology of multiple sclerosis—fact, fiction and hypothesis. *Neuropathol. Appl. Neurobiol.*, 7, 169–82.

Allen, I. V. and McKeown, S. R. (1979). A histological, histochemical and biochemical study of the macroscopically normal white matter in multiple sclerosis. *J. Neurol. Sci.*, 41, 81–91.

Alvord, E. C. Jr (1968). The pathology of parkinsonism. In Minkler, J. (ed.), *Pathology of the Nervous System*, vol. 1, McGraw-Hill, New York, chap. 85, pp. 1152–61.

Alvord, E. C. Jr, Forno, L. S., Kusske, J. A., Kauffman, R. J., Rhodes, J. S. and Goetowski, C. R. (1974). The pathology of parkinsonism: a comparison of degeneration in cerebral cortex and brain stem. *Adv. Neurol.* 5, 175–93.

Andén, N. E., Fuxe, K., Hamberger, B. and Hokfelt, T. (1966). A quantitative study on the nigro-neostriatal dopamine neuron system in the rat. *Acta Physiol. Scand.*, 67, 306–12.

Andrew, J., Fowler, C. J. and Harrison, M. J. G. (1982). Tremor after head injury and its treatment by stereotactic surgery. *J. Neurol Neurosurg. Psychiatr.*, 45, 815–19.

Bannister, R. and Oppenheimer, D. (1982). Parkinsonism, system degenerations and autonomic failure. In Marsden, C. D. and Fahn, S. (eds), *Movement Disorders*, Butterworth Scientific, London, chap. 11, pp. 174–90.

Beck, E. and Bignami, A. (1968). Some neuroanatomical observations in cases with stereotactic lesions for the relief of parkinsonism. *Brain*, 91, 589–618.

Beck, E., Daniel, P. M., Gadjusek, D. C. and Gibbs, C. J. Jr (1970). Subacute degeneration of the brain transmissible to experimental animals. A neuropathological evaluation. *Proceedings of the VIIIth International Congress of Neuropathology*, Masson, Paris, pp. 858–73.

Behrman, S., Carroll, J. D., Janota, I. and Mathews, W. B. (1969). Progressive supranuclear palsy, clinicopathological study of four cases. *Brain*, 92, 663–78.

Bird, E. D. (1978). The brain in Huntington's chorea. Editorial. *Psychol. Med.*, 8, 357–60.

Blackwood, W. (1981). Morbid anatomy. In Rose, F. C. and Capildeo, R. (eds), *Research Progress in Parkinson's Disease, Progress in Neurology Series*, part 1, Pitman Medical, London, chap. 3, pp. 25–31.

Borit, A., Rubinstein, L. J. and Urich, H. (1975). The striato-nigral degenerations. Putaminal pigments and nosology. *Brain*, 98, 101–12.

Brodal, A. (1981). *Neurological Anatomy in Relation to Clinical Medicine*, 3rd edn, Oxford University Press, Oxford.

Brownell, B. and Hughes, J. T. (1962). The distribution of plaques in the cerebrum in multiple sclerosis. *J. Neurol. Neurosurg. Psychiatr.*, 25, 315–20.

Burns, J. (1978). Immunohistological methods and their application in the routine laboratory. In Anthony, P. P. and Woolf, N. (eds), *Recent Advances in Histopathology*, vol. 10, Churchill Livingstone, Edinburgh, chap. 16, pp. 337–50.

Cavanagh, J. B. (1972). Brain abnormalities in chronic liver disease. *The Scientific Basis of Medicine, Annual Review 1972*, chap. XIII, pp. 238–47.

Cavanagh, J. B. (1979). Metallic toxicity and the nervous system. In Smith, W. T. and Cavanagh, J. B. (eds), *Recent Advances in Neuropathology*, Churchill Livingstone, Edinburgh, pp. 247–75.

Cavanagh, J. B. and Kyu, M. H. (1971). Type II Alzheimer change experimentally produced in astrocytes in the rat; and On the mechanism of Type I Alzheimer abnormality in the nuclei of astrocytes. *J. Neurol. Sci.*, 12, 63–75, 241–61.

Cooper, I. S. (1977). Neurosurgical treatment of dyskinesias. *Clinical Neurosurgery: Proceedings of the Congress of Neurological Surgeons*, vol. 24, Williams and Wilkins, Baltimore, pp. 367–90.

Corsellis, J. A. N. (1976). Aging and the dementias. In Blackwood, W. and

120   *A. Marshall*

Corsellis, J. A. N. (eds), *Greenfield's Neuropathology*, 3rd edn, Edward Arnold, London, pp. 796–848.

Corsellis, J. A. N., Bruton, C. J. and Browne, D. F. (1973). The aftermath of boxing. *Psychol. Med.*, **3**, 270–303.

Critchley, M. (1929). Arteriosclerotic Parkinsonism. *Brain*, **52**, 23–83.

Critchley, M. (1981). Arteriosclerotic pseudo-Parkinsonism. In Rose, F. and Capildeo, R. (eds), *Research Progress in Parkinson's Disease, Progress in Neurology Series*, Pitman Medical, London, chap. 6, pp. 40–2.

Cuzner, M. L. (1980). Multiple sclerosis: biochemical and immunological changes. *Neuropathol. Appl. Neurobiol.*, **6**, 405–14.

Daniel, P. M. (1972). Creutzfeldt–Jakob disease. In Dick, G. (ed.), *Host–Virus Reactions with Special Reference to Persistent Agents*, *J. Clin. Pathol.*, **25**, Suppl. 6, 97–101.

Dow, R. S. (1969). Cerebellar syndromes. In Vinken, P. J. and Bruyn, G. W. (eds), *Handbook of Clinical Neurology*, vol. 2, North-Holland, Amsterdam, pp. 392–431.

Duffy, P. E. and Tennyson, V. M. (1965). Phase and electron microscope observations of Lewy bodies and melanin granules in the substantia nigra and locus coeruleus in Parkinson's disease. *J. Neuropathol. Exp. Neurol.*, **24**, 398–414.

Ehringer, H. and Hornykiewicz, O. (1960). Verteilung von Noradrenalin und Dopamin (3-Hydroxytyramin) im Gehirn des Menschen und ihr Verhalten bei Erkrankungen des extrapyramidalen Systems. *Klin. Wochenschr.*, **38**, 1238–9.

Findley, L. J. and Gresty, M. A. (1981). Tremor. *Br. J. Hosp. Med.*, **26**, 16–32.

Forno, L. S. (1982). Pathology of Parkinson's disease. In Marsden, C. D. and Fahn, S. (eds), *Movement Disorders*, Butterworth Scientific, London, chap. 3, pp. 25–40.

Forno, L. S. and Alvord, E. C. Jr (1971). The pathology of Parkinsonism. In McDowell, F. H. and Markham, C. H. (eds), *Recent Advances in Parkinson's Disease*, Parts I and II, Blackwell Scientific, Oxford, pp. 120–61.

Greenfield, J. G. (1963). Infectious diseases of the central nervous system; and System degenerations of the cerebellum, brain stem and spinal cord. In Blackwood, W., McMenemy, W. H., Meyer, A., Norman, R. M. and Russell, D. S. (eds), *Greenfield's Neuropathology*, 2nd edn, Edward Arnold, London.

Greenfield, J. G. and Bosanquet, F. D. (1953). The brain stem lesion in Parkinsonism. *J. Neurol. Neurosurg. Psychiatr.*, **16**, 213–26.

Harriman, D. G. F. (1966). The neuropathology of Parkinsonism. *Br. J. Hosp. Med.*, **1**, 17–24.

Henson, R. A. and Urich, H. (1982). *Cancer and the Nervous System: The Neurological Manifestations of Systemic Malignant Disease*, Blackwell Scientific, Oxford.

Hersovits, E. and Blackwood, W. (1969). Essential (familial, hereditary) tremor. A case report. *J. Neurol. Neurosurg. Psychiatr.*, **32**, 509–11.

Hirano, A., Kurland, L. T., Krooth, R. S. and Lessel, S. (1961a). Parkinsonism-dementia complex, an endemic disease on the Island of Guam. 1: Clinical features. *Brain*, **84**, 642–61.

Hirano, A., Malamud, N. and Kurland, L. T. (1961b). Parkinsonism-dementia complex, an endemic disease on the Island of Guam. 2: Pathology. *Brain*, **84**, 662–79.

Holmes, G. (1904). Certain tremors in organic cerebral lesions. *Brain*, **27**, 327–75.

Hornykiewicz, O. (1982). Brain neurotransmitter changes in Parkinson's disease. In Marsden, C. D. and Fahn, S. (eds), *Movement Disorders*, Butterworth Scientific, London, chap. 4, pp. 41–58.

Hunter, D. (1975). *Diseases of Occupations*, 5th edn, English Universities Press, London, chap. 5, p. 203.

Ikeda, K., Ikeda, S., Yoshimura, T., Kato, H. and Namba, M. (1978). Idiopathic Parkinsonism with Lewy type inclusions in the cerebral cortex. A case report. *Acta Neuropathol. (Berl.)*, **40**, 263-9.

Iqbal, K., Wisniewski, H. M., Grundke-Iqbal, J. and Terry, R. D. (1977). Neurofibrillary pathology, an update. In Nandy, K. and Sherwin, I. (eds), *The Aging Brain and Senile Dementia, Advances in Behavioural Biology*, vol. 23, Plenum Press, New York, pp. 209-27.

Ishii, T. and Nakamura, Y. (1981). Distribution and ultrastructure of Alzheimer's neurofibrillary tangles in post-encephalitic Parkinsonism of Economo type. *Acta Neuropathol. (Berl.)*, **55**, 59-62.

Janota, I. (1981). Pathology of dementia. In Anthony, P. P. and MacSween, R. N. M. (eds), *Recent Advances in Histopathology*, Churchill Livingstone, Edinburgh, chap. 4, pp. 49-63.

Klatzo, I. (1979). Cerebral oedema and ischaemia. In Smith, W. T. and Cavanagh, J. B. (eds), *Recent Advances in Neuropathology*, vol. 1, Churchill Livingstone, Edinburgh, chap. 2, pp. 27-39.

Kosoka, K. (1978). Lewy bodies in the cerebral cortex. Three cases. *Acta Neuropathol. (Berl.)*, **42**, 127-34.

Kremer, M., Ritchie Russell, W. and Smyth, G. E. (1947). A midbrain syndrome following head injury. *J. Neurol. Neurosurg. Psychiatr.*, **10**, 49-60.

Krnjevic, K. (1982). GABA and other transmitters. In Palay, S. L. and Chan-Palay, V. (eds), *The Cerebellum—New Vistas, Exp. Brain Res. Suppl.*, Springer-Verlag, Berlin.

Lampert, P. W., Earle, K. M., Gibbs, C. J. and Gadjusek, D. C. (1969). Experimental Kuru encephalopathy in chimpanzees and spider monkeys. *J. Neuropathol. Exp. Neurol.*, **28**, 353-70.

Lange, H., Thomer, G., Hopf, A. and Schroeder, K. F. (1976). Morphometric studies of the neuropathological changes in choreatic diseases. *J. Neurol. Sci.*, **28**, 401-25.

Lewy, F. H. (1912). Paralysis agitans. I. Pathologische Anatomie. In Lewandowsky, M. (ed.), *Handbuch der Neurologie*, Springer, Berlin, pp. 920-33.

Lipkin, L. E. (1959). Cytoplasmic inclusions in ganglion cells associated with Parkinsonian states, a neurocellular change. Studied in 53 cases and 206 controls. *Am. J. Pathol.*, **35**, 1117-33.

McMenemy, W. H. (1966). The central nervous system. In Payling-Wright, G. and St. Clair Symmers, W. (eds), *Systemic Pathology*, vol. 2, 1st edn, Longmans, London, chap. 34, pp. 1200-2.

Marsden, C. D. (1981). Extra-pyramidal diseases. In Davison, A. W. and Thompson, R. H. S. (eds), *The Molecular Basis of Neuropathology*, Edward Arnold, London, pp. 345-83.

Marsden, C. D. (1982). Neurotransmitters and CNS disease—basal ganglia disease. *Lancet*, **2**, 1141-7.

Martin, J. P. (1968). Wilson's disease. In Vinken, P. J. and Bruyn, G. W. (eds), *Handbook of Clinical Neurology*, vol. 6, North-Holland, Amsterdam, pp. 173-217.

Matthews, J. P., Glasse, R. and Lindenbaum, S. (1968). Kuru and cannibalism. *Lancet*, **2**, 449-52.

Nashold, B. S. and Slaughter, D. G. (1969). Some observations on tremors. In Gillingham, F. J. L. and Donaldson, I. M. L. (eds), *Third Symposium on Parkinson's Disease*, E. S. and S. Livingstone, Edinburgh, pp. 241-6.

Northfield, D. W. C. (1973). *The Surgery of the Central Nervous System*, Blackwell Scientific, Oxford.

Nurick, S., Blackwood, W. and Mair, W. G. P. (1972). Giant cell granulomatous angiitis of the central nervous system. *Brain*, **95**, 133-42.

Okazaki, H., Lipkin, L. E. and Aronson, S. (1961). Diffuse intracytoplasmic ganglionic inclusions (Lewy type) associated with progressive dementia and quadraparesis in flexion. *J. Neuropathol. Exp. Neurol.*, **20**, 237–44.

Oppenheimer, D. R. (1976). Diseases of the basal ganglia, cerebellum and motor neurones; and Demyelinating diseases. In Blackwood, W. and Corsellis, J. A. N. (eds), *Greenfield's Neuropathology*, 3rd edn, Edward Arnold, London, chaps 11 and 14.

Pakkenberg, H. (1963). The globus pallidus in parkinsonism. *Acta Neuropathol. Scand.*, **4**, Suppl., 139–44.

Palay, S. L. (1982). Current status of neuroanatomical research in the cerebellum. In Palay, S. L. and Chan Palay, V. (eds), *The Cerebellum—New Vistas, Exp. Brain Res. Suppl.*, Springer-Verlag, Berlin, pp. 1–7.

Papworth, M. H. (1971). In *Primer of Medicine*, 3rd edn, Butterworths, London, p. 336.

Pearce, G. W. (1979). The neuropathology of parkinsonism. In Smith, W. T. and Cavanagh, J. B. (eds), *Recent Advances in Neuropathology*, Churchill Livingstone, Edinburgh, chap. 12, pp. 299–320.

Perry, E. K., Tomlinson, B. E., Blessed, G., Bergman, K., Gibson, P. H. and Perry, R. H. (1978). Correlation of cholinergic abnormalities with senile plaques and mental scores in senile dementia. *Br. Med. J.*, **2**, 1457–9.

Pentschew, A. (1966). Regrouping of extra-pyramidal diseases as suggested by manganese encephalopathy. *J. Neurosurg.*, **24**, 255.

Plum, B. and Hindfelt, B. (1976). The neurological complications of liver disease. In Vinken, P. J. and Bruyn, G. W. (eds), *Handbook of Clinical Neurology*, vol. 27, North-Holland, Amsterdam, pp. 349–77.

Potvin, M., Finlayson, M. H., Hinchley, E. J. and Goresky, C. A. (1976). Macroscopic and electron microscopic studies of the blood–brain barrier in acute hepatic coma following hepatectomy. *Gastroenterology*, **71**, 924.

Powell, H. C., Landon, G. N. and Lampert, P. W. (1974). Neurofibrillary tangles in progressive supranuclear palsy. *J. Neuropathol. Exp. Neurol.*, **33**, 98–106.

Rail, D., Scholtz, C. and Swash, M. (1981). Post-encephalitic Parkinsonism: current experience. *J. Neurol. Neurosurg. Psychiatr.*, **44**, 670–6.

Reynolds, E. H. (1968). Mental effects of anticonvulsants and folic acid metabolism. *Brain*, **91**, 197–214.

Rossor, M. N. (1982). Neurotransmitters and CNS disease. Dementia. *Lancet*, **2**, 1200–4.

Roy, S. and Wolman, L. (1969). Ultrastructural observations in parkinsonism. *J. Pathol.*, **99**, 39–44.

Selby, G. (1968). Parkinson's disease. In Vinken, P. J. and Bruyn, G. W. (eds), *Handbook of Clinical Neurology*, vol. 6, North-Holland, Amsterdam, pp. 143–211.

Sherlock, S. (1977). Hepatic encephalopathy. *Br. J. Hosp. Med.*, **17**, 144–59.

Shoulson, I. (1982). Care of patients and families with Huntington's disease. In Marsden, C. D. and Fahn, S. (eds), *Movement Disorders*, Butterworth Scientific, London, chap. 16, pp. 277–90.

Smith, M. C. (1966). Pathological changes associated with stereotactic lesions in Parkinson's disease. *J. Neurosurg.*, **24**, 257–63.

Smith, W. T. (1976). Nutritional deficiencies and disorders. In Blackwood, W. and Corsellis, J. A. N. (eds), *Greenfield's Neuropathology*, 3rd edn, Edward Arnold, London, chap. 5, pp. 194–232.

Snider, S. R. and Snider, R. S. (1982). Structural and functional relationship between the cerebellum and catecholamine systems. In Palay, S. L. and Chan

Palay, V. (eds), *The Cerebellum—New Vistas, Exp. Brain Res. Suppl.*, Springer-Verlag, Berlin, pp. 587–606.

Spokes, E. G., Bannister, R. and Oppenheimer, D. R. (1979). Multiple system atrophy with autonomic failure: clinical histological and neurochemical observations on four cases. *J. Neurol. Sci.*, **43**, 59–82.

Stadlan, E. M., Davison, R. and Yahr, M. (1966). The pathology of Parkinsonism. In Luthy, F. and Bischoff, A. (eds), *Proceedings of the 5th International Congress of Neuropathology*, Excerpta Medica, Amsterdam, pp. 569–71.

Strich, S. (1961). Shearing of nerve fibres, as a cause of brain damage due to head injury. *Lancet*, **2**, 443–8.

Tretiakoff, C. (1919). Contribution à l'étude de l'anatomie pathologique de locus niger de Soemmering avec quelques déductions relatives à la pathogenie des troubles du tonus musculaire et de la maladie de Parkinson. *Thèse*, Paris.

Urich, H. (1976). Diseases of peripheral nerves. In Blackwood, W. and Corsellis, J. A. N. (eds), *Greenfield's Neuropathology*, 3rd edn, Edward Arnold, London, pp. 688–770.

Weller, R. O., Swash, M., McLellan, D. C. and Scholtz, C. L. (1982). *Clinical Neuropathology*, Springer-Verlag, Berlin.

Wisniewski, H. M., Coblentz, J. M. and Terry, R. D. (1972). Pick's disease. A clinical and ultrastructural study. *Arch. Neurol. (Chic.)*, **26**, 97–108.

Wisniewski, H., Terry, R. D. and Hirano, A. (1970). Neurofibrillary pathology. *J. Neuropathol. Exp. Neurol.*, **29**, 163–76.

Yagishita, S., Itoh, Y., Amano, N. and Nakano, T. (1980). Atypical senile dementia with widespread Lewy type inclusions in the cerebral cortex. *Acta Neuropathol. (Berl.)*, **49**, 187–91.

Yahr, M. D. (1981). Introduction. In Rose, F. C. and Capildeo, R. (eds), *Research Progress in Parkinson's Disease, Progress in Neurology Series*, Pitman Medical, London, pp. 3–8.

Yates, P. O. (1976). Vascular disease of the central nervous system. In Blackwood, W. and Corsellis, J. A. N. (eds). *Greenfield's Neuropathology*, 3rd edn, Edward Arnold, London, chap. 3, pp. 86–147.

SECTION 2
NEUROPHYSIOLOGY OF TREMOR

7
Physiological and enhanced physiological tremor*

ROBERT R. YOUNG

INTRODUCTION

Physiological tremor, *sensu strictu*, is an inevitable consequence of muscle contraction. Although it is roughly an order of magnitude larger than ballisto-cardiograph tremor (passive vibrations of body parts due to the periodic force perturbations produced by contraction of the heart with ejection of blood against the arch of the aorta, etc.), physiological tremor nevertheless is difficult to see with the naked eye. Its demonstration requires either optical magnification (such as provided by a dissecting or operating microscope) or a mechanical-to-electrical transducer of some type with subsequent electronic amplification. Tremor movements can be studied directly by using a goniometer, the arms of which, attached to a potentiometer, are carefully applied to the body part being studied, with the axis of the potentiometer positioned precisely coaxial with the joint to be studied. Either velocity and acceleration of tremor movements can be derived electronically from changes in position or acceleration can be measured directly by attaching a sensitive piezoelectric accelerometer to the moving part. Although positioning this latter transducer is less critical than when one uses a goniometer, care must never-theless be taken to arrange that the acceleration being recorded is due only to movement at the joint under consideration—with an accelerometer on the dorsum of the hand, if the arm is held outstretched, a complex acceleration recording is then made which is due to summation of acceleration produced at all joints of the limb and by movements of the trunk itself.

WHAT IS PHYSIOLOGICAL TREMOR?

In any one individual, physiological tremor is not monorhythmic but consists of movements at a number of frequencies between 8 and 12 Hz, the amplitude of these movements fluctuating widely from one 'tremor beat' to the next. This

*Supported in part by the Parkinson's Disease Fund of the Massachusetts General Hospital.

low-amplitude, irregular physiological tremor is not caused by synchronisation of motoneurone discharge or other 'neural factors'. In their careful analysis of this problem, Freund and Dietz (1978) were unable to demonstrate any neural basis for these tremor movements such as is easily demonstrable for the other types of tremor to be discussed below. Allowing for the confusion resulting from earlier widespread failure to distinguish physiological tremor from enhanced physiological tremor (see below), there is general agreement that movements of physiological tremor are a reflection of mechanical properties of the muscle and limb, such as unfused twitches of motor units which are just being recruited and resonant mechanical properties of the body part.

Nevertheless, Hagbarth and Young (1979), using microneurographic techniques, demonstrated that the minute movements of physiological tremor (usually less than 0.1° at finger or wrist joints) do produce time-locked bursts of muscle spindle primary afferent activity. During each cycle of physiological tremor movement, spindle primary endings discharge more or less synchronously as the tremor movement stretches the muscle in which they lie, albeit these stretches are extremely small. Their studies employing direct recordings from human muscle spindle primary afferent fibres demonstrated non-linear, extreme sensitivity of primary endings similar to that described earlier for spindles in decerebrate cats (Matthews and Stein, 1969; Poppele and Bowman, 1970). These groups showed that, in decerebrate cats at least, spindle primary endings responded briskly to stretches of the entire muscle of less than 50 μm. Such small stretches are difficult to reproduce passively in clinical laboratories but we were able to take advantage of the tiny movements of physiological tremor to show that primary endings in normal muscle respond nearly as vigorously to movements of a fraction of a tenth of a degree as they do to movements 10 times larger. That is, normal human muscle spindle primary endings are more sensitive, as measured by number of impulses produced per unit stretch, to the onset of muscle stretch (to the acceleration?) than they are to larger stretches. This non-linear behaviour of spindle afferents has certain interesting consequences for studies of symptomatic tremor but precisely what, if any, influence these tremor-locked bursts of Ia input during physiological tremor have upon motoneurones in the already discharging pool remains to be demonstrated.

ENHANCED PHYSIOLOGICAL TREMOR

Physiological tremor, as described above, certainly is too small to produce clinical symptoms even when, as an inevitable consequence of muscle contraction, it is present in patients with various diseases of the motor system (see Young, this volume, chapter 35) just as it is in normal subjects. However, another type of physiological tremor, if by 'physiological' one means tremor in a perfectly normal subject, also occurs *both* in normal subjects and in patients with various motor disorders and *is* quite symptomatic. When a normal person is frightened, anxious, fatigued, contracting muscles very forcibly, receiving a wide variety of adrenergically active medications or subjected to several of the manoeuvres outlined below, a relatively large-amplitude, very apparent tremor is seen which disappears following the termination of these various circumstances. This tremor tends to be monorhythmic with a single peak frequency, in any one individual, between 8 and 12 Hz. A tremor of this sort can easily be produced by increasing the level of circulating adrenergic catecholamines either as a result of administration of such a medication (for the treatment of asthma or otherwise) or by increasing the endogenous release of adrenaline (as with hypoglycaemia, stage-fright or other acute or chronic anxiety states). Either the administration of thyroid hormones or their increased release from the gland itself will produce a similar tremor. Tremors of this type are also produced by various other medications (lithium, tricyclic antidepressants, levodopa, corticosteroids) or substances such as xanthines in coffee or tea which may or may not operate by increasing 'beta-adrenergic tone'.

In the past, each of these clinically relevant tremors has been named according to the circumstance in which it was seen—for example, nervous tremor, fatigue tremor, adrenergic tremor, lithium tremor, thyrotoxic tremor, and so forth. Although these names are useful insofar as they emphasise the causative factors, there are also advantages to be gained from listing these tremors under one heading (*enhanced physiological tremor*) since that emphasises, at the same time, the unity of mechanisms involved in all these tremors and their fundamental difference from simple physiological tremor and essential–familial tremor, which have often been confused with them.

With enhanced physiological tremor, the sinusoidal movements are larger in amplitude and more regular than with physiological tremor and, as Hagbarth and Young (1979) have demonstrated, muscle spindle primary endings are, as one would expect, also sensitive to these larger muscle stretches so that bursts of Ia afferent activity again mirror these tremor movements. Now, however, with a full-blown enhanced physiological tremor, there are clear-cut changes in the timing of single motor unit discharges within an active motoneurone pool so that bursts of EMG activity are seen which occur at very specific times relative to two other events. First, on the one hand, these EMG bursts begin 20 to 30 ms after the onset of Ia bursts from the stretched muscle and end a similar time after cessation of Ia bursts. In the human forearm the delay is 20–25 ms and in the lower leg about 30 ms—each of these being the monosynaptic reflex time for these areas of the body. It therefore appears that spindle afferent activity reflexly modulates the firing times in a voluntarily activated motoneurone pool, producing bursts of EMG activity time-locked to the stretch phases of an ongoing tremor. Apart from the fact that these Ia bursts synchronise already discharging motoneurones whereas larger Ia bursts following a tendon tap actually recruit otherwise inactive motoneurones, the EMG tremor bursts are the equivalent of repetitive segmental stretch reflexes. Secondly, on the other hand, these EMG bursts occur at precisely the right time, followed as they are by contraction of the muscle gradually increasing over the next 25–75 ms, so that force pulses or increased torques about the joint under study will occur during that phase of tremor movement in which the muscle is already shortening. These extra 'EMG-burst-induced' force pulses will then tend to shorten the muscle even more vigorously and, of course, the same activity will be going on in antagonistic muscles approximately 180° out of phase from the muscle under consideration. (This situation, as far as torque pulses about the joint are concerned, is analogous to a child's swing in the playground where one parent stands at either end of the swing's excursion and pushes, not particularly forcefully but with precisely correct timing, so the amplitude of the sinusoidal excursion increases.) These tremor-locked EMG bursts appear to be of spinal reflex origin, a neural mechanism which, although clearly operative in enhanced physiological tremors, is not seen in ordinary physiological tremor.

A continuum of activity therefore appears to be operative (figure 7.1) from simple physiological tremor at one end (during which the movements entrain spindle primary afferent discharges even though these do not synchronise motor unit activity) to high-amplitude enhanced physiological tremor at the other end of the spectrum (where bursts of EMG activity are evident upon simple inspection without need for statistical processing of the EMG record). Precisely where in this continuous spectrum one type of tremor switches to the other is unclear and such a question, in fact, is probably unrealistically simplistic. It seems unlikely that segmental stretch reflex mechanisms operate in an all-or-none, binary mode.

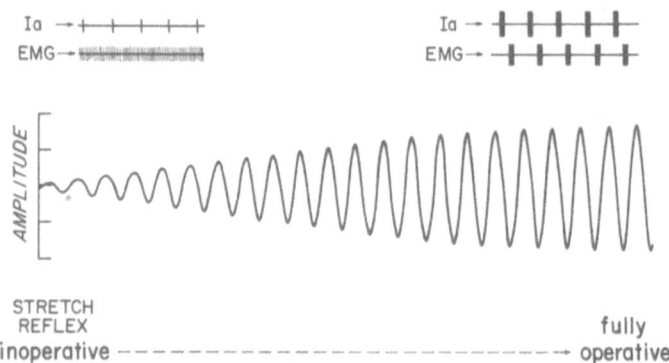

Figure 7.1 This illustrates the continuum of tremor amplitude between ordinary physiological tremor on the left and enhanced physiological tremor on the right. On the left, each stretch phase produces Ia discharges from spindles in the appropriate muscle which are time-locked to tremor movements, but these bursts of Ia activity have no demonstrable effect on the timing of discharges in the voluntarily activated motoneurone pool. As tremor amplitude increases from left to right, the segmental stretch reflex becomes increasingly operative as judged by progressive synchronisation of motoneurone discharge so that EMG bursts follow the Ia bursts at a latency compatible with mono- or oligosynaptic action. These EMG bursts are also timed appropriately so the force pulse produced by the muscle contraction following each EMG burst occurs during the subsequent shortening phase, thereby increasing the amplitude of tremor movement.

Young and Hagbarth (1980) demonstrated that various manoeuvres designed to increase activity around the segmental stretch reflex arc also produce, or increase the amplitude of, enhanced physiological tremor. These manoeuvres include voluntarily increasing central excitatory drive on the motoneurone pool, using a Jendrassik manoeuvre, vibrating muscles to increase the contrast in Ia input (between alternating shortening and lengthening phases of muscle due to physiological tremor) and stimulating the muscles adrenergically. Our hypothesis is that enhanced physiological tremor is due to increased operation of the segmental stretch reflex arc and our results, when this increase is produced by a variety of different mechanisms, support such a hypothesis. For a more detailed discussion of peripheral mechanisms which may be responsible for altered timing of stretch reflex activity ('tuning') necessary to enhance the amplitude of pre-existent physiological tremor, see Young (1983). In brief, beta-adrenergic stimulation of extrafusal muscle fibres (due to circulating and, perhaps, locally released adrenaline) shortens their twitch- and half-relaxation times, thereby producing slightly earlier stretch responses from spindles lying in parallel with these extrafusal fibres. There may also be adrenergic-induced changes in intrafusal fibre mechanical properties but they have not been clearly demonstrated in this setting. In any case, earlier (and perhaps larger) Ia input produces earlier and larger EMG bursts, the force pulses from which 'push the pendulum' of the moving body part at just the precise time necessary to increase its excursion and then maintain its larger amplitude, as illustrated in figure 7.2.

This same overall mechanism (increased operation of the segmental stretch reflex arc) will be as functional in patients with pre-existing neurological diseases (i.e. movement disorders), providing they have intact stretch reflex arcs and are able to contract muscles voluntarily, as it is in normal subjects. It must also be stressed that relatively small changes, such as anxiety about the testing situation or repeated contraction of muscle groups to be studied, can produce enhanced physiological tremor of considerable magnitude. This also applies to patients with pre-existing disorders of motor control. As Stiles (1976) has noted, and as Hagbarth and Young (1979) have more recently demonstrated, enhanced physiological tremor does not require muscle contraction to the extent that a subject feels fatigued. Simply holding a finger or the hand outstretched against gravity for a few minutes will produce enhanced physiological tremor where operation of the stretch reflex arc is easily demonstrable.

THE RELATIONSHIP OF ENHANCED PHYSIOLOGICAL TREMOR TO OTHER TREMORS

Whenever a patient with essential-familial tremor or a parkinsonian tremor is tested in a laboratory situation, the probability that the patient's anxiety level will increase is quite high even though the experimenter or technician tries to minimise the frightening or threatening nature of the study. Anxiety or 'stage-fright' have much more to do with the patient's or subject's view of the situation than with

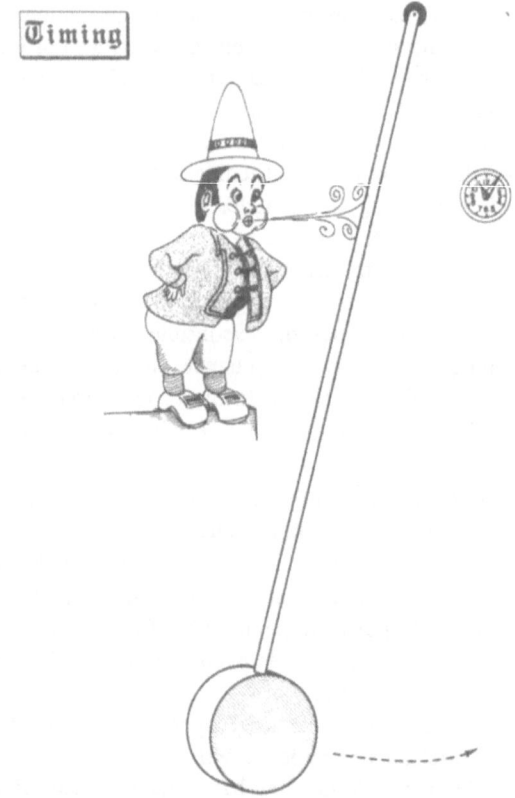

Figure 7.2 This cartoon emphasises that when dealing with simple harmonic motion (such as occurs with a child's swing, a pendulum or a tremulous hand), very weak force pulses can, providing they are delivered with precisely correct timing, increase the excursion of movement so that its eventual amplitude appears disproportionately large when compared with the magnitude of the force pulses. Similarly, relatively slight alterations in timing of the force pulses produce large changes in amplitude of the motion—an effect which may underlie the mechanisms responsible for enhanced physiological tremor.

the reality of it as viewed by the experimenter. Similarly, during a series of recordings, it is often necessary for the subject to hold the hand or arm out against gravity for several minutes or more which, itself, will produce 'fatigue' tremor as noted above. Under these or other circumstances one may speak either of 'enhanced essential (or parkinsonian) tremor' or of a combined tremor in which enhanced physiological tremor is superimposed upon essential or parkinsonian tremor. Although reasons for using one or other of these names can be debated, the point to emphasise is that studies, either of the physiological mechanisms involved or of the tremor's response to pharmacological agents, may, in fact, be telling the experimenter more about mechanisms enhancing the tremor than about the underlying tremor itself.

Over the years there have been recurrent scientific controversies as to whether 'physiological tremor' does or does not involve operation of the segmental stretch reflex arc and, as seen above, depending on one's definition of physiological versus enhanced physiological tremor, both are correct. At one end of the spectrum depicted in figure 7.1 there is no evidence of stretch reflex activity whereas at the other end that activity is obvious. Similar arguments have been raised as to whether or not essential and parkinsonian tremor amplitudes are reduced acutely by the administration of beta-adrenergic blocking agents such as propranolol. In the first example given above, confusion existed because of failure to differentiate between two different types of physiological tremor; in the second example, confusion has arisen because of failure to distinguish the pre-existing tremor, essential tremor for example, from the enhanced type which has been superimposed upon it during the experimental situation.

This latter confusion also resulted in the assertion that essential-familial tremor is an exaggeration of normal physiological tremor (Marshall, 1962) whereas all recent evidence tends to refute that hypothesis. On clinical grounds alone, patients whose essential-familial tremors have been eliminated by stereotactic ventrolateral thalamotomies are normally prone to develop enhanced physiological tremor with anxiety, fright or administration of beta-adrenergic agonists. Also as Shahani (this volume, chapter 29) has demonstrated, patients who suffer from both essential-familial tremor and Charcot-Marie-Tooth chronic progressive neuropathy of such severity that segmental stretch reflex arc activity (principally large fibre afferent activity) has failed, still have symptomatic tremor which responds nicely to chronic propranolol therapy. However, neither they nor rare deafferented patients develop enhanced physiological tremor when exposed to those circumstances, listed above, which otherwise produce it in patients or normal subjects. There are therefore a number of strong arguments to be made for the clear separation of physiological tremor from its enhanced variety and of essential-familial or parkinsonian tremor from their enhanced varieties. One hopes that future studies in these areas will attempt to differentiate these tremors, one from another. Certainly it is very difficult to evaluate the significance of most earlier investigations or clinical statements regarding 'physiological tremor' because it is usually not clear, in retrospect, which tremor or tremors were involved.

One urgent task for those of us concerned with tremor is to devise objective and quantitative methods for evaluation of tremors. Controversies such as those mentioned above can only be resolved after the mechanisms underlying each of these tremors are worked out and the type of tremor under discussion is specified in terms that can be duplicated in laboratories throughout the world.

CONCLUSIONS

Physiological tremor, *sensu strictu*, is not due to synchronisation of motoneurone discharge and does not produce clinical symptoms, but these tiny movements are very accurately monitored by primary endings of muscle spindle afferents. Under a variety of circumstances (exercise, fatigue, increased beta-adrenergic tone, fright, etc.), these bursts of Ia input begin to produce synchronisation of firing within an active motoneurone pool. The torque pulses resulting from this EMG activity are timed to produce larger-amplitude tremulous movements which, in normal subjects or patients with other types of tremor, become clinically troublesome. Such 'enhanced physiological tremor' has previously been termed physiological tremor, fatigue tremor, adrenergic tremor, nervous tremor, etc. The importance of differentiating between these 'two types of physiological tremor' has been stressed.

REFERENCES

Freund, H.-J. and Dietz, V. (1978). The relationship between physiological and pathological tremor. In Desmedt, J. E. (ed.), *Progress in Clinical Neurophysiology*, vol. 5, Karger, Basel, pp. 66–89.

Hagbarth, K.-E. and Young, R. R. (1979). Participation of the stretch reflex in human physiological tremor. *Brain*, **102**, 509–26.

Marshall, J. (1962). Observations on essential tremor. *J. Neurol. Neurosurg. Psychiatr.*, **25**, 122–5.

Matthews, P. B. C. and Stein, R. B. (1969). The sensitivity of muscle spindle afferents to small sinusoidal changes of length. *J. Physiol.*, **250**, 723–43.

Poppele, R. E. and Bowman, R. J. (1970). Quantitative description of linear behaviour of mammalian muscle spindles. *J. Neurophysiol.*, **33**, 59–72.

Stiles, R. N. (1976). Frequency and displacement amplitude relations for normal hand tremor. *J. Appl. Physiol.*, **40**, 44–54.

Young, R. R. (1983). Enhanced physiological tremor in Parkinson disease. In Yahr, M. D. (ed.), *Current Concepts of Parkinson Disease and Related Disorders*, Excerpta Medica, Princeton, NJ, in press.

Young, R. R. and Hagbarth, K.-E. (1980). Physiological tremor enhanced by manoeuvres affecting the segmental stretch reflex. *J. Neurol. Neurosurg. Psychiatr.*, **43**, 248–56.

8

Segmental reflex, muscle mechanical and central mechanisms underlying human physiological tremor

J. H. J. ALLUM

INTRODUCTION

Each discharge of an α-motoneurone produces a twitch of muscle force in the muscle fibres which comprise its motor unit. When a constant number of motoneurones activating a single muscle discharge asynchronously, one might expect the individual twitches to fuse together into a smooth contraction. However, smooth contractions are not observed in force records. Instead, small $\sim 10\,\text{Hz}$ oscillations, termed physiological tremor, are superimposed on the fused force. This tremor could be caused either by one or more neural commands which tend to synchronise motoneuronal activity and thereby produce massed twitch contractions, or because the intrinsic spring–mass system of the muscle and limb combined with that of the external load resonates as an oscillator following a muscle twitch. Alternatively, both neural and muscle mechanical mechanisms may interact to generate tremor.

Current views tend to emphasise neural mechanisms in generating tremor, and suggest that the role of muscle mechanical mechanisms is restricted to influencing the amount of muscle stretch during tremor rather than being, *per se*, tremogenic (Matthews and Muir, 1980; Cussons *et al.*, 1980). The purpose of this chapter is to add support to these views and to provide evidence that, once a motor unit generates a twitch, the ensuing segmental reflex signals cause the same or other units in the muscle to discharge after a reflex delay, thereby setting up a 'chain reaction' which enhances tremor. As an aid to the reader, the classification shown in the schema of figure 8.1 will be adopted for the present description of tremor mechanisms.

Figure 8.1 is an attempt to divide postulated mechanisms causing tremor into three broad types: first, tremor caused by central (or short-term) synchronisation; secondly, tremor caused by muscle mechanical mechanisms; and thirdly, tremor caused by segmental reflex (or long-term) synchronisation.

Central tremogenic commands, as depicted in figure 8.1 (right), refer, in a broad sense, to those mechanisms producing closely timed discharges of α-moto-

135

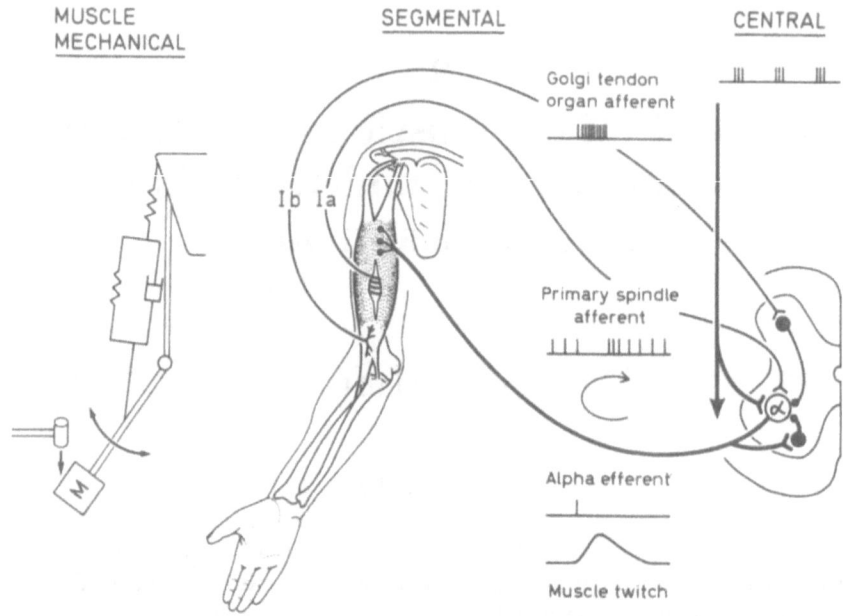

MUSCLE
MECHANICAL

SEGMENTAL

CENTRAL

Golgi tendon
organ afferent

Ib Ia

Primary spindle
afferent

Alpha efferent

Muscle twitch

Figure 8.1 Schema of proposed central, muscle mechanical and segmental reflex mechanisms underlying human physiological tremor.

neurones, technically called short-term synchronisation of α-motoneurones. By short term is meant within ±15 ms of another α-motoneurone's discharge (cf. Milner-Brown *et al.*, 1973a, 1975). Short-term synchronisation could be due to the synchronised firing of a group of cortical neurones (Allum *et al.*, 1982a) whose axons terminate in the same motoneurone pool of a muscle or to the discharge of a few cortical motoneurones whose collaterals arborise extensively within the motoneurone pool (Fetz *et al.*, 1976; Asanuma *et al.*, 1979), thereby causing synchronisation of the inputs to α-motoneurones (Moore *et al.*, 1970). Alternatively, the central drive executing a movement might set local segmental circuits with a major recurrent input to α-motoneurones into oscillations, as Elble and Randall (1976) proposed for Renshaw collateral circuits (Eccles *et al.*, 1954).

Muscle mechanical causes for tremor are shown schematically in the left part of figure 8.1. Active muscle contraction adds intrinsic muscle elasticity and viscosity to the passive muscle and tendon compliance (Joyce *et al.*, 1969). The total muscle compliance in conjunction with the limb inertia is a damped oscillatory system (as modelled in figure 8.1). Coupling an appropriate compliant load to the limb can so reduce the damping that the total system is easily set swinging by small internal or external disturbances (Joyce and Rack, 1974; Stein and Oğuztöreli, 1976).

Segmental stretch reflexes mediated by muscle afferents have been postulated as the underlying mechanism causing long-term synchronisation (over the range 15 to 100 ms) of α-motoneurones (Milner-Brown *et al.*, 1973a; Allum and Hulliger, 1982). The middle part of figure 8.1 illustrates this hypothesis. Each twitch contraction generally produces a characteristic pattern of activity in muscle spindle afferents (Ia activity is shown) and Golgi tendon organ (Ib) afferents (Binder *et al.*, 1976, 1977). When the afferent activity reaches the α-motoneurones after a transmission delay, it will either enhance or depress further α-motoneurone discharges depending on the relative strength and timing of the reflex excitatory and inhibitory pathways.

The classification scheme illustrated in figure 8.1 is not meant to exclude possible interactions between these three basic tremogenic mechanisms. Indeed, it has been convincingly argued that motor tremors result from the interaction of segmental stretch reflex and muscle mechanical mechanisms (Joyce and Rack, 1974; Stein and Oğuztöreli, 1976; Rack, 1978), and even proposed that a transcortical stretch reflex contributes to tremor (Milner-Brown *et al.*, 1975; Stein and Bawa, 1976). Figure 8.1, then, provides a basis for an empirical examination of tremor.

METHODS OF DATA ANALYSIS

Correlations between muscle EMG activity and tremor force

Most authors have recorded muscle electrical activity (EMG) and force in order to determine if rhythmic neural activity participates in tremor. Observed correlations between muscle activity and tremor force are then employed as evidence for or against the proposed tremogenic mechanisms shown in figure 8.1. The same approach will be used in this chapter, once various methods for adducing a correlation are described.

Figure 8.2 illustrates typical measurements taken during isometric contractions of the first dorsal interosseus (FDI) muscle of the human hand. Single motor unit potentials recorded with a concentric needle electrode from FDI are shown in the top traces of figure 8.2. The middle traces are surface EMG records from the same muscle after bandpass filtering, full-wave rectification and demodulation using a 10 ms time-constant averaging filter (Gottlieb and Agarwal, 1970). Force exerted by FDI is recorded at the index finger by a strain gauge (Allum *et al.*, 1978; Allum and Hulliger, 1982). The force signals are then bandpass filtered to yield the third set of traces in figure 8.2. When a subject exerts a steadily increasing force, either isometrically (figure 8.2) or against a moderately compliant spring (Matthews and Muir, 1980), the frequency of motor unit firing, the intensity of surface EMG records and the amplitude of tremor force oscillations also increase. Although the measurements shown in figure 8.2 are most commonly used as a basis for determining correlations between neural

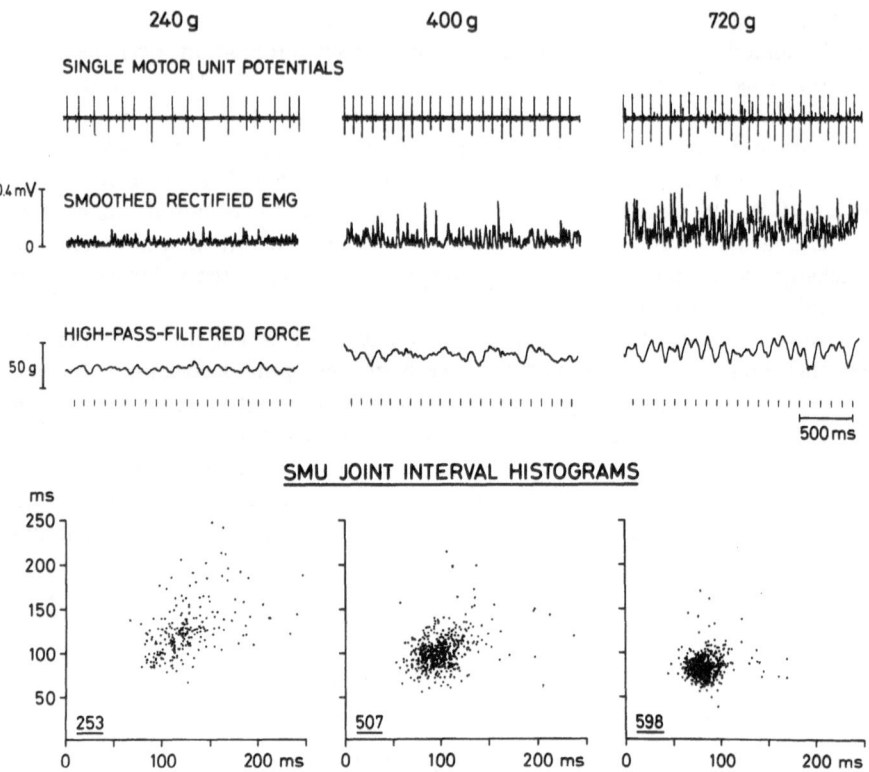

Figure 8.2 Sample records of tremor measurements during isometric contractions of the first dorsal interosseus muscle (FDI) at 240, 400 and 720 g. Longer records of simultaneously recorded single motor unit potentials are displayed as joint interval histograms. With each increase in the force exerted between thumb and index finger by the FDI muscle, the mean discharge rate of the motor unit increased and the variance in the inter-spike interval decreased. The amplitude of oscillations in the surface EMG and high-pass-filtered force records was larger as the force level was raised. Underlined numbers near the origin of each scatter plot equal the number of discharges used for the plot. (Previously unpublished records from Allum and Hulliger (1982).)

signals and tremor, the techniques of microneurography have also been utilised to record afferent nerve activity during tremor (Hagbarth and Young, 1979; Young and Hagbarth, 1980).

Spectral analysis

While, in many cases, simple inspection of surface EMG and force records suffices to demonstrate synchrony between the firing of motor units and force ripples (e.g. Elble and Randall, 1976; Hagbarth and Young, 1979), spectral analysis provides a more quantitative measure of rhythmic neural activity correlated with tremor oscillations. This is because spectral analysis permits the force oscillation to be identified as a peak along the frequency axis whose correlation with surface EMG can be tested for statistical significance via coherence analysis (Bendat and Piersol, 1971). Figure 8.3 is a sketch summarising the observations of several authors. As indicated in the figure, the coherence spectrum peaks just above

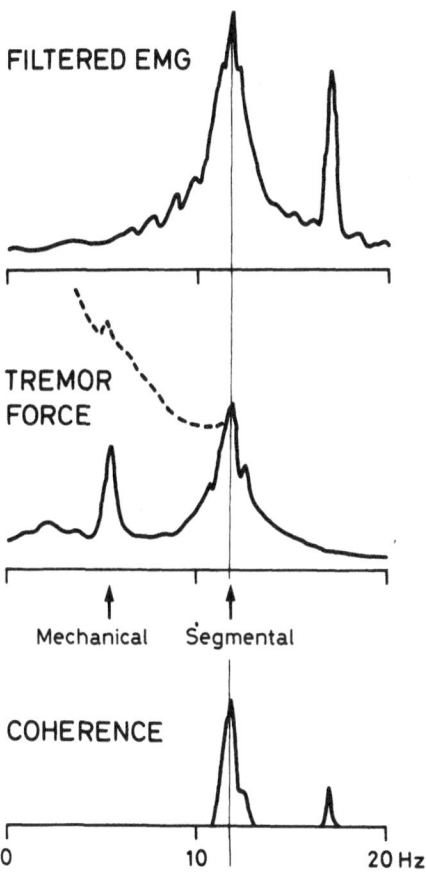

Figure 8.3 Sketch summarising common aspects of tremor spectra reported by Joyce and Rack (1974), Elble and Randall (1976), Stiles (1980), Matthews and Muir (1980), and Allum and Hulliger (1982). See text for detailed explanation.

11 Hz where the EMG and force spectra also have their maxima. This result establishes the close correlation between the moment-to-moment fluctuations in the filtered EMG records and oscillations in the simultaneously recorded force records (Elble and Randall, 1976; Stiles, 1980; Matthews and Muir, 1980; Allum and Hulliger, 1982). Indeed, the coherence values at ~11 Hz are so high that a phase-locking mechanism appears to exist between surface EMG and tremor

force. Faced with additional supporting evidence (see below), several authors have concluded that phase locking is provided by the segmental stretch reflex (Young and Hagbarth, 1980; Cussons *et al.*, 1980; Allum and Hulliger, 1982).

A second peak in the EMG spectrum is often observed between 15 and 20 Hz (Elble and Randall, 1976; Stiles, 1980; Allum and Hulliger, 1982). The coherence associated with this peak is generally small, though significant. A peak in the tremor force spectrum has not been identified in the same frequency band, probably because of the inherent attenuation, by muscle mechanical properties, of force resulting from EMG signals in this frequency range (Bawa and Stein, 1976; Allum *et al.*, 1978, figure 7).

Joyce and Rack (1974) observed two peaks in tremor force spectra. When a subject flexed his biceps against a spring of $6\,N\,mm^{-1}$, or less, spontaneous tremor occurred at the natural frequency of the mechanical system formed by the attached spring, forearm inertia and the muscle compliance. The corresponding peak in the force spectrum was well tuned (labelled 'mechanical' in figure 8.3) and not accompanied by a second peak at 11 Hz. It appears that the peaks associated with the mechanical system and that found under isometric conditions (labelled 'segmental' in figure 8.3) coalesce into a single peak if the natural frequency of the mechanical system lies between 6 and 12 Hz (Joyce and Rack, 1974; Matthews and Muir, 1980). Setting the spring constant to $13\,N\,mm^{-1}$, or greater, enhances the tendency for two peaks to occur in the force spectrum: one at ~11 Hz with a correlated peak in the EMG spectrum (Matthews and Muir, 1980) as shown in figure 8.3, and the other at the higher natural frequency of the mechanical system. That is, the mechanical peak in figure 8.3 is shifted more and more to the right of the 11 Hz peak as the mechanical natural frequency increases (Joyce and Rack, 1974). Whether or not the high-frequency, mechanical, peak is supported by neural signals is not known.

The reader is reminded that peaks in force spectra, which lie between 6 and 12 Hz, are superimposed upon low-frequency force modulations reflecting attempts by the subject to maintain the force level constant. When high-pass filtering of force records is not employed during isometric contractions, force spectra follow the course marked by the broken line in figure 8.3 (Allum *et al.*, 1978). Thus force spectra presented by different investigators are often dependent on the type of filtering used to amplify tremor peaks preferentially.

Spike-triggered averaging

To determine the delay and time course of a possible functional relationship between force changes and EMG signals during tremor, another technique, spike-triggered averaging (STA), is employed (Stein *et al.*, 1972). This technique uses single motor unit discharges (as shown in the top traces of figure 8.2) to trigger successive averages of EMG and force signals. Synchronisation of other motor units represented in surface EMG records and consistently related to the triggered unit is then apparent. The power of this technique is its ability to reveal exactly when prominent bursts of EMG activity are time-correlated to the twitch contraction of the triggered single motor unit (SMU). Thereby, supporting evidence can be accumulated for a contribution of central or short-term (Milner-Brown *et al.*, 1973a, 1975) and segmental stretch reflex or long-term (Allum and Hulliger, 1982) synchronising mechanisms in the generation of tremor. For this reason, the results of the STA technique are discussed in detail below.

MECHANISMS UNDERLYING HUMAN PHYSIOLOGICAL TREMOR

Central tremogenic mechanisms: short-term synchronisation of motor units

The hypothesis that a few unfused and occasionally synchronised motor units, discharging with rates close to their recruitment frequencies, are responsible for physiological tremor is attractive for its simplicity. According to this hypothesis, tremor oscillations are produced by a few newly recruited motor units whose discharges are brought into short-term synchrony (within ±15 ms of each other) either by a common input (of possible central origin) to the motoneurones or by chance (Allum *et al.*, 1978). It is then assumed that unfused twitches, and hence tremor oscillations, inevitably result from such synchronisation.

Newly recruited units are always the largest of all active motor units in a muscle, and their steady firing rates after recruitment are approximately the same (7 to 8.5 Hz) irrespective of their threshold force of recruitment (Milner-Brown *et al.*, 1973c; Freund *et ál.*, 1975). As newly recruited units discharge at rates close to the minimum sustainable rate, they are also the least fused of all active units. There is a rough similarity (within 3–4 Hz) between recruitment frequencies and the frequency of tremor force oscillations at all levels of maintained contraction. This fact and the correspondence between the increasing amplitude of the oscillations with increasing force level and the parallel increase in the size of the twitch contractions of newly recruited units with increasing force level provides supporting evidence for the hypothesis that short-term synchronisation underlies tremor (Allum *et al.*, 1978). Additional evidence, albeit indirect, is available when the ventral roots of cat muscles, whose afferent supply has been cut, are stimulated at frequencies close to those of recruitment. The resulting force oscillations and tremor spectra are remarkably similar to those of human physiological tremor (Allum *et al.*, 1978). Because there is not, however, a unique one-to-one relationship, this evidence is no more conclusive than that of a computer model which combines the waveforms of twitch contractions into a tremor-like force trajectory (Christakos and Lal, 1980). A more reasonable animal model for testing the correlation between naturally occurring random short-term motor unit synchrony and tremor is the behaviour of decerebrate cat soleus muscle during the tonic vibration reflex (Clark *et al.*, 1981). Here it appeared that about five of 150 soleus units firing in close synchrony could account for the tremor when Ia reflexes were blocked by 1 : 1 driving of spindle Ia afferents.

Further evidence for the correspondence between motor unit recruitment properties and the characteristics of physiological tremor is obtained by examining patients with Parkinson's disease. The motor units of parkinsonian patients have steady firing rates upon recruitment of 3–5 Hz which are significantly lower than normal rates (Dietz *et al.*, 1974). Also, the short-term synchronisation between the discharges of different motor units is pathologically greater than normal (Dietz *et al.*, 1976a,b). Consequently, the fundamental peak in the parkinsonian tremor spectrum is pronounced and occurs at a lower frequency (Allum *et al.*, 1978, figure 5) in accordance with the short-term synchronisation hypothesis.

Discussion

Two major questions need to be raised with respect to this hypothesis. First, how close is the correspondence between discharge frequencies just after units are recruited and the oscillation frequency of physiological tremor? Secondly, how many synchronised units out of all recruited units are required in order to produce tremor?

An unequivocal answer to the first question can be provided on the basis of data shown in figure 8.2 and the data used as the basis for the sketch of figure 8.3. The scatter in the joint interval histogram for 240 g (just above the threshold force for recruitment of the unit) in figure 8.2, compared to the scatter in histograms illustrated for higher force levels, indicates that, typically, motor units fire at more stable and constant rates once some rate modulation has occurred and the inter-spike intervals are 100 ms or less. Such intervals correspond more closely to the frequency of the 10–11 Hz peak in force and EMG spectra under isometric or near-isometric conditions (Joyce and Rack, 1974; Elble and Randall, 1976; Matthews and Muir, 1980; Allum and Hulliger, 1982) than the recruitment frequencies (7 to 8.5 Hz) of motor units in human hand muscles (Milner-Brown *et al.*, 1973c; Freund *et al.*, 1975; Monster and Chan, 1977). Thus it appears that units that have already undergone some rate modulation are responsible for tremor, and not those just recruited.

The second question raises the possibility that it may be difficult to assess synchronisation of motor units with previously used techniques (Dietz *et al.*, 1976a,b; Milner-Brown *et al.*, 1975), if total synchronisation is spread over many units. In any assessment of motor unit synchronisation responsible for tremor, it is important that an estimate be made of the number of units discharging with rates of 10–12 Hz. The data of Milner-Brown *et al.* (1973c) indicate that approximately 14 first dorsal interosseus motor units will be firing at 10–12 Hz when the muscle and its synergists exert a force of 0.7 kg (~20% of maximum). Twitch tensions of these units are between 5 and 20 g (Milner-Brown *et al.*, 1973b; Stephens and Usherwood, 1977). Thus, assuming an average twitch tension of 12.5 g, any three of these 14 units in total synchrony would be sufficient to generate the force oscillations observed in the trace of figure 8.2 (right).

The chances of locating two of these three synchronised units with needle elec-trodes would be about 1 in 33, and a result indicating no more than random synchronisation between motor units (Kranz and Baumgartner, 1974) may not be significant unless records have been taken from a larger number of pairs of units. If short-term synchronisation is either total, or partial and slightly more than random between units (Dietz *et al.*, 1976a,b), spike-triggered averaging (STA) of surface EMG might produce more significant results since the chance of locating one of the three totally synchronised units out of a total of 14 is, for example, at 0.7 kg just less than 1 in 4. The synchronisation of all other synchron-ised units will appear in the average surface EMG, and will thus provide more information than when only the discharge times of two separately recorded units are cross-correlated.

The STA technique relies on the difference between the shape of the triggered rectified surface EMG and the shape of the rectified motor unit potential used for triggering, to determine if short-term synchronisation occurred. Should the sur-face EMG record rise earlier, have a second maximum in any part of the interval ± 15 ms from the trigger time, or fall off later, then short-term synchronisation between motor units is assumed to be present (Milner-Brown *et al.*, 1973a, 1975). Typically, in normal subjects, units discharging near their recruitment frequencies show no significant short-term synchronisation with other units in the same muscle, although a weak trend towards increased synchronisation has been observed for larger motor units (Milner-Brown *et al.*, 1975).

Figure 8.4 illustrates how short-term synchronisation changes when a unit's discharge rate progresses from the recruitment frequency of 7 Hz (at which Milner-Brown *et al.* (1973a, 1975) examined STA surface EMG) to the tremor frequency of 11 Hz. It may be noted that the spread of the surface EMG record around the unit's discharge time (same unit and force levels as in figure 8.2) remained constant as force increased to 0.7 kg, but the height of the EMG trajectory increased. Since the unit's action potential did not change, the increased height can only be due to more units becoming synchronised with the triggered unit as rate modu-lation of the unit, with increasing force, caused it to discharge at tremor rates.

In summary, apart from the preliminary observation presented in figure 8.4, and the Milner-Brown *et al.* (1975) data for large motor units, there is little evidence to indicate a neural basis for short-term synchronisation. Rather, the available evidence tends to support the original assumption of Taylor (1962) that short-term synchronisation occurs by chance when motor units fire indepen-dently, but at the same mean frequency (Clark *et al.*, 1981).

Interactions between muscle mechanical and segmental stretch reflex mechanisms in the generation of tremor

When motor units discharge at rates lying between recruitment frequencies of 7 to 8.5 Hz and maximum steady firing rates of 20 Hz (Freund *et al.*, 1975; Monster and Chan, 1977), the peripheral mechanical system of the muscle and

SPIKE-TRIGGERED AVERAGED
SMOOTHED RECTIFIED EMG

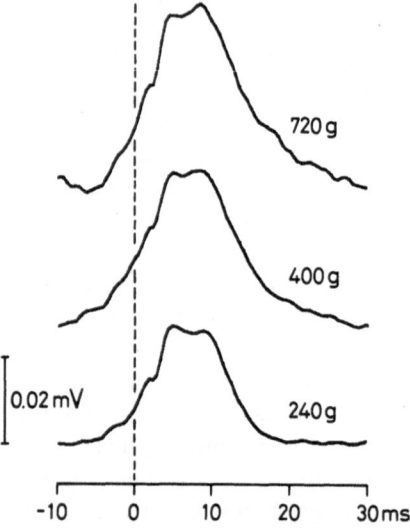

Figure 8.4 Surface EMG short-term synchronised to the same motor unit when force level was 240, 400 and 720 g. Original records are shown in figure 8.2. The trigger time on the rising slope of the triggered single motor unit action potential (not shown) is marked by the vertical broken line. To improve clarity the STA EMG records have been shifted vertically. With each force level increase, the amplitude of the surface EMG between -5 and 20 ms increased, implying that more motor units became synchronised to the triggering unit. (Previously unpublished records from Allum and Hulliger (1982).)

its load should oscillate most in response to forcing frequencies that are closest to its own natural frequency. The peripheral mechanical system comprises the limb inertia whose movements about a joint are resisted by the compliance of the agonist and antagonist muscles and the external load. Assuming that tremor arises when a chance synchronisation of motor units sets several of them discharging synchronously with rates equal to the natural frequency of the mechanical system, then changes in either intrinsic muscle compliance or the external load will alter the natural frequency of the mechanical system and the required motor unit frequency for tremor beating.

Muscle compliance consists of intrinsic elastic and viscous components whose characteristics are readily observed following a muscle stretch. The 'muscle force' trajectory, prior to 69 ms, in figure 8.5 shows the action of these components when human triceps surae muscles are stretched. Muscle force increases rapidly on stretch onset, but decreases once stretch velocity peaks. The amplitude of the initial stretch resistance increases with the level of prestretch muscle activity

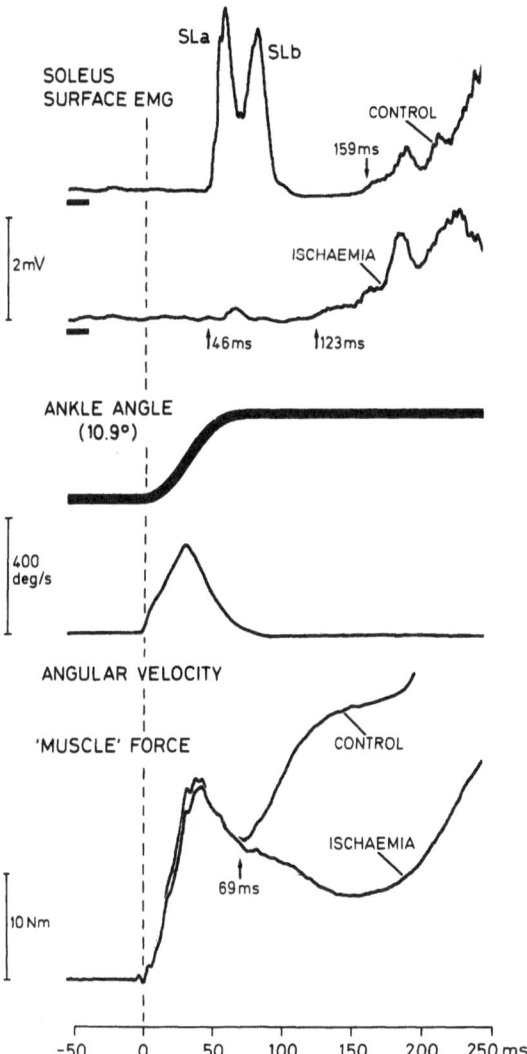

Figure 8.5 Separation of stretch reflex force into components due to intrinsic muscle compliance and force recruited by segmental reflexes. The separation was achieved by reducing the afferent response to stretch with an ischaemic block applied at the thigh and observing the change in the force response with respect to control responses. The top traces show rectified, smoothed EMG responses in the stretched soleus muscle following an $11°$ foot rotation about the ankle joint. An arrow at 46 ms marks the latency of the reflex EMG response with respect to rotation onset (peak acceleration). Absolute zero for the EMG traces is indicated by a short horizontal bar at the beginning of each trace. Incremental 'muscle' force responses from a prior torque of 8 N m are shown in the bottom set of traces. The diverging control and ischaemic force curves after 69 ms indicate the force contributed to the total stretch reflex by segmental reflex action. Each trace is the average of 10 responses. (Previously unpublished records from Allum *et al.* (1982c), from which further details may be obtained.)

(Allum *et al.*, 1982b), just as in the cat soleus muscle (Joyce *et al.*, 1969), and this result indicates that intrinsic muscle stiffness has also increased with force level. As the natural frequency of the peripheral mechanical system is dependent on the ratio of stiffness to inertia, an increase in the frequency and amplitude of tremor oscillations should result as force level is raised, provided limb inertia is held constant.

Discussion

Tremor about the human elbow joint increases in amplitude and slightly in frequency with more intense contractions of the biceps muscle (Joyce and Rack, 1974; Matthews and Muir, 1980) and is accompanied by an increase in the frequency of EMG signals driving the oscillations. This evidence supports the proposal that muscle mechanical properties must be integrated into an analysis of tremor since these can enhance or dampen out oscillations present in neural signals activating a muscle.

Continuing our examination of figure 8.5, it is clear that the preceding paragraphs have ignored reflex changes in motoneurone discharge that may affect tremor. Just as in figure 8.5 where stretch of triceps surae produces one or more bursts of EMG activity which give rise to a reflex contraction, stretch movements due to oscillation of a limb will also yield bursts of reflex EMG activity and reflex forces. Excitatory connections of muscle spindle afferents to motoneurones are the most likely cause for the early onset of EMG activity following stretch (Allum *et al.*, 1982c). In particular, muscle spindle primary afferents may well contribute to stretch responses during small tremor movements, because they are extremely sensitive to stretch acceleration even at low stretch amplitudes (Matthews and Stein, 1969; Poppele and Bowman, 1970; Poppele and Kennedy, 1974).

To explain a perpetuation of tremor force oscillations enhanced by reflex action, it is necessary to assume that the stretch in figure 8.5 was produced by the action of the antagonist tibialis anterior muscle, and not by a torque motor. The reflex recruited force must then overcome the stretch resistance of the antagonist muscle, and thereby stretch it to produce a reflex activation, which in turn will restretch the triceps muscle. Figure 8.5 illustrates that the force contributed by stretch reflex EMG activity (difference between the two force curves in figure 8.5) is about equal to that provided by intrinsic muscle stiffness, thus satisfying one condition for the development of tremor oscillations, namely, that reflex forces in the agonist must overcome intrinsic stretch resistance in the antagonist muscle and thus cause a limb movement. The period of such reflex generated oscillations would depend on the transmission delay in the segmental reflex arc, the activation delay and rise time of reflex generated force and tuning effects that the external load and muscle compliances provide. Should the reflex and activation delays equal the period associated with the natural frequency of the peripheral mechanical system, force oscillations will be sustained and in the corresponding tremor spectrum the neural and mechanical peaks would coalesce.

As described earlier (via figure 8.3), this effect is dependent on the correct choice for the external spring constant.

Two different types of indirect evidence suggest that segmental reflexes contribute to physiological tremor in the manner described above. First, when the arm is oscillated about the elbow joint at various frequencies and the work required by a motor to maintain the movement is examined, the minimum effort occurs at 10 Hz. The effort at 10 Hz is often negative, indicating that the arm does work on the motor (Joyce *et al.*, 1974; Matthews and Watson, 1981b). These authors concluded that segmental reflexes underlie the negative energy and could, therefore, sustain a tremor under appropriate external loading. Secondly, vibration applied to biceps tendon enhances both the EMG bursts and force oscillations of tremor (Cussons *et al.*, 1980). Here the supporting argument for an increased reflex contribution is based on the extreme sensitivity of muscle spindle afferents to longitudinally applied high-frequency (100 Hz) vibration (Brown *et al.*, 1967).

When applied transversely to human tendons, vibration can raise the mean firing rate of primary afferents without phase locking the afferent response to the vibration cycle (Burke *et al.*, 1976; Roll and Vedel, 1982). With an increased mean rate of Ia afferent fibres, it is assumed that their rate modulation can be deeper than normal during muscle shortening and lengthening and thus enhance the EMG response to stretch and, with it, tremor (Matthews and Watson, 1981a,b). While this line of reasoning is supported by most, but not all, experimental observations on the effect of vibration during sinusoidal stretching of biceps (Matthews and Watson, 1981b), it is not supported by the effect of vibration during controlled ramp stretches. In every muscle tested to date, vibration, without exception, reduced the early EMG response following a controlled muscle stretch (Hendrie and Lee, 1978; Allum *et al.*, 1982c; Jaeger *et al.*, 1982). More fitting to the EMG ramp stretch responses under vibratory conditions is the hypothesis that muscle spindle discharges help to damp out tremor (Goodwin *et al.*, 1978). Here it can be argued that vibration can also raise the mean Ia firing rate to such an extent that this firing rate is near the maximum possible (Roll and Vedel, 1982) and further modulation during stretch is much weaker than under control conditions. Partially saturating the spindle afferent signals by tendon vibration during tremor would then interfere with the stabilising function of Ia afferents and a larger EMG and force modulation would result as Cussons *et al.* (1980) observed. Clearly, recordings of human muscle spindle afferents during tremor and during forced stretch, with and without tendon vibration, might help to explain the different effects of vibration on EMG responses.

Massed afferent responses recorded during muscle fatigue (so-called 'enhanced' tremor) also indicate the participation of muscle spindle afferents in the generation of tremor (Hagbarth and Young, 1979; Young and Hagbarth, 1980). Accepting provisionally the argument that these microneurographic recordings were dominated by muscle spindle afferents (for detailed analysis and reservations, see Prochazka and Hulliger (1983)), it appears that each afferent burst generated the

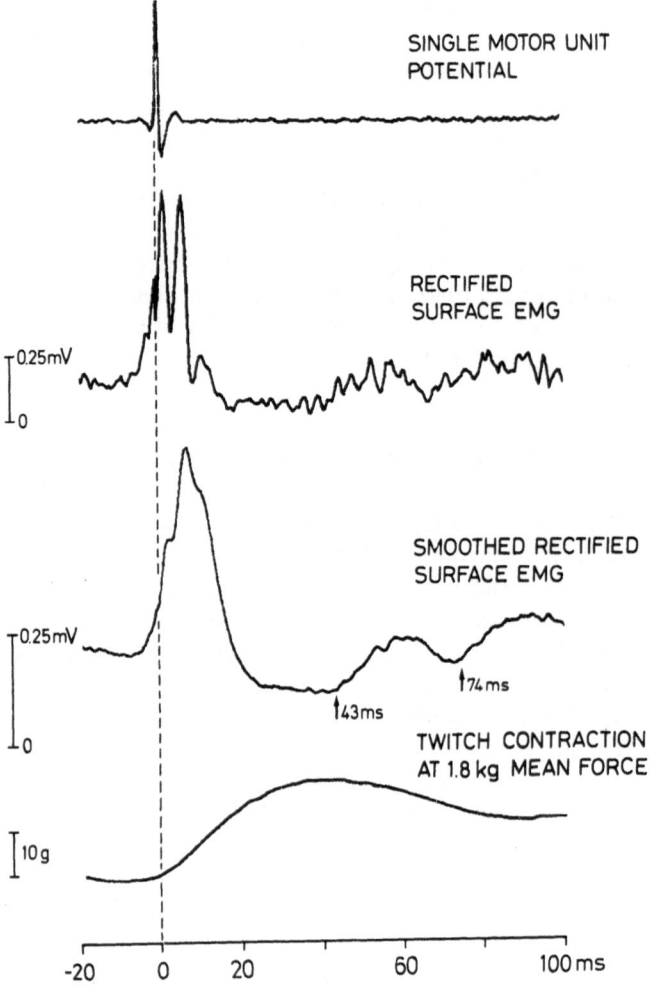

SINGLE MOTOR UNIT
POTENTIAL

RECTIFIED
SURFACE EMG

0.25mV

0

SMOOTHED RECTIFIED
SURFACE EMG

0.25mV

↑74ms

↑43ms

0

TWITCH CONTRACTION
AT 1.8 kg MEAN FORCE

10g

-20   0   20   60   100 ms

Figure 8.6 Bursts of surface EMG activity in human first dorsal interosseus muscle time-locked to twitch contractions in the same muscle. The motor unit, whose potential was used to trigger 40 times, was discharging with a modal rate of 6.5 Hz at its threshold force of 1.8 kg. Onset times for the bursts are indicated by arrows on the smoothed surface EMG trace. Zero on the EMG calibrations is the baseline for no activity. The onset of the twitch contraction prior to time zero indicates that other motor units were short-term synchronised to the triggering unit (cf. Clark *et al.*, 1978, figure 8). (Modified from Allum and Hulliger (1982, figure 1).)

succeeding EMG burst, as the delay between the two is approximately equal to the reflex transmission delay of 22 ms (Young and Hagbarth, 1980, figure 1). Unanswered by these data is the question how the afferent bursts were generated. Two possibilities arise. First, as described above, each antagonist EMG burst results in a 'twitch' force stretching the agonist muscle, thereby activating the agonist's muscle spindle afferents, and, after the reflex delay, causing an EMG burst in the same agonist muscle. Whereupon, the same process would be repeated with the agonist force stretching the antagonist muscle. Secondly, each EMG burst produces a 'twitch' contraction to which muscle spindle afferents in the same muscle respond during the falling phase of the contraction (cf. Binder *et al.*, 1976). Then, after the reflex delay, a new burst of EMG activity appears in the same muscle. That is, an interaction between agonist and antagonist muscles is not required for perpetuation of tremor. This second possibility is examined below.

Segmental tremogenic mechanisms: long-term synchronisation of motor units

The previous paragraphs have described a possible involvement of segmental reflexes in the genesis of tremor. Limb movements were assumed to be restricted by a compliant load, which nonetheless permitted external stretch of a muscle and its spindles. In this section, tremor under isometric conditions will be examined. Under these conditions afferent muscle activity can only result from internal shortening and lengthening of muscle during twitch contractions (cf. Binder *et al.*, 1976, 1977; Jansen and Rudjord, 1964). It will be suggested that the net effect of this afferent activity is to enhance tremor.

Stein and coworkers (Milner-Brown *et al.*, 1973a; Stein and Bawa, 1976) proposed that bursts of EMG activity, occurring during the falling phase of twitch contractions elicited by electrical stimulation, were generated by afferent activity and could be tremogenic. Evidence indicating massed afferent responses in response to electrical stimulation of the muscle nerve (Hagbarth and Young, 1979) complements Stein's findings. While responses to electrical stimulation may indicate the potential strength of a reflex, they provide little information on actual reflex action during naturally occurring twitch contractions of physiological tremor. To surmount this difficulty, the STA technique was employed (Allum and Hulliger, 1982).

Figure 8.6 illustrates the activity of the first dorsal interosseus (FDI) muscle time-locked to a twitch contraction occurring during the natural generation of muscle force. As shown by the third trace in the figure, the surface EMG activity paused during the rising phase of the twitch contraction, and was followed by two bursts of activity at 43 and 74 ms during the falling phase (that is, long-term synchronisation of motor units occurred). As a rule, only sections of data whose mean inter-spike interval was greater than 100 ms were employed for averaging, in order to ensure that no activity due to a second discharge of the triggering unit contributed to the EMG bursts at 43 and 74 ms. Two extra controls were employed for this purpose. First, discharges whose preceding inter-spike interval was less than 100 ms were not accepted as a trigger signal. Secondly, discharges of the triggering unit falling within the 100 ms averaging period were counted. Averaged records with a second discharge within 90 ms were removed from the data pool. The absence of motor unit potentials in the top trace of figure 8.6, at other than the trigger point, confirms the efficacy of these controls.

Discussion

Assuming the mechanisms underlying the EMG bursts are also active at higher discharge rates (see below), it is of interest to assess the relative strengths of the two bursts at 43 and 74 ms and their net effect on tremor. Force would be stabilised and tremor reduced by activity prior to 74 ms, because the early decrease in muscle activity occurs as the twitch tension is increasing and the first burst at 43 ms occurs as twitch tension begins to decrease. In contrast, if units with mean discharge rates of 10-11 Hz are responsible for tremor, the burst commencing at 74 ms would generate a destabilising force enhancing tremor providing the triggering unit occasionally discharged close to the discharge times of the 10-11 Hz units. Measurements indicate that the area under the burst at 74 ms equals, on average, 35% of that underlying the main EMG peak at zero time. The area under the burst at 43 ms was 21% of that of the main peak (Allum and Hulliger, 1982). On balance, the net effect of the two EMG bursts would appear to be tremogenic. The burst at 74 ms was still observed as the unit's firing rate increased, but it became more and more coalesced with a burst of surface EMG associated with a second discharge of the triggering unit (Allum and Hulliger, 1982, unpublished observations).

The question arises as to which segmental mechanisms could give rise to the pattern of muscle activity observed in figure 8.6 during a natural twitch contraction of tremor. It is possible that the early decreased EMG activity and the burst at 43 ms result from a decreased excitability of FDI motoneurones followed by a rebound effect, both mediated by the inhibitory connections of Renshaw cells (Eccles *et al.*, 1954; Granit *et al.*, 1957) or Golgi tendon organs (Jansen and Rudjord, 1964, Binder *et al.*, 1977). The second phase of EMG activity at 74 ms is most parsimoniously explained as the action of group Ia afferents during the falling phase of the twitch (Binder *et al.*, 1976).

The patterns of muscle afferent activity observed in human microneurographic records during electrically induced twitch tests provide a criterion for identifying afferents according to patterns expected from cat muscle Ia and Ib afferents (compare Burke *et al.*, 1976, figure 4E and Burg *et al.*, 1973, figure 2, with Matthews, 1972, figure 3.2 and Binder *et al.*, 1976, 1977). Once identified, it would be desirable to correlate EMG burst activity during a natural twitch with afferent discharges using the STA technique in two steps. First, with a motor unit discharge used as the trigger, both EMG and afferent bursts correlated to the twitch contraction waveform can be observed. Secondly, when the afferent discharge is employed as the trigger, the delay and amplitude of surface EMG activity correlated with the afferent discharge can be established. With this information the question as to which segmental pathways, associated with specific afferents, can enhance or dampen tremor would be more clearly answered.

To date, such experiments have not been completed, although bursts in massed afferent records, supposedly dominated by Ia afferents, have been reported to commence and terminate some 22 ms (one segmental reflex delay time) before the onset and offset of EMG bursts in the same muscle during 'enhanced' tremor (Hagbarth and Young, 1979; Young and Hagbarth, 1980). Here though, Prochazka and Hulliger (1983) suggest that Golgi tendon organ afferents and α-efferents may well have contributed to these massed responses because a burst of activity also occurred for the same massed afferent recordings during the rising phase of an electrically induced twitch contraction (Young and Hagbarth, 1980, figure 2B). If the massed afferent recordings were dominated by Ia afferents, such early burst activity during an electrically induced twitch should have been weak or absent. Clearly, with single afferents, the STA procedure outlined above could be profitably employed to clarify these doubts.

CONCLUSIONS

The evidence reviewed here suggests that segmental reflexes generate tremor by promoting long-term synchronisation (43 and 74 ms) between motor units. Two mechanisms were suggested for the participation of segmental reflexes in tremor. One, when the limb is free to oscillate, relied on stretch-generated contraction in one muscle of an antagonist–agonist pair to produce the next stretch in the other muscle. The second mechanism, present during isometric contractions, depended on twitch-generated afferent activity in the contracting muscle to perpetuate tremor. Each mechanism was postulated as the cause of 10-11 Hz rhythms of EMG activity significantly correlated with tremor force oscillations at the same frequency. The extent to which these two mechanisms cooperate with each other when a limb is free to move should be the subject of further research.

Neither short-term synchronisation (less than 15 ms) of motor units nor an oscillation of the peripheral mechanical system formed by the muscles and their load appear to play a major tremogenic role. Short-term synchronisation between motor units which is greater than random is exceptionally observed. Normally, the peripheral mechanical system only begins to dominate tremor when a spring load is applied to the limb.

Advances in our understanding of mechanisms generating tremor have occurred through detailed application of the STA technique. It is hoped that continued application of this technique with motor unit and muscle afferent discharges as trigger signals will provide a more quantitative basis on which to determine how muscle spindle and Golgi tendon organ afferents may, via segmental reflexes, enhance or dampen out physiological tremor, and perhaps be of later use in the diagnosis and understanding of pathological tremor forms.

ACKNOWLEDGEMENTS

The author's research cited in the chapter was supported by the Swiss National Science Foundation Grants 3.585.79 and 3.505.79, the Dr Eric-Slack-Gyr and Sandoz Foundations and Deutsche Forschungsgemeinschaft Grant SFB 70.

It is a pleasure to thank Ms R. Aegerter and B. Hofer for typing the manuscript. Dr P. B. C. Matthews provided valuable comments on the manuscript.

REFERENCES

Allum, J. H. J., Dietz, V. and Freund, H.-J. (1978). Neuronal mechanisms underlying physiological tremor. *J. Neurophysiol.*, 41, 557-71.

Allum, J. H. J., Hepp-Reymond, M. C. and Gysin, R. (1982a). Cross-correlation analysis of interneuronal connectivity in the motor cortex of the monkey. *Brain Res.*, 231, 325-34.

Allum, J. H. J. and Hulliger, M. (1982). Presumed reflex responses of human first dorsal interosseus muscle to naturally occurring twitch contractions of physiological tremor. *Neurosci. Lett.*, 28, 309-14.

Allum, J. H. J., Mauritz, K.-H. and Vögele, H. (1982b). Stiffness regulation provided by short-latency reflexes in human triceps surae muscles. *Brain Res.*, 234, 159-64.

Allum, J. H. J., Mauritz, K.-H. and Vögele, H. (1982c). The mechanical effectiveness of short latency reflexes in human triceps surae muscles revealed by ischemia and vibration. *Exp. Brain Res.*, 48, 153-6.

Asanuma, H., Zarzecki, P., Jankowska, E., Hongo, T. and Marcus, S. (1979). Projection of individual pyramidal tract neurons to lumbar motor nuclei of the monkey. *Exp. Brain Res.*, 34, 73-89.

Bawa, P. and Stein, R. B. (1976). Frequency response of human soleus muscle. *J. Neurophysiol.*, 39, 788-93.

Bendat, J. S. and Piersol, A. G. (1971). *Random Data: Analysis and Measurement Procedures*, Wiley-Interscience, New York.

Binder, M. D., Kroin, J. S., Moore, G. P., Stauffer, E. K. and Stuart, D. G. (1976). Correlation analysis of muscle spindle responses to single motor unit contractions. *J. Physiol.*, 257, 325-36.

Binder, M. D., Kroin, J. S., Moore, G. P. and Stuart, D. G. (1977). The response of Golgi tendon organs to single motor unit contractions. *J. Physiol.*, 271, 337-49.

Brown, M. C., Engberg, I. and Matthews, P. B. C. (1967). The relative sensitivity to vibration of muscle receptors of the cat. *J. Physiol. (Lond.)*, 192, 773-800.

Burg, D., Szumski, A. J., Struppler, A. and Velho, F. (1973). Afferent and efferent activation of human muscle receptors involved in reflex and voluntary contraction. *Exp. Neurol.*, 41, 754-68.

Burke, D., Hagbarth, K.-E., Lofstedt, L. and Wallin, B. G. (1976). The response of human muscle spindle endings to vibration during isometric contraction. *J. Physiol. (Lond.)*, 261, 695-711.

Christakos, C. N. and Lal, S. (1980). Lumped and population stochastic models of skeletal muscle: implications and predictions. *Biol. Cybern.*, 36, 73-85.

Clark, F. J., Matthews, P. B. C. and Muir, R. B. (1981). Motor unit firing and its relation to tremor in the tonic vibration reflex of the decerebrate cat. *J. Physiol.*, 313, 317-34.

Clark, R. W., Luschei, E. S. and Hoffman, D. S. (1978). Recruitment order, contractile characteristics and firing patterns of motor units in the temporalis muscle of monkeys. *Exp. Neurol.*, **61**, 31–52.

Cussons, P. D., Matthews, P. B. C. and Muir, R. B. (1980). Enhancement by agonist or antagonist muscle vibration of tremor at the elastically loaded human elbow. *J. Physiol.*, **302**, 443–61.

Dietz, V., Bischofberger, E., Wita, C. and Freund, H.-J. (1976a). Correlation between the discharges of two simultaneously recorded motor units and physiological tremor. *EEG Clin. Neurophysiol.*, **40**, 97–105.

Dietz, V., Freund, H.-J. and Allum, J. H. J. (1976b). Parkinsonian tremor during rest and voluntary contraction and its correlation with single motor unit activity. In Birkmayer, W. and Hornykiewicz, O. (eds). *Advances in Parkinsonism*, Roche, Basel, pp. 244–50.

Dietz, V., Hillesheimer, W. and Freund, H.-J. (1974). Correlation between tremor, voluntary contraction and firing pattern of motor units in Parkinson's disease. *J. Neurol. Neurosurg. Psychiatr.*, **37**, 927–37.

Eccles, J. C., Fatt, P. and Koketsu, K. (1954). Cholinergic and inhibitory synapses in pathway from motor axon collaterals to motoneurones. *J. Physiol.*, **126**, 524–62.

Elble, R. J. and Randall, J. E. (1976). Motor-unit activity responsible for 8- to 12-Hz component of human physiological finger tremor. *J. Neurophysiol.*, **39**, 370–83.

Fetz, E. E., Cheney, P. D. and German, D. C. (1976). Cortico-motoneuronal connections of precentral cells detected by post-spike averages of EMG activity in behaving monkeys. *Brain Res.*, **114**, 505–10.

Freund, H.-J., Budingen, H. J. and Dietz, V. (1975). Activity of single motor units from human forearm muscles during voluntary isometric contractions. *J. Neurophysiol.*, **38**, 933–46.

Goodwin, G. M., Hoffman, D. and Luschei, E. S. (1978). The strength of the reflex response to sinusoidal stretch of monkey jaw closing muscles during voluntary contraction. *J. Physiol. (Lond.)*, **279**, 81–111.

Gottlieb, G. L. and Agarwal, G. C. (1970). Filtering of electromyographic signals. *Am. J. Phys. Med.*, **49**, 142–6.

Granit, R., Pascoe, J. E. and Steg, G. (1957). The behaviour of tonic α- and γ-motoneurones during stimulation of recurrent collaterals. *J. Physiol. (Lond.)*, **138**, 381–400.

Hagbarth, K. E. and Young, R. R. (1979). Participation of the stretch reflex in human physiological tremor. *Brain*, **102**, 509–26.

Hendrie, A. and Lee, R. G. (1978). Selective effects of vibration on human spinal and long-loop reflexes. *Brain Res.*, **157**, 369–75.

Jaeger, R. J., Gottlieb, G. L., Agarwal, G. C. and Tahmoush, A. J. (1982). Afferent contributions to stretch-evoked myoelectric responses. *J. Neurophysiol.*, **48**, 403–18.

Jansen, J. K. S. and Rudjord, T. (1964). On the silent period and Golgi tendon organs of the soleus muscle of the cat. *Acta Physiol. Scand.*, **62**, 364–79.

Joyce, G. C. and Rack, P, M. H. (1974). The effects of load and force on tremor at the normal human elbow joint. *J. Physiol.*, **240**, 375–96.

Joyce, G. C., Rack, P. M. H. and Ross, H. F. (1974). The forces generated at the human elbow joint in response to imposed sinusoidal movements of the forearm. *J. Physiol.*, **240**, 351–74.

Joyce, G. C., Rack, P. M. H. and Westbury, D. R. (1969). The mechanical properties of cat soleus muscle during controlled lengthening and shortening movements. *J. Physiol.*, **204**, 461–74.

Kranz, H. and Baumgartner, G. (1974). Human alpha motoneurone discharge, a statistical analysis. *Brain Res.*, 67, 324-9.

Matthews, P. B. C. (1972). *Mammalian Muscle Receptors and Their Central Actions*, Edward Arnold, London.

Matthews, P. B. C. and Muir, R. B. (1980) Comparison of electromyogram spectra with force spectra during human elbow tremor. *J. Physiol.*, 302, 427-41.

Matthews, P. B. C. and Stein, R. B. (1969). The sensitivity of muscle spindle afferents to small sinusoidal changes of length. *J. Physiol.*, 200, 723-43.

Matthews, P. B. C. and Watson, J. D. G. (1981a). Action of vibration on the response of cat muscle spindle Ia afferents to low frequency sinusoidal stretching. *J. Physiol.*, 317, 365-81.

Matthews, P. B. C. and Watson, J. D. G. (1981b). Effect of vibrating agonist or antagonist muscle on the reflex response of sinusoidal displacement of the human forearm. *J. Physiol.*, 321, 297-316.

Milner-Brown, H. S., Stein, R. B. and Lee, R. G. (1975). Synchronization of human motor units: possible roles of exercise and supraspinal reflexes. *EEG Clin. Neurophysiol.*, 38, 245-54.

Milner-Brown, H. S., Stein, R. B. and Yemm, R. (1973a). The contractile properties of human motor units during voluntary isometric contractions. *J. Physiol.*, 228, 285-306.

Milner-Brown, H. S., Stein, R. B. and Yemm, R. (1973b). The orderly recruitment of human motor units during voluntary isometric contractions. *J. Physiol.*, 230, 359-70.

Milner-Brown, H. S., Stein, R. B. and Yemm, R. (1973c). Changes in firing rate of human motor units during linearly changing voluntary contractions. *J. Physiol.*, 230, 371-90.

Monster, A. W. and Chan, H. (1977). Isometric force production by motor units of extensor digitorum communis muscle in man. *J. Neurophysiol.*, 40, 1432-43.

Moore, G. P., Segundo, J. P., Perkel, D. H. and Levitan, H. (1970). Statistical signs of synaptic interaction in neurons. *Biophys. J.*, 10, 876-900.

Poppele, R. E. and Bowman, R. J. (1970). Quantitative description of linear behaviour of mammalian muscle spindles. *J. Neurophysiol.*, 33, 59-72.

Poppele, R. E. and Kennedy, W. R. (1974). Comparison between behavior of human and cat muscle spindles recorded in vitro. *Brain Res.*, 75, 316-19.

Prochazka, A. and Hulliger, M. (1983). Muscle afferent function during voluntary movements in cat, monkey and man. In Desmedt, J. E. (ed.), *Motor Control in Health and Disease*, Raven Press, New York, in press

Rack, P. M. H. (1978). Mechanical and reflex factors in human tremor. In Desmedt, J. E. (ed.), *Physiological Tremor, Pathological Tremors and Clonus, Progress in Clinical Neurophysiology*, vol. 5, Karger, Basel, pp. 17-27.

Roll, J. P. and Vedel, J. P. (1982). Kinaesthetic role of muscle afferents in man, studied by tendon vibration and microneurography. *Exp. Brain Res.*, 47, 177-90.

Stein, R. B. and Bawa, P. (1976). Reflex responses of human soleus muscle to small perturbations. *J. Neurophysiol.*, 39, 1105-16.

Stein, R. B., French, A. S., Mannard, A. and Yemm, R. (1972). New methods for analysing motor function in man and animals. *Brain Res.*, 40, 187-92.

Stein, R. B. and Oğuztöreli, M. N. (1976). Tremor and other oscillations in neuromuscular systems. *Biol. Cybern.*, 22, 147-57.

Stephens, J. A. and Usherwood, T. P. (1977). The mechanical properties of human motor units with special reference to their fatiguability and recruitment threshold. *Brain Res.*, 125, 91-7.

Stiles, R. R. (1980). Mechanical and neural feedback factors in postural hand tremor of normal subjects. *J. Neurophysiol.*, **44**, 40–59.

Taylor, A. (1962). The significance of grouping of motor unit activity. *J. Physiol.*, **162**, 259–69.

Young, R. R. and Hagbarth, K. E. (1980). Physiological tremor enhanced by manoeuvres affecting the segmental stretch reflex. *J. Neurol. Neurosurg. Psychiatr.*, **43**, 248–56.

9
Muscle spindle discharge patterns in tremor and clonus

KARL-ERIK HAGBARTH

INTRODUCTION

A much-debated question is to what extent the segmental stretch reflex partici-pates in the production of clonus and different types of tremor. With the techni-que of microneurography (Vallbo *et al.*, 1979) it has become possible to make recordings from muscle spindle afferents in man and such recordings combined with electromyography can help us to discriminate between those types of rhyth-mical alternating movements which are and those which are not dependent on stretch reflex oscillations.

The recordings illustrated in this chapter are taken from nerve fibres identified as group Ia muscle spindle afferents—the large-diameter, fast-conducting fibres which constitute the afferent link of the segmental stretch reflex arc. The signals in these large afferent fibres are easily discerned in microelectrode recordings, in contrast to the signals in smaller myelinated fibres which are much more difficult to detect. No one has so far succeeded in recording from or identifying the signals in the human gamma fibres—the fusimotor fibres of the spindles. However, by means of recordings from Ia afferents it is possible to study the two ways in which the spindles can be activated, either externally by passive muscle stretch or internally by fusimotor-induced intrafusal contractions.

VOLUNTARY MOVEMENT

These two types of spindle activation can be clearly seen in healthy subjects during voluntary alternating movements, where periods of contraction alternate with phases of relaxation and passive stretch. These are illustrated in figure 9.1. The upper trace in figure 9.1 shows Ia signals from a spindle in the anterior tibial muscle while the subject tries to move his foot quickly up and down, thus contracting his pretibial muscles in a rhythmical manner as seen in the bottom EMG trace. Each EMG burst is followed by a rise in torque (middle trace) and in between are the relaxation phases indicated by downward deflections. As

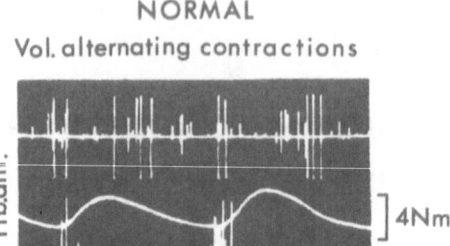

NORMAL
Vol. alternating contractions

Figure 9.1 Afferent discharges from a primary spindle ending in the anterior tibial muscle (upper trace) during rhythmical fast voluntary contractions of this muscle (the subject trying to move his foot quickly up and down). Note how the two bursts of spindle discharges that occur during each movement cycle are timed in relation to the EMG bursts in the anterior tibial muscle (bottom trace) and to the relaxation phases (indicated by downward deflections in the middle torque record). From Hagbarth *et al.* (1975a).

illustrated, the EMG bursts are accompanied by short bursts of spindle discharges, a sign indicating that these voluntary extrafusal contractions are linked with a fusimotor outflow activating the spindle endings. During the relaxation phases the spindles fire again, just as they also do during the falling phases of electrically induced muscle twitches. So, during each cycle of these rhythmical voluntary contractions the spindles tend to fire twice: once during the contraction and once during the relaxation phase. This pattern of spindle firing is also seen when recording from finger and wrist flexors during voluntary alternating hand movements.

The records in figure 9.2 (left) show examples of how spindles in relaxed human muscles (finger flexors, anterior tibial muscle, gastrocnemius) respond when exposed to passive alternating joint movements. They all respond with bursts of repetitive discharges during the stretch phases and silence during the shortening phases. For some spindle endings alternating joint movements of less than 1° are sufficient to induce this rhythmical driving. Typically, the spindles also fire during the falling phase of electrically induced muscle twitches, as shown in the records to the right. The flat EMG records (bottom traces) serve to illustrate that the subjects, as instructed, were relaxed in the receptor-bearing muscles. In this situation the EMG shows no sign of stretch reflexes appearing in response to the rhythmical afferent stretch discharges.

PASSIVE MOVEMENT

If, instead, the subject is instructed to maintain a steady voluntary contraction in the muscle, the passive alternating movements produce not only afferent spindle

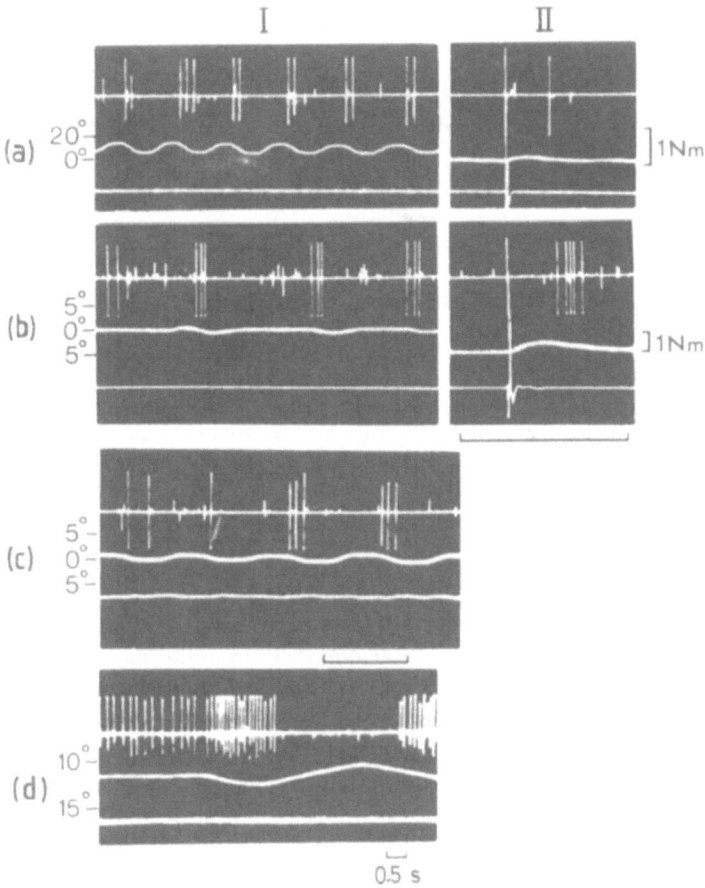

Figure 9.2 Afferent discharges from primary spindle endings in relaxed muscles exposed to passive alternating joint movements (left) and to electrically induced twitches (right). Spindles fire during the stretch phases (downward deflections in the goniometer and torque traces) and keep silent during the shortening phases. The flat EMG records from the relaxed muscles (bottom traces) show no sign of stretch reflex responses. From Hagbarth *et al.* (1975a).

discharges during the stretch phases but also a rhythmical reflex modulation of the EMG activity. The upper trace in figure 9.3 shows recurrent bursts of afferent stretch discharges from the pretibial muscles during passive alternating foot movements, and the middle trace shows the rhythmical grouping of the EMG activity. As judged by the latency between afferent and motor bursts, which is about 30 ms, the segmental stretch reflex is involved here, synchronising the motor discharges. This motor synchronising effect of passive alternating movements was shown by Hoffman 50 years ago (Hoffman, 1922). When varying the frequency of the passive alternating movements one finds that the synchronisation

NORMAL

Externally driven clonus

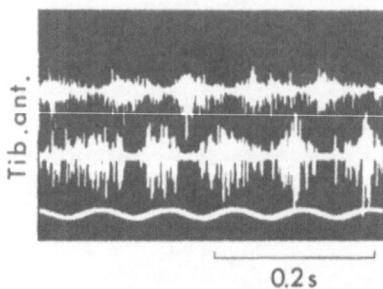

0.2 s

Figure 9.3 Multi-unit afferent stretch discharges from the anterior tibial muscle (upper trace) during passive alternating foot movements at about 10 Hz, the subject trying to maintain a steady voluntary contraction in the pretibial muscles. Note rhythmical grouping of EMG signals in these muscles (middle trace) and the delay of about 30 ms between afferent and motor bursts. See text.

becomes most pronounced somewhere between 7 and 10 Hz. It is within this frequency range that the mechanical contractions following each EMG burst happen to coincide with the passively induced shortening phases (Rack, 1978). One is likely to be disappointed if one tries by muscle power to damp a machine which is vibrating at this rate of 7–10 Hz. By adding one's own muscle power and stretch reflexes to the machine the vibrations only become greater in amplitude the more one tries to damp them. If we want to give this normal phenomenon a name, I think we can call it 'externally driven clonus'. Unlike in voluntary alternating contractions (cf. figure 9.1), in the nerve recording of figure 9.3 only the externally induced stretch discharges can be seen; there is no sign of fusimotor-induced spindle activation accompanying the EMG bursts. This seems reasonable since the segmental stretch reflex operates predominantly on the α-motoneurones, not on the fusimotor neurones.

PHYSIOLOGICAL TREMOR

In certain situations the stretch reflex in contracting muscles of healthy subjects may become sufficiently powerful to generate rhythmical movements by its own activity, without any external driving force. I am referring to the physiological finger and wrist tremor which can be enhanced by different manoeuvres and which is then accompanied by distinct rhythmical grouping of the EMG signals in the wrist and finger flexors, as seen in the bottom trace of figure 9.4. The multi-unit recording from the muscle nerve (upper trace) shows afferent stretch discharges occurring 20–25 ms before the EMG bursts and coinciding with the falling phases of the twitches (middle trace).

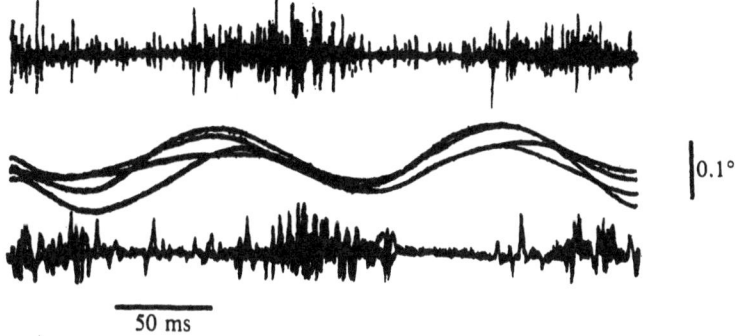

Figure 9.4 Multi-unit afferent stretch discharges from a wrist flexor muscle (upper trace) during physiological wrist tremor in a healthy subject holding the hand outstretched. Note delay of 20–25 ms between afferent impulse bursts and EMG bursts in wrist flexors. Downward deflections in goniometer trace indicate phases in the tremor cycle when wrist flexors are being stretched. From Hagbarth and Young (1979).

It is well known that physiological tremor tends to be enhanced following a prolonged voluntary contraction. Different mechanisms may be responsible for this so-called 'fatigue' enhancement of the tremor. One causative factor is probably the change in contractile properties of muscle fibres that results from long-lasting contractions. A comparison of records (a) and (b) in figure 9.5 shows that the wrist tremor was greatly enhanced when the hand had been held lifted and outstretched for about 20 min. The grouping of the afferent stretch discharges, the grouping in the EMG and the mechanical oscillations were quite pronounced at the end of this 20 min period. The traces in (d) show that such a long-lasting contraction causes a potentiation of the mechanical twitch responses to single supramaximal nerve stimuli. Such a change in the contractile properties of the muscles will enhance the oscillatory tendency of the system. If the mechanical twitches resulting from a rhythmical motor outflow become stronger and with steeper falling phases, the spindle discharges during these falling phases also become stronger and more efficient in eliciting new reflex contractions.

As shown by Marsden and Meadows (1970), changes in contractile properties of human muscles can also be induced by adrenaline and other beta-adrenergic agonists. Such drugs speed up muscle twitches and the relaxation phases become steeper. In a similar way as with 'fatigue' tremor, this will enhance the system's tendency to oscillate.

CLONUS

If we now turn to pathological types of involuntary alternating movements, we may first look at the spindle discharge patterns during sustained clonus in spastic

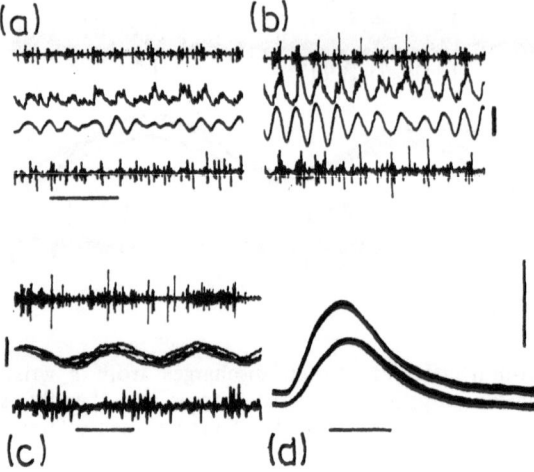

Figure 9.5 'Fatigue' enhancement of physiological wrist tremor. Top to bottom in (a) and (b): grouped afferent stretch discharges from the wrist flexors (shown in original and mean voltage neurograms), tremulous wrist movements and grouped EMG signals in wrist flexors in healthy subject soon after positioning his hand in outstretched position (a) and after having kept this position for 20 min (b). Time marker: 0.5 s. (c) Time relation between afferent stretch discharges, EMG bursts and tremulous movements during 'fatigue'. Time marker: 0.1 s. (d) Wrist flexor mechanical twitch responses to supramaximal nerve stimuli before (bottom trace) and after (top trace) a prolonged (10 min) voluntary wrist flexor contraction. Time marker: 0.1 s. From Young and Hagbarth (1980).

patients. Figure 9.6 shows a recording from a hemiplegic patient in whom sustained calf muscle clonus was easily elicited by a single Achilles tendon tap. The spindle and EMG discharges are timed in relation to each other and to the mechanical oscillations at 6–7 Hz: there is about 30 ms reflex delay between each spindle discharge and the succeedding EMG burst, and thereafter about 80–100 ms until the spindle fires again during the falling phase of the ensuing muscle contraction. The pattern is similar to that seen in 'externally driven clonus' and physiological tremor of healthy subjects. The differences is that in spastic patients the dynamic stretch reflex is strong enough to keep the oscillations going without any external drive and without any voluntary background contraction. One should realise, however, that when the clinician with his own muscle force elicits clonus in a spastic patient, he tends to get an 'externally driven clonus' in his own muscles, and this may harmonise with and enhance the clonus of the patient. A major difference between enhanced physiological tremor and clonus may be that in the former the stretch reflex merely affects the timing of discharges in an already firing motoneurone pool, whereas in the latter the spindle stretch discharges are the main generators of the rhythmical skeletomotor outflow.

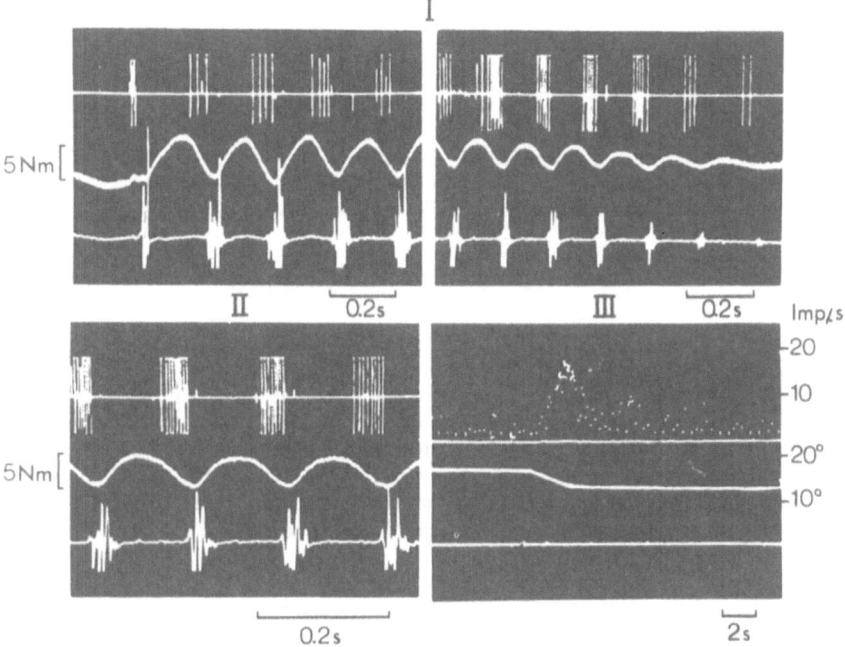

Figure 9.6 I and II: Afferent stretch discharges from a primary spindle ending in the medial gastrocnemius muscle during ankle clonus in hemiplegic patient (upper traces). Note delay of about 30 ms between spindle bursts which occur during calf muscle relaxation phases (downward deflections in torque traces) and succeeding reflex responses in calf muscle EMG (bottom traces). III: Same spindle ending responding to slow passive stretch movement. Top to bottom: instantaneous frequency plot of unit discharges, ankle joint goniometer trace, and flat EMG from relaxed calf muscles. From Hagbarth *et al.* (1975b).

PARKINSON'S DISEASE

Finally we come to the resting finger and wrist tremor in patients with Parkinson's disease. Figure 9.7 shows a recording from such a patient. In these abnormal alternating movements we can recognise a similar spindle discharge pattern as seen in the voluntary alternating movements of healthy subjects. The spindles tend to discharge twice during each movement cycle—once during the contraction and once during the relaxation phase. Since the EMG bursts are accompanied by signs of fusimotor co-activation of the spindles, the rhythmical contractions are in this case apparently not driven by the segmental stretch reflex. Even though input from the periphery can modify the phasing and amplitude of this tremor, the oscillatory movements are not critically dependent on rhythmical peripheral sensory feedback. Our findings agree with the suggestions that parkinsonian

Parkinsonian tremor

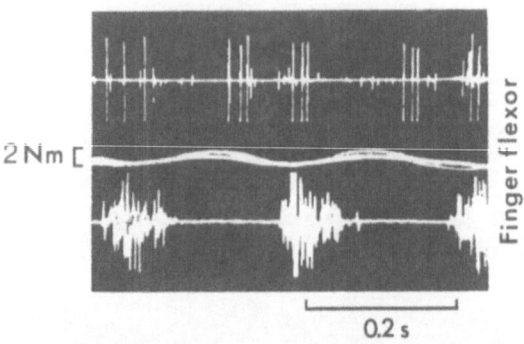

Figure 9.7 Afferent discharges from a primary spindle ending in a finger flexor muscle during resting finger tremor in a patient with Parkinson's disease. In a similar way as in voluntary alternating movements of healthy subjects (cf. figure 9.1) spindle discharges occur twice during each movement cycle: once in conjunction with the finger flexor EMG burst (bottom trace) and once during the relaxation phase (downward deflection in torque trace). From Hagbarth *et al.* (1975b).

tremor results from involuntary activation of a motor programme that is stored somewhere in the CNS and is normally utilised in the production of rapid voluntary alternating movements (Alberts, 1972).

REFERENCES

Alberts, W. W. (1972). A simple view of Parkinsonian tremor. Electrical stimulation of cortex adjacent to the Rolandic fissure in awake man. *Brain Res.*, **44**, 357-69.

Hagbarth, K.-E., Wallin, G. and Löfstedt, L. (1975a). Muscle spindle activity in man during voluntary fast alternating movements. *J. Neurol. Neurosurg. Psychiatr.*, **38**, 625-35.

Hagbarth, K.-E., Wallin, G., Löfstedt, L. and Aquilonius, S.-M. (1975b). Muscle spindle activity in alternating tremor of Parkinsonism and in clonus. *J. Neurol. Neurosurg. Psychiatr.*, **38**, 636-41.

Hagbarth, K.-E. and Young, R. R. (1979). Participation of the stretch reflex in human physiological tremor. *Brain*, **102**, 509-26.

Hoffman, P. (1922). *Die Eigenreflexe*, Springer, Berlin.

Marsden, C. D. and Meadows, J. C. (1970). The effect of adrenaline on the contraction of human muscle. *J. Physiol. (Lond.)*, **207**, 429-48.

Rack, P. M. H. (1978). Mechanical and reflex factors in human tremor. In Desmedt, J. E. (ed.), *Progress in Clinical Neurophysiology*, vol. 5, Karger, Basel, pp. 17-27.

Vallbo, Å, B., Hagbarth, K.-E., Torebjörk, H. E. and Wallin, B. G. (1979). Somatosensory, proprioceptive and sympathetic activity in human peripheral nerves. *Physiol. Rev.*, **59**, 919-57.

Young, R. R. and Hagbarth, K.-E. (1980). Physiological tremor enhanced by manoeuvres affecting the segmental stretch reflex. *J. Neurol. Neurosurg. Psychiatr.*, **43**, 248-56.

10
Rebound excitation as the physiological basis for tremor: a biophysical study of the oscillatory properties of mammalian central neurones *in vitro*

INTRODUCTION

Tremor as a sign of brain malfunction has been a topic of speculation and conjecture for over 400 years (see Capildeo, this volume, chapter 20). From a neurological point of view, the customary approach to this problem has been that of attempting to link, causally, the anatomical location and extent of central lesions to the nature of the functional abnormalities. Indeed, over the years the variances of tremor that may be seen following single or combined lesions at different sites in the CNS of man as well as of experimental animals have been described in great detail. This approach has yielded an enormous wealth of clinical information. However, the lack of a set of mechanism-related concepts serving as a common denominator for these observations has impeded the development of a truly systematic classification of tremor. Moreover, on occasion, the purely phenomenological approach has yielded conflicting views, leading to disagreement regarding both the nomenclature and the genesis of this class of motor abnormality. Thus, as underlined by Marsden (this volume, chapter 4), the categories of disagreement are many and at times quite profound, one much aired being that of the central versus peripheral nature of several of the human tremors.

From a functional point of view, therefore, the first goal in considering the genesis of tremors must be their categorisation on the basis of the underlying cellular and network pathophysiology. Indeed, the use of anatomical location to denote functional abnormality (e.g. cerebellar tremor) creates the illusion of a causal relation between the 'function' of the lesion site and the neurological symptomatology being described.

The importance of this initial point cannot be overemphasised—nomenclature should not be simply a convenient mnemonic for site of the lesion but rather it should relate to mechanism as well as to origin.

165

TREMOR AS A REFLECTION OF THE INTRINSIC OSCILLATORY PROPERTY OF NEURONES AND ITS MATCHING TO THE DYNAMIC PROPERTIES OF THE PERIPHERAL EFFECTOR SYSTEM

Tremor does not necessarily result from damage to a specific site in the neuraxis; more often it is the expression of a dynamic shift in the functional organisation of neuronal circuits or of the modification of basic electrophysiological properties of cells comprising certain nuclei. Tremor may, thus, be seen as an outward sign of the functional instability of normally quasi-unstable neuronal circuits.

This view rests on two clearly definable premises: (a) *In its function the nervous system requires the presence of close to 'tremorigenous' functional states.* Such tremorigenous states should be understood as being generated by oscillatory neuronal discharges of large sets of neuronal ensembles, and tremor itself the result of a rhythmical stereotyped and synchronous activation of given muscle groups such that involuntary cyclical movements may ensue. (b) *The dynamic properties of these central oscillatory states are matched to the dynamic properties of the external somatic effectors.*

If we choose to accept these premises, the issue of the central versus peripheral nature of particular tremors may be seen from a different perspective. Indeed, the question of whether tremor is primarily of central or peripheral origin becomes moot if we agree that central and peripheral events must resonate in unison for tremor to occur. In other words, since tremor is an emerging property, the question becomes similar to that of deciding which of the three legs determines the stability of a tripod. Tremor requires the functional synchrony of large numbers of neuronal and muscular elements functioning as oscillatory 'units'. A 'critical mass' of activity must be attained before such outward manifestation is observable. These units may not necessarily be restricted to one anatomical location or pathway or to a given neuronal system (e.g. the spino-cerebello-spinal system). They may be the result of the coupling of a parallel and distributed oscillatory property belonging to several such systems. The central issue then concerns the properties of coupled oscillators.

From these considerations a significant conclusion may be reached. In order to activate limbs with maximum efficiency, there must be a non-accidental matching of the central motor command with the dynamic properties of the limbs (as determined by their resonant frequencies). Furthermore, movement and its control are not continuous functions of time; rather they occur in steps. They are inherently unstable in a linear sense, but demonstrate non-linear stability as limited cycle oscillators (Holmes, 1979). Proceeding with this line of thought, we may consider that the oscillatory properties observed in motor systems may also be represented in the transformation of sensory input into motor execution. A corollary to the above is that, in principle, peripheral and central abnormalities may induce functional instabilities since such instabilities are only the reflection of inherent properties of the total system.

Before considering the question of the oscillatory properties of central systems we must remember that tremors may be divided into two broad groups: (a) those generated by central oscillation and its peripheral resonance counterpart (oscillatory tremors), and (b) those related to goal-directed motor activity, the so-called action or intention tremors (Holmes, 1922). It is clear that in the latter case tremors result from the inability of the nervous system to acquire an external target during a motor execution or from the inability to stabilise, in a postural sense, a certain part of the body (e.g. limbs or midline musculature). These abnormalities seem to be characterised by movements that proceed more or less normally until a definite error is detected, at which time an attempt to redirect motion produces a set of dysmetric movements simulating tremor. They can be triggered or their timing may be 'reset' by either afferent peripheral input or by corollary motor discharges that indicate that the goal is not attained (Mauritz *et al.*, 1981). Lack of goal acquisition is followed by reordering of motor intention to generate a movement vector in a different direction and thus a set of short-lived motor executions, often in opposite directions, is generated simulating true tremor (Pellionisz and Llinás, 1980). We shall consider the nature of intention tremor anon.

Research into the oscillatory behaviour of neurones has a rather short electrophysiological history. Studies in invertebrates made it evident that much of the organisation of stereotyped motor behaviour in these animals was driven by neuronal oscillators (Wilson, 1966; Szekely, 1965; Friesen and Stent, 1977; Getting *et al.*, 1980; Gorman *et al.*, 1980; Cohen *et al.*, 1982). It was postulated by Jung (1941) that the appearance of tremor in neurological diseases is attributable to the release of such primitive, stereotyped motor mechanisms. A similar type of oscillatory behaviour has been observed in mammalian CNS, most particularly following parenteral injection of harmaline (de Montigny and Lamarre, 1973, 1974; Llinás and Volkind, 1973). Initially this oscillatory behaviour was thought to be due to recurrent inhibition which would then produce the silence necessary for these cells to oscillate. However, more recently another mechanism, rebound excitation, has been demonstrated as the basis for this tremor (see below).

THE INFERIOR OLIVE:
ITS POSSIBLE RELATION TO PHYSIOLOGICAL TREMOR AND TO 'PALATAL–DIAPHRAGMATIC MYOCLONUS'

In more recent experiments using *in vitro* inferior olive slices, Yarom and I (Llinás and Yarom, 1981a,b) demonstrated that inferior olive (IO) neurones have a set of ionic currents organised such that these cells tend to oscillate. Thus, as shown in figure 10.1, the firing of IO cells is characterised by an initial fast rising action potential (a sodium spike initiated at the soma) followed by an after-depolarisation that prolongs the initial action potential for 10–15 ms. During this period the axon of the IO neurone fires repetitively. This is indicated by the small all-or-none wavelets which rise on the summit of the after-depolarisation and by the presence of multiple climbing fibre excitatory pool synaptic potentials (EPSPs) in Purkinje cells at the cerebellar level, each one of which represents a full spike in the IO

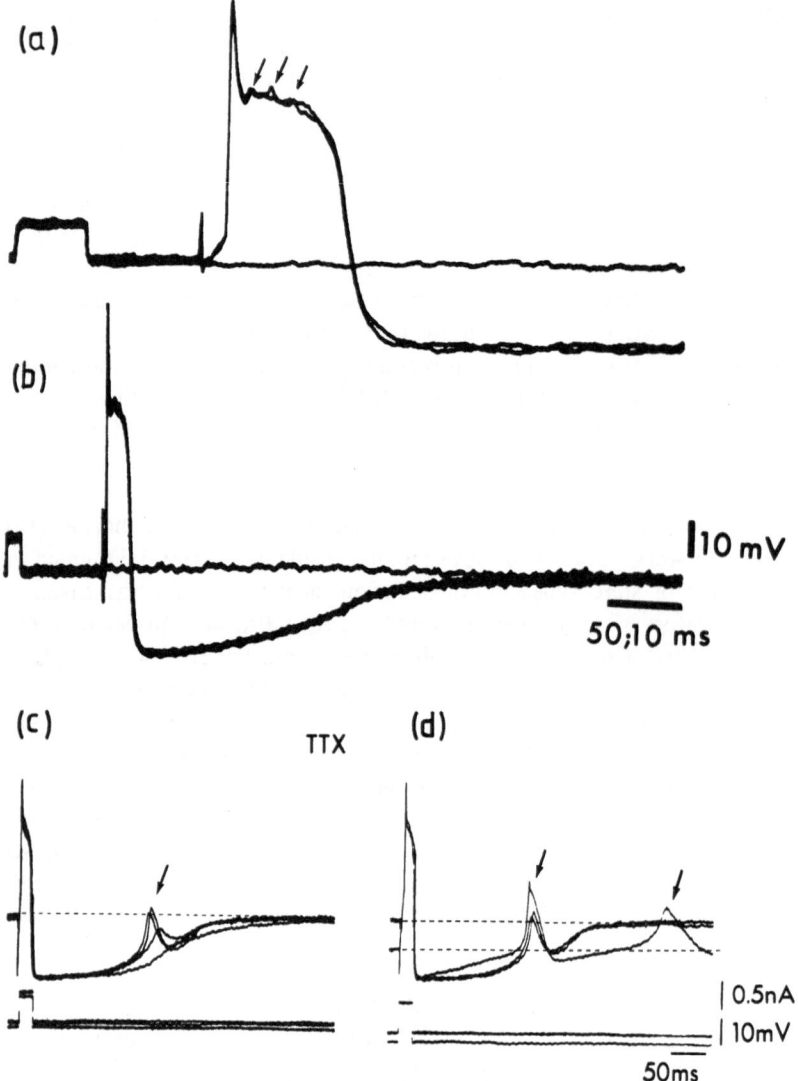

Figure 10.1 Intracellular recordings from *in vitro* inferior olive (IO) neurones in guinea-pig brainstem slice. (a) and (b) An action potential generated by antidromic invasion and displayed at two sweep speeds. In (a) note the wavelets (arrows) indicating axonal firing riding on the after-depolarisation which is due to a calcium-dependent dendritic spike. In (b) the prolonged after-hyperpolarisation is terminated by a rebound potential. (c) and (d) Direct activation of an IO neurone recorded intracellularly following tetrodotoxin blockage of g_{Na} (to prevent sodium spikes) and a slight membrane hyperpolarisation to demonstrate the 'rebound' calcium spike (arrow). In (d) a further hyperpolarisation (from upper to lower horizontal broken lines) increases the amplitude of the rebound response (arrow) such that a second rebound is observed (arrow), demonstrating the mechanism for IO cell oscillation.

axon (Eccles *et al.*, 1966b). This plateau phase is then followed by an abrupt and long-lasting after-hyperpolarisation which totally silences the spike-generating activity of the cell. The hyperpolarisation is generally terminated by an abrupt active rebound response, which overshoots the resting membrane and can generate the subsequent activation of the cell (figure 10.1c and d).

Experiments using calcium-free Ringer solutions in the bathing medium, calcium-blockers, or the substitution of barium for calcium demonstrated that the after-depolarisation–hyperpolarisation sequence which follows the initial spike is due to the activation of two membrane conductances (Llinás and Yarom, 1981a), the initial one to calcium and the latter to potassium (figure 10.2). We now know that the initial response, the after-depolarisation, is produced by activation of a voltage-dependent calcium conductance located in the dendrites. This conductance is very similar to that initially demonstrated in Purkinje cells (Llinás and Hess, 1976; Llinás and Sugimori, 1980a,b) and confirmed in dendrites of other central neurones (Schwartzkroin and Slawsky, 1977; Wong *et al.*, 1979). The initial broad calcium spike generates in IO cells a powerful increase in membrane permeability to potassium, again most powerfully in the dendrites (as noted from the amplitude and polarity of the extracellular field). During this hyperpolarising period the cell is inexcitable, its conductance being very high such that even powerful synaptic inputs are totally shunted. The membrane potential may be said to be 'clamped' at the potassium equilibrium potential. This potassium conductance is of the calcium-dependent variety and similar to that initially described in invertebrate neurones (Meech and Standen, 1975). Indeed, substitution of barium for calcium completely abolishes the after-hyperpolarisation (Llinás and Yarom, 1981b) in accordance with the finding that barium does not activate the calcium-dependent potassium conductance (Eckert and Lux, 1976).

The duration of the after-hyperpolarisation is thus modulated by the amount of calcium that enters the dendrites during the calcium action potential. Indeed, if the calcium action potential is smaller, the duration of the after-hyperpolarisation is shorter although its amplitude often reaches potassium equilibrium. Prolonged dendritic spikes generate after-hyperpolarisation with durations as long as 200–250 ms. This is an important point because it indicates that *calcium entry determines the cycle time of the oscillator* as it directly governs the duration of the after-hyperpolarisation.

The third and probably most significant factor uncovered by our *in vitro* studies with regard to neuronal oscillation was the observation that at the end of the after-hyperpolarisation the membrane potential returned to the baseline in a rather abrupt manner, often overshooting the initial resting potential. This rebound response is due to the activation of a calcium-dependent action potential generated across the somatic membrane. This rebound response is the result of a second voltage-dependent calcium conductance *which is inactive at resting membrane potential* (-65 mV). This conductance becomes de-inactivated by the membrane after-hyperpolarisation and thus, as the membrane potential returns to baseline, *a low-threshold calcium spike* is generated. Small changes in resting

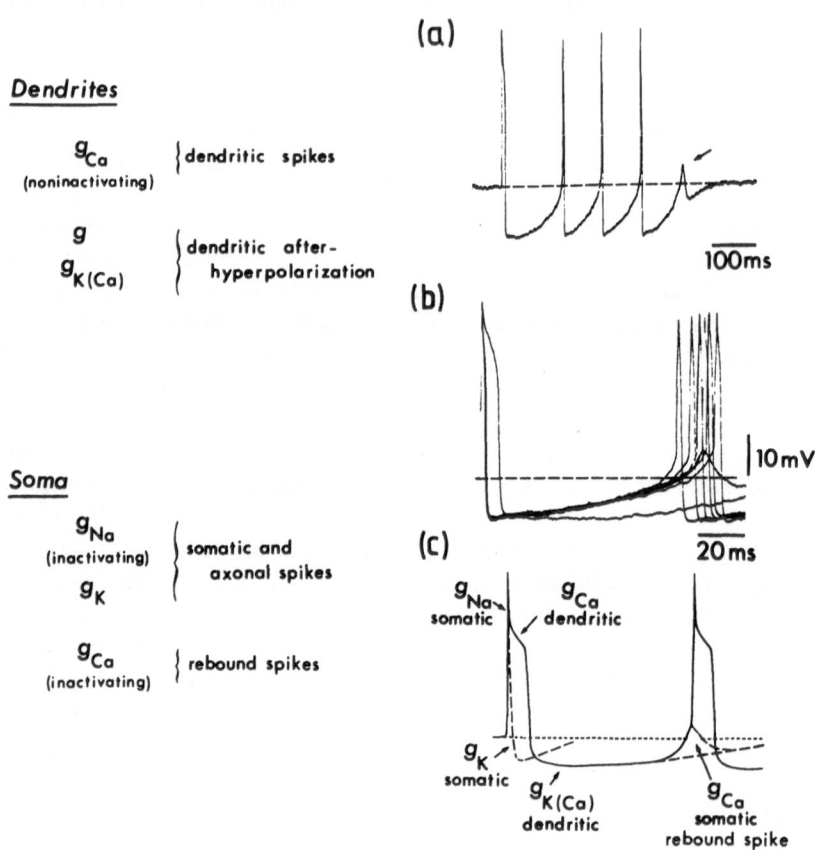

Figure 10.2 Ionic conductances in the different regions of the inferior olivary neurones and their oscillatory properties. At the left are the descriptions of ionic conductances relating to dendrites and soma. The symbols g_{Ca} and g_K relate to the calcium and potassium conductances which are voltage-dependent; $g_{K(Ca)}$ relates to calcium-dependent conductance change at the dendritic level. At the somatic level, sodium and potassium conductances (g_{Na} and g_K) generate the action potential. The rebound spikes are generated by g_{Ca} (inactivating). (a) This illustrates the oscillatory properties of a single inferior olivary cell recorded intracellularly *in vitro* following harmaline administration to enhance the oscillatory behaviour. The components of the action potential in (a) are shown in (c) and relate to the different ionic conductances. Note in (a) that the last action potential generates a rebound (arrow) which is subthreshold for the generation of the full spike after which the membrane potential returns to rest. This oscillatory behaviour, which can last for many seconds *in vitro* and has a rather set frequency, as shown in (b) by means of superimposed traces, is generated by the sequence of events shown in (c). (Llinás and Yarom, unpublished observations.)

membrane potential can increase the rebound potential sufficiently to produce a sodium spike, which in turn can set forth the whole sequence of events once again and thus generate the oscillatory firing of the neurone, with a frequency of 5–10 Hz.

Harmaline tremor

From a behavioural point of view, among the most spectacular tremors that can be induced pharmacologically in mammals is that generated by the administration of harmaline (figure 10.2), an alkaloid of *Pegamus harmala*. Such a tremor had already been reported before the turn of the century by Neuner and Tappeiner (1894). Its effect on decerebrated cats, where it can produce a 10–12 Hz tremor, was reported by Villablanca and Riobo (1970) and by Lamarre *et al.* (1971) and de Montigny and Lamarre (1973). The latter authors were the first to indicate an inferior olive and Purkinje cell involvement in this tremor. Intracellular recording from Purkinje cells confirmed and enlarged this observation by demonstrating that harmaline tremor was accompanied by all-or-none Purkinje cell EPSPs which could be reversed by direct depolarisation (Llinás and Volkind, 1973). The reversal of this large synaptic potential was the hallmark of activation of Purkinje cells by the axons of the inferior olivary cells, the so-called climbing fibres (Eccles *et al.*, 1966a).

Because this oscillatory firing reflects intrinsic conductance changes in each inferior olivary neurone, the basic frequency of this oscillation cannot be easily modified. IO cells are limited cycle oscillators. Indeed, under normal conditions IO cells cannot be made to discharge with frequencies higher than 10–12 Hz. During each cycle the IO axons generate short bursts of repetitive firing. These bursts are spaced in time by the rather powerful after-hyperpolarisation that separates the calcium plateaux. At the cerebellar cortical level the activation of the IO is seen as a burst of climbing fibre inputs which have a basic frequency of 1–2 Hz (Llinás, 1981). Today we know that the application of harmaline hyperpolarises IO neurones and produces an exaggerated rebound response even in the *in vitro* brainstem slice preparation (Yarom and Llinás, 1981).

In this preparation, and also in some preparations in the absence of harmaline, it can often be observed that the resting membrane potential of IO neurones tends to oscillate in an almost perfect sinusoidal manner (figure 10.3). This sinusoidal modulation of membrane potential is observed throughout the IO slice and is not related necessarily to IO firing. The frequency in this case (5 Hz) is the same for neighbouring cells and there is total coherence in the oscillation of different neurones. This oscillatory property varies from 5 to 10 Hz in different preparations, probably reflecting the metabolic state of the preparation. Regardless of variability, this ensemble property does suggest an underlying chemical oscillatory mechanism (Neu, 1980) modulating membrane conductance and does emphasise, given its synchrony amongst cells, the importance of their electrotonic coupling.

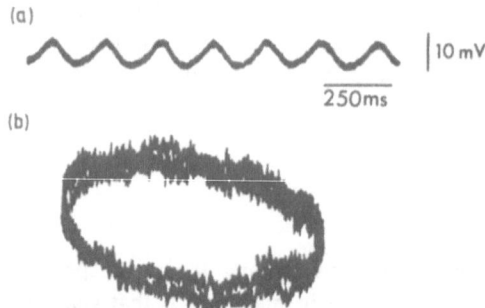

Figure 10.3 Oscillatory properties of the membrane potential in inferior olivary cells *in vitro*. In (a) spontaneous oscillations of the membrane potential in intracellularly recorded inferior olivary cells are shown. Three traces are superimposed to demonstrate the constancy of the waveform. In (b) is shown a Lissajous figure generated by pairing the oscillatory events in the inferior olive in the y axis of the cathode ray tube with a 5 Hz sinusoid in the x axis to demonstrate the constant periodicity of the harmonic oscillations of this potential. (Llinás and Yarom, unpublished observations.)

Another issue of significance here is that this activity in the IO results in a synchronous activation of motoneurones even after deafferentation either by application of curare or following dorsal root section (Llinás and Volkind, 1973). Also, destruction of the IO totally abolishes this tremor (Llinás *et al.*, 1975). Thus, IO activity can be demonstrated to be the necessary and sufficient requisite for the generation of tremor following harmaline administration.

The similarity in frequency between harmaline tremor and physiological or 'enhanced' physiological tremor provokes speculation on the possibility that the inferior olive may play a part in the generation of physiological tremor. Under normal circumstances, when a limb is held in posture, there is a physiological tremor which consists of more or less random twitch contractions of muscle fibres filtered by the passive viscoelastic and inertial characteristics of the limb. The pattern of twitch contractions of individual units is about 8 Hz, as determined by the recruitment rate of motor units. Units at higher frequencies tend to fuse, so the dominant tremor frequency observed is about 8 Hz. With increase in tone the tremor may become 'enhanced'; the amplitude increases and the frequency shifts upwards to 9–10 Hz. In this state the tremor is determined largely by cyclic reactivation of the stretch reflex (Halliday and Redfearn, 1956; Neilson and Lance, 1978; cf. Marsden, 1978; Marshall, 1970). Harmaline tremor, which synchronises muscle twitch contractions at similar frequencies, may be revealing to us that the olive produces oscillations that are the CNS counterpart of those of spinal cord mechanisms. If this view is correct, it follows that under normal circumstances the inferior olive synchronises CNS functions with respect to the more rigidly organised spinal and peripheral machinery. Under abnormal circumstances the olive may play a part in either sustaining enhanced physiological tremor or indirectly generating tremor itself.

Palatal myoclonus

Another aspect of tremor relating to the function of the inferior olive is that of palatal myoclonus. The presence of palatal myoclonus following damage of the central tegmental tract has been described in both man and primates (Spencer, 1886; Guillain and Mollaret, 1931; Alajouanine *et al.*, 1937; Hermann and Brown, 1967). The involuntary movements can involve the soft palate and other midline musculature systems as well as eye muscles, and even far distal limb musculature is often involved (Alajouanine *et al.*, 1937; Ell *et al.*, this volume, chapter 32). The movements in different parts of the body have the remarkable feature that they can be perfectly synchronous (Tahmoush *et al.*, 1972). While the basic mechanism for this low-frequency myoclonus (100 to 150/min) has not been determined directly, it is most likely due to the basic mechanism described above for olivary tremor. These motor abnormalities are generally accompanied by the well known IO hypertrophy syndrome which occurs with olivary deafferentation in humans as well as in primates (Wisotzkey and Cole, 1974) and cats (Verhaart and Voogd, 1962). Histologically the hypertrophy seems to be due to an increased size of the IO cells which can be seen at electron microscopic level to have increased their diameter (Koeppen *et al.*, 1980). In addition, the cells show a greater number of gap junctions (J. Voogd, personal communication), suggesting a larger degree of electrotonic coupling than that usually observed (Llinás *et al.*, 1974, Llinás and Yarom, 1981a). One would be tempted to speculate that the myoclonal dyskinesia would be related to IO deafferentation, the low frequency of the tremor being due to the increased neuronal area and concomitant increase in calcium conductance, and the peculiar distribution of the tremors being related to distribution of increased coupling in the olive. A basic point of interest here, which explains the synchronous nature of palatal myoclonus, is that it indicates, as will be reviewed below, that the IO is a phasic motor triggering system serving to activate muscle groups coherently in time (Llinás, 1970).

THE THALAMUS: ITS OSCILLATORY PROPERTIES

A second example of an oscillator neurone has been recently described in mammalian thalamus by similar *in vitro* studies of guinea-pig brain slices. Here Jahnsen and I reported that thalamic neurones are capable of demonstrating ionic mechanisms similar to those encountered in IO cells (Llinás and Jahnsen, 1982). This oscillatory behaviour is present in all parts of the thalamus including the lateral geniculate nucleus. Ionic conductances generated in these cells are similar to those in the IO in that a strong rebound calcium spike can be obtained at membrane potential level negative to −60 mV (figure 10.4). This rebound phenomenon, as with the IO cell, is resistant to blockage of the Na conductance by tetrodotoxin, and together with the hyperpolarising potassium conductance is capable of generating oscillatory responses at frequencies close to 10 Hz in the *in vitro* slice. When depolarised, the distribution of the electrical activity in these

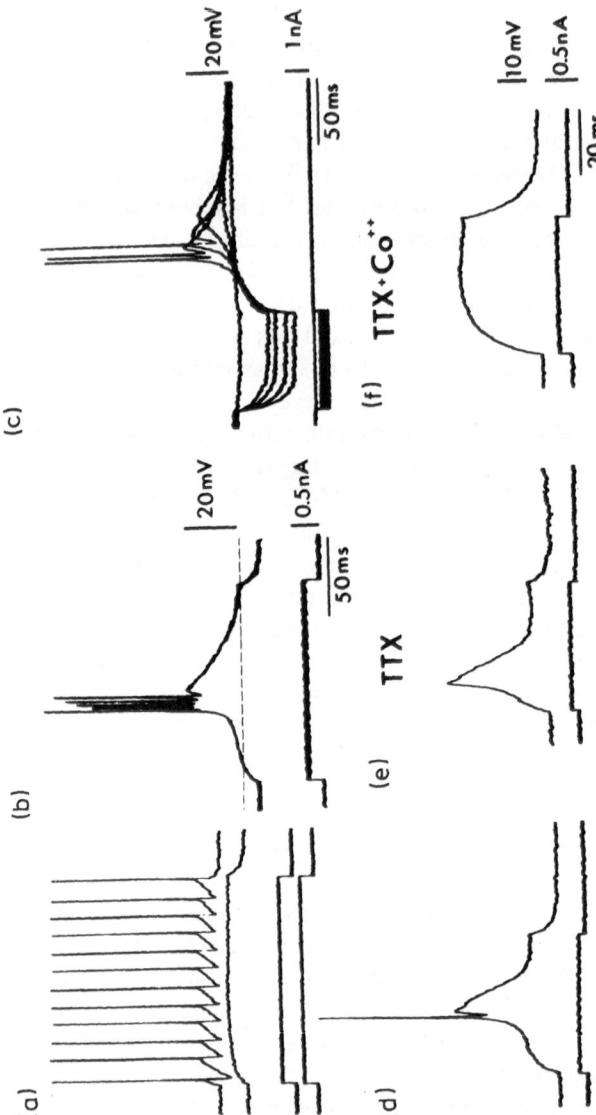

Figure 10.4 Intracellular recordings from thalamic neurones *in vitro*. (a) Subthreshold depolarisation of the cell at resting level produces, after a DC depolarisation, repetitive firing of the cell during the same current pulse. (b) After DC hyperpolarisation, similar current pulses as in (a) produce a single high-frequency spike burst. (c) Rebound burst response after hyperpolarising pulses of different amplitudes. Note the slow return to baseline, indicating an 'early' potassium conductance. (d) Slow all-or-none response generating fast spike, from a cell slightly hyperpolarised from rest potential. (e) After blockage of sodium conductance with tetrodotoxin, the fast action potential is blocked but the slow response remains unchanged. (f) Addition of $COCl_2$ to the bathing solution abolishes completely the slow response seen in (e) even when the current pulse is increased in amplitude by 2.5 times (Modified from Llinás and Jahnsen (1982).)

cells is somewhat different from that of IO neurones. Indeed, while a calcium conductance is present in the dendrites, it is not as powerful as that in the IO. Somatic firing may not activate the after-depolarisation/after-hyperpolarisation sequence as in the IO and thalamic cells can fire at high frequencies if tonically depolarised. Two other currents present in these thalamic cells are an early potassium conductance similar to that described by Hagiwara *et al.* (1961) and by Connor and Stevens (1971) in invertebrate neurones and a non-inactivating sodium conductance similar to that seen in Purkinje cells (Llinás and Sugimori, 1980a). However, the issue here is that we have at least two groups of cells capable of distinct oscillatory behaviour in the absence of recurrent inhibition; that is to say, the oscillatory properties are inherent in the individual cells.

As in the IO then, the ionic conductances and their spatial distribution in the thalamic cells are arranged such that these neurones can behave as intrinsic oscillators. As opposed to the IO neurones, thalamic cells have two distinct functional states. When the cells are depolarised, they can transmit information in a continuous manner. If the cells are hyperpolarised, they behave as oscillators with a period of about 9 Hz (Llinás and Jahnsen, 1982). This switching arrangement (from tonic to phasic responses) has so far been seen only in thalamic neurones. It is quite probable, however, that such properties may exist in many other neurones of the CNS.

DISCUSSION AND CONCLUSIONS

Significance of oscillatory properties of neurones to the problem of tremor—the question of rebound excitation

The issue to be considered at this time is the following. Several cell types in the CNS, as exemplified by the thalamus and IO cells, are capable of intrinsically determined oscillatory activations whose frequencies are very close to those observed in motor tremors in patients and experimentally in animals. Furthermore, particular nuclei may be singled out in relation to a particular form of tremor. It is in fact very possible that the IO and associated nuclei may be directly related to the so-called 8-10 Hz physiological tremor observed in higher vertebrates, while other forms of behaviour such as the alpha rhythm would probably be related to the thalamus. In both cases the main theme is the activation of cells via a rebound excitatory phenomenon.

It must be remembered that anodal break 'rebound' responses (postanodal excitation) are a general property of excitable tissues. They are observable to varying degrees in most excitable elements from axons to central dendrites. At this juncture then, an important point must be made: rebound excitation is a general phenomenon usually produced by de-inactivation of sodium channels following a hyperpolarisation. Indeed, at normal resting level a certain percentage of these channels are in the inactivated state and can be reincorporated into the active channel pool by hyperpolarising the membrane. In special cases, such as in the IO and the thalamus, new ionic mechanisms (de-inactivation of g_{Ca}) greatly exaggerate this tendency to rebound depolarisation. The importance of rebound excitation in these cases is clear; it is the most reliable way to activate a neurone since its activation is preceded by a hyperpolarisation that ensures the maximal level of electroresponsive readiness during the rebound. The hyperpolarising of the membrane may be equated metaphorically with the stretching of a bow, the rebound as the release of the arrow. Synchronisation is then attained by the simultaneous release of arrows, and the interval by the time necessary to stretch the bow once again.

Role of the inferior olive in the coordination of movement

In order to recruit the necessary motoneuronal pools along the neuraxis, a mechanism capable of transforming the oscillatory behaviour of single neurones into a synchronised oscillation of a population of such neurones is necessary. In the IO such a mechanism may be subserved by the electrical coupling between IO neurones (Llinás *et al.*, 1974; Llinás and Yarom, 1981a,b). This coupling is most probably related to the presence of gap junctions (Bennett and Goodenough, 1978) at the olivary glomeruli as well as directly between dendrites (Sotelo *et al.*, 1974; King, 1976; Gwyn *et al.*, 1977; Rutherford and Gwyn, 1977). The coupling would ensure that the oscillatory behaviour of single cells becomes synchronous such that the IO may generate a phasic modulation of the motoneurones in brainstem and spinal cord via vestibulo- and reticulospinal pathways (de Montigny and Lamarre, 1973; Llinás and Volkind, 1973). Its main function then would be to synchronise the activation of groups of muscles throughout the body in order to generate organised motor responses. In fact, the ability of the upper CNS to recruit in a synchronous manner different groups of motoneuronal pools is essential in the generation of even the simplest coordinated movement. Organised movement requires that sets of muscles must be thrown into action at very specific moments in time and in a preset order. The idea that the climbing fibre may play a role as a 'phasic motor control system' in every way similar to the concept of physiological tremor in the sense of behaving as a pacemaker activity upon which the onset of motion can be generated was proposed many years ago (Llinás, 1970) and has received a measure of support by simultaneous recording from motoneurones in the spinal cord (Llinás and Berthoz, unpublished observations; Y. Lamarre, personal communication). The results of such experiments indicate that during harmaline tremor synaptic potentials can be recorded in flexor and extensor motoneurones, regardless of their size, and are not restricted to the small tonic motoneurones as initially reported by Lamarre and Weiss (1973). The lack of activation of the larger motoneurones is now known to be due to their rather low membrane resistance, as they are among the largest of the motoneuronal elements.

Parkinsonian tremor

In the case of the thalamus, oscillatory properties may also be implicated not only in the generation of the alpha rhythm but in the generation of tremor such as, for instance, that of Parkinson's disease (e.g. Lamarre, 1975). As indicated by our own results (Llinás and Jahnsen, 1982), the oscillatory behaviour of the thalamus could, in principle, be generated by their partial deafferentation as occurs, for example, following damage to the dentate nucleus (Carrea and Mettler, 1947; Goldberger and Growdon, 1971; cf. Lamarre and Dumont, 1972) or its cooling (Brookes *et al.*, 1973). Partially deafferented thalamic cells would thus tend to fire in an oscillatory manner with a frequency close to 6 Hz, a frequency similar to the tremor observed in parkinsonism. This, by the way, is successfully treated surgically by thalamotomy, implicating the oscillatory properties of thalamic cells in the generation of Parkinson's tremor (cf. Andrew, this volume, chapter 25).

Tremors due to ataxia

The intention tremor

In order to understand the intention tremor (especially that produced by damage to those parts of the cerebellum relating to the organisation of motor coordination), one must consider the fact that a system may be thrown into oscillation if motor intentions require an abrupt change in the direction of movement (Holmes, 1922). For example, in cerebellar ataxia where patients are dysmetric, tremor-like movement may develop as the system is forced to generate precise movements under conditions where, due to lesion, the patient is inherently incapable of such fine control. This tremor, resulting from the attempt at correcting a dysmetric movement, may be difficult to distinguish from others because the maximal speed for correction may be quite close to tremor frequency. Indeed, as remarked in this volume (chapter 12) by Freund, echoing Jung: 'Nobody can move faster than he trembles'. Tremor in these cases may have frequency similar to oscillatory tremor, as they both represent top speeds. Their mechanisms are nevertheless very different. Oscillatory tremors would be produced by abnormal tuning of the sensorimotor system, while intention tremors would be produced by an abnormally high input to the oscillatory systems forcing the system to work at peak level.

The question of central or peripheral origin for tremor in humans

We have reviewed the possible electrophysiological basis for the pathophysiology of tremor. Physiological and parkinsonian tremor were offered as possible examples of how tremor may be related to single-cell electrophysiology and to the property of neuronal circuits. Tremors of this variety seem to be generated by central

oscillatory mechanisms capable of modulating motoneuronal systems in conjunction with peripheral systems, such as the spindle loop, which may reinforce the
central oscillator. According to this view, tremor is produced neither by neuronal
oscillation nor by the gamma loop alone, but rather by the matching of these two
systems to produce a positive reinforcing feedback which has the proper frequency to become self-sustaining. We must thus conclude that the *tremor is an
emerging property*. It must be remembered, nevertheless, that the rhythm of the
oscillation is probably produced by the supraposition of a rebound response in a
central oscillator which, in turn, sends an intermittent and powerful descending
barrage onto the motoneurones. In addition, the motoneurones themselves may
also have, to a lesser extent, such rebound ability due either to intrinsic membrane properties, to their order of recruitment (Allum *et al.*, 1978) or to rebound
following direct or Renshaw cell inhibition (Elble and Randall, 1976).

An intriguing point here would be to determine whether the loop time via the
periphery is properly tuned to the oscillatory properties of these central nuclei.
In the case of the 'parkinsonian' patients, on the other hand, central oscillators
are probably powerful enough to ensure that even under deafferented conditions
a tremor response may be clearly seen (Hagbarth *et al.*, 1975). In short then, if
one is to be concerned with both sides of the issue, one must ultimately conclude
that tremor seems to be basically a central phenomenon which can be strongly
modulated by peripheral loops.

The question of localisation versus mechanism

I would like to emphasise the importance of developing a more physiological
neurology rather than continuing to emphasise the anatomical locations exclusively. Indeed, historically, the ultimate aim of this area of endeavour has been
the localisation of the lesion or lesions generating the pathological condition.
Unfortunately, what the neurologist observes in real life and what the patient
suffers are functional abnormalities rather than anatomical problems. It is then
of the essence that we try to understand the physiological mechanisms by which
particular neurological conditions are generated.

In the context of such functional mechanisms we can advance with great
strides if we are not forced to classify the neurological patient on the basis of
common sites of lesion but rather on the basis of common functional abnormality. I do not advocate that neurologists forget 200 years of effort relating to
localisation but rather that localisation be placed in the context of functional
properties of the nervous system. Indeed if one is to consider the abnormal
function that occurs in olivary neurones or in thalamic neurones, one cannot
consider such abnormalities in isolation. Rather, the new properties of the motor
system in the presence of abnormal activity are the real phenomena to be understood. For instance, deafferentation ultimately increases oscillatory tendencies
of given nuclei which in time would drive the motor system into an unbalanced
state. This may indeed be what occurs following the injection of neuroleptics

or in the presence of social pressure or increased exercise or weakness, all of which would tend to drive the system to instability (Shahani and Young, 1978).

If we assume that oscillator systems are the proper way to activate motor sequences and such step activation serves, for instance, to break inertia as do burst cells in the ocular system (Zee, this volume, chapter 31), we are then truly on our way to understanding the biophysical basis for tremor. We would then be in the very happy situation of being able to define the conductance requirements which must be modified to control abnormal activity in neuronal oscillation.

ACKNOWLEDGEMENTS

Research was supported by United States Public Health Service Grant NS13742 from the National Institute of Neurological and Communicative Disorders and Stroke.

REFERENCES

Alajouanine, T., Thurel, R. and Hornet, T. (1937). Un cas anatomoclinique de myoclonies vélopharyngées et oculaires. *Rev. Neurol.*, **64**, 853–72.

Allum, J. H. J., Dietz, V. and Freund, H. J. (1978). Neuronal mechanisms underlying physiological tremor. *J. Neurophysiol.*, **41**, 557–71.

Bennett, M. V. L. and Goodenough, D. A. (1978). Gap junctions, electrotonic coupling and intercellular communication. *Neurosci. Res. Prog. Bull.*, **16** (3), 377–463.

Brooks, V. B., Kozlovskaya, I. B., Atkin, A., Horvath, F. E. and Uno, M. (1973). Effects of cooling dentate nucleus on tracing task performance in monkeys. *J. Neurophysiol.*, **36**, 974–95.

Carrea, R. M. E. and Mettler, F. A. (1947). Physiological consequences following extensive removals of the cerebellar cortex and deep cerebellar nuclei and effect of secondary cerebral ablations in the primate. *J. Comp. Neurol.*, **87**, 169–288.

Cohen, A. H., Holmes, P. J. and Rand, R. H. (1982). The nature of the coupling between segmental oscillators of the lamprey spinal generator for locomotion: a mathematical model. *J. Math. Biol.*, **13**, 345–69.

Connor, J. A. and Stevens, C. F. (1971). Prediction of repetitive firing behavior from voltage clamp data on an isolated neuron soma. *J. Physiol. (Lond.)*, **213**, 31.

Eccles, J. C., Llinás, R. and Sasaki, K. (1966a). The excitatory synaptic action of climbing fibres on Purkinje cells of the cerebellum. *J. Physiol. (Lond.)*, **182**, 268–96.

Eccles, J. C., Llinás, R., Sasaki, I. and Voorhoeve, P. E. (1966b). Interaction experiments on the responses evoked in Purkinje cells by climbing fibers. *J. Physiol. (Lond.)*, **182**, 297–315.

Eckert, R. and Lux, H. D. (1976). A voltage-sensitive persistent calcium conductance in neuronal somata of *Helix*. *J. Physiol. (Lond.)*, **254**, 129–51.

Elble, R. J. and Randall, J. E. (1976). Motor-unit activity responsible for the 8- to 12-Hz component of human physiological finger tremor. *J. Neurophysiol.*, **39**, 370–83.

Friesen, O. and Stent, G. S. (1977). Generation of a locomotory rhythm by a neural network with recurrent cyclic inhibition. *Biol. Cybern.*, **28**, 27-40.

Getting, P. A., Lennard, P. R. and Hume, R. I. (1980). Central pattern generator mediating swimming in *Tritonia*. I. Identification and synaptic interactions. *J. Neurophysiol.*, **44**, 151-64.

Goldberger, M. E. and Growdon, J. H. (1971). Tremor at rest following cerebellar lesions in monkeys: effects of L-dopa administration. *Brain Res.*, **2**, 183-7.

Gorman, A. L. F., Hermann, A. and Thomas, M. V. (1980). The neuronal pacemaker cycle. In Koester, J. and Byrne, J. H. (eds), *Molluscan Nerve Cells: From Biophysics to Behavior, Cold Spring Harbor Reports in the Neurosciences*, vol. 1, Cold Spring Harbor Laboratory, pp. 169-80.

Guillain, G. and Mollaret, P. (1931). Deux cas de myoclonies synchronés et rythmées vélo-pharyngolaryngo-oculo-diaphragmatiques: le probleme anatomique et physio-pathologique de ce syndrome. *Rev. Neurol. (Paris)*, **2**, 545-66.

Gwyn, D. G., Nicholson, G. P. and Flumerfelt, B. A. (1977). The inferior olivary nucleus in the rat: a light and electron microscopic study. *J. Comp. Neurol.*, **174**, 489-520.

Hagbarth, K. E., Wallin, G., Lofstedt, L. and Aquilonius, S. M. (1975). Muscle spindle activity in alternating tremor of Parkinsonism and in clonus. *J. Neurol. Neurosurg. Psychiatr.*, **38**, 636-41.

Hagiwara, S., Kusano, K. and Saito, N. (1961). Membrane changes of *Onchidium* nerve cell in potassium-rich media. *J. Physiol. (Lond.)*, **155**, 470.

Halliday, A. M. and Redfearn, J. W. T. (1956). An analysis of the frequency of finger tremor in healthy subjects. *J. Physiol., (Lond.)*, **134**, 600-11.

Hermann, C. Jr and Brown, J. W. (1967). Palatal myoclonus: a reappraisal. *J. Neurol. Sci.*, **5**, 473-92.

Holmes, G. (1922). The Croonian lectures on the clinical symptoms of cerebellar disease and their interpretation. *Lancet*, **100**(1), 1177-82, 1231-7; **100**(2), 59-65, 111-15.

Holmes, P. J. (1979). A nonlinear oscillator with a strange attractor. *Phil. Trans. R. Soc. Lond. A*, **292**, 419-48.

Jung R. (1941). Physiologische untersuchungen ueber den Parkinsontremor und andere zitterformen beim menschen. *Z. Ges. Neurol. Psychiatr.*, **173**, 263-330.

King, J. S. (1976). The synaptic cluster (glomerulus) in the inferior olivary nucleus. *J. Comp. Neurol.*, **165**, 387-400.

Koeppen, A. H., Barron, K. D. and Dentinger, M. P. (1980). In Courville, J., *et al.* (eds), *The Inferior Olivary Nucleus: Anatomy and Physiology*, Raven Press, New York, p. 309ff.

Lamarre, Y. (1975). Tremorgenic mechanisms in primates. In Meldrum, B. S. and Marsden, C. D. (eds), *Advances in Neurology*, vol. 10, Raven Press, New York, pp. 23-34.

Lamarre, Y. and Dumont, M. (1972). In Goldsmith, E. I. and Moor-Jankowski, J. (eds), *Medical Primatology*, Karger, Basel, pp. 274-81.

Lamarre, Y., Montigny, C. de, Dumont, M. and Weiss, M. (1971). Harmaline-induced rhythmic activity of cerebellar and lower brain stem neurons. *Brain Res.*, **32**, 246-50.

Lamarre, Y. and Weiss, M. (1973). Harmaline-induced rhythmic activity of alpha and gamma motoneurons in the cat. *Brain Res.*, **63**, 430-4.

Llinás, R. (1970). Neuronal operations in cerebellar transactions. In Schmitt, F. O. (ed.), *The Neurosciences: Second Study Program*, Rockefeller Univ. Press, New York, pp. 409-26.

Llinás, R. (1981). Microphysiology of the cerebellum. In Brooks, V. B. (ed.), *Handbook of Physiology*, vol. II, *The Nervous System*, part II, American

Physiology Society, Bethesda, MD, chap. 17, pp. 831–976.

Llinás, R., Baker, R. and Sotelo, C. (1974). Electrotonic coupling between neurons in cat inferior olive. *J. Neurophysiol.*, **37**, 560–71.

Llinás, R. and Hess, R. (1976). Tetrodotoxin-resistant dendritic spikes in avian Purkinje cells. *Proc. Natl Acad. Sci. (USA)*, **73**, 2520–3.

Llinás, R. and Jahnsen, H. (1982). Electrophysiology of mammalian thalamic neurons *in vitro*. *Nature*, **297**, 406–8.

Llinás, R. and Sugimori, M. (1980a). Electrophysiological properties of *in vitro* Purkinje cell somata in mammalian cerebellar slices. *J. Physiol. (Lond.)*, **305**, 171–95.

Llinás, R. and Sugimori, M. (1980b). Electrophysiological properties of *in vitro* Purkinje cell dendrites in mammalian cerebellar slices. *J. Physiol. (Lond.)*, **305**, 197–213.

Llinás, R. and Volkind, R. A. (1973). The olivo-cerebellar system: functional properties as revealed by harmaline-induced tremor. *Exp. Brain. Res.*, **18**, 69–87.

Llinás, R., Walton, K., Hillman, D. E. and Sotelo, C. (1975). Inferior olive: its role in motor learning. *Science*, **190**, 1230–1.

Llinás, R. and Yarom, Y. (1981a). Electrophysiology of mammalian inferior olivary neurons *in vitro*. Different types of voltage-dependent ionic conductances. *J. Physiol. (Lond.)*, **315**, 549–67.

Llinás, R. and Yarom, Y. (1981b). Properties and distribution of ionic conductances generating electroresponsiveness of inferior olivary neurons *in vitro*. *J. Physiol. (Lond.)*, **315**, 569–84.

Marsden, C. D. (1978). The mechanisms of physiological tremor and their significance in pathological tremors. In Desmedt, J. E. (ed.), *Progress in Clinical Neurophysiology*, vol. 5, *Physiological Tremor, Pathological Tremors and Clonus*, Karger, Basel, pp. 1–16.

Marshall, J. (1970). Tremor. In Vinken, P. J. and Bruyn, G. W. (eds), *Handbook of Clinical Neurology*, vol. 6, North-Holland, Amsterdam, pp. 809–25.

Mauritz, K. H., Schmitt, C. and Dichgans, J. (1981). Delayed and enhanced long latency reflexes as the possible cause of postural tremor in late cerebellar atrophy. *Brain*, **104**, 97–116.

Meech, R. W. and Standen, N. B. (1975). Potassium activation in *Helix aspersa* neurons under voltage clamp: a component mediated by calcium influx. *J. Physiol.*, **249**, 211–39.

Montigny, C. de and Lamarre, Y. (1973). Rhythmic activity induced by harmaline in the olivo-cerebellar-bulbar system of the cat. *Brain Res.*, **53**, 81–95.

Montigny, C. de and Lamarre, Y. (1974). Activity in the olivo-cerebello-bulbar system of the cat during ibogaline- and oxotremorine-induced tremor. *Brain Res.*, **82**, 369–73.

Neilson, P. D. and Lance, J. W. (1978). Reflex transmission characteristics during voluntary activity in normal man and patients with movement disorders. In Desmedt, J. E. (ed.), *Progress in Clinical Neurophysiology*, vol. 5, *Physiological Tremor, Pathological Tremors and Clonus*, Karger, Basel, pp. 263–99.

Neu, J. C. (1980). Large populations of coupled chemical oscillators. *SIAM J. Appl. Math.*, **38**(2), 305–16.

Neuner, A. and Tappeiner, H. (1894). Ueber bei Wirkungen der Alkaloide von *Peganum harmala*, insbesonders des Harmalins. *Arch. Exp. Pathol. Pharmakol.*, **36**(I), 69.

Pellionisz, A. and Llinás, R. (1980). Tensorial approach to the geometry of brain function. Cerebellar coordination via metric tensor. *Neuroscience*, **5**, 1125–36.

Rutherford, J. G. and Gwyn, D. G. (1977). Gap junctions in the inferior olivary nucleus of the squirrel monkey, *Saimiri sciureus. Brain Res.*, **128**, 374–8.

Schwartzkroin, P. A. and Slawsky, M. (1977). Probable calcium spikes in hippocampal neurons. *Brain Res.*, **135**, 157–61.

Shahani, B. T. and Young, R. R. (1978). Action tremors: a clinical neurophysiological review. In Desmedt, J. E. (ed.), *Progress in Clinical Neurophysiology*, vol. 5, *Physiological Tremor, Pathological Tremors and Clonus*, Karger, Basel, pp. 129–37.

Sotelo, C., Llinás, R. and Baker, R. (1974). Structural study of the inferior olivary nucleus of the cat: morphological correlates of electrotonic coupling. *J. Neurophysiol.*, **37**, 541–9.

Spencer, H. R. (1886). Pharyngeal and laryngeal 'nystagmus'. *Lancet*, **2**, 702.

Szekely, G. (1965). Logical network for controlling limb movements in Urodela. *Acta Physiol. Acad. Sci. Hung.*, **27**, 285–9.

Tahmoush, A. J., Brooks, J. E. and Keltner, J. L. (1972). Palatal myoclonus associated with abnormal ocular and extremity movement: a polygraphic study. *Arch. Neurol.*, **27**, 431–40.

Verhaart, W. J. C. and Voogd, J. (1962). Hypertrophy of the inferior olives in the cat. *J. Neuropathol. Exp. Neurol.*, **21**, 92–104.

Villablanca, J. and Riobo, F. (1970). Electroencephalographic and behavioral effects of harmaline in intact cats and in cats with chronic mesencephalic transection. *Psychopharmacologia*, **17**, 302–13.

Wilson, D. M. (1966). Central nervous mechanisms for the generation of rhythmic behavior in arthropods. *Symp. Soc. Exp. Biol.*, **209**, 199–228.

Wisotzkey, H. and Cole, M. (1974). Reversible neurofilamentous change with deafferentation of the inferior olive in the monkey. *J. Neuropathol. Exp. Neurol.*, **33**, 187.

Wong, R. K. S., Prince, D. A. and Basbaum, A. I. (1979). Intradendritic recordings from hippocampal neurons. *Proc. Natl Acad. Sci. (USA)*, **76**, 986–90.

Yarom, Y. and Llinás, R. (1981). Oscillatory properties of inferior olive cells. A study of guinea pig brain stem slices *in vitro. Soc. Neurosci. Abst.*, **7**, 864.

11
Animal models of physiological, essential and parkinsonian-like tremors

YVES LAMARRE

INTRODUCTION

The purpose of this chapter is to review briefly and to summarise our work of the last decade in which we have studied animal models of tremor. By using different experimental approaches such as brain lesions, electrophysiological recordings and the use of tremogenic drugs like harmaline, we have been able to distinguish three types of experimental tremor and to study their neural mechanisms (Lamarre, 1979). First, a mechanism involving the olivo-cerebellar system generates a tremor at 8-12 Hz which might be regarded as a model of physiological or normal tremor. Secondly, a mechanism also involving the olivo-cerebellar system can generate a tremor at 6-8 Hz which shows some of the characteristics of the so-called essential tremor observed in human patients. Finally, a third mechanism at the thalamo-cortical level appears to generate a parkinsonian-like tremor at the frequency of 3-6 Hz.

OLIVO-CEREBELLAR TREMOR AT 8-12 Hz

Harmaline and ibogaline generate muscle tremor at 8-12 Hz via the olivo-cerebello-bulbar system (de Montigny and Lamarre, 1973, 1974; Llinás and Volkind, 1973). These drugs produce repetitive firing of the inferior olivary neurones by facilitating their normal tendency for rhythmic activity and synchronisation (Llinás and Yarom, 1981). Tremogenic impulses travel via reticulo- and vestibulo-spinal pathways to produce rhythmic co-activation of α- and γ-motoneurones (Lamarre and Weiss, 1973). This tremor is usually synchronous in antagonistic muscles and also in muscles of different limbs (Lamarre and Mercier, 1971).

Figure 11.1 illustrates the activity recorded simultaneously from the cerebellar vermian cortex in lobule VIII (trace 1) and from the contralateral caudal half of the medial accessory olive (trace 2) following administration of ibogaline (2.5 mg kg^{-1} i.v.). Each contralateral olivary discharge is associated with a climbing fibre response in the cerebellar cortex where there is no simple spike activity.

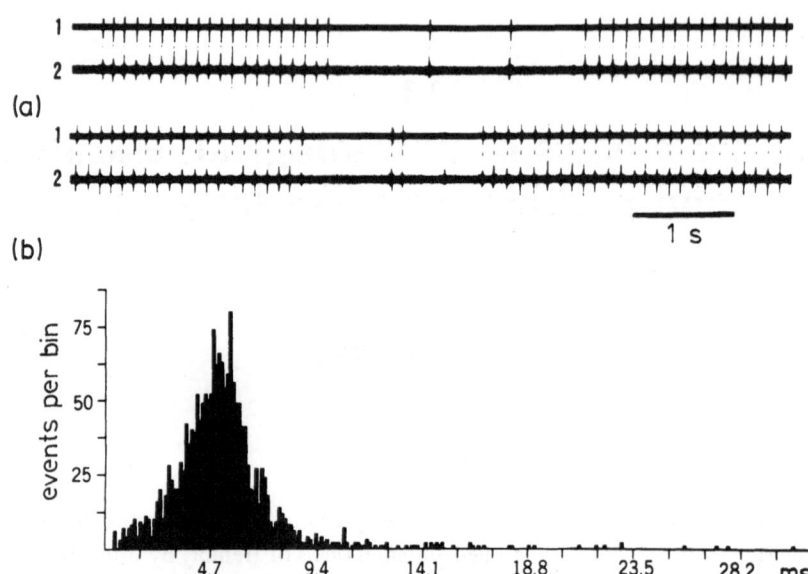

Figure 11.1 (a) Simultaneous extracellular recordings from lobule VIII of the cerebellar cortex (trace 1) and contralateral caudal half of the medial accessory olive (trace 2) following administration of ibogaline. (b) Cross-correlogram of Purkinje and olivary cells shown above where time zero corresponds to the occurrence of the olivary spikes. The analysis was made on a 13.5 min period of recording (2000 olivary spikes) using a bin width of 125 μs. (From de Montigny and Lamarre (1974). *Brain Res.*, **82**, 369–73. Reproduced by permission of Elsevier Biomedical Press BV, Amsterdam.)

The cross-correlogram indicates that the olivary discharge precedes the Purkinje cell activity by about 5 ms, which is compatible with the olivo-cerebellar conduction time (Eccles *et al.*, 1966).

Figure 11.2 shows simultaneous recordings in the left cerebellar cortex (trace 1), bulbar reticular formation on both sides (traces 2 and 3) and left hamstring muscles (trace 4), in a decerebrate cat injected with harmaline (5 mg kg^{-1} i.v.). The traces in (a) and (b) were obtained respectively before and after complete paralysis of the animal. The rhythmic activity in the cerebellum and in the reticular formation persists unchanged at about 8 Hz after tremor was abolished by Flaxedil (20 mg kg^{-1} i.v.).

In figure 11.3(a) we show recordings from single fusimotor (small spike, conduction velocity 27 m s^{-1}) and alpha (conduction velocity 86 m s^{-1}) units in a filament of medial gastrocnemius nerve following administration of harmaline in a decerebrate and paralysed cat. The rhythmic bursting of the gamma spikes occurs at a frequency of about 9 Hz. The repetitive firing of the alpha spike is not sustained but is phase-locked with the rhythmic gamma bursting as demonstrated in the cross-correlogram in (b). From such recordings, it is quite clear

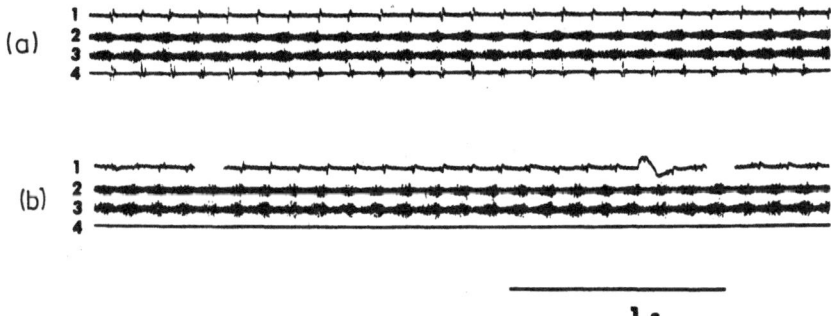

Figure 11.2 Recordings in the cerebellar cortex (trace 1), medullary reticular formation on both sides (traces 2 and 3) and hamstring muscles ipsilateral to the cerebellar recording (trace 4). In (a) the rhythmic activity at about 8 Hz in the cerebellum is phase-locked with the high-frequency bursts in the reticular formation and with the muscle tremor. The rhythmic activity in the cerebellum and brainstem continues, unmodified, after complete paralysis of the animal as shown in (b). Interruptions of trace 1 in (b) indicate attempts to modify the activity by pinna reflex.

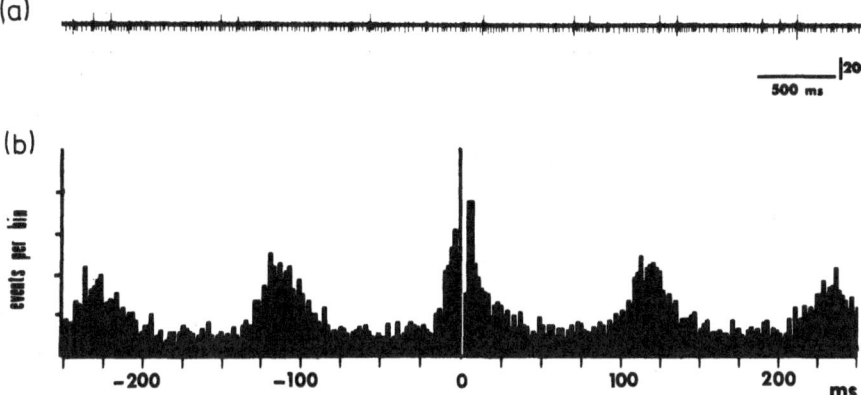

Figure 11.3 (a) Recording from single fusimotor (small spike, conduction velocity 27 m s^{-1}) and alpha (conduction velocity 86 m s^{-1}) units in a filament of medial gastrocnemius nerve following administration of harmaline. The repetitive firing of the alpha spike is not sustained but is phase-locked with the rhythmic bursts of the gamma spikes. (b) Cross-correlogram of alpha and gamma spikes with the alpha spike occurring at time zero on the abscissa. The rhythmic gamma bursts begin some 15–20 ms before the occurrence of the alpha spike. (From Lamarre and Weiss (1973). *Brain Res.*, **63**, 430–4. Reproduced by permission of Elsevier Biomedical Press BV, Amsterdam.)

that harmaline tremor involves rhythmic co-activation of α- and γ-motoneurones as was also demonstrated during parkinsonian tremor (Habgarth *et al.*, 1975).

Harmaline tremor can be antagonised by small doses of diazepam. However, we found that diazepam, at doses that suppress muscle tremor, did not block the harmaline-induced rhythmic activity in the olivo-cerebello-bulbar system. On the other hand, the rhythmic activity of motoneurones was suppressed at the same time as the muscle tremor (Busby and Lamarre, 1980).

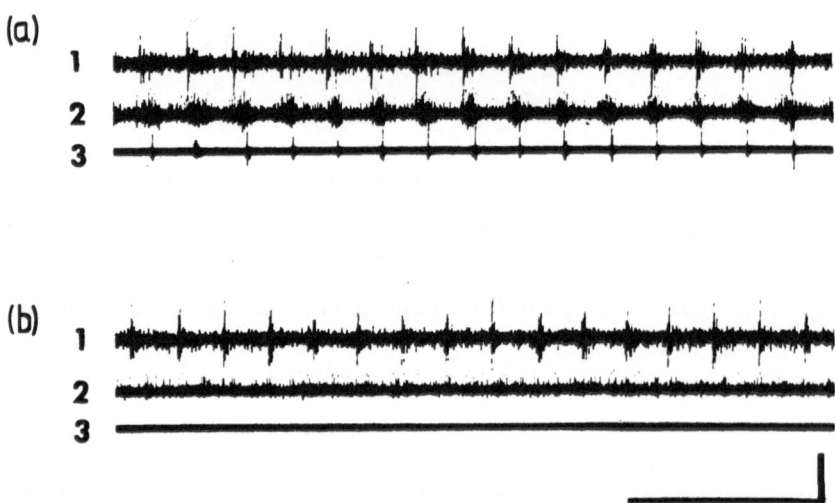

Figure 11.4 Activity recorded in the anterior lobe of the cerebellum (trace 1), ventral root filament from L3 (trace 2) and quadriceps muscle on the same side as the ventral root (trace 3). (a) Following harmaline injection, 1.5 mg kg^{-1} i.v. (b) Same as in (a) but 1 min after diazepam injection, 0.5 mg kg^{-1} i.v. Rhythmic activity at 8.5 Hz is abolished after diazepam administration in the muscle and the ventral root but not in the cerebellum. Calibration: 500 ms; 300 μV (traces 1 and 2) and 800 μV (trace 3). (From Busby and Lamarre (1980). In Courville *et al.* (eds), *The Inferior Olivary Nucleus: Anatomy and Physiology*. Reproduced by permission of Raven Press, New York.)

Figure 11.4 illustrates the results of one of these experiments. Recordings were obtained simultaneously from the anterior vermis of the cerebellar cortex (trace 1), ventral root filament from L3 (trace 2) and the quadriceps muscle on the same side (trace 3). The rhythmic activity at 8.5 Hz was abolished after diazepam administration (0.5 mg kg^{-1} i.v.) in the muscle and in the ventral root but not in the cerebellum. Similar results were obtained with diphenylhydantoin (10 mg kg^{-1} i.v.). We believe that these results demonstrate that diazepam and diphenylhydantoin antagonise harmaline tremor by acting at the level of the spinal cord.

OLIVO-CEREBELLAR TREMOR AT 6-8 Hz

In intact monkeys, harmaline can also induce a fast tremor in the 8-12 Hz range via the olivo-cerebellar system (Lamarre *et al.*, 1975). When injected into monkeys with brainstem lesions (ventromedial tegmentum and/or lateral cerebellar system), the frequency range of the drug-induced tremor varied from 3 to 12 Hz (Lamarre and Dumont, 1972; Lamarre *et al.*, 1975). Careful analysis of the tremor characteristics has revealed some differences between animals with spontaneous tremor produced by the lesion (Poirier, 1960) and those with tremor induced or exaggerated by harmaline (Poirier *et al.*, 1966). In the absence of harmaline, the spontaneous tremor produced by midbrain tegmentum lesion shows normally a reciprocal organisation and has a regular frequency of about 5 Hz (range 3-6 Hz in 22 monkeys) (Cordeau *et al.*, 1960; Lamarre and Cordeau, 1967). It often involves hand muscles at rest. Tremor frequencies in the range 6-8 Hz were seen only in animals injected with harmaline after lesion of the brainstem and/or lateral cerebellar system (dentate or brachium conjunctivum). This tremor, rarely seen in finger muscles, most often involved the proximal musculature such as deltoid, trapezius and periscapular muscles. It always showed a strong postural component and persisted, sometimes exaggerated, during movement. In some of these animals we could observe two distinct tremor frequencies in the same muscles: a slower tremor at 4-5 Hz which was at times replaced by a faster tremor at 7.0-8.0 Hz (Lamarre and Dumont, 1972).

Figure 11.5 illustrates tremor at two frequencies in the left biceps (upper trace) and left triceps (lower trace) in a monkey with right brainstem lesions

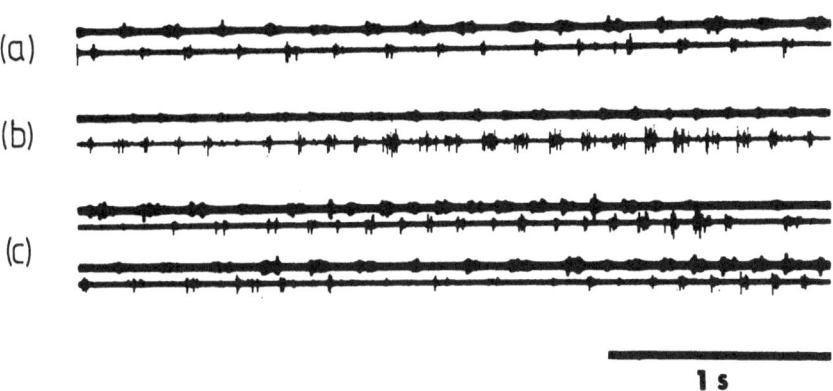

Figure 11.5 EMG recordings showing tremor at two frequencies in the left biceps (upper trace) and left triceps (lower trace) in a monkey with right brainstem lesions and harmaline. The frequency is 4.5 Hz in (a) and 7.0 Hz in (b). The two recordings in (c) are continuous and show abrupt change from slow to fast tremor. (From Lamarre and Dumont (1972). In Goldsmith and Moor-Jankowski (eds), *Medical Primatology*. Reproduced by permission of S. Karger AG, Basel.)

and harmaline. The frequency is 4.5 Hz in (a) and 7.2 Hz in (b). The two recordings in (c) are continuous and show a rather abrupt change from slow to fast tremor. Figure 11.6 presents autocorrelograms of the biceps activity shown in figure 11.5: (a) and (b) were computed respectively during episodes of slow and fast tremor only, whereas (c) and (d) were computed during episodes when the two frequencies occurred. The slow tremor predominates in (d) while the fast one predominates in (c).

The 6–8 Hz tremor observed only in lesioned monkeys injected with harmaline appears to be generated by the olivo-cerebellar system. This is based on recordings as well as on lesion experiments.

Figure 11.7 shows recordings in the lateral part of the left principal olive (upper trace) and contralateral triceps EMG (lower trace) in a monkey with

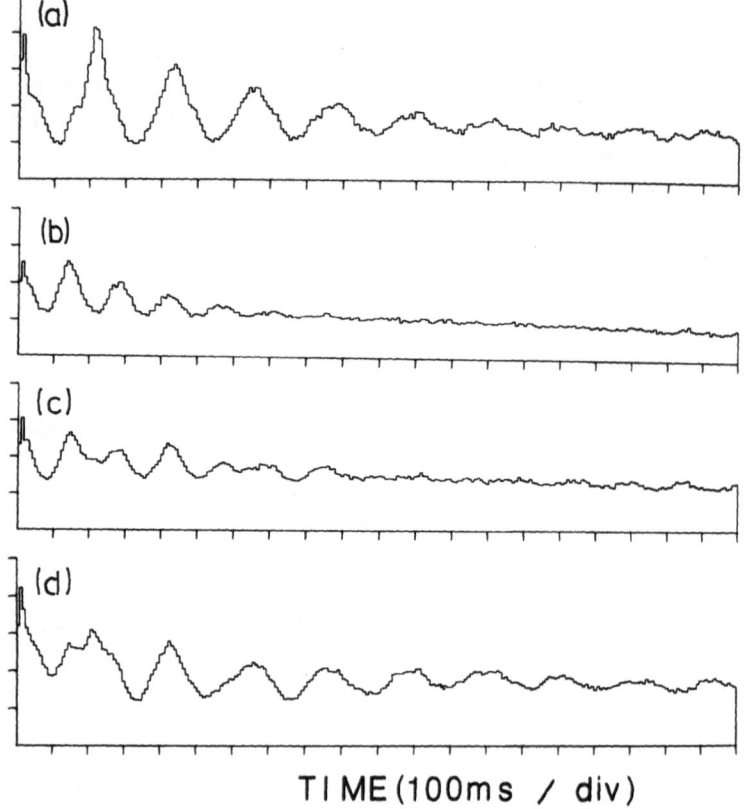

TIME (100ms / div)

Figure 11.6 Autocorrelograms of biceps activity shown in figure 11.5. (a) Episode of slow tremor only at 4.6 Hz. (b) Episode of fast tremor at 7.0 Hz. (c) and (d) Episodes when both tremors are present with predominance of the fast (c) and slow (d) components. Bin width: 8 ms. Time of analysis: 19 min in (a) and (b); 7 min in (c) and (d).

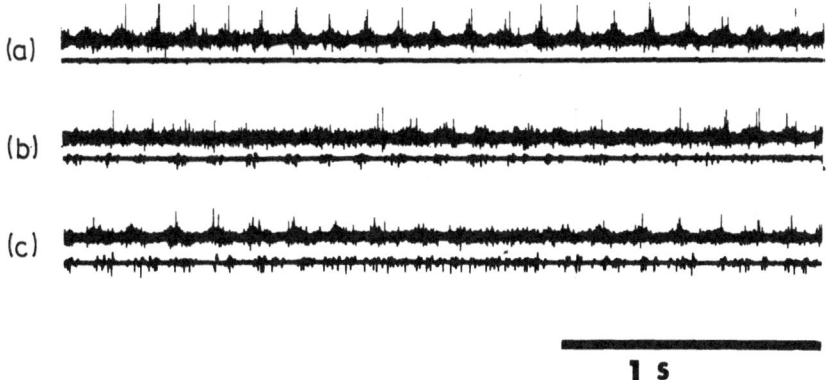

1 s

Figure 11.7 Recordings in the left inferior olive (upper trace) and contralateral triceps EMG (lower trace) in a monkey with left brainstem lesion and harmaline. The olivary spikes are superimposed on large rhythmic field potentials at about 7.0 Hz. In (a) the olivary discharge is sustained with relatively no peripheral tremor. In (b) the olivary rhythm is not sustained even though muscle tremor is present at about 7.0 Hz. Traces (c) show a short arrest of olivary rhythmic activity associated with a similar arrest of the peripheral tremor. (From Lamarre and Dumont (1972). In Goldsmith and Moor-Jankowski (eds), *Medical Primatology*. Reproduced by permission of S. Karger AG, Basel.)

left brainstem lesion and harmaline. The olivary spikes are superimposed on large rhythmic field potentials at about 7.0 Hz. In (a) the olivary discharge is sustained with relatively no peripheral tremor. In (b) the olivary rhythm is not sustained even though muscle tremor is present at about 7.0 Hz. Traces in (c) show a short arrest of olivary rhythmic activity associated with a similar arrest of the peripheral tremor.

Rhythmic climbing fibre responses in the cerebellar vermis at the same frequency as the 6-8 Hz muscle tremor were also recorded in three lesioned animals. One animal injected with harmaline was also paralysed, thus indicating that the rhythmic activity was not evoked from the periphery.

THALAMO-CORTICAL MECHANISM

In monkeys with brainstem lesion and total ablation of the cerebellum and subsequent degeneration of olivary neurones, tremor frequencies higher than 6 Hz were not observed, either spontaneously or after harmaline administration. On the other hand, cerebellectomy did not abolish the spontaneous tremor at 4-6 Hz previously induced by mesencephalic lesions. Thus, such a tremor, which shows the greatest similarity to the classical parkinsonian rest tremor, does not seem to be generated by the olivo-cerebellar system. Based on the results of lesion and recording experiments (Jasper *et al.*, 1972; Joffroy and Lamarre, 1971; Lamarre and Cordeau, 1967; Ohye *et al.*, 1970), we were led to believe that a thalamo-cortical mechanism could be involved in the production of this experimental parkinsonian-like tremor (Lamarre and Joffroy, 1979).

Figures 11.8 and 11.9 illustrate some of these results. Neurones were recorded in the ventral lateral portion of the thalamus of trembling monkeys before and during arrest of tremor movements by cooling of the ipsilateral motor cortex. Cells were found, such as the one in figure 11.8, which fired in bursts at the tremor frequency (a) and which continued to fire at the same frequency even when tremor was arrested by local cortical cooling (b).

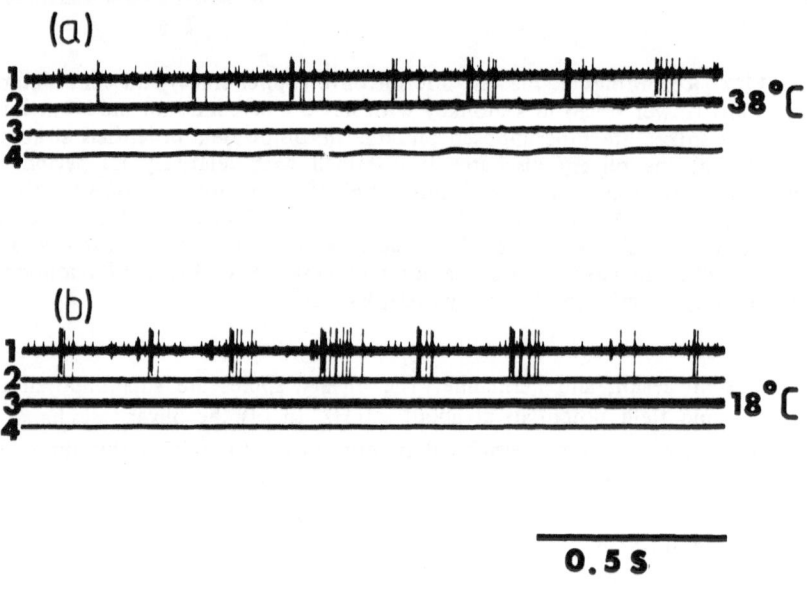

Figure 11.8 (a) Thalamic unit firing in bursts at 4 Hz (trace 1) during 4 Hz tremor in the contralateral arm, as indicated in the needle EMG from the biceps muscle (trace 2) and by the strain-gauge transducer (trace 4). (b) The thalamic firing pattern is undisturbed when tremor is arrested after cooling of the ipsilateral motor cortex to 18°C. (From Jasper *et al.* (1972). In Frigyesi *et al.* (eds), *Cortico-thalamic Projections and Sensorimotor Activities.* Reproduced by permission of Raven Press, New York.)

Figure 11.9 shows the activity of a neurone recorded in the arm area of the motor cortex contralateral to the deafferented upper limb (C2 to T3). This cell, which did not respond to passive movements of the limbs, shows a striking relation-ship with the tremor bursts recorded in the contralateral triceps. From these observations, we conclude that peripheral feedback is not necessary for the appearance of thalamo-cortical rhythmic activity related to tremor, and that such activity might itself result in the appearance of tremor.

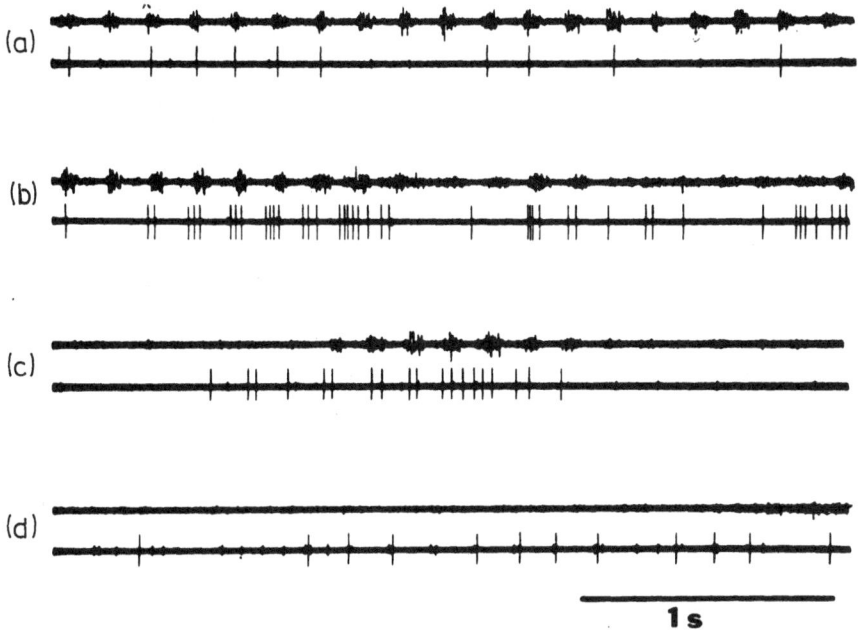

Figure 11.9 Activity of a motor cortex neurone in monkey during tremor in the contralateral deafferented arm. The upper trace is the contralateral triceps EMG. (From Lamarre and Joffroy (1979). In Poirier *et al.* (eds), *Advances in Neurology*, vol. 24. Reproduced by permission of Raven Press, New York.)

DISCUSSION

The experimental results that have been reviewed so far seem to indicate that there exist at least two independent systems capable of generating peripheral tremor: an olivo-cerebellar system and a thalamo-cortical system. The efferent pathways of the olivo-cerebellar system lead mainly through the fastigial nucleus and via the vestibulo- and reticulo-spinal pathways in the ventral half of the spinal cord. In intact animals, harmaline and some related drugs produce tremor at 10 Hz by exciting cells in the inferior olivary complex which cause repetitive firing in the climbing fibres and activate Purkinje cells and cerebellar and brain-stem nuclei. This tremor is usually synchronous (no alternation) in the antagonists. It is tempting to hypothesise that this harmaline tremor induced in normal animals may be an exaggeration of an 8–12 Hz physiological tremor.

In monkeys with a lesion of the dentato-rubro-olivary system, harmaline injection produces a tremor of larger amplitude, slower rate (6–8 Hz), often not alternating and showing characteristics of an action tremor. We believe that this experimental tremor could be analogous to some symptomatic essential tremors seen in human patients and also that it involves the olivo-cerebellar system and bulbo-spinal pathways coursing through the ventral funiculi of the spinal cord.

Such tremors could still be present in monkeys with complete interruption of the direct cortico-spinal fibres (Poirier *et al.*, 1972; Ohye *et al.*, 1970). Why harmaline would activate the inferior olive at a slower frequency (6–8 Hz instead of 8–12 Hz) after lesion of the dentato-rubro-olivary system in primates is not known.

After complete destruction of the olivo-cerebellar system, tremor can still be observed at a frequency of about 5 Hz following lesion of the midbrain ventro-medial tegmental area. This is a spontaneous rest tremor occurring regularly, and alternating in antagonistic muscles and often involving mainly the distal muscula-ture. This experimental tremor appears to be the best replica of the classical parkinsonian tremor. It is associated with rhythmical activity at the thalamo-cortical level and also in the cortico-spinal system (Lamarre and Dumont, 1972). It disappears after lesion of the lateral thalamus, motor cortex and internal capsule (Cordeau *et al.*, 1960; Jasper *et al.*, 1972).

Lesions in the medial tegmentum of the midbrain disrupt several nervous mechanisms among which is the nigro-striatal dopaminergic system (Poirier and Sourkes, 1965). The role of this system in the genesis of parkinsonian-like tremor remains to be clarified and other ascending pathways may also be involved. Harmaline can exaggerate this spontaneous tremor which, however, remains at a frequency below 6 Hz (Lamarre and Joffroy, 1979). If the brainstem lesion also involves the dentato-olivary fibres, harmaline may generate the other tremor through the olivo-cerebellar system at higher frequencies (6–8 Hz) and this may be recorded in the same muscle displaying the slower tremor at 4–6 Hz. Similar shifts in tremor frequency have been observed in parkinsonian patients and there is some evidence that two distinct mechanisms may be involved (Lamarre, 1975; Lance *et al.*, 1963; Shahani and Young, 1976; Findley *et al.*, 1981). It is possible that, in human patients, the same fundamental perturbations of the mechanisms of neuronal synchronisation occur in the inferior olive as well as at the thalamo-cortical level. It is our belief that further studies of these tremor models may lead to deeper understanding of the physiopathology of tremors in man.

CONCLUSIONS

Three types of tremor can be distinguished in the monkey. One type appears in normal animals following harmaline injection (frequency range 8–12 Hz) and is characterised by synchronous activation of antagonistic muscle pairs. It is produced by the olivo-cerebellar system. The second type of tremor, also produced by the stimulation of the olivo-cerebellar system by harmaline, occurs only in monkeys with lesion of the dentate nucleus and has a slower frequency (6–8 Hz) and most of the time is synchronous in antagonistic muscles. The third type of tremor can appear spontaneously following lesion of the ventromedial teg-mentum of the midbrain. This parkinsonian-like tremor occurs at rest at the frequency of 4–6 Hz and is characterised by alternating activity in antagonistic muscles. It appears to be generated at the thalamo-cortical level.

ACKNOWLEDGEMENTS

This research was supported by the Medical Research Council of Canada.

REFERENCES

Busby, L. and Lamarre, Y. (1980). In Courville, J., de Montigny, C. and Lamarre, Y. (eds), *The Inferior Olivary Nucleus: Anatomy and Physiology*, Raven Press, New York, pp. 315-20.

Cordeau, J.-P., Gybels, J., Jasper, H. H. and Poirier, L. J. (1960). Microelectrode studies of unit discharges in the sensori-motor cortex. Investigations in monkeys with experimental tremor. *Neurology*, 10, 591-600.

de Montigny, C. and Lamarre, Y. (1973). Rhythmic activity induced by harmaline in the olivo-cerebello-bulbar system of the cat. *Brain Res.*, 53, 81-95.

de Montigny, C. and Lamarre, Y. (1974). Activity in the olivo-cerebello-bulbar system of the cat during ibogaline- and oxotremorine-induced tremor. *Brain Res.*, 82, 369-73.

Eccles, J. C., Llinás, R. and Sasaki, K. (1966). The excitatory synaptic action of climbing fibres on Purkinje cells of the cerebellum. *J. Physiol. (Lond.)*, 182, 268-96.

Findley, L. J., Gresty, M. A. and Halmagyi, G. M. (1981). Tremor, the cogwheel phenomenon and clonus in Parkinson's disease. *J. Neurol. Neurosurg. Psychiatr.*, 44 (6), 534-46.

Hagbarth, K. E., Wallin, G., Löfstedt, L. and Aquilonius, S. M. (1975). Muscle spindle activity in alternating tremor of Parkinsonism and in clonus. *J. Neurol. Neurosurg. Psychiatr.*, 38, 636-41.

Jasper, H. H., Lamarre, Y. and Joffroy, A. J. (1972). In Frigyesi, T., Rinvik, E. and Yahr, M. D. (eds), *Cortico-thalamic Projections and Sensorimotor Activities*, Raven Press, New York, pp. 461-73.

Joffroy, A. J. and Lamarre, Y. (1971). Rhythmic unit firing in the precentral cortex in relation with postural tremor in a deafferented limb. *Brain Res.*, 27, 386-9.

Lamarre, Y. (1975). In Meldrum, B. S. and Marsden, C. D. (eds), *Advances in Neurology*, vol. 10, Raven Press, New York, pp. 23-34.

Lamarre, Y. (1979). In Massion, J. and Sasaki, K. (eds), *Cerebro–Cerebellar Interactions*, Elsevier/North-Holland Biomedical Press, Amsterdam, pp. 249-59.

Lamarre, Y. and Cordeau, J.-P. (1967). Etude du mécanisme physio-pathologique responsable, chez le Singe, d'un tremblement expérimental de type parkinsonien. *Actual. Neurophysiol.*, 7, 141-66.

Lamarre, Y. and Dumont, M. (1972). In Goldsmith, E. I. and Moor-Jankowski, J. (eds), *Medical Primatology*, Karger, Basel, pp. 274-81.

Lamarre, Y. and Joffroy, A. J. (1979). In Poirier, L. J., Sourkes, T. L. and Bédard, P. J. (eds), *Advances in Neurology*, vol. 24, Raven Press, New York, pp. 109-22.

Lamarre, Y., Joffroy, A. J., Dumont, M., de Montigny, C., Grou, F. and Lund, J. P. (1975). Central mechanisms of tremor in some feline and primate models. *Can. J. Neurol. Sci.*, 2, 227-33.

Lamarre, Y. and Mercier, L. A. (1971). Neurophysiological studies of harmaline-induced tremor in the cat. *Can. J. Physiol. Pharmacol.*, 49, 1049-58.

Lamarre, Y. and Weiss, M. (1973). Harmaline-induced rhythmic activity of alpha and gamma motoneurons in the cat. *Brain Res.*, 63, 430-4.

Lance, J. W., Schwab, R. S. and Peterson, E. A. (1963). Action tremor and the cogwheel phenomenon in Parkinson's disease. *Brain*, 86, 95–110.

Llinás, R. and Volkind, R. A. (1973). The olivo-cerebellar system: functional properties as revealed by harmaline-induced tremor. *Exp. Brain Res.*, 18, 69–87.

Llinás, R. and Yarom, Y. (1981) Properties and distribution of ionic conductances generating electroresponsiveness of mammalian inferior olivary neurones *in vitro. J. Physiol.*, 315, 569–84.

Ohye, C., Bouchard, R., Larochelle, L., Bédard, P., Boucher, R., Raphy, B. and Poirier, L. J. (1970). Effect of dorsal rhizotomy on postural tremor in the monkey. *Exp. Brain Res.*, 10, 140–50.

Poirier, L. J. (1960). Experimental and histological study of midbrain dyskinesia. *J. Neurophysiol.*, 23, 534–51.

Poirier, L. J., Bédard, P., Langelier, P., Larochelle, L., Parent, A. and Roberge, A. G. (1972). Les circuits neuronaux impliqués dans la physiopathologie des syndromes parkinsoniens. *Rev. Neurol.*, 127, 37–50.

Poirier, L. J. and Sourkes, T. L. (1965). Influence of the substantia nigra on the catecholamine content of the striatum. *Brain*, 88, 181–2.

Poirier, L. J., Sourkes, T. L., Bouvier, G., Boucher, R. and Carabin, S. (1966). Striatal amines, experimental tremor and the effect of harmaline in the monkey. *Brain*, 89, 37–52.

Shahani, B. T. and Young, R. R. (1976). Physiological and pharmacological aids in the differential diagnosis of tremor. *J. Neurol. Neurosurg. Psychiatr.*, 39, 772–83.

12
Determinants of tremor rate

H.-J. FREUND, H. HEFTER, V. HÖMBERG and K. REINERS

THE DEVELOPMENT OF TREMOR CONCEPTS

Tremor is an inevitable side-effect of any muscle activity. The physiological tremor accompanying any movement or isometric muscle contraction is not usually perceived. Only after augmentation by fatigue, emotion or shivering does it become apparent and it may even be present at rest. Strong tremors represent a typical feature of certain lesions of the extrapyramidal system.

The large amplitudes and regular beating of such pathological or augmented physiological tremors were of considerable influence on the development of tremor concepts. The rate of this rhythmicity was measured and, prior to the introduction of spectral analysis, was referred to as the tremor rate. Since Horsley and Schaeffer (1886) the rate of physiological tremor has been known to be in the 8–12 Hz range.

The refinement of tremor measurements by new technology revealed that physiological tremor is a necessary by-product of any muscle action. Spectral analysis of tremor records introduced by Halliday and Redfearn (1956) demonstrated that physiological tremor is not a single regular frequency but a mixture of different frequencies. The 'tremor rate' appeared only as a small local peak in the 6–12 Hz range, often not prominent with respect to the remainder of the spectrum. On the basis of these results physiological tremor could no longer be regarded as a rhythmic process.

In order to understand the controversies in the development of tremor concepts it is necessary to discuss the role of synchronisation for tremor generation.

MECHANISMS UNDERLYING SYNCHRONISATION

The recording of neuronal tremor force during stationary isometric contractions of a small hand muscle and its relation to motor unit discharges recorded simultaneously in the tremor-generating muscle showed that tremor is also present without physiological synchronisation between the motor units (Dietz et al., 1976). Synchronisation in this context is referring to a long-term periodicity which has later been called input synchronisation and has to be distinguished from short-term synchronisation (Sears and Stagg, 1976). These two types of synchronisation between motoneurones are due to different mechanisms.

Short-term synchronisation

This refers to the rise in the firing probability of a motoneurone pool as a consequence of a substantial number of common presynaptic fibres. Its strength depends on the amount of common input and is reflected by a narrow central peak (±3 ms) in the cross-correlogram or pre- and post-stimulus time histogram (Moore *et al.*, 1966). It simply reflects this type of connectivity between cells and can also be detected in cross-correlograms of simultaneously recorded motor unit discharges (Dietz *et al.*, 1976).

Input synchronisation

This is reflected by long-term changes in firing probability as it appears in slower periodicities. It is the consequence of synchronised inputs to the motoneurone as they arise if an input cell has interconnections with other input cells which also synapse on that motoneurone. It is this 'input synchronisation' which is usually meant in discussions on tremor. It leads to the well known grouping of motor unit discharges as it appears in EMG recordings during coarser tremor. Whereas short-term synchronisation always exists between the motor units of a muscle, input synchronisation may or may not be present. A characteristic difference between the two types of synchronisation is that short-term synchronisation is not dependent on the firing rate, so that it is present between cells irrespective of their actual firing rates. In contrast, long-term synchronisation can only be observed for motor units discharging at their lowest rates.

For simplicity, we will use synchronisation from here on in the sense of 'input' synchronisation.

THE PROBLEM OF TREMOR RATE

Looking at power spectra of physiological tremor, it is difficult to detect a distinct peak indicative of 'the tremor rate'. Since physiological tremor contains a broad band of frequencies it does not seem justified to use the term 'tremor rate' at all. It is only in augmented tremors that a clear peak appears in the power spectrum corresponding to the regular rhythm in the tremor recording. In a strict sense the term 'tremor rate', representing a dominant frequency, can only be used for augmented tremor.

The reason for the transition from irregular to regular tremor lies in the synchronisation of motor units: the resulting rhythmic EMG bursts have been attributed to a servo-loop oscillation in the stretch reflex arc (Hammond *et al.*, 1956). But it has been proved only recently by microneurography from human subjects

(Hagbarth and Young, 1979) that the muscle spindles are not excited in 'non-activated' physiological tremor but that they become activated by grouped motor unit discharges in 'activated' physiological tremor. The two phenomena accompanying spindle activation and thereby motor unit synchronisation are more regularity and higher amplitudes of tremor, reflected by the appearance of a distinct peak in the power spectrum of the tremor record. This is illustrated by typical examples of power spectra obtained from a non-activated (a) and activated (b) physiological tremor shown in figure 12.1. Tremor was recorded by means of

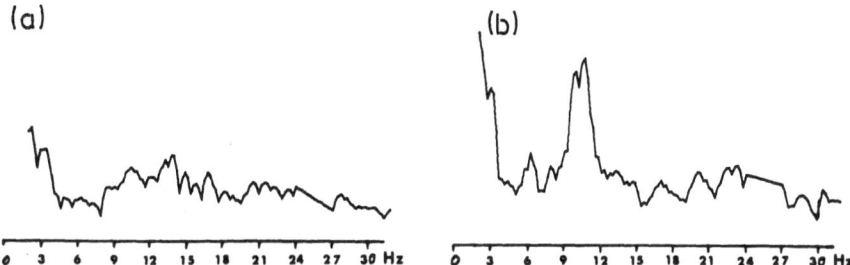

Figure 12.1   Averaged force spectra of two normal subjects maintaining a constant isometric force of about 6 N for 17 s (index finger extension). A broad band of physiological tremor is present in the spectra of the subject in (a). A more distinct peak of activated physiological tremor is apparent in the spectra of the subject in (b).

high-gain AC-couples force transducers during extension of the forefinger (6 N). When tremor is recorded with accelerometers instead of force transducers, the low-frequency part of the spectrum is reduced but the higher-frequency part including the tremor peak is similar.

The synchronisation between two motor units recorded simultaneously from the tremor-producing muscle leads to a change in the cross-correlogram with respect to non-activated tremor. This is shown in figure 12.2. Part (b) shows a correlogram with a small narrow peak derived from a recording during non-activated physiological tremor, whereas part (a) shows a broad peak in a parkinsonian patient. This difference reflects the change from short-term to long-term (input) synchronisation.

THE RELATIONSHIP BETWEEN TREMOR RATE AND MOTOR UNIT FIRING RATES

The characteristic feature of (input) synchronisation—no matter whether in activated physiological or in pathological tremor—is the fact that it occurs invariably between those motor units discharging at the slowest rates. During an isotonic movement or during an isometric contraction, the motor units in a particular muscle discharge at various frequencies depending on the angle of movement or the acquired force level. This range of firing rates is reflected in the power spectrum

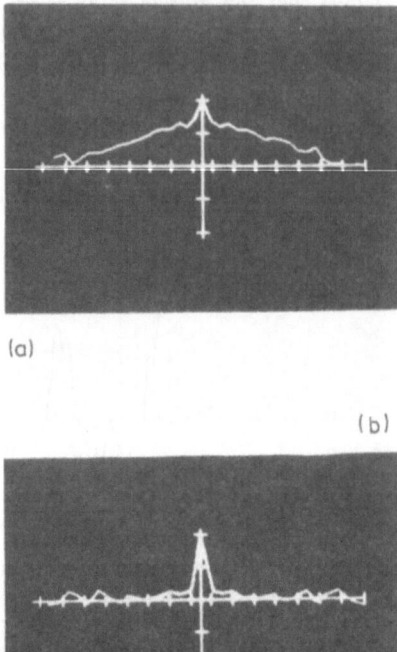

(a)

(b)

Figure 12.2 Pre- and post-stimulus time histograms (cross-correlograms) with 1 ms bin width of two simultaneously recorded motor units in the first dorsal interosseus muscle. Note the small narrow peak during non-activated physiological tremor in a normal subject (b) compared to the broad peak in a parkinsonian patient (a) due to a long-term synchronisation. Calibration is 10 ms/division on the abscissa.

by a corresponding frequency band. Freshly recruited motor units start firing at rates between 6 and 10 Hz. Input synchronisation to these motor units was apparent after systemic examination of tremor spectra obtained from normal subjects and from patients with various kinds of pathological tremor, and from the correlation of these tremor peaks with the onset firing rates of motor units recorded from the tremor-producing muscle (Reiners *et al.*, 1981).

Synchronisation between motor units firing at their onset rates can easily be recognised on the power spectra. This is illustrated in figure 12.3 by the consecutive power spectra of tremor force recorded during a slowly increased ramp contraction of the index finger from a patient with essential tremor. The peak at 8 Hz is prominent throughout the 17 s recording and remains preserved when more motor units fire at higher rates during the higher force levels at the end of

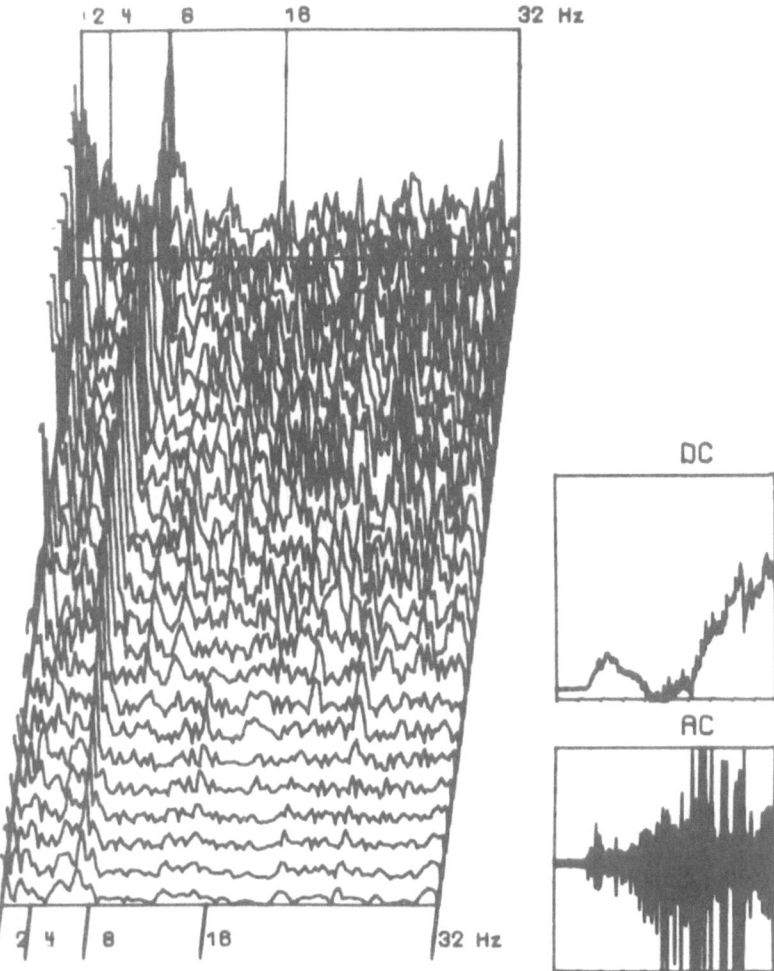

Figure 12.3 Series of force tremor spectra during a slow increase of isometric extension of the forefinger, recorded from a subject with essential tremor. Note that the distinct peak around 8 Hz increases in amplitude with increasing force.

the recording. This is due to the fact that the high-threshold units recruited later also start firing at 8 Hz as the low-threshold units do at lower force levels. This constancy of the onset firing rates of motor units with different thresholds is well known from single unit studies. Although fewer high-threshold units become recruited at higher force levels, their contractions are much stronger than those of lower-threshold units.

THE TREMOR RATE IN PATHOLOGICAL TREMOR

The essential tremor shown in figure 12.3 reveals the same spectral distribution as physiological tremor, and the peak due to synchronisation of motor units around 8 Hz is similar to that in activated physiological tremor. In contrast to this, the pathological tremors in extrapyramidal motor disorders and also in some cases with essential tremor show consistently that this peak appears at frequencies lower than 8 Hz. This shift of the peak towards lower frequencies is observed in these conditions irrespective of the type of tremor. The tremor at rest in Parkinson's disease, the action tremor in Wilson's disease or the intention tremor in patients with dentate lesions all show tremor peaks at low frequencies. This is illustrated by the power spectra in figure 12.4. Both sets of consecutive spectra are derived from force records of the index finger during a stationary muscle contraction. The records show that the abnormal synchronisation at an abnormally low rate is also prominent during steady muscle contractions, although the parkinsonian tremor shown in (a) was primarily a tremor at rest and the cerebellar tremor shown in (b) was a typical intention tremor. In both cases, the peaks were in the 5–6 Hz range and very prominent with respect to the remainder of the spectrum. The gain in these recordings had to be reduced as compared with the spectra of physiological tremor because of the large peak amplitudes.

When the slowest discharge rates of the motor units are measured in these patients they show either the same low rate as the tremor peak, or multiples of it. The latter is the consequence of repetitive firing of the motor units so that the units show double or triple discharges during strong tremor beats.

From our material of power spectra from patients with various extrapyramidal tremors we can conclude that the characteristic feature of these tremors is the appearance of the tremor peak at low frequencies that can *never* be observed in isometric contractions of normal subjects. Associated with the shift towards lower frequencies is the increase in amplitude due to the abnormal strong synchronisation. Similar phenomena were observed in animal experiments. Destruction of subcortical motor nuclei in cats (Gilman *et al.*, 1976) or transient dysfunction of cerebellar nuclei or of parts of the basal ganglia in monkeys (Meyer-Lohmann *et al.*, 1975) by cooling leads to the appearance of a coarse, slow tremor. In the cooling experiments, tremor rate decreases with temperature and motor unit tremor amplitude increases. The subsequent rise in temperature reverses these effects back to normal.

The linkage between the slowing of tremor rate and the augmentation in tremor amplitude raises the question about the mechanism underlying these changes. In neuronal terms, these phenomena correspond to a slowing of the onset firing rates (or burst repetition rate) and to an increase of synchronisation. The question why this happens as a consequence of a central lesion in the cerebellum, basal ganglia, nucleus ruber or some other subcortical motor nuclei is the key problem for the understanding of the pathophysiology of these tremors. It brings us back to the question why input synchronisation is restricted to the frequency of the onset firing rates, whereas short-term synchronisation is frequency independent.

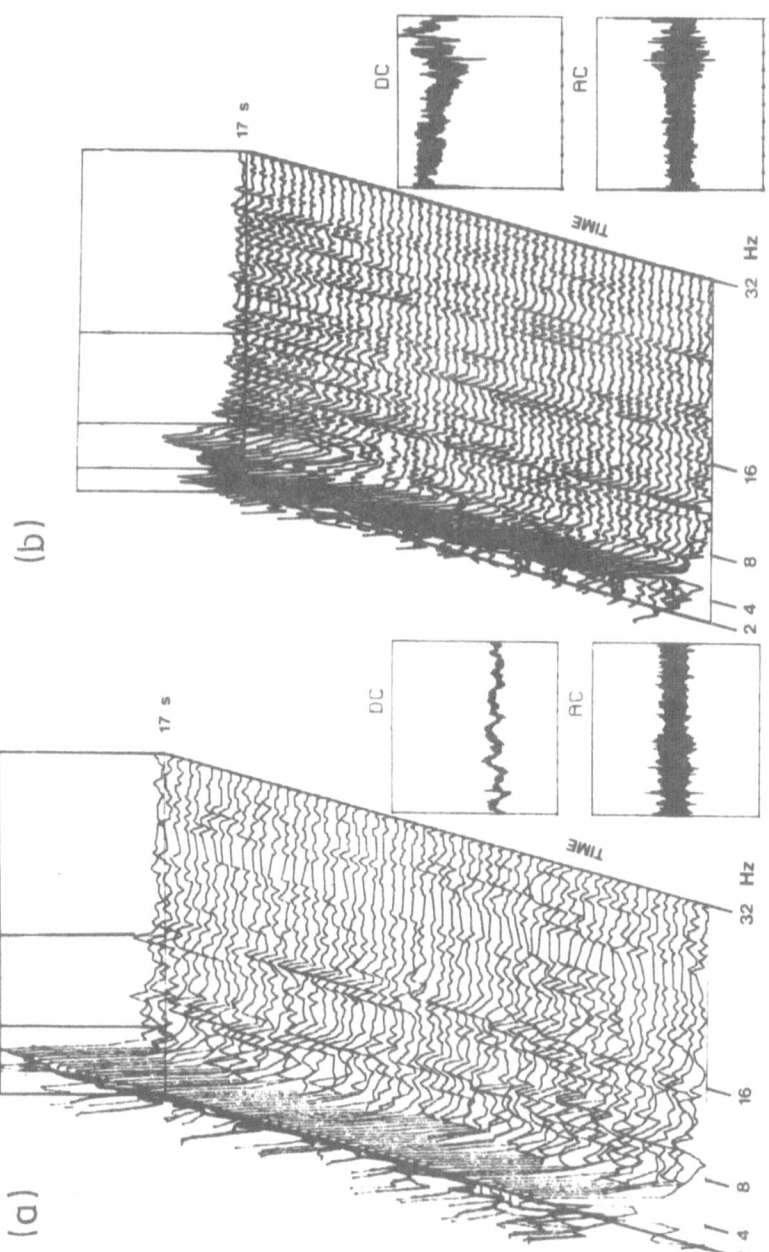

Figure 12.4 Series of overlapping force tremor spectra during maintained stationary contraction of extensor indices muscle in two patients with extrapyramidal tremor. Both parkinsonian (a) and cerebellar (b) show marked peaks at frequencies around 4 Hz.

DISCUSSION ON THE DETERMINANTS OF TREMOR RATE

When the synchronisation between motor units exceeds a certain threshold, the muscle spindles become activated (Hagbarth and Young, 1979). The excitation of the spindles is best triggered off by the almost unfused twitch contractions produced by the motor units firing at the lowest rates. The higher the motor unit firing rates, the more fused are the resulting contractions. Owing to this damping effect, the effectiveness of motor unit discharges in eliciting spindle excitation decreases with increasing rate. At higher rates a stronger synchronisation would have to occur between the motor units before spindle activation could be accomplished. Thus the lowest discharge rates have the highest efficiency in exciting muscle spindles and thus force synchronisation to that slow rate at which the synchronisation of the fewest motor units brings the servo-loop into play via spindle activation. The frequency of the servo-loop oscillation would thus be determined by the onset firing rate of the motor units.

Such a conclusion stands in contrast to the conventional assumption that the rate of the servo-loop oscillation is dependent on the length of the servo-loop. This argument has often been a matter of controversy. At least there are a number of observations which are difficult to explain on this basis. The most difficult point is the lack of any systematic examination of the dependence of the rate of augmented tremor on the length of the servo-loop. The effects of cooling extremities, growth of arm length in children and of deafferentation have been extensively discussed in that context.

The causal relationship between the motor unit onset firing rates and tremor rate makes the length of servo-loop as the determinant of tremor rate even more difficult to understand. It is an interesting feature of motor units that the onset rates for maintained firing lie in the range between 6 and 12 Hz in the different limb muscles. It is impossible to produce maintained firing rates below this range. This onset firing range is obviously not governed by servo-loop mechanisms, because the muscle spindles become non-activated during such muscle contractions. When the servo-loop comes into play by synchronisation under conditions with augmented tremor, the servo-loop oscillation does not impose a change in the onset rates according to their loop time.

A difficulty would arise in explaining the slowing of tremor rate in pathological tremors. The lesions that usually lead to the appearance of such coarse slow tremors are located in the CNS and do not alter the loop time. Conduction time or the length of the servo-loop cannot therefore be responsible for the pathological slowing of rate in pathological tremor. What other mechanism then can cause such a shift in rate? At this point we would like to discuss some recent experiments of our group on the maximal rate of alternating voluntary movements. Augmented tremor represents the fastest possible involuntary movement. Its rate reflects and is indicative of the motor unit onset firing rates. When the rates of the fastest possible alternating finger movements that can be performed for a short time by human subjects were measured, they approximated the tremor rates of the subject and finger examined (Reiners et al., 1981). Nobody can move faster than he trembles. The investigation of the frequency-limiting factors and the functional capacity of these movements showed that the full range of the functional capacity—angle of movement or range of force—can be preserved until ~3 Hz. Faster movements can only be performed at smaller amplitudes. This damping of amplitude has mechanical reasons.

When tremor represents the fastest involuntary movement, the increase in amplitude of this rapid alternating movement with decreasing rate shows a close resemblance to its voluntary counterpart. Because of the mechanical constraints, fast alternating movements are subject to considerable mechanical damping. When the tremor rate becomes slower under pathological conditions, the same number of motor units discharging synchronously produce larger amplitudes because of less mechanical damping; larger amplitudes generate a more powerful spindle activation which in turn leads to a stronger synchronisation. The neuronal mechanisms causing the development of 'pathological' tremor after lesions in some central motor nuclei are not known.

A further difficulty of such an explanation arises from experiments on muscle spindle recordings from parkinsonian patients (Hagbarth *et al.*, 1975) where no increased spindle activation could be seen during tremor. The slow burst activity at corresponding rates in thalamic nuclei also persists where afferent or efferent pathways are interrupted (Gilman *et al.*, 1976). These results provide evidence that the slow, synchronous central rhythms underlying pathological tremor may be independent from peripheral feedback. Whatever the mechanism is, in the normal subject these central nuclei must prevent the development of pathological synchronisation. Otherwise our motoneurone pools would synchronise as in the pathological cases. When synchronisation is not prevented, an increase of loop gain by decreasing mechanical damping as achieved by slowing of onset firing and therefore tremor rates could be a positive feed-forward mechanism optimising the loop gain. Such a hypothesis implies that the tremor rate under these pathological conditions or in the cooling experiments would be determined by a gain setting mechanism. The difficulty of this assumption is the fact that large-amplitude tremors do not always become slower. Tremor amplitude in patients with essential tremor is also increased but the rate remains normal.

Another alternative is the consideration of different loops involved in the generation of physiological and pathological tremor. The short loop would explain rates around 8 Hz whereas the involvement of disinhibited long loops in pathological conditions would explain rates of around 4 Hz as a result of long loop time. The difficulty of this assumption is the fact that the slowing of tremor in the course of the disease or of cooling occurs continuously and not as a sudden change from one loop time to the other.

CONCLUSION

The neurophysiological mechanisms leading to the slowing of tremor rates are not understood. Further studies will be needed to elucidate this problem, which is a central issue in tremor research.

REFERENCES

Dietz, V., Bischofsberger, E., Wita, C. and Freund, H.-J. (1976). Correlation between discharges of two simultaneously recorded motor units and physiological tremor. *EEG Clin. Neurophysiol.*, **40**, 97–105.

Gilman, S., Carr, D. and Helenberg, J. (1976). Kinematic effects of deafferentation and cerebellar ablation. *Brain*, **102**, 311–30.

Hagbarth, K. E., Wallin, G., Burke, D., Löfstedt, L. and Aquilonius, S.-M. (1975). Muscle spindle activity in alternating tremor of Parkinsonism and in clonus. *J. Neurol. Neurosurg. Psychiatr.*, **38**, 636–41.

Hagbarth, K. E. and Young, R. R. (1979). Participation of the stretch reflex in human physiological tremor. *Brain*, **102**, 509–26.

Halliday, A. M. and Redfearn, J. W. T. (1956). An analysis of the frequencies of finger tremor in healthy subjects. *J. Physiol. (Lond.)*, **134**, 600–11.

Hammond, P. H., Merton, P. H. and Sutton, C. G. (1956). Nervous gradation of muscular contraction. *Br. Med. Bull.*, **12**, 214–18.

Horsley, V. and Schaeffer, E. H. (1886). Experiments on the character of the muscular contractions which are evoked by excitation of the various parts of the motor tract. *J. Physiol. (Lond.)*, **7**, 96–110.

Meyer-Lohmann, J., Conrad, B., Matsunami, K. and Brooks, V. B. (1975). Effects of dentate cooling on precentral unit activity following torque pulse injections into elbow movements. *Brain Res.*, **94**, 237–51.

Moore, G. P., Perkel, D. H. and Segundo, J. P. (1966). Statistical analysis and functional interpretation of neuronal spike data. *Am. Rev. Physiol.*, **28**, 493–522.

Reiners, K., Hefter, H. and Freund, H.-J. (1981). Vergleiche der Frequenzeigenschaften motorischer Einheiten und des Muskels bei Willkürbewegungen. *Pflügers Arch.*, **389**, Suppl. R 57.

Sears, T. A. and Stagg, D. (1976). Short-term synchronization of intercostal motoneurone activity. *J. Physiol. (Lond.)*, **263**, 357–81.

SECTION 3
ESSENTIAL TREMOR

13
Essential tremor: introductory remarks

L. J. FINDLEY

Essential tremor, with its senile and familial varieties, is a common and geographic-ally ubiquitous disorder of unknown aetiology. The prevalence and spectrum of disability of this disorder are difficult to gauge, but from information from com-munities in the United States, Scandinavia and New Guinea the prevalence is variably quoted as being from 0.4 to 5.6% of the population. This 10-fold differ-ence in prevalence can be attributed to differences in the genetic structure of the communities studied and variations in the epidemiological techniques employed (see Rautakorpi et al., this volume, chapter 14). Sevitt (1974) has estimated that there are 80 000 consultations annually for essential tremor in the United Kingdom and 1.4 million consultations annually for senile tremor. The sex incidence is quoted as being equal by Critchley (1949); however, some studies have shown an increased incidence in females (Sevitt, 1974) and others have shown an increase in males (Critchley, 1972).

Essential tremor is considered to be dominantly inherited but with variable penetrance (Critchley, 1949). In our own series of 200 patients, one-third have a family history of tremor. Sex chromosome abnormalities have been reported in some patients (Bangman et al., 1973).

The tremor can commence at any age and frequently becomes exacerbated in the senium (Critchley, 1949). It commonly begins in the hands and arms with slow progression in some patients to involve head, chin, tongue, face, trunk and legs. In our experience one-quarter of patients have involvement of the head, which is usually of the 'yes–yes' type. Occasionally the tremor can be confined to single structures such as the head or voice (Hatchinski, 1975). The frequency of the tremor between individuals is quoted as ranging from 5 to 9 Hz (Shahani and Young, 1978). The frequency of symptomatic tremor in an individual limb of an affected patient does not vary and the characteristic waveform of the motion is sinusoidal. When well developed, the tremor is generated from recipro-cal activation of antagonistic muscles although periods of co-contraction may be observed. The amplitude of a tremor (measured at the peak frequency) may undergo up to a three-fold change on different days of recording; however the sudden, spontaneous, wide fluctuations in amplitude seen in parkinsonian rest tremor are not characteristic of essential tremor. The tremor is present typically in posture, attenuating during movement but becoming obvious again at the termination of movement. It can occasionally be seen at rest, particularly in the elderly, which is a feature that may cause difficulty in making the differential diagnosis with respect to Parkinson's disease (see Salisachs and Findley, this volume, chapter 15). When present at rest, the amplitude of the tremor is invariably smaller than the amplitude in posture.

Essential tremor is often prefixed with the word 'benign', which reflects its slowly progressive natural history but belies the fact that individual patients can be so severely affected that they are physically and socially handicapped. There is a small subset of patients with essential tremor who suffer with generalised *gross* tremor, which is totally disabling and may pervade all activities.

There has been a tendency to consider essential tremor as a single homogeneous entity; however, recent studies have distinguished subtypes which differ either on behavioural characteristics (Marsden *et al.*, 1983; Marsden, this volume, chapter 4) or on pharmacological responsivity (Calzetti *et al.*, 1983). Essential tremor has usually been considered monosymptomatic; however, it is now recognised that the tremor is frequently accompanied by some rigidity (see Salisachs and Findley, this volume, chapter 15), is associated with other movement disorders such as torticollis (Critchley, 1972), can manifest in Charcot-Marie-Tooth disease (Salisachs, 1970) and has been associated with nystagmus by Nettleship (1911) and Van Bogaert and De'Savitsch (1937) [we have never noted an eye movement disorder in patients with essential tremor]. In addition a higher incidence of essential hypertension and vascular disease has been reported in patients with essential tremor (Rautakorpi *et al.*, this volume, chapter 14; Rajput *et al.*, 1982). The pathophysiology of essential tremor is not understood and the few morbid anatomical studies that have been undertaken have failed to reveal any structural basis (Herskovits and Blackwood, 1969).

REFERENCES

Bangman, F. A. Jr, Higgins, J. V. and Mann, J. D. (1973). Sex chromosome anomalies in ET. *Neurology*, 23, 623–5.

Calzetti, S., Findley, L. J., Gresty, M. A., Perucca, M. D. and Richens, A. (1983). The effects of a single oral dose of propranolol on essential tremor: a double blind controlled study. *Ann. Neurol.*, 13, 165–71.

Critchley, E. (1972). Clinical manifestations of essential tremor. *J. Neurol. Neurosurg. Psychiatr.*, 35, 365–72.

Critchley, M. (1949). Observations on essential (heredofamilial) tremor. *Brain*, 72, 113–39

Hatchinski, V. C. (1975). The nature of primary vocal tremor. *Can. J. Neurol. Sci.*, 2, 195–7.

Herskovits, E. and Blackwood, W. (1969). Essential (familial, hereditary) tremor. A case report. *J. Neurol. Neurosurg. Psychiatr.*, 32, 509–11.

Marsden, C. D., Obeso, J. and Rothwell, J. C. (1983). Benign essential tremor is not a single entity. In Yahr, M. D. (ed.), *Current Concepts in Parkinson's Disease*, Excerpta Medica, Amsterdam, in press.

Nettleship, E. (1911). On some cases of hereditary nystagmus. *Trans. Ophthalmol. Soc. UK*, 31, 159–62.

Rajput, A. H., Beard, K. P. O. M. and Kurland, L. T. (1982). An epidemiologic survey of essential tremor in Rochester MN. *Neurology*, 32, 128-34.

Salisachs, P. (1970). Charcot-Marie-Tooth disease associated with essential tremor. *J. Neurol. Sci.*, 28, 17-40.

Sevitt, I. (1974). A comparison of propranolol and benzhexol in essential tremor. *Practitioner*, 213, 91-4.

Shahani, B. T. and Young, R. R. (1978). Action tremors: a clinical neurophysiological review. In Desmedt, J. E. (ed.), *Physiological Tremor, Pathological Tremors and Clonus, Progress in Clinical Neurophysiology*, vol. 5, Karger, Basel, pp. 129-37.

Van Bogaert, L. and De'Savitsch, E. (1937). Sur une maladie congenitale et hérédo-familiale comportant un tremblement rythmique de la tête, des globes oculaires, et des membres supérieurs. *Encephale*, 32(1), 113-30.

14
Epidemiology of essential tremor

I. RAUTAKORPI, R. J. MARTTILA and U. K. RINNE

INTRODUCTION

Essential tremor probably occurs in all parts of the world and in different types of population, but there are only limited data available concerning its epidemiology, and the prevalence estimates vary to a considerable degree. This chapter discusses the problems encountered in epidemiological studies of essential tremor and outlines the epidemiological features of this disorder.

CASE ASCERTAINMENT

The disability caused by essential tremor is often mild, and its progression is usually slow. It therefore causes only a slight inconvenience to many patients, in whom it may be regarded not as a disease but as a harmless symptom (Critchley, 1949; Larsson and Sjögren, 1960). Essential tremor is dominantly inherited. Many patients have noticed one or even more of their relatives trembling and the tremor does not evoke any embarrassment or undue concern. On the other hand, there are patients who are distressed by the presence of tremor and try to conceal it. For these reasons, patients with essential tremor rarely present themselves for medical treatment. In the series of Larsson and Sjögren (1960) only one out of 210 patients had contacted a hospital for treatment for tremor, and in our series only 10% had actively sought medical advice (Rautakorpi et al., 1982).

Even if the patient has sought appropriate medical advice, there is still the possibility that the disorder may not be recognised as such. The mild tremor that the patient complains of may be interpreted as constitutional, e.g. an infirmity due to old age. It may be seen as a symptom of some other disease, or the patient may be considered 'neurotic or alcoholic' (Critchley, 1949; Magee, 1965; Paulson, 1976). If the tremor is more severe, it is commonly misdiagnosed as Parkinson's disease (Pollock and Hornabrook, 1966; Hoehn and Yahr, 1967; Marttila and Rinne, 1976a; Rautakorpi, 1978; Salisachs and Findley, this volume, chapter 15).

The registration of patients with essential tremor is thus incomplete, and the generally available registration systems, such as hospitals, physicians' records, insurance or pension establishments, cover only a small proportion of the patients.

This renders the community survey method (Kurtzke and Kurland, 1976) invalid for the investigation of the epidemiology of essential tremor. The cases collected by this method tend to be highly selective, consisting mainly of patients with considerable physical, social or psychic disability, or patients with interesting or exceptional features, e.g. an advanced state of the disease, localisation of tremor, or occurrence throughout a family. Patients with mild tremor are seldom reached by community surveys unless the patient's occupation demands the utmost skill in the use of the hands, when even mild tremor may lead to his seeking medical aid at an early stage.

A more feasible method for investigating the epidemiology of essential tremor is a population-based approach, either a total population survey or a survey by random sampling. These methods are, however, rather laborious, and have to be restricted to limited geographical areas and populations. Generalisation from the results of such surveys may not always be justified.

The diagnosis of essential tremor is a clinical diagnosis which depends basically on the observation of postural or action tremor in the extremities and/or head, and the absence of other diseases associated with tremor, or tremor caused by drugs. In the epidemiological studies of essential tremor so far completed, there seems to be considerable variation in diagnostic criteria. There have been no fixed standards concerning the degree of tremor, duration of tremor, or degree of disability caused by tremor required to justify a diagnosis of essential tremor.

For our population-based survey (Rautakorpi *et al.*, 1982), we formulated clear criteria for diagnosis of essential tremor (table 14.1). Our criteria require

Table 14.1 Diagnostic criteria for essential tremor.

(1) Patient has a history of oft-recurring tremor (at least several times a week) or constant tremor in the extremities and/or head
(2) In clinical examination, patient has postural or action tremor in the extremities and/or head, sometimes with a slight intentional component
(3) Patient has no systemic or neurological disease known to be associated with tremor
(4) Patient does not use any drugs known to cause tremor
(5) Occurrence of similar tremor in family supports the diagnosis

nothing more than a thorough medical history of the patient and a clinical, neurological and general medical examination. It has been our experience that by applying these criteria it is possible in most cases to make a clear diagnosis. The differential diagnosis of essential tremor is discussed elsewhere in this volume, but, as far as our diagnostic criteria are concerned, the greatest difficulty is encountered in trying to distinguish enhanced physiological tremor from the early stages of essential tremor. However, occasionally enhanced physiological tremor is excluded by the first criterion; moreover, in our own experience, there is often a recognisable factor leading to recurring enhancement of physiological tremor, e.g. neurotic behaviour, thyrotoxicosis or sympathomimetic drugs. A more rigorous distinction between essential tremor and enhanced physiological tremor can be made if one includes only cases with constant tremor, but there are then inevitably some affected patients who are not recognised.

PREVALENCE

There are five epidemiological studies of essential tremor available: two from Scandinavia (Larsson and Sjögren, 1960; Rautakorpi, 1978; Rautakorpi *et al.*, 1982), one from New Guinea (Hornabrook and Nagurney, 1976) and two from the USA (Haerer *et al.*, 1981; Rajput *et al.*, 1982). The differences between the populations studied, some of them ethnically and genetically isolated, and the various epidemiological approaches and diagnostic criteria applied probably account in part for the over 10-fold variation in the prevalence estimates, ranging from 0.4 to 5.6% of the population aged over 40 years old (table 14.2).

Table 14.2 Epidemiological studies of essential tremor.

Country	Prevalence (%)		Reference
	Total population	Over-40-year-old population	
Sweden	1.7	3.73	Larsson and Sjögren (1960)
New Guinea	0.35	1.64*	Hornabrook and Nagurney (1976)
Finland	–	5.55	Rautakorpi (1978), Rautakorpi *et al.* (1982)
USA	–	0.45 white female 0.41 white male 0.41 black female 0.33 black male	Haerer *et al.* (1981)
USA	0.31	–	Rajput *et al.* (1982)

*Range in different districts 0.14–2.24%.

The first figures concerning the occurrence of essential tremor were reported by Larsson and Sjögren in 1960. These investigators made a survey of a rural area in northern Sweden where they had observed a large number of essential tremor cases during an earlier study. Case ascertainment was carried out by means of a field investigation and thorough interviews with a large number of the patients' relatives and also other persons. The total number of registered cases of essential tremor was 210 in a population of 5522 persons; by the end of the study period, 105 were living and 105 were deceased. This yielded a prevalence of 1.7% in the total population and in the population aged over 40 years old, which comprised 34% of the total population, the prevalence was 3.7%. A clinical examination was performed on 80 of the 105 patients who were still alive. Most of the patients had been born and still resided in one part of the area, and all had a lineage to one or more of nine ancestral couples. The diagnosis of essential tremor was based on earlier clinical descriptions of the disorder, and the report does not include any comments on differential diagnostic problems.

The area investigated in New Guinea by Hornabrook and Nagurney (1976) was divided into a number of ethnically and linguistically isolated districts, where the communities had been living in isolation for between 500 and 2000 years.

The field officers first screened the population and subsequently those persons suspected of having a neurological disease were examined. Altogether 175 cases of essential tremor were diagnosed, the diagnosis being based on the occurrence of monosymptomatic tremor. The prevalence varied in different districts from 0.14 to 2.24% of the population aged over 40 years. In the whole study area, the prevalence in that age group was 1.64%, and in the total population, 0.35%. The age structure of the population was different from those in the other studies; the population aged over 40 years was only 21% of the total population.

For the reasons stated above, we adopted a population-based two-phase approach in our investigation of the epidemiology of essential tremor in Finland (Rautakorpi *et al.*, 1982). The study was carried out in two rural communes in south-west Finland with a total population of 8759 persons. In the first phase, the persons with tremor were identified in the over-40-year-old population (3304 persons; 38% of the total population) by a personal interview (persons aged 40–64 years) or by a postal enquiry (persons aged over 64 years). Answers were obtained from 3080 persons (93.2%). In 253 (8.2%) tremor had occurred often or fairly often, in 595 (19.3%) occasionally, and 2232 persons (72.5%) had never experienced tremor. In the second phase, all those who had reported tremor as occurring often or fairly often were invited to a clinical examination. Of the 247 persons living and still resident in the area, 222 (89.9%) attended the examination. In addition, a sex- and age-matched sample of 202 persons reporting occasional tremor were asked to come for a clinical examination. Of the 198 persons alive, 151 (76.3%) participated.

On the basis of a clinical examination carried out by one of the present investigators (IR), and by employing the diagnostic criteria mentioned above (table 14.1), out of a total of 222 persons with continuous or frequently recurring tremor, 171 patients were diagnosed as having essential tremor. An additional 19 cases of essential tremor were found among the 151 persons with occasional tremor. Since there is some diagnostic overlap among the patients with occasional tremor, i.e. between those with essential tremor in an early stage and those with enhanced physiological tremor, the prevalence rates were calculated on the basis of the 171 patients with constant essential tremor, the persons who responded to the enquiry being used as the population base. The minimum prevalence was then 5.55% of the population aged over 40 years (table 14.3). The prevalences did not differ in the two communes, but the prevalence among males was higher than that among females in both places (table 14.3).

To show how many cases are lost if epidemiological methods relying on the available registration systems are used, we calculated the prevalence of essential tremor on the basis of those cases which could have been identified by analysing hospital or physicians' records, or patients who had previously been diagnosed as having essential tremor. Of our patients, 19 had sought medical advice for tremor and prior to our study five of them had been diagnosed as having essential tremor. The frequency of essential tremor calculated according to the 19 traceable patients would be 0.62% of the over-40-year-old population, and respectively 0.16% for diagnosed cases.

Table 14.3 Prevalences of essential tremor in a Finnish population.

	Population aged over 40 years	*Number of patients*	*Prevalence (%)*
Commune (a)			
Female	908	39	4.30
Male	715	46	6.43
Total	1623	85	5.24
Commune (b)			
Female	827	43	5.20
Male	630	43	6.83
Total	1457	86	5.90
Both communes			
Female	1735	82	4.73
Male	1345	89	6.62
Total	3080	171	5.55

In Copiah County, USA, Haerer *et al.* (1981) carried out a door-to-door enquiry in order to make a survey of neurological disorders. Over 99% of eligible households participated. All persons over the age of 39 years who had responses suggesting essential tremor were examined by a neurologist. The criteria for a positive diagnosis were as follows: gradual onset, disease in the family or present for at least 10 years, serious interference with handwriting, daily activities or speech. Moreover, all other types of tremor had to be excluded. There was no difference in the prevalence observed in white or black populations, both being about 0.4% of the population aged over 39 years. This prevalence is some 10 times lower than that found in our study in Finland. However, if the criteria of Haerer *et al.* are applied to our material, only about one in five of the cases would be included, because 12–24% had markedly or severely incapacitating tremor according to a global clinical rating, or when their condition was estimated by handwriting, drawing and pegboard tests (Rautakorpi, 1978).

Using the records of the Mayo Clinic, Rajput *et al.* (1982) made a list of all patients with tremor observed over a 45-year period. In this case the patients were not examined personally and the diagnosis of essential tremor was based on medical records. The observed prevalence rose gradually with time, and the most recent prevalence was 0.31% of the total population.

Age-specific prevalence

Studies that include age-specific prevalences reveal an increase in the prevalence of essential tremor with advancing age (table 14.4). The prevalence is low under the age of 30 years, and essential tremor most often begins after that age. Only in 14% of essential tremor cases in Sweden was the age at onset less than 30 years (Larsson and Sjögren, 1960). In our study, the first symptoms had occurred before the age of 30 years in 24% of the patients (Rautakorpi, 1978).

Table 14.4   Comparison of age-specific prevalences (%) of essential tremor.

Age groups	Larsson and Sjögren (1960)	Hornabrook and Nagurney (1976)	Rautakorpi et al. (1982)
0–29	0.10	0	
30–39	0.65	0.07	
40–49	1.00	0.58	2.20
50–59	3.93	1.67	5.06
60–69	⎫ 5.45		6.84
70–79	⎬	⎫ 4.11	12.60 ⎫
80–	⎭ 8.33	⎭	11.84 ⎬ 12.47

Essential tremor seems to be concentrated in the age groups above 50 years (table 14.4), and the highest prevalences have been observed in persons over 70—8.3% in Sweden and 11.5% in Finland. In New Guinea, the highest prevalence was 4.1%, in the age group over 60 years.

SEX DISTRIBUTION

In New Guinea more females than males were found to have essential tremor, the female : male ratio being 2.06. In the USA, too, slightly more females than males had essential tremor, the ratios being 1.07 for white and 1.24 for black populations respectively (Haerer *et al.*, 1981). In Scandinavia, however, the situation was the reverse. In Sweden the female : male ratio was 0.50 (Larsson and Sjögren, 1960), and in Finland 0.71 (Rautakorpi, 1978). Since the differences in age structure between the female and male populations may bias the ratios based on the total population, it would be better to judge the distribution between sexes according to age- and sex-specific prevalences. As will be seen from table 14.5, the prevalence of essential tremor among males in Finland clearly exceeds the prevalence among females of all age groups except the oldest and this also suggests that essential tremor is more common among men.

Table 14.5   Age- and sex-specific prevalences (%) of essential tremor in Finland.

Age groups	Female	Male	Total
40–49	1.43	3.02	2.20
50–59	3.34	7.20	5.06
60–69	5.62	8.55	6.84
70–79	11.25	15.04	12.60
80–	13.79	5.56	11.84
Total	4.73	6.62	5.55

RELATION TO OTHER DISEASES

The assumption that essential tremor is genetically related to or a *forme fruste* of Parkinson's disease (Critchley, 1949; Mjönes, 1949; Barbeau and Pourcher, 1982) has not been supported by epidemiological studies of either disorder, though Hornabrook and Nagurney (1976) found slight evidence that these two disorders may be in some way linked. On the other hand, Larsson and Sjögren (1960) found no patient with Parkinson's disease in the families of essential tremor patients. The patients in our own epidemiological study, when compared to a sex- and age-matched control sample from the same population, were found to have a similar proportion of parkinsonian relatives (Rautakorpi, 1978). In the same way, there is no accumulation of essential tremor cases among relatives of patients with Parkinson's disease (Duvoisin *et al.*, 1969; Marttila and Rinne, 1976b). Furthermore in our case control evaluation, there was no evidence of association of any other neurological disorder with essential tremor, but the patients with essential tremor had cardiovascular diseases, including arterial hypertension, coronary heart disease and cerebrovascular disease, significantly more often than did the controls. The explanation of this association is not known at present. It may depend on the occurrence of a selection bias in the control group, or alternatively on a genetic linkage between essential tremor and certain risk factors of cardiovascular diseases.

CONCLUSIONS

Essential tremor is epidemiologically a somewhat inaccessible disorder. Owing to the incomplete registration of patients, reliable data about its occurrence can be obtained only by population-based surveys and by applying adequate diagnostic criteria. Although the epidemiological profile of essential tremor is just now emerging, the available data show that essential tremor is a common disorder. The highest prevalences, 3.7 and 5.6% of the over-40-year-old population, have been observed in Sweden and Finland, respectively. Essential tremor is mainly concentrated in the age groups above 40 years, with the highest prevalence in the seventh decade. The sexes may be affected differently in different populations, both male and female preponderance having been reported. There is no convincing evidence of the association of essential tremor with any other neurological disease, including Parkinson's disease, but some data suggest that there may be increased risk of cardiovascular disease in patients with essential tremor.

ACKNOWLEDGEMENT

This study was supported by the Sigrid Jusélius Foundation, Finland.

REFERENCES

Barbeau, A. and Pourcher, E. (1982). New data on the genetics of Parkinson's disease. *Can. J. Neurol. Sci.*, 9, 53–60.

Critchley, M. (1949). Observations on essential (heredofamilial) tremor. *Brain*, 72, 113–39.

Duvoisin, R. C., Grearing, F. R., Schweitzer, M. D. and Yahr, M. D. (1969). A family study of parkinsonism. In Barbeau, A. and Brunette, J. R. (eds), *Progress in Neurogenetics*, International Congress Series No 175, Excerpta Medica, Amsterdam, pp. 492–6.

Haerer, A. F., Anderson, D. W. and Schoenberg, B. S. (1981). Prevalance of essential tremor in the biracial adult population of Copiah County, Mississippi. *Ann. Neurol.*, 10, 93–4.

Hoehn, M. M. and Yahr, M. D. (1967). Parkinsonism: onset, progression and mortality. *Neurology*, 17, 427–42.

Hornabrook, R. W. and Nagurney, J. T. (1976). Essential tremor in Papua New Guinea. *Brain*, 99, 659–72.

Kurtzke, J. F. and Kurland, L. T. (1976). The epidemiology of neurological disease. In Baker, A. B. and Baker, L. H. (eds), *Clinical Neurology*, vol. 3, Harper and Row, New York, pp. 1–80.

Larsson, T. and Sjögren, T. (1960). Essential tremor. A clinical and genetic population study. *Acta Psychiatr. Neurol. Scand.*, Suppl. 144.

Magee, K. R. (1965). Essential tremor: diagnosis and treatment. *Clin. Med.*, 72, 33–41.

Marttila, R. J. and Rinne, U. K. (1976a). Epidemiology of Parkinson's disease in Finland. *Acta Neurol. Scand.*, 54, 81–102.

Marttila, R. J. and Rinne, U. K. (1976b). Arteriosclerosis, heredity, and some previous infections in the etiology of Parkinson's disease. A case-control study. *Clin. Neurol. Neurosurg.*, 79, 45–56.

Mjönes, H. (1949). Paralysis agitans. *Acta Psychiatr. Neurol.*, Suppl. 54.

Paulson, G. W. (1976). Benign essential tremor in childhood. Symptoms, pathogenesis and treatment. *Clin. Pediatr.*, 15, 65–75.

Pollock, M. and Hornabrook, R. W. (1966). The prevalence, natural history and dementia of Parkinson's disease. *Brain*, 89, 429–48.

Rajput, A. H., Beard, K. P. O. M. and Kurland, L. T. (1982). Epidemiologic survey of essential tremor in Rochester, MN. *Neurology*, 32, 128.

Rautakorpi, I. (1978). *Essential Tremor. An Epidemiological, Clinical and Genetic Study*, Research Reports from the Department of Neurology, No. 12, University of Turku, Finland.

Rautakorpi, I., Takala, J., Marttila, R. J., Sievers, K. and Rinne, U. K. (1982). Essential tremor in a Finnish population. *Acta Neurol. Scand.*, 66, 58–67.

15
Problems in the differential diagnosis of essential tremor

P. SALISACHS and L. J. FINDLEY

INTRODUCTION

Essential tremor is a common disorder and is usually considered to be mono-symptomatic. An increasingly common problem in clinical practice is in distinguishing essential tremor from the tremor arising in association with Parkinson's disease, particularly as it presents in the elderly patient (Raymond, 1876; Marshall, 1968).

On theoretical grounds there should be little difficulty in differential diagnosis; however, in a recent hospital study of 115 patients, many of whom had been treated for Parkinson's disease diagnosed largely on the basis of tremor before entering hospital, on detailed inpatient review 20% were found to have benign essential (senile) tremor (Rautakorpi, 1978). As essential tremor is usually considered to be dominantly postural or action in type, whereas the tremor of Parkinson's disease is usually thought of as dominantly a tremor of rest, such difficulties in diagnosis would seem unlikely. In addition to the appearance of tremor, the other signs usually attributed to extrapyramidal disease, in particular the cogwheel rigidity and hypokinesia, should facilitate the diagnosis. However, Critchley (1956) in his article 'Neurological changes in the aged' emphasised that a degree of rigidity and bradykinesia may be a 'common' feature in the elderly individual and does not necessarily reflect disturbance of basal ganglia function. In addition objective studies of large numbers of tremulous parkinsonian patients by Lance et al. (1963) and more recently by Findley et al. (1981) have shown that the presence of a symptomatic postural tremor is as common as the classical resting tremor. In addition, the asymmetrical manifestation of tremor in the limbs, which is frequently considered to be a hallmark of Parkinson's disease, can also be found in cases of essential tremor, particularly early in the natural history of the disease (Rautakorpi, 1978). These features must necessarily increase the difficulties for the clinician dealing with the elderly tremulous patient. Indeed, even in young patients with essential tremor, cogwheel rigidity can be brought out by synkinetic movement of the opposite limb (Salisachs, 1978). This phenomenon is termed Froment's sign (Froment and Gardere, 1926) and prior to

219

Salisachs' (1978) study was considered to be pathognomonic of extrapyramidal disorder. Thus, throughout the age ranges in a population of patients presenting with tremor, the clinical signs can be 'equivocal' in attempting a differential diagnosis (Davis and Kunkle, 1951; Doshay, 1961; Pollock and Hornabrook, 1966; Hoehn and Yahr, 1967; Duvoisin, 1972).

CHARACTERISTICS OF TREMOR IN 'ESSENTIAL' TREMOR AND PARKINSON'S DISEASE

The studies of tremor in Parkinson's disease by Lance *et al.* (1963) and Findley *et al.* (1981) have shown that the symptomatic postural tremor can vary widely in frequency from patient to patient. However, there is a modal frequency of 6 Hz. The distribution of tremor frequency in the more symptomatic hand of 38 patients with essential tremor is shown in figure 15.1. The distribution shows

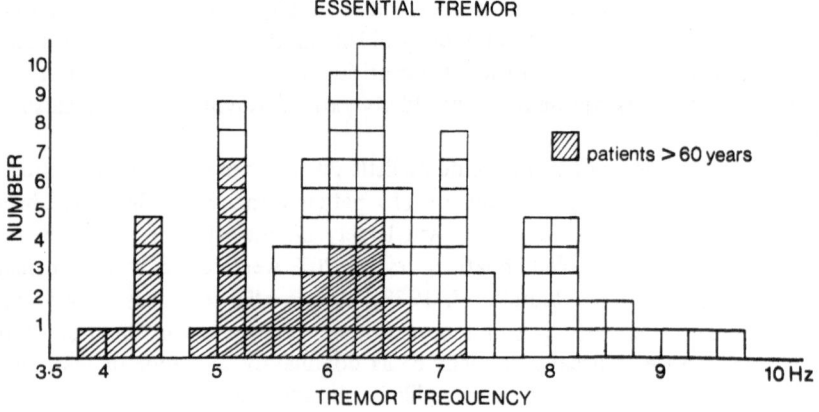

Figure 15.1 Histogram of tremor frequency recorded from the more symptomatic hand in 38 patients with essential tremor. The shaded area is a subset consisting of patients aged over 60 years; although they do not have tremor at the higher frequencies, there is still a popular representation at frequencies around 6 Hz.

that the range of frequency of essential tremor of the hand varies between 4 and 9 Hz with a modal frequency of 6–6.5 Hz. The shaded histogram representing the frequencies of patients older than 60 years has absent values at the higher frequencies but still has popular values around 6 Hz. Thus on the basis of frequency analysis alone it is not possible to separate patients with symptomatic, predominantly postural, tremor arising from basal ganglia disorder from those with essential tremor.

When the resting tremor is dominant in Parkinson's disease, differential diagnosis should not be difficult. When tremor at rest does present in essential tremor it is invariably of lesser amplitude than the postural tremor and almost identical in frequency (less than 0.5 Hz dfference). But when resting tremor dominates in a parkinsonian patient, the tremor on posture is usually much smaller in amplitude and at a significantly higher frequency (Findley *et al.*, 1981). It seems that, although frequency alone is not a sufficiently reliable criterion for differential diagnosis, the observation of an alteration of frequency with movement of the limb from a resting position into posture is of considerable help in establishing the diagnosis of Parkinson's disease. This characteristic is shown in figure 15.2, which compares the behavioural characteristics of tremor in patients with essential tremor and Parkinson's disease.

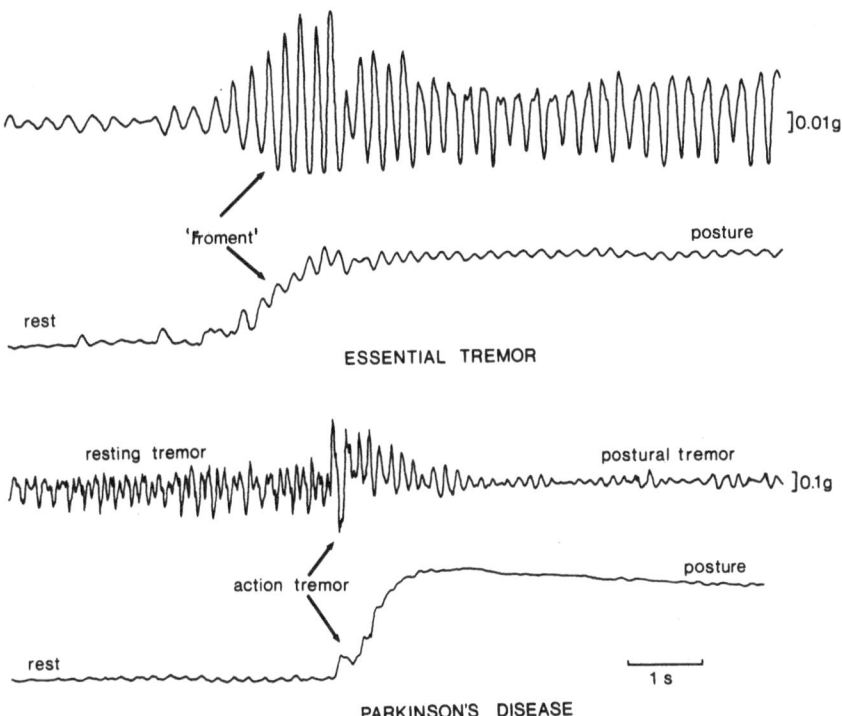

Figure 15.2 Accelerometric and displacement recordings of resting, action (hand lifting into posture) and postural tremor in a patient with essential tremor compared with a patient with Parkinson's disease. The patient with Parkinson's disease has a large-amplitude tremor at 4.5 Hz. The patient with essential tremor has minimal movement at rest. In the middle of the traces the hand is raised into posture. During the movement there are a series of large transients in the waveform which are the action tremors in both patients. When in posture the patient with essential tremor shows a waveform with a frequency of 7 Hz. The patient with Parkinson's disease has a small-amplitude tremor at 6 Hz which is quite different in quality from the resting tremor.

RIGIDITY

Cogwheel rigidity (Negro, 1928), i.e. the tremulous interruption of passive movement about a joint, and the similar phenomenon brought out by active movement
of an opposite limb during the examination, i.e. 'signe de Froment', have for a
long time been considered pathognomonic of disorders of the basal ganglia. In a
study of 17 patients with uncomplicated essential tremor (Salisachs, 1978), 16
showed an unequivocally positive Froment's sign. In cases of essential tremor
studied by Findley (unpublished work), this sign was present in at least 50% of
patients and there seemed to be a fairly equal distribution of this sign across the
age ranges. Recordings of the 'signe de Froment' from a pateint with a five-
year history of essential tremor of familial type are shown in figure 15.3. Apart
from postural and action tremor, the only other clinical findings was a positive
Froment's sign. The 'signe de Froment' has many characteristics in common with
the cogwheel phenomenon. The vibratory interruption during passive movement
of the hand which corresponds to the sign has an identical frequency to that of
the postural and action tremors. This is also the major characteristic of the cogwheel phenomenon in Parkinson's disease (Findley *et al.*, 1981), i.e. cogwheel
rigidity is a manifestation of the postural tremor of the disease and not of the
resting tremor.

(a)

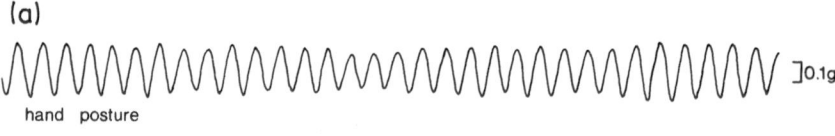

hand posture

(b)

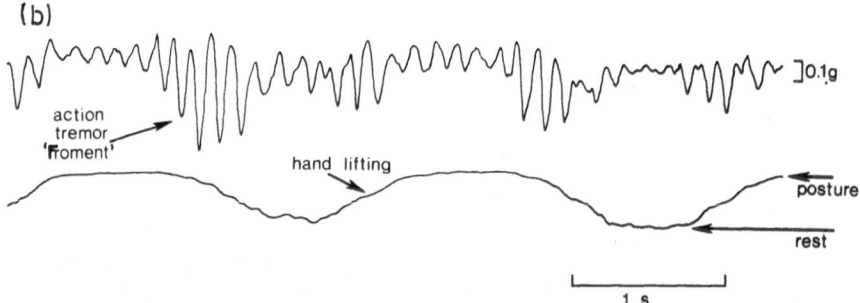

Figure 15.3 Recordings of postural tremor of the hand and the Froment's sign
in a patient with essential tremor. (a) Accelerometric recording of postural tremor.
(b) Accelerometric and displacement recordings of the hand being lifted from rest
to posture.

DISCUSSION

Thus the so-called pathognomonic signs of Parkinson's disease overlap considerably with those of essential tremor, particularly in the elderly. This is particularly true when Parkinson's disease presents in a predominantly tremulous form which usually has a more benign course and is often without the other 'soft' supportive signs such as positive glabellar tap. In some patients with Parkinson's disease, using objective recording techniques it is possible to distinguish two separate tremor frequencies arising in the same limb and even supported by the same muscle (Gresty and Findley, 1983). These two frequencies correspond to the resting and postural tremors of the disease. Normally they occur in mutual exclusion but occasionally they overlap as one or the other vies, as it were, for dominance. It has been argued that the ability to demonstrate two separate tremors at different frequencies is strong evidence for basal ganglia disease. If one is unable to demonstrate these sorts of findings then, bearing in mind that other clinical signs are common to both disorders, the differential diagnosis of essential tremor from Parkinson's disease remains a considerable problem in some patients.

CONCLUSION

Problems in the differential diagnosis of patients with essential tremor arise particularly in the elderly, tremulous patient in whom the possibility of an extrapyramidal syndrome must be considered. Errors in diagnosis can occur for several reasons. First, some patients with Parkinson's disease do have a tremor that is similar in character to essential tremor in that it is predominantly postural. Conversely, a few of the essential tremors observed have a resting component. In addition, rigidity and bradykinesia can be a common finding in otherwise normal elderly people. In particular, cogwheel rigidity, a phenomenon considered a hallmark of parkinsonism, may be found in the majority of essential tremor patients in the form of a positive Froment's sign. Measurements of tremor reveal that in the majority of parkinsonian patients the postural and resting tremors have different frequencies and behavioural characteristics. If these features can be demonstrated, then a confident diagnosis of Parkinson's disease can be made. Unfortunately, there still remain occasional patients in whom there is insufficient evidence for a firm diagnosis.

REFERENCES

Critchley, M. (1956). Neurological changes in the aged. *J. Chronic Dis.*, **3**, 459–77.
Davis, C. H. and Kunkle, E. C. (1951). Benign essential (heredofamilial) tremor. *Arch. Intern. Med.*, **87**, 808–16.
Doshay, L. J. (1961). Senile tremor versus Parkinson's disease. *Postgrad. Med.*, **30**, 550–4.

Duvoisin, R. C. (1972). Clinical diagnosis of the dyskinesias. *Med. Clin. N. Am.*, 56, 1321–41.

Findley, L. J., Gresty, M. A. and Halmagyi, G. M. (1981). Tremor, the cogwheel phenomenon and clonus in Parkinson's disease. *J. Neurol. Neurosurg. Psychiatr.*, 44, 534–46.

Froment, J. and Gardere, H. (1926). La rigidité et la rue dentée Parkinsoniene s'effacent au repos. *Rev. Neurol.*, 1, 52–3.

Gresty, M. A. and Findley, L. J. (1983). Postural and resting tremor in Parkinson's disease. In Hassler, R. G. and Christ, J. F. (eds), *Parkinson-Specific Motor and Mental Disorders, Advances in Neurology*, vol. 40, Raven Press, New York, pp. 361–4.

Hoehn, M. M. and Yahr, M. D. (1967). Parkinsonism: onset, progression and mortality. *Neurology (Minneap.)*, 17, 427–42.

Lance, J. W., Schwab, R. S. and Peterson, E. A. (1963). Action tremor and the cogwheel phenomenon in Parkinson's disease. *Brain*, 86, 95–110.

Marshall, J. (1968). Tremor. In Vinken, P. J. and Bruyn, G. W. (eds), *Handbook of Clinical Neurology*, vol. 16, North-Holland, Amsterdam, pp. 809–25.

Negro, C. (1928). Le phénomène de la rue dentée. *Encephale*, 23, 203–20.

Pollock, M. and Hornabrook, R. W. (1966). The prevalence, natural history and dementia of Parkinson's disease. *Brain*, 89, 429–48.

Rautakorpi, I. (1978). *Essential Tremor. An Epidemiological, Clinical and Genetic Study* (Thesis), Research Reports from the Department of Neurology, No. 12, University of Turku, Finland.

Raymond, F. (1876). *L'Hémichorée, l'Hémianesthésie et les Tremblements Symptomatiques*, A. Delahaye, Paris, p. 115.

Salisachs, P. (1978). Dos signos clinicos no conocidos del tremblor esencial. *Med. Clin. (Barcelona)*, 70, 120–1.

16
Beta-adrenoceptor involvement in tremor production: possible defects in essential tremor

S. KILFEATHER, A. MASSARELLA, P. TURNER
and L.J.FINDLEY

INTRODUCTION

Recent pharmacological studies on patients with essential tremor (ET) and physio-logical tremor have largely centred on the tremolytic action of the beta-adreno-ceptor antagonists (β-blockers) and the tremor-enhancing action of the beta-agonists (β-agonists). These studies have indicated possible 'tremogenic' areas vulnerable to β-blockade and involvement of peripheral beta-adrenoceptors (β-adrenoceptors) in the production of augmented physiological tremor (APT) (Bowman, 1980). β-Blockers have become the drugs of choice in the management of ET (Wilson *et al.*, this volume, chapter 17) and the tremor associated with other clinical conditions, such as hyperthyroidism (Turner, 1974). The mode of action of β-blockers in treatment of ET has not been established, but loci of activity in the central nervous system (CNS), in the periphery and at both β_1- and β_2-adrenoceptor subtypes could be involved.

APT observed in fear and isoprenaline infusion is similar to the tremulous activity associated with hyperthyroidism and the β-blocker withdrawal syndrome (BWS). Increases in β-adrenoceptor responsiveness in several tissues in both hyper-thyroidism and BWS could underlie the production of tremor and other symptoms associated with abnormally elevated adrenergic activity in these conditions.

Larsen (1980) suggested that altered β-adrenoceptor responsiveness could arise in the periphery affecting the reflex servo-loop in patients with ET. While it is possible that an isolated β-adrenoceptor defect of this kind can exist and contribute to tremogenesis, there is, at present, no indication of such a defect in the ET states. Tremolytic activity of β-blockers could be achieved at loci on tremogenic pathways that are sensitive to β-blockade but do not possess abnormally respon-sive β-adrenoceptors. Concerning possible general β-adrenoceptor defects in ET, there are no other signs of increased β-adrenoceptor responsiveness to suggest a general increase in catecholamine activity in the periphery. In a recent, as yet unpublished, retrospective survey of 119 ET patients from the Mayo Clinic seen

225

over a nine-year period, 26% were reported to have hypertension, in contrast to the lower prevalence (7%) of hypertension in the local normal population (Rajput, personal communication). While this finding is suggestive of an association between sympathetic mechanisms and ET, confirmation of this finding awaits results of further prospective epidemiological studies.

In this chapter the possible roles of β-adrenoceptors in tremogenesis and in β-blocker tremolytic action are discussed. In addition, results of an investigation of general β-adrenoceptor responsiveness in ET are presented.

CATECHOLAMINE ACTION IN SKELETAL MUSCLES AND THE PRODUCTION OF AUGMENTED PHYSIOLOGICAL TREMOR

Marsden et al. (1967a) demonstrated that tremolytic activity of propranolol after intra-arterial isoprenaline in a peripheral artery was localised distally to the site of infusion. Thus, β-adrenoceptors responsible for production of APT exist in the periphery and are probably those present on the skeletal muscles and spindles. Several clinical studies have identified the β_2-adrenoceptor as the β-adrenoceptor subtype responsible for production of APT, by demonstrating that β_1-selective antagonists (cardioselective β-blockers) are relatively ineffective in reducing the amplitude of APT (Larsson and Svedmyr, 1977). This view is supported by work on isolated muscle preparations, which suggests that the β_2-adrenoceptor on the skeletal muscle fibres is responsible for mediation of β-agonist effects on skeletal muscle contractility. These effects on skeletal muscle contraction properties differ according to the class of fibre under exposure. In fast-twitch fibres they increase tension and duration of twitch, and the reverse holds in slow-twitch fibres (Bowman, 1980). Non-selective agonists, such as isoprenaline, and β_2-adrenoceptor-selective agonists, such as terbutaline, are potent stimulators of contraction in isolated fast-fibre striated muscle, but the β_1-selective agonists tazozol, H80/60 and H133/22 do not evoke this contractile response (Waldeck, 1977; Al-Jeboory and Marshall, 1978). Furthermore, the β_2-adrenoceptor selective β-blocker ICI 118 551 completely abolishes the relaxant effects of isoprenaline on the soleus muscle (Smith et al., 1983).

Bowman and Zaimis (1958) suggested that disrupted integration of slow- and fast-twitch muscle activity could give rise to catecholamine-induced APT, and indeed changes in mechanical properties of skeletal muscle can give rise to changes in the physiological tremor through the reflex arc (Marsden, 1978).

In addition to direct actions on muscle fibres, catecholamines can facilitate transmission at the neuromuscular junction, but this is believed to be mediated through α-adrenoceptors (Bowman, 1980) and its role in supporting β-adrenoceptor-mediated APT is not known.

Spindle involvement in tremor production may extend only as far as synchronisation of motoneurone discharge in response to an underlying tremor or muscle perturbation. This view is illustrated by the single case reported by Marsden *et al.* (1967b), in which deafferentation of one arm resulted in reduction of the physiological tremor amplitude and widening of the tremor frequency band. This indicates that muscle spindles play at least some part in 'timing' of tremor frequency and maintenance of amplitude, while spinal or supraspinal mechanisms predominate in generation of the underlying tremor.

The presence of sympathetic innervation at the muscle spindle demonstrated by various workers (Banker and Girvin, 1971; Santini and Ibata, 1971; Ballard, 1978; Barker and Saito, 1981) supports the concept of catecholamine influence over spindle sensitivity, and the significance of this action in production of catecholamine-induced APT. Since circulating catecholamines have limited access to the spindle interior (McInnes, 1980), their actions must be mediated through receptors on the spindle capsule surface. In general, noradrenergic terminals innervate a predominantly β_1-adrenoceptor population in the periphery. Demonstration of sympathetic innervation at muscle spindle capsules, therefore, implies that additional β-agonist tremogenic action could be achieved at β_1-adrenoceptors at this site. This view is not supported, however, by the findings of Hodgson *et al.* (1969), who reported that adrenaline and isoprenaline, but not noradrenaline, could increase the tension of tonic contractions of human calf muscles evoked by vibration of the Achilles tendon, a response known to be generated by activity in the primary afferent endings of the muscle spindles (Matthews, 1972). The findings of Hodgson *et al.* (1969) imply that the β_2-adrenoceptor subtype predominates in mediation of this response, since noradrenaline has relatively low affinity for the β1-adrenoceptor subtype.

Close examination of spindle activity during isoprenaline infusion and sympathetic stimulation suggests that sympathetic innervation does not exert significant influence over spindle sensitivity to contraction. During isoprenaline infusion in man, Young and Hagbarth (1980) demonstrated enhanced afferent 'tremor' with grouping of spindle afferent signals during the stretch phase of spindle discharge. These changes resulted in elevation of contraction amplitude, as a consequence of increased synchronisation of motor unit discharge. No apparent change in spindle sensitivity during isoprenaline infusion was observed in this study, however, suggesting that catecholamines do not influence spindle sensitivity. This is in agreement with the observation made by Phillips *et al.* (1973) that propranolol demonstrated no apparent effect on muscle spindle activity. Also, Hunt *et al.* (1982), during stimulation of the lumbar sympathetic trunk innervating cat hindlimb spindles, observed only a slight and inconsistent rise in spindle discharge frequency and a possible facilitation of fusimotor action, but without a change in spindle sensitivity to stretch. These results suggest that the sympathetically innervated muscle β-adrenoceptors exert only minor effects on spindles. More studies of this kind are required to evaluate the exact role, if any, of the sympathetic innervation of the muscles in tremogenesis and the possibility of subtle effects on spindle sensitivity emerging under conditions of increased β-adrenoceptor responsiveness.

BETA-ADRENOCEPTOR DEFECTS AND SYMPTOMATIC AUGMENTED PHYSIOLOGICAL TREMOR

Some conditions with which symptomatic tremor occurs and where there is evidence for enhanced β-adrenoceptor-mediated responses are listed below:

Catecholamine infusion
Emotional stress
Phaeochromocytoma
Methylxanthine administration
Thyrotoxicosis
Beta-blocker abstinence (withdrawal) syndrome
Morphine and alcohol abstinence syndromes

APT or tremulous activity observed during catecholamine infusion, emotional stress and phaeochromocytoma is undoubtedly the result of peripheral β-adrenoceptor exposure to high plasma catecholamine levels, giving rise to the effects on muscle and spindle function as previously described.

APT is also a common side-effect of the xanthine derivatives used as bronchodilators in the treatment of obstructive airways diseases. The main actions of these compounds are mediated through the following mechanisms: mobilisation of intracellular calcium (Ca^{2+}), adenosine antagonism and inhibition of cyclic nucleotide phosphodiesterase (Bergstrand, 1980; Fredholm et al., 1979; Ralf, 1980; Svedmyr and Simonsson, 1978). APT induced by these compounds could arise from a combination of these effects on fast and slow muscle fibres. Ca^{2+} mobilisation has been shown to inhibit β-agonist-stimulated cyclic adenosine monophosphate (cAMP) accumulation in the rat uterus (Meisheri and McNeill, 1979) and mouse diaphragm (Gross and Kelly, 1981), but also potentiates β-agonist facilitation of skeletal muscle contraction in fast fibres (Bianchi, 1961; Thorpe and Seeman, 1971; Jeppsson et al., 1982). In slow fibres, however, Ca^{2+} mobilisation opposes the depressant effects of β-adrenoceptor stimulation and this would account for the inability of theophylline to potentiate the depressant effects of β-adrenoceptor agonists on the soleus muscle observed by Jeppsson et al. (1982). Methylxanthines could induce tremulous activity, therefore, by upsetting the balance of fast- and slow-fibre mechanical properties through Ca^{2+} mobilisation and inhibition of cAMP catabolism. Further investigation of the adenosine antagonistic properties of xanthine derivatives may provide additional information concerning mechanisms involved in the development of APT during treatment with these compounds.

Thyrotoxicosis

The density of peripheral β-adrenoceptors in the hyperthyroid state has been shown to be increased in several tissues, including the heart (McConnaughey et al.,

1979) and lymphocytes (Ginsberg *et al.*, 1981). The β-adrenoceptor population of the lymphocyte consists mainly of the β_2-subtype (Brodde *et al.*, 1981), whereas those of the heart are predominantly of the β_1-subtype (U'Prichard *et al.*, 1978). The influence of the hyperthyroid state is not, therefore, confined to either of the known β-adrenoceptor subtypes or a single tissue. In electromechanical studies of hyperthyroid cardiac tissue, Wei *et al.* (1982) have shown that induction of hyperthyroidism causes a reduction in the threshold of contractile response to the facilitatory effect of catecholamines on development of twitch tension in this tissue. Guarnieri *et al.* (1980) and Stiles and Lefkowitz (1981) have produced evidence indicating that enhanced β-adrenoceptor responsiveness is responsible for the electromechanical changes observed by Wei *et al.* (1982) in hyperthyroidism. It is possible that similar changes in β-adrenoceptors could occur on skeletal muscles and spindles. Buur *et al.* (1982) have shown that chronic treatment with the β-adrenoceptor agonist terbutaline induces a state of hyporesponsiveness of guinea-pig soleus muscle to the effects of adrenaline and terbutaline on cAMP accumulation, sodium and potassium transport and subtetanic contractions. Furthermore, they observed a distinct correlation between the depression of muscle contraction and cAMP accumulation, suggesting that a reduction in β-adrenoceptor responsiveness was responsible for the reduced relaxation response. This demonstrates the capacity of altered skeletal muscle β-adrenoceptor responsiveness to interfere with the normal contractile responses of the muscle to circulating adrenaline.

Increased β-adrenoceptor responsiveness at the muscles and spindles could, therefore, be responsible for the production of APT in hyperthyroidism, and would account for the effectiveness of β-blockers in the reduction of tremor and other symptoms of adrenergic overactivity in this condition.

Beta-blocker abstinence (withdrawal) syndrome (BWS)

BWS is a well documented phenomenon, which can occur when chronic treatment with β-blockers is suddenly withdrawn. The condition is characterised by increasingly severe anginal attacks, arrhythmias, myocardial infarction, APT and occasionally sudden death (Slome, 1973; Diaz *et al.*, 1973; Alderman *et al.*, 1974; Mizgala and Counsell, 1976; Boudoulas *et al.*, 1977; Harrison and Alderman, 1976; Frishman and Silverman, 1979; Nattel *et al.*, 1979; Pedersen *et al.*, 1979). Chronic administration of propranolol has been associated with an increase in β-adrenoceptor density in rat ventricles (Glaubiger and Lefkowitz, 1977), and increased ventricular inotropic responsiveness to isoprenaline in the dog *in vivo* (Webb *et al.*, 1981) and the rat *in vitro* (Kennedy and Donnelly, 1982). In the study by Webb *et al.* (1981), plasma noradrenaline levels showed no apparent change before, during, or after propranolol administration in dogs exhibiting ventricular hyperresponsiveness after propranolol withdrawal, indicating that this hyperadrenergic state is not due to reflex increases in circulating noradrenaline.

In man, elevated β-adrenoceptor-mediated responses have also been demonstrated after propranolol withdrawal (Boudoulas *et al.*, 1977; Aarons *et al.*, 1980). Aarons *et al.* (1980) demonstrated an elevation in lymphocyte β_2-adrenoceptors in association with chronic propranolol administration, indicating that the β-adrenoceptor defect is general, probably extending throughout the periphery and CNS, as indeed may be the case with hyperthyroidism. Similarly in this condition a β-adrenoceptor defect could exist in skeletal muscles and spindles, giving rise to tremulous activity associated with sudden withdrawal of propranolol administration.

Morphine and alcohol abstinence syndromes

Tremulous activity is experienced during the morphine and alcohol abstinence syndromes together with other symptoms indicative of elevated sympathetic drive. The increase in plasma catecholamine levels observed during withdrawal from chronic administration of alcohol in man (Ogata *et al.*, 1971; Sellers *et al.*, 1978), and the significant benefit obtained from treatment of alcohol withdrawal tremor with β-blockers (Zilm *et al.*, 1975), suggest that the tremor is derived from normal muscle responses to raised plasma catecholamine levels. Moreover, anxiety and stress experienced during withdrawal would contribute to the adrenergic activity observed. Investigation of central β-adrenoceptors during chronic administration and withdrawal of alcohol and morphine suggests that changes in β-adrenoceptor responsiveness could also be involved in the expression of these abstinence syndromes.

cAMP has been shown to be important in maintenance of the morphine abstinence syndrome (Collier, 1980) and this implies that receptor-mediated activation of adenylate cyclase could be involved. From studies of β-adrenoceptor density and adenylate cyclase responsiveness to catecholamines in the rat brain, several groups have reported findings that are consistent with the view that chronic administration of alcohol and morphine causes changes in β-adrenoceptor density and responsiveness. These reports suggest that an increase in responsiveness develops during administration of these compounds (Lorens *et al.*, 1978; Hamburg and Tallman, 1981), or during the development of the morphine (Kuriyama *et al.*, 1978, 1981) and alcohol (Israel *et al.*, 1972; Kuriyama and Israel, 1973; French *et al.*, 1975, 1977; Banerjee *et al.*, 1978; Kuriyama *et al.*, 1981) abstinence syndromes. All reports agree, however, that an increase in β-adrenoceptor density is present at the withdrawal stage and could be associated with the abstinence syndrome. Furthermore, increases in β-adrenoceptor density have been observed in the superior cervical ganglion after chronic administration of morphine (Mattio and Kirby, 1982), and these authors have proposed that changes in β-adrenoceptor density in the periphery may also contribute to the abstinence syndrome.

The relevance of these central β-adrenoceptor changes to expression of tremor and other symptoms of the abstinence syndromes is not clear, since changes in other receptor systems have also been observed as a consequence of chronic administration of morphine and alcohol. Hyporesponsiveness of cerebral dopaminergic receptors has been observed during withdrawal from chronic administration of morphine (Puri *et al.*, 1976, 1978) and ethanol (Hoffman and Tabakoff, 1977; Tabakoff *et al.*, 1978). Of greater significance, however, is the increase in α_2-adrenoceptor density observed by Hamburg and Tallman (1981) in the rat cortex during chronic administration of morphine, which may account for the benefit obtained from the α_2-adrenoceptor agonist clonidine during morphine abstinence and the marked similarity between the morphine and clonidine abstinence syndromes (Reid *et al.*, 1977). Furthermore, there is little understanding at present of the relationship between these receptor changes and the dramatic changes in membrane phospholipid composition observed during chronic administration of central depressants (Goldstein, 1979). It would be of value, therefore, to examine local membrane lipid composition while investigating possible changes in receptor functional status in areas concerned with tremogenesis during administration and withdrawal of central depressants. Initial studies of effects of such membrane changes on membrane receptor density have been reported (Heron *et al.*, 1982).

BETA-ADRENOCEPTORS IN ESSENTIAL TREMOR

Beta-adrenoceptor antagonist activity in essential tremor

There is some evidence to suggest that maximum tremolytic action of β-blockers in ET after oral administration is achieved after a delay of hours or sometimes a day, and this could be related to accumulation in central or peripheral compartments (Young *et al.*, 1975). More recent studies, however, have shown that a maximum response to a single oral dose of propranolol is observed without such a delay (Calzetti *et al.*, 1981). Nevertheless, the greater ease with which more lipophilic β-blockers penetrate the blood–brain barrier and accumulate in the CNS suggests that tremolytic activity of these compounds could be achieved centrally or in peripheral sites that are less accessible than skeletal muscle β-adrenoceptors. Furthermore, it is possible that membrane-stabilising activity may enhance the tremolytic action achieved through β-blockade, especially with lipophilic compounds such as propranolol.

Several attempts have been made to establish the relative importance of peripheral and central actions of propranolol in treatment of ET from measurement of tremolytic activity and plasma drug levels. Of the four studies conducted so far which seek a relationship between plasma propranolol level and degree of tremor reduction, such a relationship could only be demonstrated in one (McAllister *et al.*, 1977), in which the propranolol was administered intravenously. In the other studies propranolol was administered orally and tremor was monitored after chronic administration (Jefferson *et al.*, 1979b; Sorensen *et al.*, 1981; Calzetti *et al.*, 1983b). The apparent absence of a relationship in the oral studies could be attributed to several factors relevant to the pharmacodynamics of propranolol. A wide variation in the tremor response to propranolol is common on oral regimens. This may be influenced by the complex relationship between anxiety and physiological tremor, or by the normal fluctuation in tremor amplitudes, which as yet has been little explained. Evaluation of responses to propranolol is complicated, therefore, by variation in anxiety levels, individual response to propranolol and the effects of these factors on plasma catecholamine levels. Less obvious factors include differing degrees of tolerance to propranolol within the subject group, and the production of its active metabolite 4-hydroxypropranolol. Possibly the most important factor, however, is accumulation of propranolol and its active metabolite in the CNS and peripheral areas, where they could produce significant β-blockade and non-specific activity, which would be difficult to relate to their plasma levels (Turner, 1983).

There is insufficient evidence available at present, therefore, to estimate the relative importance of central and peripheral tremolytic activity of propranolol. Further studies of the time course of development of β-blocker tremolytic action during intravenous infusion will be of value in this respect.

Despite the considerable level of membrane-stabilising activity (MSA) exhibited by propranolol, several reports indicate that MSA is of little significance in its tremolytic activity. Studies of propranolol on isolated muscles have demonstrated that the MSA of propranolol is observed at much higher plasma concentrations than are required to produce significant β-blockade. Therapeutic benefit of propranolol in treatment of tremor is obtained at plasma levels of up to 0.1 mg l^{-1} (Nies and Shand, 1975; McAllister et al., 1977; Jefferson et al., 1979b; Sorensen et al., 1981), whereas the MSA of propranolol appears at plasma concentrations of 10 mg l^{-1} in cardiac muscle (Coltart and Meldrum, 1971) and 5 mg l^{-1} in skeletal muscle (Larsen, 1978). Accumulation of β-blockers in the CNS or peripheral sites, more accessible to lipophilic compounds, could result in significant reduction of tremor through a non-specific membrane effect in addition to the tremolytic effect of the more rapidly developed β-blockade, and this event cannot be ruled out as a mode of action in the CNS or periphery (Calzetti et al., 1983b; Calzetti and Findley, this volume, chapter 18). Sotalol, however, exhibits virtually no MSA, but demonstrates considerable tremolytic activity (Jefferson et al., 1979a; Rangel-Guerra, 1974; Rinne and Kaitaniemi, 1974). The effectiveness of sotalol in treatment of essential tremor, therefore, indicates that β-blockade rather than a non-specific membrane effect is responsible for a major part of the peripheral tremolytic action of the β-blockers and that penetration into the CNS is not a prerequisite to tremolytic activity in ET.

Involvement of both beta$_1$- and beta$_2$-adrenoceptor subtypes in beta-blocker tremolytic action

Although therapeutic benefit of cardioselective β-blockers, which have a greater affinity for the β_1-adrenoceptor subtype, has been demonstrated in ET, several studies indicate that they remain inferior to the non-cardioselective β-blockers

(Jefferson *et al.*, 1979a; Larsen *et al.*, 1982; Dietrichson and Espen, 1981; Leigh *et al.*, 1981; Calzetti *et al.*, 1981, 1982, 1983a). However, the tremolytic activity of the cardioselective compounds in ET implies that β_1-adrenoceptor blockade in addition to blockade of the non-innervated β_2-subtype is of value in β-blocker tremolytic action in ET. Furthermore, atenolol, a relatively hydrophilic cardioselective compound that accumulates in very low levels in the CNS (van Zweiten and Timmermans, 1979; Neil-Dwyer *et al.*, 1981; Taylor *et al.*, 1981), produces significant tremolytic action in ET, indicating that ET is sensitive to β_1-adrenoceptor blockade in the periphery. Some reservation should be exercised, however, when attributing the tremolytic action of relatively hydrophilic compounds exclusively to a peripheral action, since Taylor *et al.* (1981) have demonstrated that atenolol can attain levels in the cerebrospinal fluid on oral dosing that may be adequate for β-blockade.

GENERAL BETA-ADRENOCEPTOR RESPONSIVENESS IN ESSENTIAL TREMOR

Based on an apparent relationship between frequency and amplitude of ET and responsiveness to propranolol, Calzetti *et al.* (1982, 1983a) proposed that ET states were not homogeneous. Recently, an extensive classification of ET has been made (Marsden *et al.*, 1983), describing four types of ET. The first and second groups within this classification, namely Type I and Type II, encompass essential tremors which have been reported to be responsive to β-blockers. Type I ET in common with APT is characterised by a relatively high tremor frequency band (8–12 Hz) and low amplitude, and is sensitive to the driving influence of an external torque motor. Type I ET is, therefore, behaviourally indistinguishable from APT observed during emotional stress and catecholamine infusion. Despite the marked similarity between the Type I ET and APT, however, the absence of other peripheral signs of a β-adrenoceptor defect in ET, and the unlikelihood of such a defect being confined to the skeletal muscles or spindles, may suggest that the cause of Type I ET lies in central 'control' of physiological tremor or in defective spindle reflex responses.

Type II ET is characterised by larger amplitude and a lower frequency band (5–7 Hz), and is not responsive to entrainment by an external oscillator. This insensitivity of Type II tremors to peripheral entrainment indicates that tremogenic mechanisms in the CNS predominate in production of this class of tremor. Furthermore, when enhanced by catecholamines, the ET states with lower frequency exhibit increased tremor amplitude, but without alteration to the tremor frequency. On closer examination of changes within the reflex arc during isoprenaline infusion, Young and Hagbarth (1980), demonstrated that isoprenaline increases the amplitude of afferent signals and muscle unit synchrony produced through the reflex arc in response to isolated twitches, without affecting the tremor frequency. The absence of a shift in frequency towards that of physiological tremor and APT in this case suggests that peripheral β-adrenoceptors affected by catecholamines during, or shortly after, catecholamine infusion may only mediate an increase in the underlying tremor amplitude, rather than a modification of the tremor frequency. A peripheral β-adrenoceptor defect in Type II ET is not suspected, therefore, since enhanced responsiveness of the β-adrenoceptors as the major tremogenic defect should give rise to a tremor similar to that of APT or Type I ET.

Here, we present results of an investigation of general β-adrenoceptor responsiveness in patients with Type I and II ET. The β_2-adrenoceptor population of the peripheral blood lymphocyte was used as a model of the general condition of β-adrenoceptors, and lymphocyte membrane β-adrenoceptor density and isoprenaline-induced cAMP accumulation in intact lymphocytes were measured as indices of receptor responsiveness.

Peripheral blood lymphocyte beta$_2$-adrenoceptor as a model of general beta-adrenoceptor status

The assumed universal flexibility of receptor density and responsiveness enables extrapolation between certain tissues when predicting the response of identical receptor regulating mechanisms to alterations in the level of exposure to agonists or antagonists. Thus receptor systems of peripheral blood cells including the lymphocyte have been used to investigate similar receptor systems elsewhere in less accessible areas of the periphery (Greenacre and Conolly, 1978; Greenacre et al., 1978; Frazer et al., 1981; Aarons and Molinoff, 1982). The virtual absence of the β_1-subtype on the lymphocyte has not precluded the use of the lymphocyte β-adrenoceptor population as a model of drug-induced changes of β_1-adrenoceptors elsewhere in the periphery (Aarons and Molinoff, 1982). When using the lymphocyte to assess general β-adrenoceptor function in the untreated disease states, however, the possibility of isolated tissue-specific receptor defects must be considered, and therefore only conclusions concerning general β-adrenoceptor status can be made in this case.

Extrapolation between tissues concerning the effects of drug exposure on mechanisms regulating events distal to receptors is more complex. Contractile actinomycin filaments are present in many non-muscle cells, and in lymphocytes they are utilised in mitogenesis and motility (Fechheimer and Cebra, 1982). There are, however, several mechanisms regulating contraction in all cells and their degree of operation depends upon the conditions within the cell. Thus the phosphorylation of myosin is not as important in regulation of contraction of skeletal muscle as it is in smooth muscle and non-muscle cells (Alderstein et al., 1982). It is important, therefore, when extrapolating from biochemical parameters to monitor an event that is known to occur consistently after drug-receptor interaction in the cell types under consideration. In this study we have used the conventional approach to the question of events distal to agonist-β-adrenoceptor interaction by measuing cAMP accumulation subsequent to the stimulation of adenylate cyclase activity with isoprenaline in the intact lymphocyte plasma membrane. Verification of the sensitivity of the technique used to determine lymphocyte β-adrenoceptor responsiveness and its capacity to detect differences between normal and patient groups has been made in previous studies (Kirby *et al.*, 1980; Kovacs *et al.*, 1983).

Methodology

Patients

Patients exhibiting either Type I or II ET were accepted into the study. Patients with signs of cardiovascular disorder (apart from hypertension), respiratory or other neurological disorders were excluded from the study. All patients were untreated and had received no medication for at least two weeks prior to investigation. Details of the three groups are presented in table 16.1.

Table 16.1 Patient data.*

	Age range (years)	Age mean (years)	Tremor frequency (Hz)	Tremor magnitude (milli-g)†	Tremor duration (years)
Normal subjects (6 male, 4 female)	20–55	30.5 ± 9.8	–	–	–
Type I ET (2 male, 6 female)	17–50	26.0 ± 11.1	8.58 ± 0.98	15.7 ± 12.4	7.4 ± 5.6
Type II ET (9 male, 2 female)	19–86	54.7 ± 20.0	6.10 ± 0.77	69.0 ± 83.3	19.9 ± 24.3

*All values are means ± standard deviation (SD).
†g = acceleration due to gravity (981 cm s^{-2}).

Tremor recording

The tremor was measured on the basis of the mean of 150 acceleration spectra (bandwidth 0–25 Hz, dF 0.1 Hz) derived from 1.5 min time record of tremor. Magnitude was characterised in terms of peak amplitude of the dominant frequency band of the spectrum. The type of ET was distinguished by the fact that Type I was readily entrained by the application of external perturbations of similar magnitude to the tremor itself. In contrast Type II was resistant to entrainment unless the externally applied forces were excessively large (Gresty and Findley, this volume, chapter 2).

Cell preparation

Peripheral blood was heparinised (20 units ml^{-1}) and immediately diluted with an equal volume of phosphate-buffered saline (PBS) supplemented with glucose (5.55×10^{-3} M). Diluted plasma was removed by centrifugation for 30 min at 150g and 20°C. The remaining cells were rediluted with PBS to replace the volume of diluted plasma removed. Lymphocytes were separated by a modification of the method of Böyum (1968). Diluted blood (14 ml) was then layered over Ficoll-paque (10 ml; Pharmacia Fine Chemicals) and centrifuged for 30 min at 400g and 20°C. The lymphocyte bufficoat was removed and diluted with five volumes of PBS. The lymphocyte suspension was then centrifuged for 10 min at 150g and 12°C. The remaining cell pellet was rediluted with six volumes of PBS and recentrifuged for 30 min at 400g and 12°C. The cells were resuspended in PBS and cell counting was performed using Turk's stain. In all cases granulocyte contamination was less than 1% and the platelet:lymphocyte ratio was no greater than 3.

Isoprenaline incubation

Lymphocytes (2×10^6 ml^{-1}) were incubated with isoprenaline (10^{-9} to 10^{-4} M) and isobutylmethylxanthine (5×10^{-4} M) for 15 min at 37°C. Incubation was terminated by immediately freezing in acetone and dry ice. EDTA was added to a final concentration of 5×10^{-3} M. The incubation mixture was then immersed in boiling water for 5 min. The cell debris was removed by centrifugation at $2 \times 10^3 g$ for 30 min at 20° C and the supernatant was removed for cAMP assay and stored frozen at -25°C. cAMP content was assayed with a modification of the method of Brown *et al.* (1971) in which 100 μl of supernatant samples were incubated with 25 μl (1.8×10^{-8} M) of ^{3}H-cAMP (40 Ci mmol^{-1}) and 200 μl of a bovine adrenal extract prepared as previously described (Brown *et al.*, 1971), for 2 h at 1-4°C. The bound fraction was separated with addition of 500 μl of a charcoal suspension (20 mg activated charcoal/ml, 3 mg bovine serum albumin/ml) at 1-4°C and centrifuged at $2.5 \times 10^3 g$ for 10 min at 1-4°C.

Receptor binding studies

Previously frozen lymphocytes were homogenised ice cold with an Ultraturrax homogeniser for 30 s. The membrane suspension was centrifuged for 30 min at $1.5 \times 10^4 g$ and 1-2°C. The supernatant was discarded and replaced with incubation buffer (Tris, 0.01 M ; NaCl, 0.154 M, bovine serum albumin, 5×10^{-6} ml^{-1}) at 1°C. Membranes of 2×10^5 lymphocytes were incubated with [^{125}I]-iodocyanopindolol (ICYP) (10-100 pM) in 200 μl at 37°C for 1 h. Non-specific binding was determined by inclusion of ($\pm$)isoprenaline, HCl (2×10^{-4} M) and ascorbic acid (10^{-3} M) in the incubation. Incubations were terminated by dilution with 10 ml of incubation buffer at 37°C and immediately filtered through Whatman GF/C filters. The filters were then washed with 10 ml of incubation buffer at 37°C and counted in a gamma counter (Nuclear Enterprises NE1600).

Results

cAMP responses

The lymphocyte responses of the patients and normal subjects to isoprenaline are presented in figure 16.1. Analysis of variance applied to the dose–response curves indicates that no significant difference exists between the three groups with respect to their lymphocyte β-adrenoceptor responsiveness.

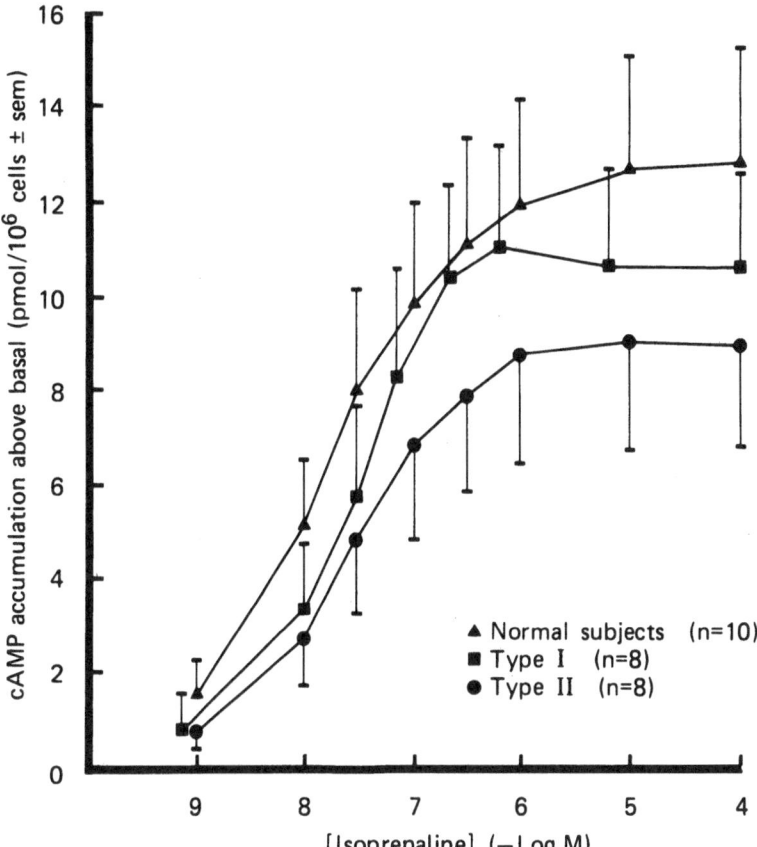

Figure 16.1 Lymphocyte dose–response curves to isoprenaline. Lymphocytes were incubated with isoprenaline (10^{-9} to 10^{-4} M) and isobutylmethylxanthine (5×10^{-4} M) at 37°C for 15 min. Ordinate axis shows cAMP accumulation above basal levels in normal subjects, Type I ET and Type II ET.

Receptor binding studies

The results of receptor binding studies are presented in figure 16.2. Analysis of the K_d and receptor density with Wilcoxon's test showed no difference in the affinity or receptor density between the patient and normal groups.

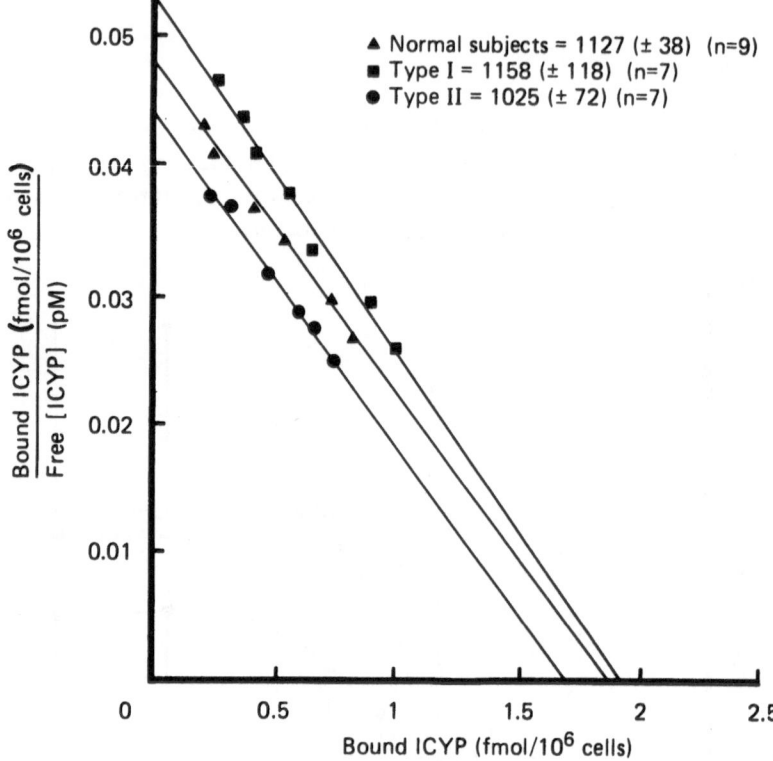

Figure 16.2 Scatchard analysis of β-adrenoceptor binding data. Lymphocyte membranes were incubated with [^{125}I]-iodocyanopindolol (ICYP) (10–100 pM) at 37°C for 1 h. The abscissal intercept provides an estimate of B_{max} (number of β-adrenoceptor binding sites per cell ± s.e.m.) for normal subjects, Type I ET and Type II ET.

CONCLUSIONS

The role of β-adrenoceptors in the generation of ET is not as well understood as in APT observed during catecholamine infusion and fear, where peripheral β_2-adrenoceptors are responsible for mediation of the tremogenic action of circulating β-adrenoceptor agonists. As expected, our results suggest that a general β-adrenoceptor defect is not involved in the production of Type I and II ET states. Furthermore, preliminary results of measurements of plasma catecholamine levels, not presented here, in patients investigated for β-adrenoceptor defects confirm that elevated catecholamine levels are not responsible for the production of the Type I ET, which according to the recent classification by Marsden *et al.* (1983) exhibits characteristics similar to that of APT. In view of the large difference between the mean ages of the control group and Type II ET patients, confirmation of these results should be obtained by comparison with age- and sex-matched controls.

While the lymphocyte β-adrenoceptor has proved useful in reflecting the response of β-adrenoceptors in less accessible areas to chronic drug administration, our demonstration of unaltered lymphocyte β-adrenoceptors does not exclude the possibility of an isolated tissue-specific β-adrenoceptor defect. This is particularly relevant to β-adrenoceptors at spinal or supraspinal levels, which do not share a common plasma environment with peripheral blood lymphocytes and skeletal muscles. The benefit obtained from β_2-adrenoceptor blockade in ET suggests that a large proportion of tremolytic activity could be achieved at these sites in the periphery and that adrenaline maintains optimal muscle mechanical properties during tremogenesis in ET. The possibility that central β-adrenoceptors could mediate facilitation of tremogenic signals should not be ignored, however, since β-blockade at the innervated β_1-subtype accounts for the benefit obtained from the cardioselective compounds such as atenolol. Additional information concerning central β-adrenoceptor involvement in ET may be provided by investigation of the widespread β-adrenoceptor hyperresponsiveness observed in the hyperthyroid state and BWS, which could extend into central areas.

Consensus opinion maintains that APT observed during periods of fear is of little biological value, because of the reduction in dexterity that this response causes. Rennie *et al.* (1982), however, demonstrated that adrenaline exerts a facilitatory action on skeletal muscle contractility, which is greatly prolonged during motoneurone-stimulated muscle contraction, and suggested that this may be of value in 'flight-or-fight situations'. APT could, therefore, be a manifestation of an adaptive mechanism, the purpose of which is to prime the skeletal muscles for execution of reactions under stress. Similarly, the paucity of literature concerning the role of sympathetic innervation at the muscle spindle suggests that it is of little physiological importance in terms of its effects on spindle sensitivity. Sympathetic innervation at the spindles could, however, serve a metabolic function, as Hunt *et al.* (1982) suggested. Furthermore, its role may be dependent upon high plasma adrenaline levels produced during stress, with which noradrenaline could exert a permissive effect on muscle mechanics through α-adrenoceptors.

REFERENCES

Aarons, R. D. and Molinoff, P. B. (1982). Changes in the density of beta adrenergic receptors in rat lymphocyte, heart and lung after chronic treatment with propranolol. *J. Pharmacol. Exp. Ther.*, 221(2), 439–43.

Aarons, R. D., Nies, A. S., Gal, J., Hegstrand, L. R. and Molinoff, P. B. (1980). Elevation of beta-adrenergic receptor density in human lymphocytes after propranolol administration. *J. Clin. Invest.*, 65, 949–51.

Alderman, E. L., Coltart, D. J., Wettach, G. E. and Harrisson, D. C. (1974). Coronary artery syndrome after sudden propranolol withdrawal. *Ann. Intern. Med.*, 81, 625–7.

Alderstein, R. S., deLanerolle, P., Sellers, J. R., Pato, M. D. and Conti, M. A. (1982). In Kakiuchi, S., Hidaka, H. and Means, A. R. (eds), *Calmodulin and Intracellular Ca²⁺ Receptors*, Plenum Press, London, pp. 313–29.

Al-Jeboory, A. A. and Marshall, R. J. (1978). Correlation between the effects of salbutamol on contractions and on cyclic AMP content of isolated fast-

and slow-contracting muscles of the guinea-pig. *Naunyn-Schmeideberg Arch. Pharmacol.*, **305**, 201–6.

Ballard, K. J. (1978). Typical noradrenergic endings in a muscle spindle of the cat. *J. Physiol. (Lond.)*, **285**, 61–2.

Banerjee, P. S., Sharma, V. K. and Khanna, J. M. (1978). Alterations in beta-adrenergic binding during ethanol withdrawal. *Nature*, **276**(5686), 407–9.

Banker, B. Q. and Girvin, J. P. (1971). The ultrastructural features of the mammalian muscle spindle. *J. Neuropathol. Exp. Neurol.*, **30**, 155–95.

Barker, D. and Saito, M. (1981). Autonomic innervation of receptors and muscle fibres in cat skeletal muscle. *Proc. R. Soc. Lond. B*, **212**, 317–32.

Bergstrand, H. (1980). Phosphodiesterase inhibition and theophylline. *Eur. J. Resp. Dis.*, **61**, Suppl. 109, 37–44.

Bianchi, C. P. (1961). The effect of caffeine on radiocalcium movement in frog sartorius. *J. Gen. Physiol.*, **44**, 845–58.

Boudoulas, H., Lewis, R. P., Kates, R. E. and Dalamangas, G. (1977). Hypersensitivity to adrenergic stimulation after propranolol withdrawal in normal subjects. *Ann. Intern. Med.*, **87**, 433–6.

Bowman, W. C. (1980). Effects of adrenergic activators and inhibitors on the skeletal muscles. *Handb. Exp. Pharmacol.*, **54**(II), 47–128.

Bowman, W. C. and Zaimis, E. (1958). The effects of adrenaline, noradrenaline and isoprenaline on skeletal muscle contractions in the cat. *J. Physiol. (Lond.)*, **144**, 92–107.

Böyum, A. (1968). Isolation of mononuclear cells and granulocytes from human blood. *Scand. J. Clin. Invest.*, **21**, Suppl 97, 77.

Brodde, O. E., Engel, G., Hoyer, D., Bock, K. D. and Weber, F. (1981). The β-adrenergic receptor in human lymphocytes: subclassification by the use of a new radioligand, (±)-[125]iodocyanopindolol. *Life Sci.*, **29**, 2189–98.

Brown, B. L., Albano, J. D. M., Ekins, R. P., Sgherzi, A. M. and Tampion, W. (1971). A simple and sensitive saturation assay method for the measurement of adenosine $3',5'$-cyclic monophosphate. *Biochem. J.*, **121**, 561–2.

Buur, T., Clausen, T., Holmberg, E., Johansson, U. and Waldeck, B. (1982). Desensitisation by terbutaline of beta-adrenoceptors in the guinea-pig soleus muscle: biochemical alterations associated with functional changes. *Br. J. Pharmacol.*, **76**, 313–17.

Calzetti, S., Findley, L. J., Gresty, M. A., Perucca, E. and Richens, A. (1981). Metoprolol and propranolol in essential tremor: a double blind study. *J. Neurol. Neurosurg. Psychiatr.*, **44**, 814–19.

Calzetti, S., Findley, L. J., Perucca, E. and Richens, A. (1982). Controlled study of metoprolol and propranolol during prolonged administration in patients with essential tremor. *J. Neurol. Neurosurg. Psychiatr.*, **45**, 893–7.

Calzetti, S., Findley, L. J., Perucca, E. and Richens, A. (1983a). Effect of a single oral dose of propranolol on essential tremor. A double blind controlled study. *Ann. Neurol.*, **13**, 165–71.

Calzetti, S., Findley, L. J., Perucca, E. and Richens, A. (1983b). The response of essential tremor to propranolol: evaluation of clinical variables governing its efficacy on prolonged administration. *J. Neurol. Neurosurg. Psychiatr.*, **46**, 393–8.

Collier, H. O. J. (1980). Cellular site of opiate dependence. *Nature*, **283**, 625–9.

Coltart, D. J. and Meldrum, S. J. (1971). The effect of racemic propranolol, dextropropranolol and racemic practolol on the human and canine transmembrane action potentials. *Arch. Intern. Pharmacodyn.*, **192**, 188–97.

Diaz, R. G., Somberg, J. C., Freeman, E. and Levitt, B. (1973). Withdrawal of propranolol and myocardial infarction. *Lancet*, **1**, 1068.

Dietrichson, P. and Espen, E. (1981). Effects of timolol and atenolol on benign essential tremor: placebo controlled studies based on quantitative tremor recording. *J. Neurol. Neurosurg. Psychiatr.*, **44**, 677–83.

Fechheimer, M. and Cebra, J. J. (1982). Phosphorylation of lymphocyte myosin catalyzed *in vitro* and in intact cells. *J. Cell Biol.*, **93**, 261–8.

Frazer, J., Nadeau, J., Robertson, D. and Wood, A. J. J. (1981). Regulation of human leucocyte beta receptors by endogenous catecholamines. *J. Clin. Invest.*, **67**, 1777–84.

Fredholm, B. B., Brodin, K. and Strandberg, K. (1979). On the mechanism of action of relaxation of the tracheal muscle by theophylline and other cyclic nucleotide phosphodiesterase inhibitors. *Acta Pharmacol. Toxicol. (Kbh.)*, **45**, 336–44.

French, S. W., Palmer, D. S. and Kenneth, D. W. (1977). Changes in receptor sensitivity of the cerebral cortex and liver during ethanol ingestion and withdrawal. In Gross, M. M. (ed.), *Advances in Experimental Medicine and Biology*, 85A, *Alcohol Intoxication and Withdrawal*, Plenum Press, New York, IIIa: Biological aspects of ethanol.

French, S. W., Palmer, D. S., Narod, M. E., Reid, P. E. and Ramey, C. W. (1975). Noradrenergic sensitivity of the cerebral cortex after chronic ethanol ingestion and withdrawal. *J. Pharmacol. Exp. Ther.*, **194**, 319–26.

Frishman, W. and Silverman, R. (1979). Clinical pharmacology of the new beta blocking drugs. Part 3. Comparative clinical experience and new therapeutic implications. *Am. Heart J.*, **98**, 119–31.

Ginsberg, A. M., Clutter, W. E., Shah, S. D. and Cryer, P. E. (1981). Triiodothyronine-induced thyrotoxicosis increases mononuclear leukocyte beta-adrenergic receptor density in man. *J. Clin. Invest.*, **67**, 1785.

Glaubiger, G. and Lefkowitz, R. J. (1977). Elevated beta-adrenergic number after chronic propranolol treatment. *Biochem. Biophys. Res. Commun.*, **78**, 720–5.

Goldstein, D. B. (1979). Speculations on membrane lipid adaptation as a mechanism for drug tolerance and dependence. In Sharp, C. W. and Abood, L. G. (eds), *Membrane Mechanisms of Drugs Abuse*, Alan R. Liss, NewsYork, pp. 151–66.

Greenacre, J. K. and Conolly, M. E. (1978). Desensitisation of the beta-adrenoceptor of lymphocytes from normal subjects and patients with phaeochromocytoma: studies *in vivo*. *Br. J. Clin. Pharmacol.*, **5**, 191–7.

Greenacre, J. K., Schofield, P. and Conolly, M. E. (1978). Desensitisation of the beta-adrenoceptor of lymphocytes from normal subjects and asthmatic patients *in vitro*. *Br. J. Clin. Pharmacol.*, **5**, 199–206.

Gross, S. R. and Kelly, M. (1981). Ca^{2+} inhibition of isoproterenol responses in mammalian skeletal muscle. *J. Pharmacol. Exp. Ther.*, **217**, 271–7.

Guarnieri, T., Filburn, C. R., Beard, E. S. and Lakatta, E. G. (1980). Enhanced contractile response and protein kinase activation to threshold levels of beta-adrenergic stimulation in hyperthyroid rat heart. *J. Clin. Invest.*, **65**, 861–8.

Hamburg, M. and Tallman, J. F. (1981). Chronic morphine administration increases the apparent number of alpha$_2$-adrenoceptors in the rat brain. *Nature*, **291**, 493–5.

Harrison, D. C. and Alderman, E. L. (1976). Discontinuation of propranolol therapy—cause of rebound angina pectoris and acute coronary events. *Chest*, **69**, 1–2.

Heron, D. S., Shinitsky, M., Zamir, N. and Samuel, D. (1982). Adaptive modulations of brain membrane lipid fluidity in drug addiction and denervation supersensitivity. *Biochem. Pharmacol.*, **31** (14), 2435–8.

Hodgson, H. J. F., Marsden, C. D. and Meadows, J. C. (1969). The effect of adrenaline on the response to muscle vibration in man. *J. Physiol. (Lond.)*, **202**, 98P.

Hoffman, P. L. and Tabakoff, B. (1977). Alterations in dopamine receptor sensitivity by chronic ethanol treatment. *Nature*, **268**, 551–3.

Hunt, C. C., Jami, L. and Laporte, Y. (1982). Effects of stimulating the lumbar sympathetic trunk on cat hindlimb muscle spindles. *Arch. Ital. Biol.*, **120**(4), 371–84.

Israel, M. A., Kimura, H. and Kuriyama, K. (1972). Changes in activity and hormonal sensitivity of brain adenylate cyclase following chronic ethanol administration. *Experientia*, **28**, 1322–3.

Jefferson, D., Jenner, P. and Marsden, C. D. (1979a). Relationship between plasma propranolol and relief of essential tremor. *J. Neurol. Neurosurg. Psychiatr.*, **42**, 831–7.

Jefferson, D., Jenner, P. and Marsden, C. D. (1979b). Beta-adrenoceptor antagonists in essential tremor. *J. Neurol. Neurosurg. Psychiatr.*, **42**, 904–9.

Jeppsson, A. B., Johansson, U. and Waldeck, B. (1982). Dissociation between the effects of some xanthine derivatives on the tracheal smooth muscle and on the skeletal muscle. *Acta Pharmacol. Toxicol.*, **51**, 115–21.

Kennedy, R. H. and Donnelly, T. E. Jr (1982). Cardiac responsiveness after acute withdrawal of chronic propranolol treatment in rats. *Gen. Pharmacol.*, **13**, 231–9.

Kirby, J. D. T., Lima, D. R. A., Dowd, P. M., Kilfeather, S. and Turner, P. (1980). Prostacyclin increases cyclic nucleotide responsiveness of lymphocytes from patients with systemic sclerosis. *Lancet*, **2**, 453.

Kovacs, I. B., Dowd, P. M., Kirby, J. D. T. and Turner, P. (1983). Cyclic adenine nucleotide levels in lymphocytes from patients with systemic sclerosis: efficiency of prostacyclin infusions. *Postgrad. Med. J.*, **59**, 241–3.

Kuriyama, K. and Israel, M. A. (1973). Effect of ethanol administration on cyclic $3',5'$-adenosine monophosphate metabolism in brain. *Biochem. Pharmacol.*, **22**, 2919–22.

Kuriyama, K., Muramatsu, M., Aiso, M. and Ueno, E. (1981). Alteration in beta-adrenergic binding in brain, lung and heart during morphine and alcohol dependence and withdrawal. *Neuropharmacology*, **20**, 659–66.

Kuriyama, K., Nakagawa, K., Naito, K. and Muramatsu, M. (1978). Morphine induced changes in cyclic AMP metabolism and protein kinase activity in the brain. *Jpn. J. Pharmacol.*, **28**, 73–84.

Larsen, A. (1978). Effects of pindolol, sotalol and the optical isomers of propranolol on muscle action potentials and depolarising–secretion coupling in the rat. *Acta Physiol. Scand.*, **102**, 357–63.

Larsen, A. (1980). *Beta-blockers, Tremor and Neuromuscular Transmission* (Academic dissertation), Department of Neurology, University of Helsinki, Finland.

Larsen, T. A., Teravainen, H. and Calne, D. B. (1982). Atenolol vs propranolol in essential tremor: a controlled, quantitative study. *Acta Neurol. Scand.*, **66**, 547–54.

Larsson, S. and Svedmyr, N. (1977). Tremor caused by sympathomimetics is mediated by beta$_2$-adrenoceptors. *Scand. J. Resp. Dis.*, **58**, 5–10.

Leigh, P. N., Marsden, C. D., Twomey, A. and Jefferson, D. (1981). Beta-adrenoceptor antagonists and essential tremor. *Lancet*, **1**, 1106.

Llorens, C., Martres, M. P., Baudry, M. and Schwartz, J. C. (1978). Hypersensitivity to noradrenaline in cortex after chronic morphine: relevance to tolerance and dependence. *Nature*, **274**, 603–5.

McAllister, R. G. Jr, Markesbery, W. R., Ware, R. W. and Howell, S. M. (1977). Suppression of essential tremor by propranolol: correlation of effect with drug plasma levels and intensity of beta-adrenergic blockade. *Ann. Neurol.*, **1**, 160–6.

McConnaughey, M. M., Jones, L. R., Watanabe, A. M., Besch, H. R. Jr, Williams,

L. T. and Lefkowitz, R. J. (1979). Thyroxine and propylthiouracil effects on alpha- and beta-adrenergic receptor number, ATPase activities, and sialic acid content of rat cardiac membrane vesicles. *J. Cardiovasc. Pharmacol.*, 1, 609–23.

McInnes, A. (1980). *The Muscle Spindle, its Blood Supply and the Sympathetic Nervous System*, Ph.D. Thesis, University of Glasgow.

Marsden, C. D. (1978). The mechanisms of physiological tremor and their significance for pathological tremors. In Desmedt, J. E. (ed), *Progress in Clinical Neurophysiology*, vol. 5, Karger, Basel, pp. 1–17.

Marsden, C. D., Foley, T. H., Owen, D. A. L. and McAllister, R. C. (1967a). Peripheral beta-adrenoceptors associated with tremor. *Clin. Sci.*, 33, 53–65.

Marsden, C. D., Meadows, J. C., Lange, G. W. and Watson, R. S. (1967b). Effect of deafferentation on human physiological tremor. *Lancet*, 30, 700–2.

Marsden, C. D., Obeso, J. A. and Rothwell, J. C. (1983). Benign essential tremor is not a single entity. In Yahr, M. D. (ed.), *Current Concepts in Parkinson's Disease*, Excerpta Medica, Amsterdam, pp. 31–46.

Matthews, P. B. C. (1972). *Mammalian Muscle Receptors and Their Central Actions*, Edward Arnold, London.

Mattio, T. G. and Kirby, M. L. (1982). Effects of chronic morphine administration on catecholamines and beta-adrenergic receptors of the superior cervical ganglion and iris of the rat. *Life Sci.*, 30, 1432–42.

Meisheri, K. D. and McNeill, J. H. (1979). Role of Ca^{2+} in isoprenaline induced increases in cAMP levels in rat uterus. *Am. J. Physiol.*, 237, C257–63.

Mizgala, H. F. and Counsell, J. (1976). Acute coronary syndromes following abrupt cessation of oral propranolol therapy. *Can. Med. Assoc. J.*, 114, 1123–6.

Nattel, S., Rangno, R. E. and Van Loon, G. (1979). Mechanism of propranolol withdrawal phenomena. *Circulation*, 59, 1158–62.

Neil-Dwyer, G., Bartlett, J. and Cruickshank, J. M. (1981). Beta-blockers and the blood brain barrier. *Br. J. Clin. Pharmacol.*, 11, 549–53.

Nies, A. S. and Shand, D. G. (1975). Clinical pharmacology of propranolol. *Circulation*, 52, 6–14.

Ogata, M., Mendelson, J. H., Mello, N. K. and Majchrowitz, E. (1971). Adrenal function and alcoholism, II. Catecholamines. *Psychosomatic Med.*, 33, 159–80.

Pedersen, L. O., Mikkelsen, E., Nielsen, L. J. and Christensen, N. J. (1979). Abrupt withdrawal of beta-blocking agents in patients with arterial hypertension. Effects on blood pressure, heart rate and plasma catecholamines and prolactin. *Eur. J. Clin. Pharmacol.*, 15, 215–17.

Philips, S. J., Richens, A. and Shand, D. G. (1973). Adrenergic control of tendon jerk reflexes in man. *Br. J. Pharmacol.*, 47, 595–605.

Puri, S. K., Spaulding, T. C. and Mantione, C. R. (1978). Dopamine antagonist binding: a significant decrease with morphine dependence in the rat striatum. *Life Sci.*, 23, 637–42.

Puri, S. K., Volicer, L. and Cochin, J. (1976). Changes in striatal adenylate cyclase activity following acute and chronic morphine treatment and during withdrawal. *J. Neurochem.*, 27, 1551–4.

Rall, T. W. (1980). Central nervous system stimulants; the xanthines. In Goodman Gilman, A., Goodman, L. S. and Gilman, A. (eds), *The Pharmacological Basis of Therapeutics*, Macmillan, New York.

Rangel-Guerra, R. (1974). Treatment of benign essential tremor with a beta-adrenergic blocking agent (sotalol). In Snart, A. G. (ed.), *Advances in Beta-adrenergic Blocking Therapy—Sotalol*, International Congress Series 341, Excerpta Medica, Amsterdam, V62–66.

Reid, J. L., Wing, L. M. H., Dargie, H. J., Hamilton, C. A., Davies, D. S. and Dollery, C. T. (1977). Clonidine withdrawal in hypertension. *Lancet*, 1, 1171–4.

Rennie, M. J., Fell, R. D., Ivy, J. L. and Holloszy, J. O. (1982). Adrenaline reactivation of muscle phosphorylase after deactivation during contractile activity. *Biosci. Rep.*, **2**, 323-31.

Rinne, U. K. and Kaitaniemi, P. (1974). Sotalol in treatment of essential tremor. In Snart, A. G. (ed.), *Advances in Beta-adrenergic Blocking Therapy—Sotalol*, International Congress Series 341, Excerpta Medica, Amsterdam, V56-61.

Santini, M. and Ibata, Y. (1971). The fine structure of thin unmyelinated axons within muscle spindles. *Brain Res.*, **33**, 289-302.

Sellars, E. M., Cooper, S. D. and Roy, M. L. (1978). Variations in serum dopamine-betahydroxylase in normal subjects and chronic alcoholics. *Can. J. Physiol. Pharmacol.*, **56**, 806-11.

Slome, R. (1973). Withdrawal of propranolol and myocardial infarction. *Lancet*, **1**, 1068.

Smith, H. J., Halliday, S. E. and Rouse, W. (1983). The effects of a $beta_2$-selective adrenergic receptor antagonist (ICI 118,551) on twitch tension in cat soleus muscle. *J. Pharmacol. Exp. Ther.*, **224**, 228-30.

Sorensen, P. S., Paulson, O. B., Steiness, E. and Jansen, E. C. (1981). Essential tremor treatment with propranolol: lack of correlation ·between clinical effect and plasma propranolol levels. *Ann. Neurol.*, **9**, 53-7.

Stiles, G. L. and Lefkowitz, R. J. (1981). Thyroid hormone modulation of agonist-beta-adrenergic receptor interactions in the rat heart. *Life Sci.*, **28**, 2529-36.

Svedmyr, N. and Simonsson, B. G. (1978). Drugs in the treatment of asthma. *Pharmacol. Ther. (B)*, **13**, 397-440.

Tabakoff, B., Hoffman, P. L. and Ritzma, R. F. (1978). Dopamine receptor function after chronic ingestion of alcohol. *Life Sci.*, **23**, 643-8.

Taylor, E. A., Jefferson, D., Carroll, J. D. and Turner, P. (1981). Cerebrospinal fluid concentrations of propranolol, pindolol and atenolol in man: evidence for central actions of beta-adrenoceptor antagonists. *Br. J. Clin. Pharmacol.*, **12**, 549-59.

Thorpe, W. R. and Seeman, P. (1971). The site of action of caffeine and procaine in skeletal muscle. *J. Pharmacol. Exp. Ther.*, **179**, 324-30.

Turner, P. (1974). Beta-adrenergic receptor blocking drugs in hyperthyroidism. *Drugs*, **7**, 48-54.

Turner, P. (1983). In Turner, P. and Shand, D. G. (eds), *Recent Advances in Clinical Pharmacology*, vol. 3, Churchill Livingstone, Edinburgh, pp. 223-34.

U'Prichard, D. C., Bylund, D. B. and Snyder, S. H. (1978). $(\pm)$-$(^3$H)epinephrine and $(-)$-$(^3$H)dihydroalprenol binding to $beta_1$- and $beta_2$-noradrenergic receptors in brain, heart and lung membranes. *J. Biol. Chem.*, **253**, 5090-102.

van Zweiten, P. A. and Timmermans, P. B. M. W. M. (1979). Comparison between the acute hemodynamic effects and brain penetration of atenolol and meto-prolol. *J. Cardiovasc. Pharmacol.*, **1**, 85-96.

Waldeck, B. (1977). Analysis of the beta-adrenoceptor mediated effects on slow-contracting skeletal muscle. *J. Pharm. Pharmacol.*, **29**, 550-4.

Webb, J. G., Newman, W. H., Walle, T. and Daniell, H. B. (1981). Myocardial sensitivity to isoproterenol following abrupt propranolol withdrawal in conscious dogs. *J. Cardiovasc. Pharmacol.*, **3**, 622-35.

Wei, J. Y., Spurgeon, H. A. and Lakatta, E. G. (1982). Electromechanical responsiveness of hyperthyroid cardiac muscle to beta-adrenergic stimulation. *Am. J. Physiol.*, **243**, Endocr. Metab. Suppl. 6, E114-22.

Young, R. R., Growdon, J. H. and Shahani, B. T. (1975). Beta-adrenergic mechanisms in action tremor. *New Engl. J. Med.*, **293**, 950-3.

Young, R. R. and Hagbarth, K. (1980). Physiological tremor enhanced by manoeuvers affecting the segmental stretch reflex. *J. Neurol. Neurosurg. Psychiatr.*, **43**(3), 248-56.

Zilm, D. H., Sellers, E. M., Macleod, S. M. and Degani, N. (1975). Propranolol effect on tremor in alcohol withdrawal. *Ann. Intern. Med.*, **83**, 234-5.

17
Essential tremor: treatment with beta-adrenoceptor blocking drugs

J. F. WILSON, R. W. MARSHALL and A. RICHENS

INTRODUCTION

Essential tremor is a chronic disorder of movement. It shows a familial tendency and is more common in patients over the age of 50 years. The characteristics of the disease are well documented (for reviews see Critchley, 1972; Murray, 1981). Although patients suffering from clearly separate tremor-producing conditions such as Parkinson's disease may occasionally be present in a group of essential tremor patients, when accurately diagnosed essential tremor is a monosymptomatic illness. That is not to say, however, that essential tremor patients are a homogeneous group. The variability in responsiveness to drug therapy that will be described suggests that a review of the current single classification may be in order. The tremor is an action or postural tremor, being absent when a limb is at rest. It can be seen in a limb held in a fixed position against gravity, the usual arrangement used during accelerometer recordings of tremor (Wilson *et al.*, 1982). Patients may show additional intention tremors which increase in amplitude towards the end of intention movements. The tremor occurs in short bursts which correlate with electromyographic activity. The frequency of the tremor covers a range from some 6 to 12 Hz but an individual patient shows a generally stable frequency or pattern of frequencies when measured repeatedly over a period of time. Emotional and physical stress aggravate the tremor and this aspect of the disease presumably accounts for the limited effectiveness of anxiolytic agents such as chlordiazepoxide in the treatment of tremor (Critchley, 1972). The disease may progress over a period of years but typically involves only the upper limbs and head. It must be emphasised, however, that the underlying pathological process is unknown.

SITE OF ORIGIN OF ESSENTIAL TREMOR

There are lines of evidence that point to a central component in the aetiology of

245

essential tremor. The success of surgical thalamotomy (Andraw, 1981) in the treatment of the severest cases supports this view. The widely known action of small amounts of ethanol in reducing tremor is also thought to act via the central nervous system (Growdon *et al.*, 1975). Evidence of the relative importance of this central component in essential tremor comes from studies of the length of the neuronal reflex loops involved in the disease (Lee and Stein, 1981). By applying a mechanical displacement to a tremulous limb the previous authors were able partially to reset the phase of essential tremor. Physiological tremor, which is largely a peripheral phenomenon resulting from oscillations in spinal reflex loops or from partial fusion of motor units, resets almost totally following mechanical displacement (Lippold, 1970, 1971; Joyce and Rack, 1974). Parkinsonian tremor, in contrast, hardly resets at all (Lee and Stein, 1981). The latter is generated by an oscillator high in the brain and is thereby buffered from the external mechanical perturbations by longer and multisynaptic pathways. The intermediate phase resetting index noted in essential tremor patients is consistent with the involvement of the higher central pathways in essential tremor but demonstrates a strong spinal reflex component to the disease. The important point to note from these investigations is that essential tremor arises solely neither from peripheral nor from central mechanisms but apparently has contributions from more than one anatomical site. Variations in the relative contribution from these sites may explain the heterogeneity that is starting to be reported amongst essential tremor patients (Findley *et al.*, 1981; Findley and Gresty, 1981; Calzetti *et al.*, 1983a,b). Tremors originating predominantly in higher centres may be those responsible for high-amplitude and low-frequency tremor whilst spinal ones might tend towards the high-frequency, low-amplitude pattern. Calzetti *et al.* (1983b) have proposed a diagnostic separation based on these differences. This may prove to be of therapeutic value since they demonstrated a significant correlation between responsiveness to propranolol and tremor amplitude, the high-frequency, low-amplitude tremors being unresponsive to treatment. These developments serve to reinforce the importance to the clinician of accurate quantification of tremor, a need that can now be filled by the application of relatively inexpensive, self-contained microcomputer-based systems to tremor measurement (Wilson *et al.*, 1982).

THERAPY WITH PROPRANOLOL

The introduction of the β-adrenoceptor blocking drugs in the early 1960s led to a flurry of activity in studying the antagonism of the pharmacological effects of adrenaline. It soon became clear that drugs like propranolol effectively inhibited the tremogenic effects of infused adrenaline (Owen and Marsden, 1965; Marsden *et al.*, 1967). As both emotional tension and administration of adrenaline increased parkinsonian tremor (Barcroft *et al.*, 1952; Constas, 1962), it seemed sensible to investigate the action of β-adrenoceptor blockers in Parkinson's disease. Early attempts concluded that propranolol could be effective in reducing tremor in some cases (Herring, 1964; Owen and Marsden, 1965; Strang, 1965; Vas, 1966). Trials of β-adrenoceptor blocking agents in other spontaneous tremors including essential tremor were thus encouraged, though the assumed unifying principle that physiological, drug-induced and pathological tremors all share a common adrenergic mechanism was far from justified. Of the two original reports concerning the effects of propranolol in essential tremor, one was stimulated by the successes with parkinsonian tremor (Sevitt, 1971) whilst the second was a chance observation in an essential tremor patient being treated for a cardiac condition (Winkler and Young, 1971). More extensive controlled trials followed, which by the mid-1970s had demonstrated that racemic propranolol had a beneficial effect in essential tremor (Gilligan, 1972; Gilligan *et al.*, 1972; Murray, 1972, 1976; Pakkenberg, 1972; Barbeau, 1973; Dupont *et al.*, 1973; Morgan *et al.*, 1973; Sevitt, 1974; Winkler and Young, 1974; Tolosa and Loewenson, 1975; Young *et al.*, 1975; McClure and Davis, 1976; Teräväinen *et al.*, 1976).

A synthesis of the main conclusions from these numerous studies with propranolol would be that essential tremor can be suppressed in many patients by single oral or intravenous doses of propranolol for a period of a few hours. The failure by Young *et al.* (1975) to produce an effect by the intravenous route and their observation that 24 h or so was needed for a response to oral therapy has not been substantiated. Significant effects following intravenous (McAllister *et al.*, 1977; Abila *et al.*, 1983) and single oral (Calzetti *et al.*, 1981) administration have subsequently been reported to confirm the observations of Morgan *et al.* (1973). The diagnostic test proposed by Young *et al.* (1975) to differentiate essential from catecholamine-induced tremors on the basis of the failure of essential tremor to respond to intravenous propranolol dosage is thus untenable.

There is general agreement over the dose levels required in chronic oral therapy. Some patients occasionally respond in a dosage range up to some 60 mg/day but the majority require doses of at least 120 or 240 mg/day in divided doses. Daily treatment with up to 800 mg of propranolol has been thought worth while (McAllister *et al.*, 1977). A common feature of the studies has been the variable benefit that occurred between individual essential tremor patients. In a large proportion of the reports patients were present who failed to respond significantly. There were also reports where the effect of propranolol was no better than the undoubted placebo response in suppressing essential tremor (Balla, 1973; Foster *et al.*, 1973; Scopa *et al.*, 1973; Sweet *et al.*, 1974). The latter complete failures of propranolol have been ascribed variously to inadequate evaluation techniques, to the use of different doses or dosage regimes and to the timing of tremor measurements relative to the doses.

The inter-patient variability in response has attracted more detailed consideration. Three investigations have been described in which tremor responses were correlated to measurements of the plasma level of propranolol. McAllister *et al.* (1977) produced stable plasma concentrations by propranolol infusions and noted a dose-related tremolytic action but against a background of a large inter-subject variability in sensitivity to propranolol. The other two studies used variable oral doses of propranolol as the basis of their experimental design (Jefferson *et al.*,

1979a; Sørensen *et al.*, 1981). In the latter study increasing doses of propranolol caused increases in tremor reduction but the measured plasma levels of propranolol were very variable between subjects and no correlation between anti-tremor effect and plasma level could be demonstrated. The study by Jefferson *et al.* also failed to show a significant correlation between plasma propranolol concentration and tremor reduction against a similar wide variation in plasma level between patients on the same oral dose. They were, however, unable to demonstrate any dose-related effects as maximum responses were achieved with their lower doses. One simple deduction that follows from these findings is that monitoring of plasma levels will be of little value in patient management. There remains therefore in essential tremor patients a great variation in therapeutic response to propranolol that cannot be explained by differences in plasma concentrations.

The recent reports by Findley, Calzetti and coworkers referred to in the previous section offer the first significant step towards an understanding of the wide inter-subject variability in responsiveness to β-blocker therapy. The heterogeneity in response would be explicable if patients were taken from a population that showed a range of causal factors in tremor production of which only some were open to manipulation by β-adrenoceptor blocking drugs. Their proposed means of identifying β-blocker sensitive patients deserves further investigation.

COMPARATIVE EFFECTS OF BETA-ADRENOCEPTOR BLOCKING DRUGS

The introduction of a range of β-adrenoceptor blocking drugs with differing properties for use principally in cardiology has enabled certain aspects of their action in essential tremor to be assessed. The main differences between the β-adrenoceptor blockers has been in their intrinsic sympathomimetic activity, membrane-stabilising activity, lipid solubility and cardioselectivity (table 17.1). The latter refers to the subdivision of β-adrenoceptors into β_1- and β_2-subtypes (Lands *et al.*, 1967). The β_1-subtype is associated with the heart whilst the β_2-subtype is that present in bronchus, blood vessels and other peripheral sites. The question arises as to what can be deduced about the nature of the β-adrenoceptors involved in the suppression of essential tremor from the comparative use of these agents. In order to assess whether the tremolytic receptors are of the β_2-subtype for example, experiments are designed so that β-blockers with differing cardio-selectivities are dosed in such a way that their β_1-activities on the heart are identical, so that any differences in potency on essential tremor can be correlated with their relative β_2-activity. Similar arguments apply to comparisons of membrane-stabilising or other activities. Comparisons are rather more complex than this simple design would indicate, however, as each property cannot be tested in isolation. Only by consideration of relative potencies across a series of compounds can we hope to dissect out the importance and potential interaction of the several properties of β-adrenoceptor blockers.

Further difficulties in performing this already complex task need to be considered. Comparisons will clearly be complicated by the heterogeneity in patients

Table 17.1   Properties of some β-adrenoceptor blocking drugs.

Drug	Cardioselective	Intrinsic sympathomimetic activity	Membrane-stabilising activity	Lipid solubility partition coefficient, n-octanol/buffer, pH 7.4, 37°C	Plasma protein binding (%)	Metabolism (%)	Elimination half-life of active drug (h)
propranolol	no	no	yes	20.2	90	> 95	2–3
timolol	no	slight	slight	1.2	65	~ 50	4–6
pindolol	no	yes	yes	0.8	60	~ 60	3–4
sotalol	no	no	no	0.04	5	0	8–13
metoprolol	yes	no	yes	1.0	15	~ 85	3–4
atenolol	yes	no	no	0.02	10	< 10	6–9

in their sensitivity to β-adrenoceptor blockers, which has already been discussed. Trials must therefore use full crossover designs to allow the inter-patient variability to be compensated for in data analysis. The selection of equipotent doses in terms of one of the β-blocker actions also requires consideration. To take the selection of equivalent cardiac β_1-activity as an example, the reflex effects on the heart resulting from variable β_2-activity in the vasculature are not taken into account. The quantitative assessment of the β_1-blocking activity on the heart free from parasympathetic interference can also be far from straightforward. Measures based on the difference between supine and standing heart rate, the Valsalva manoeuvre or glyceryl trinitrate stimulation have all been questioned (for a review see McDevitt, 1977) and cardiac stimulation based on maximal exercise would seem to be the preferred technique. The latter is, however, not practicable with elderly essential tremor patients. Our own solution to this particular problem (Abila *et al.*, 1983) has been to perform initial comparative studies of β-adrenoceptor blockers in healthy volunteers in order to determine the relative potency of the β-blockers in antagonising the increase in heart rate produced by maximal exercise. We then used the equipotent doses so determined in studies with essential tremor patients and backed up the procedure by measurements in the patients with one of the less physically exacting heart rate measures. Unfortunately criteria such as these have not always been met in comparative studies so that interpretation of the published data still fails to provide clear answers to many of the important questions.

Membrane-stabilising activity

Propranolol is by far the most widely used β-adrenoceptor blocker in the treatment and study of essential tremor and as such provides the reference against which the other β-blockers are compared. In addition to its non-cardioselective β-blocking effect, propranolol also possesses membrane-stabilising properties that may contribute to its therapeutic activity. Comparison with other non-cardioselective agents such as sotalol or timolol, which have respectively no or slight membrane-stabilising activity, should throw light on this possibility. In placebo-controlled trials, sotalol at 160 or 240 mg/day dose levels significantly reduced tremor (Rangel-Guerra, 1974; Rinne and Kaitaniemi, 1974) as did 10 mg doses of timolol (Dietrichson and Espen, 1979). In the only comparative study involving propranolol to be published (Jefferson *et al.*, 1979b), sotalol in oral doses designed to produce a similar degree of blockade of cardiac β-adrenoceptors was of equivalent potency to propranolol in reducing tremor. In a comparison with the cardioselective agent metoprolol, which like propranolol possesses some membrane-stabilising activity, sotalol was more potent (Leigh *et al.*, 1981). The difference in cardio-selectivity is probably more important than the membrane-stabilising activity difference in this study. In our own study (Abila *et al.*, 1983) with intravenous administration, sotalol and timolol, at doses producing the same antichronotropic effect, were significantly less potent than propranolol in reducing essential tremor though both were significantly better than placebo. We would agree with Jefferson *et al.* (1979b), however, that the membrane-stabilising effect of propranolol is probably unimportant in practice, the reduced potency of sotalol and timolol in our own study being related to differences in lipid solubility.

Intrinsic sympathomimetic activity

Pindolol is a β-adrenoceptor blocking drug that retains some ability to stimulate rather than to block adrenoceptors. Like propranolol it is non-cardioselective and would appear to have few important differences in its spectrum of activity compared with propranolol other than an increased water solubility. In the one major study with pindolol (Teräväinen *et al.*, 1977) it was shown to be less potent than propranolol but it produced an increase in tremor amplitude when compared to placebo. The intrinsic sympathomimetic activity would thus appear to be capable of producing disadvantageous effects on tremor. The very small degree of adrenergic stimulation produced by timolol may contribute in the same way to its reduced potency compared to propranolol described above.

Cardioselective activity

Two cardioselective agents, atenolol and metoprolol, have been investigated by several groups in the hope of identifying the subtype of adrenoceptor responsible for the action of the β-blockers in essential tremor. These two drugs differ in respect of their lipid solubility, metoprolol being relatively lipid-soluble and atenolol water-soluble. Atenolol was no better than placebo in one study at a once daily dose of 100 mg (Dietrichson and Espen, 1981) but has usually been effective at this dose (Jefferson *et al.*, 1979b; Larsen and Teräväinen, 1981; Leigh *et al.*, 1981). These studies have shown atenolol to be less potent than propranolol, timolol and sotalol when used at doses giving equivalent β_1-effects on the heart. Our intravenous study (Abila *et al.*, 1983) confirmed these findings; atenolol though better than placebo was significantly less potent than the three non-cardioselective agents. Jefferson *et al.* (1979b), Dietrichson and Espen (1981) and Leigh *et al.* (1981) all concluded that these data indicated that the main receptors mediating the anti-tremor effect were of the β_2-subtype, though a role for β_1-sites could not be excluded since atenolol was beneficial.

The results of studies with metoprolol have been much less clear-cut. Several investigators claimed an improvement in essential tremor patients in uncontrolled trials (Britt and Peters, 1979; Riley and Pleet, 1979; Ljung, 1979; Newman and Jacobs, 1980; Turnbull and Shaw, 1980) and so the predominance of β_2-receptors in essential tremor was brought into question. Claims and counterclaims followed as to whether the 100 or 150 mg/day dose of metoprolol was indeed cardio-selective (Jefferson and Marsden, 1980; Ljung, 1980). The consensus view is that cardioselectivity is at least partially lost at doses higher than 100–150 mg/day. The availability of results from controlled trials has not clarified matters. In a single-dose study comparing metoprolol and propranolol at equipotent doses for the β_1-cardiac effects, the two β-blockers produced statistically similar reductions in essential tremor (Calzetti *et al.*, 1981). The authors concluded that, although some degree of non-cardioselectivity with metoprolol was possible, the action of the drug would seem to be mediated in part by β_1-receptors. Chronic dosing trials, however, gave different results. In a two-week trial in which the relative β_1-effects were not adequately controlled, metoprolol was no better than placebo (Leigh *et al.*, 1981), a result confirmed independently in a fully controlled two-week study using 150 and 300 mg/day metoprolol doses (Calzetti *et al.*, 1982). In both these studies propranolol was still effective. Only in the one-week study by Larsen and Terävainen (1981) was a significant effect of metoprolol reported to correlate with the original uncontrolled clinical observations. The relative potencies of the three β-blockers used were propranolol > atenolol > metoprolol > placebo. It is difficult to put these data into a clear perspective, the effectiveness of metoprolol especially in chronic use being equivocal. The apparent loss of activity in the longer term seems unlikely to be the result of a rapid clearance of the drug combined with inappropriate tremor assessment timings as the pharmaco-kinetic clearance parameters of metoprolol are close to those of propranolol (table 17.1), which was always active in these studies. The development of toler-ance to the tremolytic response is possible, though the heart rate response did not show it.

A definite answer to the identity of the β-adrenoceptor subtype responsible for the effect of β-blockers in essential tremor is thus elusive. The data are sugges-tive of some important β_2-selective sites but β_1- or possibly non-selective sites would also seem to exist. The recent introduction of specific β_2-selective blockers such as ICI 118 551, which has already been reported to be effective on drug-induced tremor (Arnold *et al.*, 1982), should facilitate the investigation of this problem.

Lipid solubility

The relative lipid solubility of the β-adrenoceptor blockers has been used as a tool to provide information as to the possible site of the β-adrenoceptors involved in essential tremor. The claim usually made is that lipid solubility will differentiate between peripheral and central sites on the basis that the blood–brain barrier reduces the rate and amount that the less lipid-soluble drugs penetrate into the brain. There is evidence that the blood–brain barrier does indeed exert such an action. The water-soluble compound atenolol has been shown to achieve much lower central levels compared to plasma concentrations than more lipid-soluble compounds such as propranolol or metoprolol (van Zwieten and Timmermans, 1979; Neil-Dwyer *et al.*, 1981; Taylor *et al.*, 1981). The distinction is by no means absolute as some have implied; the more water-soluble compounds attain concentrations that may be of the order of one-tenth of the concentrations of the more lipid-soluble agents. Two points should be noted in passing. First, the lipid solubility values in table 17.1 should be compared on a logarithmic scale, the steps from 10 to 1 and from 1 to 0.1 being equal changes in lipid solubility. Secondly, the concentration gradient driving the drug into the central compartment is the free plasma concentration (Neil-Dwyer *et al.*, 1981). Since one might assume that the free drug concentration in plasma will be directly related to the peripheral effects of the drug, then in an experimental design where β-blocker doses have been adjusted to give equal β_1-antichronotropic responses, the free drug concentrations should also be equivalent. No corrections are therefore necessary for the different degrees of plasma protein binding seen between the various β-blockers (table 17.1).

There is unfortunately a fundamental weakness in the above scheme. It is not currently possible to say whether other deep compartments exist in the periphery which would present a similar lipid barrier as the brain to the penetration of β-adrenoceptor blockers. It may be that the β-adrenoceptors mediating the tremolytic response are located in their own slowly accessible compartment within the skeletal musculature. Distinctions based on relative lipid solubility can thus only point to the existence of such a deep compartment, and other evidence would be needed to deduce its location.

The most telling comparisons for the lipid solubility difference will be between propranolol and sotalol of the non-cardioselective agents and between metoprolol and atenolol from the cardioselective series. As described above, sotalol was equipotent with propranolol in a chronic dosage study (Jefferson *et al.*, 1979b). In the two comparative trials with metoprolol and atenolol, the more lipid-soluble drug metoprolol was less effective in chronic use (Larsen and Teräväinen, 1981; Leigh *et al.*, 1981). All authors therefore concluded that the central actions were not of primary importance in essential tremor. The problems already considered in relation to the chronic use of metoprolol may, however, make the latter two comparisons suspect. It should also be noted that in chronic dosing studies information on differences due to the differential rate of drug penetration into deep compartments will not be produced; only that resulting from equilibrium drug concentrations will be available. Differences in total brain content due to lipid solubility could conceivably be balanced out by the local environment of the receptor being more favourable to the water-soluble drugs. Interpretation of data is certainly not easy. We have therefore attempted in our recent studies (Abila *et al.*, 1983) to follow the dynamic changes in tremor following intravenous administration of different β-blockers and to compare the rate of onset of this response with that of the antichronotropic response (figure 17.1). Whereas the cardiac effect had reached a peak by 15 min after injection, the reduction in tremor continued to develop more slowly, reaching a peak 1 h after injection in the case of propranolol. The β-adrenoceptors involved in essential tremor are thus located in a deeper, less accessible compartment than the cardiac β-adrenoceptors but as noted above we cannot say whether this is the central nervous system or not. Our data were not adequate to detect the hoped for differences in rate of onset of the tremolytic response with the different β-blockers but did show significant differences in peak tremolytic response, the order being propranolol >

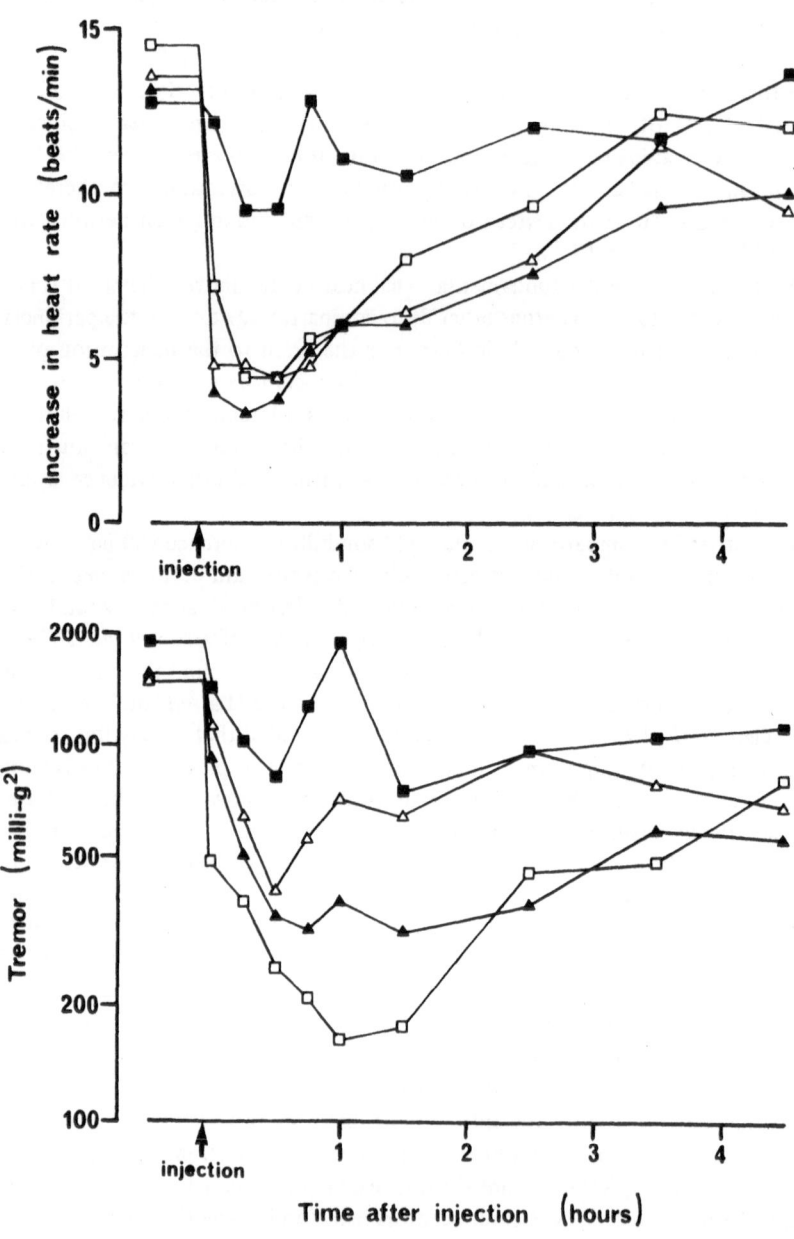

Figure 17.1 Variations in the increase in heart rate on standing and in hand tremor after intravenous administration of saline (■), 0.1 mg kg^{-1} propranolol (□), 0.54 mg kg^{-1} sotalol (▲) and 0.13 mg kg^{-1} atenolol (△). Points are means from five patients with essential tremor.

sotalol > atenolol > placebo. A correlation of the tremor-inhibiting response with both lipid solubility and with cardioselectivity can thus be made, and both these aspects of a β-adrenoceptor blocker could therefore contribute to its potency.

MECHANISM OF ACTION OF BETA-ADRENOCEPTOR BLOCKING DRUGS

It is perhaps self-evident that the effectiveness of the β-adrenoceptor blocking drugs in the therapy of essential tremor presupposes the existence of some β-adrenoceptors that are being activated by an endogenous transmitter. This assumes that the non-selective actions of the β-blockers such as membrane-stabilising or intrinsic sympathomimetic activity are not important in the response, as the evidence reviewed above would confirm. There are then only a limited number of possibilities for the origin and site of action of this endogenous transmitter.

Catecholamines are well known to be present in the circulation. Adrenaline originates mainly from the adrenal medulla whereas noradrenaline levels are maintained in addition by sympathetic neurone discharge (de Prada and Zuercher, 1979). Evidence obtained from studies of the tremor response produced by the application of exogenous sympathomimetic amines has demonstrated the existence of tremogenic receptors capable of responding to such circulating amines (Owen and Marsden, 1965; Marsden *et al.*, 1967; Larsson and Svedmyr, 1977; Perucca *et al.*, 1981). These data further demonstrate that the receptors are of the β_2-subtype and respond within seconds to adrenaline but not to noradrenaline. The location of these receptors has not been fully determined but they would not seem to be innervated by sympathetic nerves (Marsden *et al.*, 1969). Two popular suggestions as to their location, on the intrafusal fibres of the muscle spindles (Calma and Kidd, 1962; Smith, 1963; Paintal, 1964) and in the extrafusal muscle fibres themselves (Bowman and Nott, 1969; Marsden and Meadows, 1970), are both possible. The receptors on the muscle spindles would act by increasing the gain in the spinal reflex loop (Lippold, 1970, 1971; Young and Hagbarth, 1980), though the failure of propranolol to affect tendon jerk reflexes (Phillips *et al.*, 1973) is evidence against an important role for β-adrenoceptors in this site in normal drug-free subjects. The receptors on the extrafusal muscle fibres would act by shortening the twitch duration of the muscle, leading to a reduction in fusion of incomplete tetanic contractions and hence postural tremor (Bowman and Nott, 1969; Marsden and Meadows, 1970). It seems likely that the exacerbation of essential tremor produced by stress is mediated through increases in circulating adrenaline acting through these peripheral β_2-adrenoceptors. This component of the tremor would be blocked by the β_2-receptor antagonists. What has not been proved, however, is that these sites with their circulating amine drive are one and the same as those involved in mediating the effects of β-adrenoceptor blockers on the underlying essential tremor. As noted by Marsden *et al.* (1967) and Perucca *et al.* (1981), infusion of catecholamines caused increases in tremor after some 90 s whilst intravenous propranolol blocked isoprenaline-induced tremor within 1 min (Young *et al.*, 1975). The receptors mediating these drug-induced tremor changes are thus readily accessible and contrast with those involved in the β-blocker action in essential tremor which seem to be located in a relatively inaccessible compartment (Abila *et al.*, 1983).

Moving to the second potential source for an adrenergic transmitter, the role played by neurones of the sympathetic nervous system must be considered. It is generally held that the skeletal muscle fibres do not receive a direct sympathetic innervation but that the muscle spindles receive a noradrenergic supply (Banker and Girvin, 1971). The same mechanism of action for neuronally released catecholamines on tremor as discussed for circulating amines acting on muscle spindles would then apply. The receptors involved in such a mechanism being located in relation to neuronal endings may then be less accessible to circulating amines and could appear to be in a deeper compartment. As the pharmacology of the system follows the standard sympathetic pattern with noradrenaline as the transmitter, the receptors will be of the β_1-subtype.

The remaining possible source of the endogenous transmitter is within the central nervous system. The anatomy of the extensive noradrenaline-containing systems and the relatively few adrenaline-containing neurones has been well documented (Moore and Bloom, 1979). Noradrenergic neurones synapse directly with both α- and γ-motoneurones in the spinal cord and aminergic terminals are to be found in several of the higher centres involved in motor control. The evidence for central components from both higher and spinal reflex levels in essential tremor has been reviewed above and an aminergic contribution to this mechanism is therefore possible. There is as yet no evidence as to whether central adrenoceptors can be classified into the subtypes used so successfully in the periphery. Any central receptors involved in essential tremor could thus be β_1-, β_2- or nonspecific in their selectivity.

To summarise, the tremor produced by stress in essential tremor patients is almost certainly controlled by the β-adrenoceptor blockers acting through non-innervated β_2-adrenoceptors on either the muscle fibres or muscle spindles. A role for these receptors in the β-adrenoceptor blocker control of the underlying essential tremor cannot be discounted. In addition, there appear to be other less accessible innervated β-adrenoceptors which mediate a major part of the tremolytic response in essential tremor. These receptors may be located in a deep peripheral compartment associated with muscle spindles or may be in the central nervous system at one or more locations. The selectivity of the less accessible β-adrenoceptors is not known, though peripheral innervated receptors would be expected to be of the β_1-subtype.

SUGGESTIONS FOR TREATMENT

Within the group of patients diagnosed as having essential tremor there are those who will fail to respond or who will respond poorly to β-adrenoceptor blockade. The suggested diagnostic classification for identifying these patients requires further development (Calzetti *et al.*, 1983b). There is no evidence to suggest that any differential benefit is to be obtained from using a different β-blocker in these cases. For patients responsive to β-adrenoceptor blockers, the first choice of agent must be propranolol, no other agent having been shown to be more effective. The dose should start at 40 mg twice daily and may be increased to the maximum tolerated dose in order to derive the greatest benefit. In patients suffering concurrently from conditions such as chronic obstructive airways disease, cardiac failure or peripheral vascular disease, it is wise to avoid β-blockers completely; in these patients primidone may represent a useful alternative (see Findley *et al.*, this volume, chapter 19). The introduction of the specific β_2-selective agent ICI 118 551 may provide a new approach, particularly in patients in whom cardiovascular disease precludes the use of a β_1-adrenoceptor blocker.

REFERENCES

Abila, B., Marshall, R. W., Wilson, J. F. and Richens, A. (1983). Do β-adrenoceptor blockers have peripheral or central effect in essential tremor? *Br. J. Clin. Pharmacol.*, **16**, 210P.

Andrew, J. (1981). Surgery for involuntary movements. *Br. J. Hosp. Med.*, **26**, 522–8.

Arnold, J. M. O., Johnston, G. D., Harron, D. W. G., Shanks, R. G. and McDevitt, D. G. (1982). The effect of ICI 118 551 on isoprenaline-induced β-adrenoceptor responses in man. *Br. J. Clin. Pharmacol.*, **15**, 133–4P.

Balla, J. I. (1973). Treatment of essential tremor with propranolol. *Lancet*, **1**, 205.

Banker, B. Q. and Girvin, J. P. (1971). The ultrastructural features of the mammalian muscle spindle. *J. Neuropathol. Exp. Neurol.*, **30**, 155–95.

Barbeau, A. (1973). Traitement du tremblement essentiel familial par le propranolol. *Union Méd. Can.*, **102**, 899–902.

Barcroft, H., Peterson, E. and Schwab, R. S. (1952). Actions of adrenaline and noradrenaline on the tremor of Parkinson's disease. *Neurology*, **2**, 154–60.

Bowman, W. C. and Nott, M. W. (1969). Actions of sympathomimetic amines and their antagonists on skeletal muscle. *Pharmacol. Rev.*, **21**, 27–72.

Britt, C. W. and Peters, B. H. (1979). Metoprolol for essential tremor. *New Engl. J. Med.*, **301**, 331.

Calma, I. and Kidd, G. L. (1962). The effect of adrenaline on muscle spindles in cat. *Arch. Ital. Biol.*, **100**, 381–93.

Calzetti, S., Findley, L. J., Gresty, M. A., Perucca, E. and Richens, A. (1981). Metoprolol and propranolol in essential tremor: a double-blind, controlled study. *J. Neurol. Neurosurg. Psychiatr.*, **44**, 814–19.

Calzetti, S., Findley, L. J., Gresty, M. A., Perucca, E. and Richens, A. (1983a). Effect of a single oral dose of propranolol on essential tremor. A double-blind controlled study. *Ann. Neurol.*, **13**, 165–71.

Calzetti, S., Findley, L. J., Perucca, E. and Richens, A. (1982). Controlled study of metoprolol and propranolol during prolonged administration in patients with essential tremor. *J. Neurol. Neurosurg. Psychiatr.*, **45**, 893–7.

Calzetti, S., Findley, L. J., Perucca, E. and Richens, A. (1983b). The response of essential tremor to propranolol: evaluation of clinical variables governing its efficacy on prolonged adminstration. *J. Neurol. Neurosurg. Psychiatr.*, **46**, 393–8.

Constas, C. (1962). The effects of adrenaline, noradrenaline and isoprenaline on Parkinsonian tremor. *J. Neurol. Neurosurg. Psychiatr.*, **25**, 116–21.

Critchley, E. (1972). Clinical manifestations of essential tremor. *J. Neurol. Neurosurg. Psychiatr.*, 35, 365–72.

Dietrichson, P. and Espen, E. (1979). The effect of timolol vs placebo in benign essential tremor. In *Proceedings of the Timolol Intercontinental Symposium*, Stockholm, October, 1979, Merck Sharp & Dohme International.

Dietrichson, P. and Espen, E. (1981). Effects of timolol and atenolol on benign essential tremor: placebo-controlled studies based on quantitative tremor recording. *J. Neurol. Neurosurg. Psychiatr.*, 44, 677–83.

Dupont, E., Hansen, H. J. and Dalby, M. A. (1973). Treatment of benign essential tremor with propranolol. *Acta Neurol. Scand.*, 49, 75–84.

Findley, L. J., Calzetti, S., Gresty, M. A. and Paul, E. A. (1981). Amplitude of benign essential tremor and response to propranolol. *Lancet*, 2, 479–80.

Findley, L. J. and Gresty, M. A. (1981). Tremor. *Br. J. Hosp. Med.*, 26, 16–32.

Foster, J. B., Longley, B. P. and Stewart-Wynne, E. G. (1973). Propranolol in essential tremor. *Lancet*, 1, 1455.

Gilligan, B. S. (1972). Propranolol in essential tremor. *Lancet*, 2, 980.

Gilligan, B. S., Veale, J. L. and Wodak, J. (1972). Propranolol in the treatment of tremor. *Med. J. Aust.*, 1, 320–2.

Growdon, J. H., Shahani, B. T. and Young, R. R. (1975). The effect of alcohol on essential tremor. *Neurology*, 25, 259–62.

Herring, A. B. (1964). Action of pronethalol on Parkinsonian tremor. *Lancet*, 2, 892.

Jefferson, D., Jenner, P. and Marsden, C. D. (1979a). Relationship between plasma propranolol concentration and relief of essential tremor. *J. Neurol. Neurosurg. Psychiatr.*, 42, 831–7.

Jefferson, D., Jenner, P. and Marsden, C. D. (1979b). β-Adrenoreceptor antagonists in essential tremor. *J. Neurol. Neurosurg. Psychiatr.*, 42, 904–9.

Jefferson, D. and Marsden, C. D. (1980). Metoprolol in essential tremor. *Lancet*, 1, 427.

Joyce, G. C. and Rack, P. M. H. (1974). The effects of load and force on tremor at the normal human elbow joint. *J. Physiol.*, 240, 375–96.

Lands, A. M., Arnold, A., McAuliff, J. P., Luduena, F. P. and Brown, T. G. (1967). Differentiation of receptor systems activated by sympathomimetic amines. *Nature*, 214, 597–8.

Larsen, T. A. and TerävÄinen, H. (1981). Beta-blockers in essential tremor. *Lancet*, 2, 533.

Larsson, S. and Svedmyr, N. (1977). Tremor caused by sympathomimetics is mediated by beta$_2$-adrenoreceptors. *Scand. J. Resp. Dis.*, 58, 5–10.

Lee, R. G. and Stein, R. B. (1981). Resetting of tremor by mechanical perturbations: a comparison of essential tremor and Parkinsonian tremor. *Ann. Neurol.*, 10, 523–31.

Leigh, P. N., Marsden, C. D., Twomey, A. and Jefferson, D. (1981). Beta-adrenoceptor antagonists and essential tremor. *Lancet*, 1, 1106.

Lippold, O. C. J. (1970). Oscillation in the stretch reflex arc and the origin of the rhythmical 8–12 c/s component of physiological tremor. *J. Physiol.*, 206, 359–82.

Lippold, O. (1971). Physiological tremor. *Sci. Am.*, 224, 65–73.

Ljung, O. (1979). Treatment of essential tremor with metoprolol. *New Engl. J. Med.*, 301, 1005.

Ljung, O. (1980). Metoprolol in essential tremor. *Lancet*, 1, 1032.

McAllister, R. G., Markesbery, W. R., Ware, R. W. and Howell, S. M. (1977). Suppression of essential tremor by propranolol: correlation of effect with drug plasma levels and intensity of beta-adrenergic blockade. *Ann. Neurol.*, 1, 160–6.

McClure, C. G. and Davis, J. N. (1976). The effect of D-propranolol on action tremors. *Trans. Am. Neurol. Assoc.*, **101**, 269–70.

McDevitt, D. G. (1977). The assessment of β-adrenoceptor blocking drugs in man. *Br. J. Clin. Pharmacol.*, **4**, 413–25.

Marsden, C. D., Foley, T. H., Owen, D. A. L. and McAllister, R. G. (1967). Peripheral β-adrenergic receptors concerned with tremor. *Clin. Sci.*, **33**, 53–65.

Marsden, C. D. and Meadows, J. C. (1970). The effect of adrenaline on the contraction of human muscle. *J. Physiol.*, **207**, 429–48.

Marsden, C. D., Meadows, J. C. and Lowe, R. D. (1969). The influence of noradrenaline, tyramine and activation of sympathetic nerves on physiological tremor in man. *Clin. Sci.*, **37**, 243–52.

Moore, R. Y. and Bloom, F. E. (1979). Central catecholamine neurone systems: anatomy and physiology of the norepinephrine and epinephrine systems. *Annu. Rev. Neurosci.*, **2**, 113–68.

Morgan, M. H., Hewer, R. L. and Cooper, R. (1973). Effect of the beta adrenergic blocking agent propranolol on essential tremor. *J. Neurol. Neurosurg. Psychiatr.*, **36**, 618–24.

Murray, T. J. (1972). Treatment of essential tremor with propranolol. *Can. Med. Assoc. J.*, **107**, 984–6.

Murray, T. J. (1976). Long-term therapy of essential tremor with propranolol. *Can. Med. Assoc. J.*, **115**, 892–4.

Murray, T. J. (1981). Essential tremor. *Can. Med. Assoc. J.*, **124**, 1559–65.

Neil-Dwyer, G., Bartlett, J., McAinsh, J. and Cruickshank, J. M. (1981). β-Adrenoceptor blockers and the blood–brain barrier. *Br. J. Clin. Pharmacol.*, **11**, 549–53.

Newman, R. P. and Jacobs, L. (1980). Metoprolol in essential tremor. *Arch. Neurol.*, **37**, 596–7.

Owen, D. A. L. and Marsden, C. D. (1965). Effect of adrenergic β-blockade on Parkinsonian tremor. *Lancet*, **2**, 1259–62.

Paintal, A. S. (1964). Effects of drugs on vertebrate mechanoreceptors. *Pharmacol. Rev.*, **16**, 341–80.

Pakkenberg, H. (1972). Propranolol in essential tremor. *Lancet*, **1**, 633.

Perucca, E., Pickles, H. and Richens, A. (1981). Effect of atenolol, metoprolol, and propranolol on isoproterenol-induced tremor and tachycardia in normal subjects. *Clin. Pharmacol. Ther.*, **29**, 425–33.

Phillips, S. J., Richens, A. and Shand, D. G. (1973). Adrenergic control of tendon jerk reflexes in man. *Br. J. Pharmacol.*, **47**, 595–605.

de Prada, M. and Zuercher, G. (1979). Radioenzymatic assay of plasma and urinary catecholamines in man and various animal species: physiological and pharmacological applications. In Albertini, A., de Prada, M. and Peskar, B. A. (eds), *Radioimmunoassay of Drugs and Hormones in Cardiovascular Medicine*, Elsevier/North-Holland Biomedical Press, Amsterdam.

Rangel-Guerra, R. (1974). Treatment of benign essential tremor with a beta-adrenergic blocking agent (sotalol). In Snart, A. G. (ed), *Advances in Beta-adrenergic Blocking Therapy – Sotalol*, International Congress Series 341, Excerpta Medica, Amsterdam, V62–6.

Riley, T. and Pleet, A. B. (1979). Metoprolol tartrate for essential tremor. *New Engl. J. Med.*, **301**, 663.

Rinne, U. K. and Kaitaniemi, P. (1974). Sotalol in the treatment of essential tremor. In Snart, A. G. (ed.), *Advances in Beta-adrenergic Blocking Therapy – Sotalol*, International Congress Series 341, Excerpta Medica, Amsterdam, V56–61.

Scopa, J., Longley, B. P. and Foster, J. B. (1973). Beta-adrenergic blockers in benign essential tremor. *Curr. Ther. Res.*, **15**, 48–51.

Sevitt, I. (1971). The effect of adrenergic beta-receptor blocking drugs on tremor. *Practitioner*, **207**, 677–8.

Sevitt, I. (1974). A comparison of propranolol and benzhexol in essential tremor. *Practitioner*, **213**, 91–6.

Smith, C. M. (1963). Neuromuscular pharmacology, drugs and muscle spindles. *Annu. Rev. Pharmacol.*, **3**, 223–42.

Sørensen, P. S., Paulson, O. B., Steiness, E. and Jansen, E. C. (1981). Essential tremor treated with propranolol: lack of correlation between clinical effect and plasma propranolol levels. *Ann. Neurol.*, **9**, 53–7.

Strang, R. R. (1965). Clinical trial with a beta-receptor antagonist (propranolol) in Parkinsonism. *J. Neurol. Neurosurg. Psychiatr.*, **28**, 404–6.

Sweet, R. D., Blumberg, J., Lee, J. E. and McDowell, F. H. (1974). Propranolol treatment of essential tremor. *Neurology*, **24**, 64–7.

Taylor, E. A., Jefferson, D., Carroll, J. D. and Turner, P. (1981). Cerebrospinal fluid concentrations of propranolol, pindolol and atenolol in man: evidence for central actions of β-adrenoceptor antagonists. *Br. J. Clin. Pharmacol.*, **12**, 549–59.

Terävainen, H., Fogelholm, R. and Larsen, A. (1976). Effect of propranolol on essential tremor. *Neurology*, **26**, 27–30.

Terävainen, M. D., Larsen, A. and Fogelholm, R. (1977). Comparison between the effects of pindolol and propranolol on essential tremor. *Neurology*, **27**, 439–42.

Tolosa, E. S. and Loewenson, R. B. (1975). Essential tremor: treatment with propranolol. *Neurology*, **25**, 1041–4.

Turnbull, D. M. and Shaw, D. A. (1980). Metoprolol in essential tremor. *Lancet*, **1**, 95.

Vas, C. J. (1966). Propranolol in Parkinsonian tremor. *Lancet*, **1**, 182–3.

Wilson, J. F., Marshall, R. W., Dunstan, F. D. J. and Richens, A. (1982). A microcomputer based technique for the assessment of hand tremor in man. *Br. J. Clin. Pharmacol.*, **15**, 158P.

Winkler, G. F. and Young, R. R. (1971). The control of essential tremor by propranolol. *Trans. Am. Neurol. Assoc.*, **96**, 66–8.

Winkler, G. F. and Young, R. R. (1974). Efficacy of chronic propranolol therapy in action tremors of the familial, senile or essential varieties. *New Engl. J. Med.*, **290**, 984–8.

Young, R. R., Growdon, J. H. and Shahani, B. T. (1975). Beta-adrenergic mechanisms in action tremor. *New Engl. J. Med.*, **293**, 950–3.

Young, R. R. and Hagbarth, K. E. (1980). Physiological tremor enhanced by manoeuvres affecting the segmental stretch reflex. *J. Neurol. Neurosurg. Psychiatr.*, **43**, 248–56.

van Zwieten, P. A. and Timmermans, P. B. M. W. M. (1979). Comparison between the acute hemodynamic effects and brain penetration of atenolol and metoprolol. *J. Cardiovasc. Pharmacol.*, **1**, 85–96.

18
D,L-Propranolol and D-propranolol in essential tremor

S. CALZETTI and L. J. FINDLEY

INTRODUCTION

The β-adrenoceptor antagonist D,L-propranolol is the drug of first choice in the symptomatic control of essential tremor (ET) but the mechanism that mediates the tremolytic effect has not been established. Some authors believe that the drug exerts its effect mainly by blocking central and/or peripheral β-adrenergic receptors (Young *et al.*, 1975; Jefferson *et al.*, 1979), but other mechanisms of action unrelated to blockade of β-adrenoceptors have also been postulated (Young *et al.*, 1975; Koch-Weser, 1975). In particular, the possible role of the membrane-stabilising action (MSA) (quinidine-like) is unclear. While an early report claimed that D-propranolol (the D-isomer retaining the MSA of the racemic mixture but virtually devoid of β-adrenoceptor blocking properties) is as effective as D,L-propranolol (McClure and Davis, 1976), a more recent study failed to confirm these findings (Teräväinen and Larsen, 1981). In a previous study (Calzetti *et al.*, 1983) we have demonstrated that a single oral dose of D,L-propranolol (120 mg) significantly reduces the amplitude of ET within 2 h following its administration. The present study was designed to assess under controlled conditions the comparative tremolytic efficacy of D-propranolol and D,L-propranolol on acute administration.

SINGLE ORAL DOSE STUDY

Patients

Fourteen patients with moderately disabling to severe ET (10 male and four female), aged between 16 and 75 years, who were attending the outpatient clinics at the National Hospital for Nervous Diseases, Queen Square, London, gave their informed consent to participate in the study. The diagnosis was established on the basis of the clinical history and detailed general and neuro-logical examination accompanied by ancillary laboratory investigations. All patients had been symptomatic for at least one year (range 1 to 50 years) prior to the study. The patients were selected on the basis of tremor amplitude of the more involved hand, which according to a previous study (Calzetti *et al.*, 1983) was expected to be responsive to acute administration of D,L-propranolol. In five patients there was a family history of tremor affecting hands and/or head. Nine patients were not receiving any drug therapy for tremor at the time of the study. Three patients on chronic treatment with propranolol and two with primidone agreed to have their treatment discontinued and remained drug-free for at least two weeks prior to and until completion of the study. Patients with a history of excessive alcohol intake, congestive cardiac failure, heart block, diabetes mellitus and asthma were excluded.

Protocol

The study was double-blind and placebo-controlled. Each patient was studied on three different occasions separated by an interval of at least one week. The tests were performed at the same time of the day for each individual patient, approximately 3 h after a light meal. The patients were instructed to abstain from smoking and from taking alcohol or caffeinated beverages for at least 12 h before testing. After 15 min rest, piezoresistive linear accelerometers (Endevco 7625-10) were taped to the dorsal surface of each hand in the second interspace 1 cm proximal to the metacarpophalangeal joints, their sensitive axis orientated in the vertical plane. Hand tremor was assessed with the patient seated, the forearms supported up to the wrist and the hands unsupported outstretched horizontally in a pronated posture. Three separated tremor recordings of about 1 min duration were obtained at 5 min intervals, and to minimise the effect of fatigue the hands were allowed to rest freely between recordings. Accelerometric signals were amplified and recorded simultaneously on paper and magnetic tape for subsequent analysis. Measurement of pulse rate was obtained after a 10 min period of rest in the supine position and repeated after 1, 2 and 3 min of standing. After recordings of tremor and pulse rate, the patients were given a single oral dose of D,L-propranolol (120 mg), D-propranolol (120 mg) or identical placebo capsules together with 50 ml plain water. The order of treatments was randomised. Recording of tremor and supine and standing pulse rate were repeated 1.5 h following treatment, at a time when the serum level of both D,L-propranolol and D-propranolol was expected to be approaching the maximum. The inhibition of standing tachycardia was used as an index of the degree of cardiac β-blockade (Carruthers *et al.*, 1974). Venous blood samples for the determination of serum D,L-propranolol and D-propranolol concentration were taken at the completion of the tests.

Serum D,L-propranolol and D-propranolol concentration was determined by high-pressure liquid chromatography according to the method described by Nygard *et al.* (1979).

Tremor analysis was performed on-line using a Hewlett-Packard 5420 A signal analyser. For each condition, i.e. before and after treatment, the program averaged 150 autospectra, each derived from overlapping 10.24 s samples of tremor. Fifty samples were taken from the beginning of each of the three separate recordings and approximately 45 s of tremor recording contributed to the analysis of each condition. The spectra, averaged thus, were displayed for measurement in the form of 'autospectra' in which the root-mean-square (r.m.s) magnitude of the frequency components was plotted as a function of the frequency. For a simple characterisation of the tremor, measurements were taken of the frequency (Hz) of the dominant peak and of its magnitude scaled in r.m.s. acceleration, the unit of acceleration being taken as $1g$ ($g = 981$ cm s^{-2}). As it was found that the dominant tremor frequency did not vary significantly before and after treatment, the magnitude of acceleration is proportional to the amplitude of hand displacement, that is,

$$\text{amplitude of displacement} = \frac{\text{acceleration} \times 981}{4\pi^2 \times \text{frequency}^2} \quad \text{cm r.m.s.}$$

In each patient only the data obtained from the more involved hand were used for the computation of the results.

Changes in tremor magnitude were compared by using Wilcoxon's test for paired differences. Analysis of pulse rate was performed by using the Student's 't' test for paired data.

RESULTS

The frequency of the dominant peak of hand tremor of the patients studied ranged from 4.3 to 8.0 Hz. In any individual patient the frequency of tremor was similar in all baseline recordings and did not change significantly after the three treatments. The pretreatment peak magnitude of tremor ranged from 8.38 milli-g to 679.36 milli-g and showed considerable variation within any individual patient on different occasions of recording. However, within any single pretreatment recording session there was little fluctuation in tremor magnitude. Because of this, only the percentage change of baseline tremor magnitude was used to compare the effect of the different treatments.

After administration of placebo the magnitude of tremor decreased in six patients, remained unchanged in three (i.e. showed a decrease of less than 15%) and increased in five. Administration of D-propranolol was associated with a decrease of tremor magnitude in 10 patients, an increase in three patients, whereas one patient remained unchanged. Following administration of D,L-propranolol the tremor showed a decrease in 12 patients and increased in two (figure 18.1). None of the patients had tremor magnitude suppressed within the range of physiological tremor. The mean percentage decrease of baseline tremor magnitude was by 11.65 ± 8.63 s.e.m. (NS) following placebo, by 16.23 ± 16.2 s.e.m. (NS) following D-propranolol, and by 36.95 ± 8.17 s.e.m. ($p < 0.01$) following D,L-propranolol. D-Propranolol and D,L-propranolol pro-

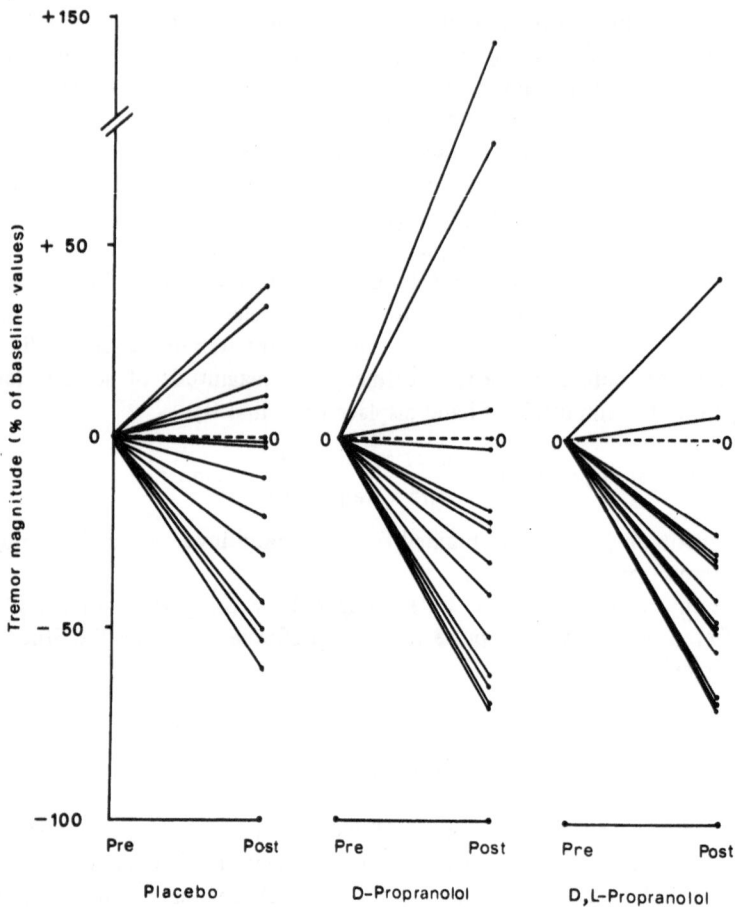

Figure 18.1 Effect of placebo, D-propranolol (120 mg) and D,L-propranolol (120 mg) on magnitude of postural hand tremor in individual patients.

duced a percentage decrease of tremor magnitude greater than that produced by placebo in nine and 10 patients, respectively. When all the patients were considered, D,L-propranolol but not D-propranolol produced a percentage reduction of baseline tremor magnitude significantly greater than that observed after administration of placebo ($p < 0.05$) (figure 18.2). However, when the effects of D,L-propranolol and D-propranolol were compared, the former did not prove significantly superior to the latter. Of the 12 patients who responded to D,L-propranolol, nine responded to the D-isomer, whereas of the 10 patients who showed a response to D-propranolol, eight responded to the racemic mixture. In seven of 14 patients the percentage decrease of baseline tremor magnitude was greater following D-propranolol than D,L-propranolol.

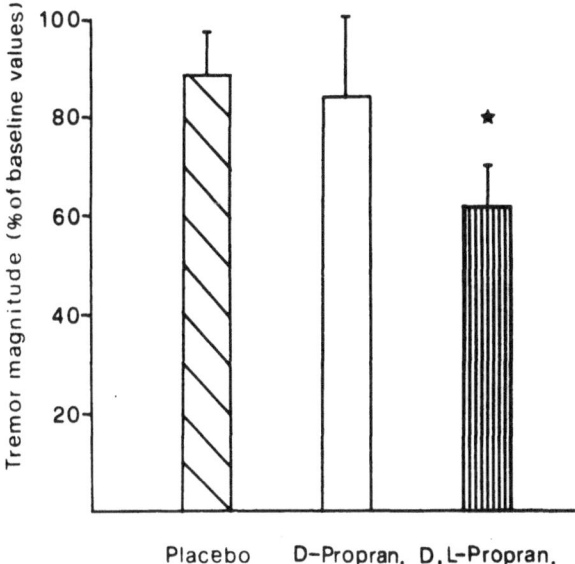

Figure 18.2 Percentage change in tremor magnitude after administration of a single oral dose of placebo, D-propranolol (120 mg) and D,L-propranolol (120 mg) in the patients studied. Bars represent the mean change + s.e.m. (*$p < 0.05$ as compared with placebo).

There was no difference in the pulse rate recorded at 1, 2 and 3 min after standing, and therefore the mean of the three values was taken for further calculations. Baseline values of supine and standing pulse rate did not differ significantly between treatments. D,L-Propranolol diminished the normal increase in pulse rate on standing ($p < 0.01$) whereas both placebo and D-propranolol had no effect. The inhibition of standing tachycardia produced by D,L-propranolol was significantly greater than that produced by D-propranolol and placebo ($p < 0.01$) (figure 18.3).

Serum concentration of D-propranolol (14 patients) was found to vary between 52.0 ng ml^{-1} and 254.2 ng ml^{-1} (median 90.3 ng ml^{-1}), whereas serum concentration of D,L-propranolol (13 patients) ranged between 48.9 ng ml^{-1} and 283.2 ng ml^{-1} (median 111.0 ng ml^{-1}) (figure 18.4). There was no significant difference in serum concentration of D-propranolol and D,L-propranolol in the patients studied.

DISCUSSION

The studies so far conducted in order to evaluate the role of MSA in the relief of ET produced by D,L-propranolol have led to conflicting results. McClure and

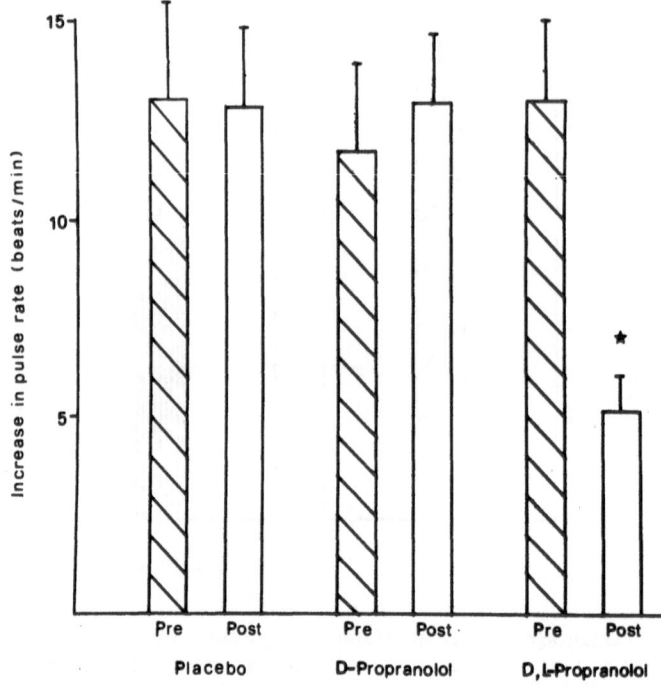

Figure 18.3 Increase in pulse rate on standing before and after administration of placebo, D-propranolol (120 mg) and D,L-propranolol (120 mg). Bars represent the mean + s.e.m. (*$p < 0.01$ as compared with pre-drug values and placebo).

Davis (1976) found D-propranolol (120 mg daily) as effective as D,L-propranolol at the same dosage in three patients, but the study was not double-blind and not placebo-controlled. More recently Teräväinen and Larsen (1981) failed to demonstrate any significant effect of D-propranolol following prolonged administration in a double-blind controlled study, suggesting that MSA is not of therapeutic value in this condition. The results of this study are in line with those of Teräväinen and Larsen indicating that the acute tremolytic action of propranolol in ET is largely (and possible entirely) mediated by its β-blocking properties. It is relevant in this context to mention that both sotalol and timolol, two β-adrenoceptor antagonists devoid of MSA, have been found to be effective in the same disorder (Rinne and Kaitaniemi, 1974; Jefferson et al., 1979; Dietrichson and Espen, 1981). The fact that in this study nine out of 14 patients were better on D-propranolol than on placebo may represent a chance finding or may indicate that the MSA of the drug contributes to some extent to the overall clinical response. In this regard it should be admitted that D,L-propranolol exerts its acute anti-tremor effect on ET by two mechanisms of action, one mediated by specific blockade of β-adrenoceptors and the other by an action independent of blockade of these adrenoceptors and

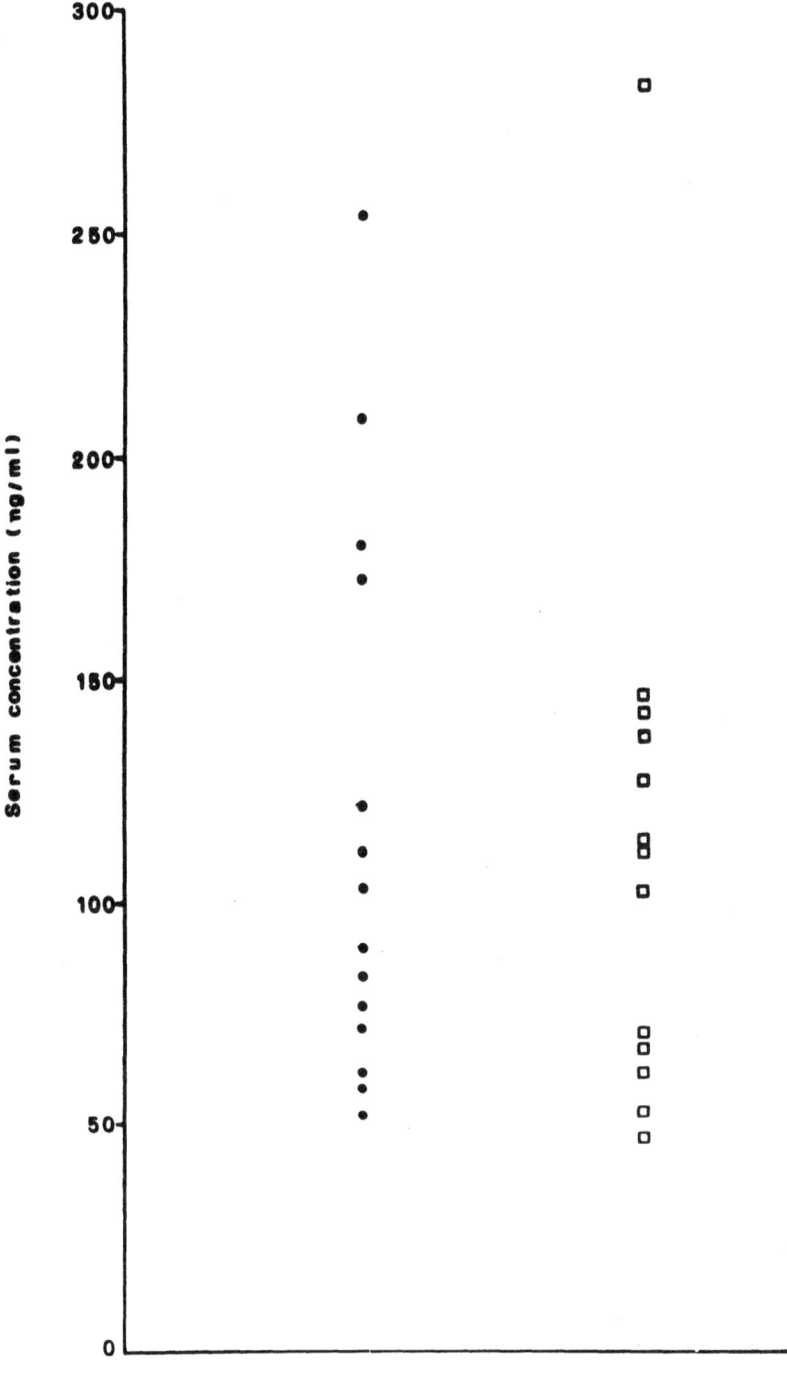

Figure 18.4 Serum concentration of D-propranolol (14 patients) and D,L-propranolol (13 patients) after a single oral dose of 120 mg of D-propranolol and D,L-propranolol.

possibly related to MSA of the drug. The racemic mixture, which possesses both pharmacological properties, reached a statistically significant effect, whereas D-propranolol, nearly devoid of β-blocking activity, failed to.

Another possibility that cannot be excluded is that the effect observed following D-propranolol could be partly ascribed to its minimal β-blocking property, which is reported to be about one-hundredth of that exhibited by the L-isomer (Larsen, 1980). However, at the dosage used in this study (120 mg), it seems unlikely that D-propranolol would have shown a sufficient degree of blockade of the β-receptors to account for the tremolytic effect observed. This is also indirectly supported by the finding that D-propranolol failed in the same patients to inhibit the standing tachycardia, taken as an index of cardiac β-blockade.

In rat phrenic nerve–diaphragm preparation used as a model of cholinergic synapse and excitable membranes, the acute reduction of the electrical excitability and the depression of the presynaptic action potentials in the muscles produced by D,L-propranolol have been postulated to be mediated by a mechanism related to the membrane-stabilising effect of the drug (Larsen, 1980). However, whether these properties could be partly responsible for the tremolytic effect of the drug in humans remains to be established. Although the concentration of propranolol achieved in those *in vitro* experiments was higher than that required in clinical practice to observe a therapeutic benefit, it cannot be excluded that when the 'safety margin' of neuromuscular transmission is lower, as in some central or peripheral nervous system disease states, a significant effect may become evident even at lower concentration of the drug.

The results of this study were confined only to the acute effect of D-propranolol and therefore further studies are necessary to verify whether these findings hold true following prolonged administration of D,L-propranolol and D-propranolol.

The fact that D,L-propranolol reduced ET following a single oral dose administration confirms that a 'long-latency' central action of the drug is not necessary for its anti-tremor effect to become evident (Calzetti *et al.*, 1983). More likely a 'short-latency' peripheral and/or central mechanism of action is involved.

REFERENCES

Calzetti, S., Findley, L. J., Gresty, M. A., Perucca, E. and Richens, A. (1983). Effect of a single oral dose of propranolol on essential tremor. A double-blind controlled study. *Ann. Neurol.*, **13**, 165-71.

Carruthers, S. G., Ghosal, A. G., McDevitt, D. G., Nelson, J. K. and Shanks, R. G. (1974). The assessment of beta-adrenoceptor blocking drugs in hyperthyroidism. *Br. J. Clin. Pharmacol.*, **1**, 93-8.

Dietrichson, P. and Espen, E. (1981). Effect of timolol and atenolol on benign essential tremor: placebo-controlled studies based on quantitative tremor recording. *J. Neurol. Neurosurg. Psychiatr.*, **44**, 677-83.

Jefferson, D., Jenner, P. and Marsden, C. D. (1979). Beta-adrenoceptor antagonists is essential tremor. *J. Neurol. Neurosurg. Psychiatr.*, **42**, 904-9.

Koch-Weser, J. (1975). Non-beta-blocking actions of propranolol. *New Engl. J. Med.*, **293**, 988-9.

Larsen, A. (1980). *Beta-blockers, Tremor and Neuromuscular Transmission. A Clinical and Experimental Study* (Academic dissertation), University of Helsinki, Finland.

McClure, C. G. and Davis, J. N. (1976). The effect of D-propranolol on action tremors. *Trans, Am. Neurol. Assoc.*, **101**, 269–70.

Nygard, G., Shelver, W. M. and Wahba Khalil, S. K. (1979). Sensitive high pressure liquid-chromatographic determination of propranolol in plasma. *J. Pharmacol. Sci.*, **68**, 379–81.

Rinne, U. K. and Kaitaniemi, P. (1974). Sotalol in the treatment of essential tremor. In Snart, A. G. (ed.), *Advances in Beta-adrenergic Blocking Therapy – Sotalol*, International Congress Series 341, Excerpta Medica, Amsterdam, V56–61.

Teräväinen, H. and Larsen, A. (1981). Beta-blockers in the treatment of benign essential tremor. *12th World Congress of Neurology*, Kyoto, Japan, International Congress Series 548, Excerpta Medica, Amsterdam, Abstr. no. 130, pp. 41–2.

Young, R. R., Growdon, J. H. and Shahani, B. T. (1975). Beta-adrenergic mechanisms in action tremor. *New Engl. J. Med.*, **293**, 950–3.

19
Primidone in essential tremor

L. J. FINDLEY, S. CALZETTI and L. CLEEVES

INTRODUCTION

Essential tremor, with its senile and familial varieties, is a common disorder (Marshall, 1968; Critchley, 1949; Rautakorpi *et al.*, this volume, chapter 14) which, although usually prefixed with the adjective 'benign', frequently produces significant disability. As yet there is no satisfactory drug available that can predictably control essential tremor. Alcohol can be effective in reducing or abolishing the tremor in some patients (Growdon *et al.*, 1975). However, this is an impracticable therapy and the effect is not specific to essential tremor. At present beta-adrenoceptor antagonists, in particular propranolol, have proven to have the most therapeutic benefit in attenuating the tremor (Morgan *et al.*, 1973; Winkler and Young, 1974; Tolosa and Loewenson, 1975; McAllister *et al.*, 1977; Calzetti *et al.*, 1982).

Propranolol is considered the drug of first choice in this condition but the clinical responsiveness to the drug is unpredictable and not completely satisfactory. Indeed, we have never seen a large-amplitude essential tremor completely suppressed by propranolol, even with doses exceeding 300 mg daily. Some of the variability of responsiveness noted may reflect the heterogeneity now recognised in this disorder (Marsden, this volume, chapter 4). In addition to the limitation on the effectiveness of propranolol in more severe essential tremors, it is contra-indicated in some groups of patients, in particular those with obstructive airways disease, cardiac failure and peripheral vascular disease. Thus the beta-adrenoceptor antagonists have limited efficacy in the suppression of essential tremor and it is clearly desirable to seek alternative drugs.

In a recent, open, prospective, clinical study in 20 patients with essential tremor, O'Brien *et al.* (1981) confirmed the previously anecdotal observation that the tremor of 12 patients showed a 'good to dramatic' response to primidone. Six patients were unable to tolerate the drug because of vertigo and nausea and it was commented that these side-effects occurred with smaller doses than is normal when this drug is used in its more common role as an anticonvulsant in epileptic patients. Unfortunately the trial was not double-blind and placebo-controlled and objective measurements of tremor were not performed.

In this chapter we report the results of a double-blind controlled study of primidone in a group of patients with moderate to severe essential tremor of the hands. Some preliminary findings of this study were reported by Findley and Calzetti (1982).

METHODOLOGY

Patients

Twenty-three patients were admitted to the trial. All exhibited uncomplicated, moderate to severe essential tremor, i.e. monosymptomatic, postural tremor of both hands. None were receiving other medications during the time of this trial. The relevant clinical characteristics of the patients ($n = 18$) who were able to complete the study are shown in table 19.1. Five patients could not continue, owing to immediate side-effects (*vide infra*).

Table 19.1 Patient data.

Age (years)	Successful completions	Family history	Duration of symptoms (years)	Tremor on placebo	Frequency (Hz)
Mean: 57	18	5	Mean: 12	Acceleration: 14–675 milli-g*	Range: 4.1–
Range: 15–82			Range: 2–40	Displacement: 0.03–0.62 cm	8.1

*g is the acceleration of gravity, 9.81 m s^{-2}

Protocol

The study was double-blind and placebo-controlled. In a separate open pilot study with primidone commencing 250 mg daily, an unacceptable incidence of side-effects occurred. The patients therefore were warned of possible side-effects and started on 62.5 mg of primidone daily, i.e. one-quarter of the standard tablet, and increased by 62.5 mg daily up to a maximum of 250 mg three times daily or until the tremor was completely suppressed or side-effects necessitated a reduction in dosage. Patients were warned of possible side-effects at the commencement of the trial.

Tremor was assessed at the end of a five-week period on drug or placebo to allow for a steady state of serum primidone and phenobarbitone to be reached. Measurements of tremor were made according to a standard procedure which we have adopted for similar trials (Calzetti *et al.*, 1981a). The patients were instructed to refrain from alcohol, smoking or taking caffeinated beverages for 12 h before each assessment. For each assessment the patient sat comfortably in a carver chair and was given several minutes in this situation before any measurements were taken so that he could become reaccustomed to the laboratory environment, which he would have already visited on several occasions. For each assessment three, 1 min long, samples of tremor were recorded from the hands, which were extended beyond the arms of the chair in pronation with the forearms supported to the wrists. In between these samples the patient rested his hands in a dependent posture. Tremor was transduced with miniature DC piezoresistive accelerometers (Endevco 7250-10), which were taped to the dorsum of the hands in the second interspace, 1 cm proximal to the metacarpophalangeal joints and oriented so that their sensitive axis was in the vertical plane coincident with the direction of flexion and extension of the hand.

Tremor magnitude was quantified using a spectrum analyser which calculated the average magnitude spectra of 150 overlapping 10.24 s records of tremor. These were taken equally from the middle portions of each of the three, 1 min, samples. Each 10.24 s record was digitally filtered, windowed and subjected to fast Fourier transformation. The derived spectra had a bandwidth of 25 Hz and frequency resolution better than 0.1 Hz. Spectral magnitudes were calibrated in units of root-mean-square (r.m.s.) 'g'. For all subjects *symptomatic* tremor magnitude spectra exhibited a single finely tuned peak (e.g. shown in figure 19.1a) and thus tremor could be characterised by the frequency and magnitude of the dominant peak in the spectrum. As it was found that the dominant frequency of symptomatic tremor did not differ significantly on placebo or drug, then the magnitude of tremor acceleration in the two conditions is proportional to displacement according to the relationship:

$$\text{magnitude of displacement} = \frac{\text{magnitude of acceleration}}{4\pi^2 \text{ frequency}^2}$$

Additional evaluations of tremor symptomaticity included a clinical assessment of postural and intention tremor of the hands and performance tests (handwriting, drawing and tracing an Archimedes' spiral). An arbitrary scale from 0 to 5 (maximum severity) was used to quantitate the results. The performance tests were evaluated by three different assessors and the final score for each patient was the mean of the ratings of three independent assessors. There was also a patient's self-assessment on a similar arbitrary scale from 0 to 5 which included abilities at daily living activities and family opinion about change in tremor.

At the end of each tremor assessment, venous blood samples were obtained for the estimation of serum primidone and phenobarbitone (enzyme mediated immunoassay).

RESULTS

As the amplitude of tremor in the two hands was invariably dissimilar, and the magnitude of tremor in the less involved hand could be minimal, only results obtained from the more affected hand are presented. This selectivity is further

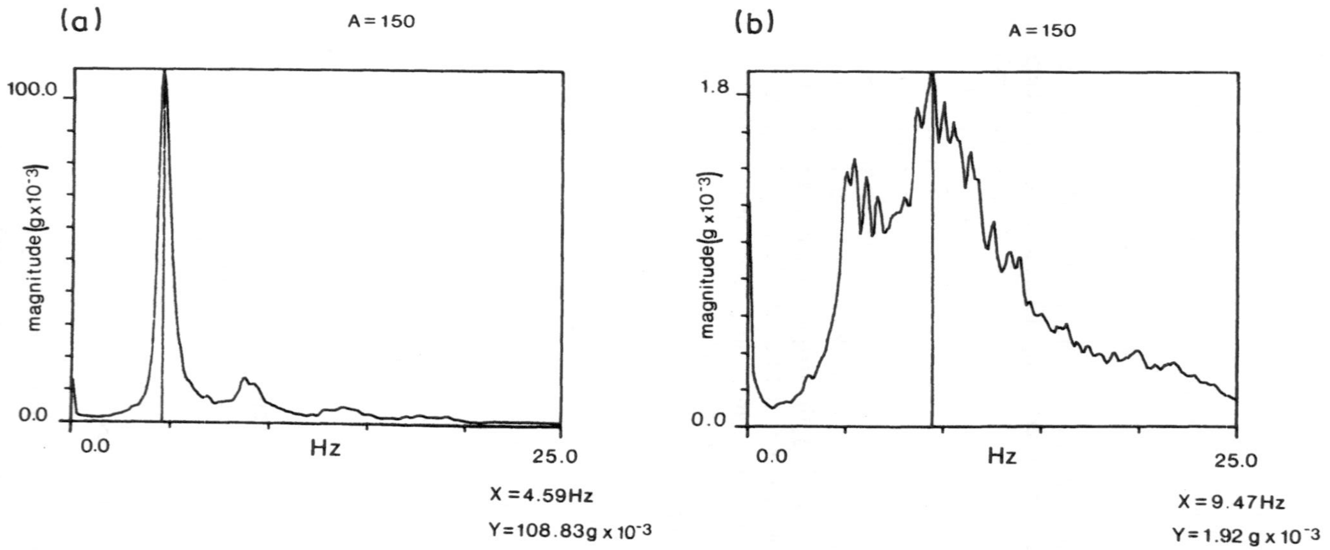

Figure 19.1 Examples of average spectra of tremor magnitude under placebo (a) and primidone (b) recorded from the right hand of a 69-year-old man with a four-year history of bilateral postural tremor of the hands. The placebo spectrum shows a large-magnitude tremor at a mean fundamental frequency of 4.59 Hz with a magnitude at this frequency of 108 milli-g r.m.s. (equivalent to approximately 1 m s^{-2}). On primidone (250 mg t.d.s.) the spectrum of his tremor had a different appearance. The dominant peak in the spectrum was 9.47 Hz with a magnitude of 1.92 milli-g (note that the scale of the y-axis in (b) is one-fiftieth that in (1)). The spectrum of (b) also shows a significant peak in the region of 4.6 Hz which has a magnitude of 1.4 milli-g. The magnitude of both these peaks is within the range of magnitudes that we record for frequency components of asymptomatic physiological tremor using this method of transduction and analysis. Our interpretation is that the pathological tremor has been suppressed greatly in amplitude so that the physiological tremor becomes evident. The small peak at 4.6 Hz represents a small residual trace of the pathological tremor. The improvements on self-assessment, clinical assessment and performance tests were equally dramatic. This patient experienced no side-effects although serum primidone was 100 μmol l^{-1}, which demonstrates that 'susceptibility' to the drug in some patients is an important factor responsible for toxic effects.

validated by the observation that, in this study, on the two occasions of assessment, the order of difference in magnitude between the tremors in the two hands remained unchanged. The dominant, peak frequency of the more affected hand ranged between 4.1 and 8.1 Hz with a median frequency of 6.2 Hz. There was no significant change in frequency of any symptomatic tremor whilst treated with either primidone or placebo. The magnitude of tremor on placebo ranged between 14 and 675 milli-*g* r.m.s. with a median magnitude of 33 milli-*g* r.m.s.

When differences in magnitude were calculated as the absolute change, in 16 of the 17 patients who completed the study, primidone reduced tremor magnitude to levels significantly below those recorded under placebo ($p < 0.01$, Wilcoxon's test for paired differences). The median reduction of tremor amplitude on primidone, compared with placebo, was 27 milli-*g* r.m.s. (see figure 19.2). The percentage reduction in tremor amplitude by primidone compared with placebo was 56% (range of +12.7% to −98.7%), which is significant at the 0.01 level (Wilcoxon's test for paired differences).

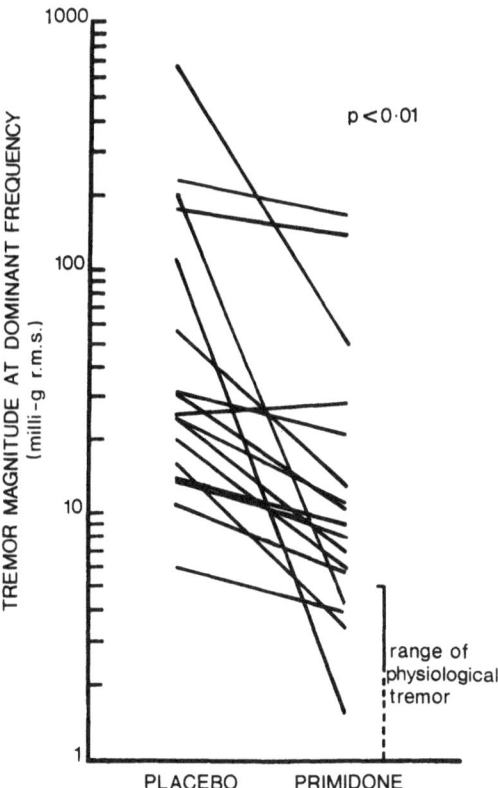

Figure 19.2 Absolute levels and changes of tremor recorded under drug and placebo in 17 patients with essential tremor. Each sloping line represents the results on a single patient and connects the magnitudes of tremor recorded under placebo and drug respectively.

One patient showed an increase in tremor amplitude on primidone. He was a 15-year-old male who had a history of bilateral tremor from early childhood. There was no family history of tremor. The frequency of tremor of the more affected hand was identical on drug and placebo at 6.9 Hz with an amplitude, on placebo, of 25 milli-g r.m.s. This tremor was also unresponsive to propranolol 100 mg t.d.s., baclofen 30 mg t.d.s. and tizanidine (a new drug that selectively depresses polysynaptic reflexes) 2 mg given as a single oral dose (McClellan and Hassan, 1980).

Two severely affected patients had their tremor suppressed to non-symptomatic levels, which were within the levels of magnitude of physiological tremor recorded in our laboratory (see figure 19.2). In one patient there was an apparent shift in the dominant frequency of tremor. Inspection of the spectrum revealed that the pathological tremor was still marginally present at the same frequency as before but had been suppressed in amplitude to a level that was less than the amplitude of the peak frequency of physiological tremor which then dominated the spectrum (see figure 19.1).

The reduction in tremor magnitude, as measured objectively, was reflected in the results from the clinical evaluation and the patient's self-assessment, each of which showed a significant improvement on primidone compared with placebo ($p < 0.05$, Wilcoxon's test). The performance tests also show parallel significant differences ($p < 0.05$, Wilcoxon's test). An example of the changes in handwriting, under the two conditions, of a moderately affected patient who kept a diary are shown in figure 19.3. One may note that following the withdrawal of primidone there is a continual decline in the quality of the patient's writing over a period of some 10 days. In contrast, with change from placebo to primidone in the same patient there is a prompt response with a detectable improvement in handwriting with the first day (figure 19.4).

There was no correlation, involving either absolute or percentage change in tremor magnitude on primidone, with patient's age, duration of tremor symptoms, family history, and frequency and magnitude of tremor on placebo (Spearman rank correlation).

All patients showing a positive response to primidone in terms of attenuation of tremor magnitude maintained this response at follow-up one year later.

Owing to dose-related side-effects, only 13 patients reached the maximum permitted dosage. The mean daily dosage was 625 mg, range 125–750 mg. Serum phenobarbitone concentrations ranged between 5 and 87 μmol l^{-1} (mean 49 μmol l^{-1}) and serum primidone concentrations ranged between 18 and 100 μmol l^{-1} (mean 53 μmol l^{-1}). There was no correlation between the reduction in tremor magnitude on primidone and either the serum phenobarbitone or primidone concentration. Dose-limiting side-effects occurred in four patients but only during the primidone phase. They consisted of a variable combination of sedation, tiredness, nausea and vertigo and were attenuated with reduction in dosage.

Five patients were unable to complete the trial, owing to an acute 'toxic' reaction which occurred with the initial 62.5 mg dose of primidone. This

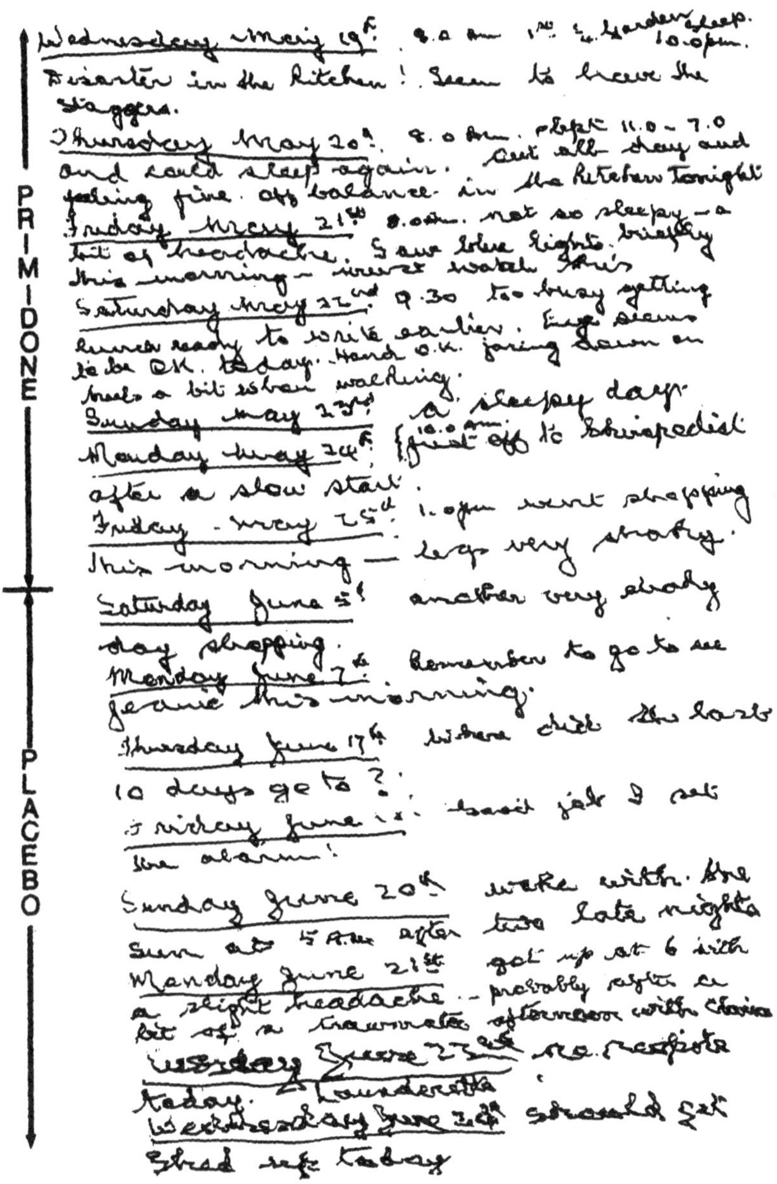

Figure 19.3 Examples of handwriting, sampled on successive days, of a patient who was changed from primidone to placebo and who kept a written record during the trial. On withdrawal of primidone there was a progressive deterioration in legibility over a period of nine days, which is perhaps most consistent with the known pharmacokinetics of the phenobarbital derivative.

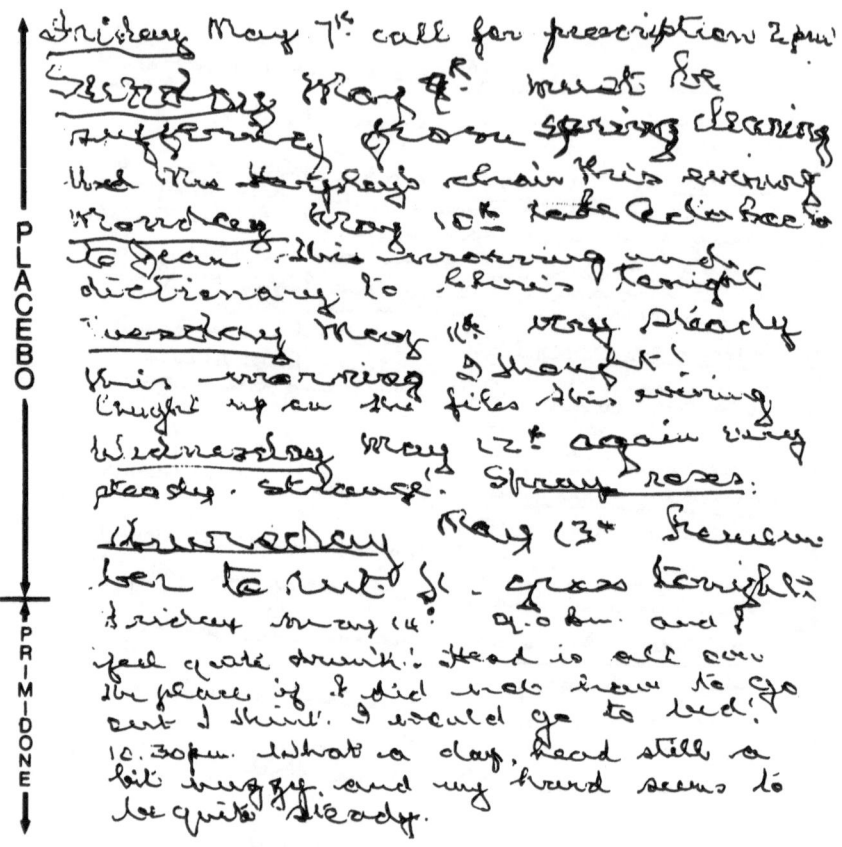

Figure 19.4 Examples of handwriting, sampled on successive days, of a patient who was changed from placebo to primidone. The character of the writing changes within 24 h of the introduction of primidone.

produced acute nausea, vomiting, ataxia and giddiness forcing the patient to bed. The duration of these symptoms usually varied between 12 and 24 h after the first and only dose. Following a single 62.5 mg dose, severe symptoms persisted for three days in one patient.

DISCUSSION

The results of this study are in agreement with the findings of the clinical trial of O'Brien *et al.* (1981) in that primidone consistently attenuates essential tremor and may therefore be considered an alternative form of medication to beta-adrenoceptor antagonists. The median reductions in tremor magnitude on primidone were comparable to that achieved in another controlled trial of prolonged administration of propranolol (240 mg daily) (Calzetti *et al.*, 1982). In contrast with propranolol, however, in some patients with very large-amplitude tremors, primidone reduced tremor magnitudes to within the range of non-symptomatic physiological tremor (see figures 19.1 and 19.2). We have not seen this 'total' suppressive effect with beta-adrenoceptor antagonists in patients with large-amplitude tremors. The response to primidone in terms of the objective assessments of tremor amplitude are paralleled by the results obtained from the performance tests, self-rating and clinical assessments of tremor.

It is clear that primidone would offer an alternative treatment in patients in whom beta-adrenoceptor antagonists are contra-indicated, and may be considered the drug of first choice in patients with tremors of large amplitude as, in these patients, one can sometimes see a dramatic effect. O'Brien *et al.* noted from clinical observation that some patients on primidone derived additional benefit from the introduction of propranolol. From our experience with the practical management of patients with essential tremor we would concur with these observations although the additive effects of the two drugs have not been objectively studied.

The mechanism of action of primidone in its effect on essential tremor and in its production of acute toxic and dose-related side-effects is not understood. Primidone is an established anticonvulsant drug in common use. It is well absorbed from the upper gastrointestinal tract with peak drug serum concentration attained within 3 to 5 h. About 25% remains as primidone and is excreted unconjugated by the kidneys. It is converted to two active metabolites, phenylethylmalonamide (PEMA) (approximately 50%), which is also unconjugated and has a half-life of 24 to 48 h, and phenobarbital (approximately 5%), of which some 50% is bound to protein and has a half-life of about 120 h. Thus phenobarbital accumulates during chronic administration and requires approximately three weeks to reach steady-state plasma levels.

In the study of O'Brien *et al.* (1981), from primidone withdrawal tests in two patients followed by PEMA substitution, it was felt that the efficacy of the drug was largely due to the derived PEMA but that primidone itself had some effect. However, Calzetti *et al.* (1981b), in a double-blind controlled study of PEMA in essential tremor, with dosages up to 800 mg daily, found the drug to be totally inert in terms of its effect on tremor magnitude. In addition, none of the patients developed any side-effects and yet achieved PEMA serum levels that would be expected from 1500 mg of primidone daily (twice the maximum dose allowed in the current trial).

A possibility would seem to be that the derived phenobarbital is the metabolite responsible for the suppressant effect of primidone on essential tremor. It is well known that all sedative and tranquillising drugs do have a beneficial effect on tremor. Phenobarbitone in particular has been used widely in patients with tremulous states, although in most instances it does not have a 'dramatic' effect. Procaccianti *et al.* (1981), in an open study, showed that patients with essential tremor benefited from phenobarbitone. In a follow-up, controlled study, although phenobarbitone (dose $1.3 \, \text{mg} \, \text{kg}^{-1}$) was shown effectively to attenuate tremor significantly below baseline, it was not stated whether this effect was significantly greater than the effect of placebo. More recently Baruzzi *et al.* (1983) found that phenobarbital (about 1.3 mg kg^{-1}) was significantly better than placebo and equipotent to propranolol (about 1.7 mg kg^{-1}) in reducing essential tremor in a double-blind controlled study that utilised accelerometric measurements of tremor and patients' subjective evaluations. In the present study there was no correlation between tremor response and either the serum primidone or phenobarbitone levels. It is not known how much the parent drug and/or the derived phenobarbitone individually contribute to the suppressive effect of primidone in essential tremor or whether a therapeutic range of plasma concentrations of primidone or derived phenobarbitone can be established for the management of essential tremor.

As phenobarbital is derived directly from primidone, it is difficult in studies *in vivo* to obtain evidence of their respective, separate and independent pharmacological actions. However, there is evidence that primidone, as regards its anticonvulsant activity, has independent activity from phenobarbital (Baumel *et al.*, 1973; Woodbury and Pippenger, 1982), and in normal therapeutic concentrations their mechanisms of action may well be entirely different. In this respect it is proposed either that phenobarbitone functions with a GABA-like action or that it enhances the effects of GABA, producing postsynaptic inhibition (Harvey, 1980). In contrast, in the case of primidone, because of the similarities between its pharmacological effects and those of phenytoin and carbamazepine in experimental models of epilepsy, and the similarity of their relative efficacies in the control of complex partial seizures, it is anticipated that one mechanism of action of primidone is through effects on the neuronal membrane, particularly with respect to alterations of ionic fluxes (Woodbury and Pippenger, 1982). It has been proposed that the oscillatory properties of central neurones, which are determined by the characteristics of their transmembranous ionic fluxes, are responsible for some forms of pathological tremor (see Llinás, this volume, chapter 10). We could therefore hypothesise that the effects of primidone on transmembranous ionic fluxes are the mechanism of action in the suppression of essential tremor. This could explain the very prompt responses that can be seen with the first dose, and it would be of interest to know whether other anticonvulsants with similar properties show similar effects on tremor.

From pilot studies we were aware that using larger doses of primidone (i.e. commencing at 125 mg twice daily and increasing by 125 mg daily) all patients developed unacceptable dose-related side-effects of nausea, vomiting and ataxia. By using the low-dose incremental regimen in this trial, these side-effects were considerably reduced, but even so four of the 17 patients who completed the trial showed dose-limiting side-effects of primidone. Thus we would recommend a slowly incremental regimen to be adopted when the drug is used in patients with essential tremor. Primidone, when used in essential tremor, shows a higher incidence of side-effects than when used as an anticonvulsant. It has been argued that this is due to delayed metabolism of the drug because of the absence of hepatic enzyme induction in patients previously unexposed to anticonvulsant drugs. Perhaps with prior exposure to a more acceptable anticonvulsant, to induce hepatic enzymes, these side-effects could be reduced (Feely, 1981).

Acute side-effects occurred in the five patients who were unable to complete the trial. These all occurred immediately on taking the first 62.5 mg of primidone and consisted of severe nausea, vomiting and ataxia which lasted 12 to 24 h, and in one patient for three days. The symptoms began before any metabolism of the drug could have occurred. The mechanism of this dramatic and acute intoxication is not understood and seems to be a much rarer event in epileptics treated with primidone. From the trial of Calzetti *et al.* (1981b) showing that large doses of PEMA did not produce any side-effects and the low incidence of side-effects with phenobarbitone itself, one may conclude that the parent drug, primidone, is responsible for such ill-understood effects.

CONCLUSIONS

Primidone is effective in attenuating tremor of the hands in patients with benign essential tremor. In some patients the effects can be dramatic, with large-amplitude tremors suppressed to within the physiological range. Primidone provides an alternative form of therapy to propranolol, particularly with tremors of large amplitude. This effect is mediated either by the parent drug, primidone, or by its derivative, phenobarbital, or by both. Both acute and dose-related side-effects may occur, which are caused by primidone and not by the derived metabolites. Prior treatment with a hepatic-enzyme-inducing drug may reduce the incidence and severity of these acute side-effects. Further controlled trials of phenobarbitone to assess its efficacy in essential tremor are indicated.

REFERENCES

Baruzzi, A., Procaccianti, G., Martinelli, P., Riva, R., Denoth, E., Montanaro, N. and Lugaresi, E. (1983). Phenobarbital and propranolol in essential tremor: a double-blind controlled clinical trial. *Neurology (Cleveland)*, 33, 296–300.

Baumel, I. P., Gallagher, B. B., DiMicco, H. and Goico, H. (1973). Metabolism and anticonvulsant properties of primidone in the rat. *J. Pharmacol. Exp. Ther.*, 186, 305–14.

Calzetti, S., Findley, L. J., Gresty, M. A., Perucca, E. and Richens, A. (1981a). Metoprolol and propranolol in essential tremor: a double blind controlled study. *J. Neurol. Neurosurg. Psychiatr.*, 44, 814–19.

Calzetti, S., Findley, L. J., Perucca, E. and Richens, A. (1982). Controlled study of metoprolol and propranolol during prolonged administration in patients with essential tremor. *J. Neurol. Neurosurg. Psychiatr.*, 45, 893–7.

Calzetti, S., Findley, L. J., Pisani, F. and Richens, A. (1981b). Phenylethylmalonamide in essential tremor. A double blind controlled study. *J. Neurol. Neurosurg. Psychiatr.*, 44, 932–4.

Critchley, M. (1949). Observations on essential (heredofamilial) tremor. *Brain*, 72, 113–39.

Feely, M. P. (1981). Benign familial tremor treated with primidone. *Br. Med. J.*, 282, 740–1.

Findley, L. J. and Calzetti, S. (1982). Double-blind controlled study of primidone in essential tremor: preliminary results. *Br. Med. J.*, 285, 608–9.

Growdon, J. H., Shahani, B. T. and Young, R. R. (1975). The effect of alcohol on essential tremor. *Neurology (Minneap.)*, 25, 259-62.

Harvey, S. C. (1980). Hypnotics and sedatives. In Gilman, A. G., Goodman, L. S. and Gilman, A. (eds), *The Pharmacological Basis of Therapeutics*, Macmillan, New York, pp. 339-75.

McAllister, R. J. Jr, Markesbery, W. R., Ware, R. W. and Howell, S. M. (1977). Suppression of essential tremor by propranolol: correlation of effect with drug plasma levels and intensity of beta blockade. *Ann. Neurol.*, 1, 160-6.

McClellan, D. L. and Hassan, N. (1980). A double blind comparison of single doses of DS 103-282, baclofen and placebo in the suppression of spasticity. *J. Neurol. Neurosurg. Psychiatr.*, 43, 1132-6.

Marshall, J. (1968). Tremor. In Vinken, P. J. and Bruyn, G. W. (eds), *Handbook of Clinical Neurology*, vol. 6, North-Holland, Amsterdam, pp. 809-25.

Morgan, M. H., Hewer, R. L. and Cooper, R. (1973). Effect of the beta adrenergic blocking agent, propranolol, on essential tremor. *J. Neurol. Neurosurg. Psychiatr.*, 36, 618-24.

O'Brien, M. D., Upton, A. R. and Toseland, P. A. (1981). Benign familial tremor treated with primidone. *Br. Med. J.*, 282, 178-80.

Procaccianti, G., Agostino, B., Martinelli, P., Pazzaglia, P. and Lugaresi, E. (1981). Benign familial tremor treated with primidone. *Br. Med. J.*, 283, 558.

Tolosa, E. S. and Loewenson, R. B. (1975). Essential tremor, treatment with propranolol. *Neurology (Minneap.)*, 25, 1041-4.

Winkler, G. F. and Young, R. R. (1974). Efficacy of chronic propranolol therapy in action tremors of the familial senile or essential varieties. *New Engl. J. Med.*, 290, 984-8.

Woodbury, D. M. and Pippenger, C. E. (1982). Primidone. Mechanisms of action. In Woodbury, D. M., Kiffin Penry, J. and Pippenger, C. E. (eds), *Antiepileptic Drugs*, Raven Press, New York, pp. 449-52.

SECTION 4
THE TREMORS OF PARKINSON'S DISEASE

20
Parkinson's disease complex — restyling an old overcoat!

RUDY CAPILDEO

The fashion for attaching eponyms to any new symptom, sign or disease has become far less prevalent in recent years. Their continued use, particularly when teaching medical students or impressing patients, suggests a degree of erudition that the user seldom has. Very few physicians have read the original description upon which the eponym is based and as a result misquote and add their own interpretation. In this way, eponyms may 'grow up' with new symptoms or signs added, whilst some might be subtracted. These changes usually occur over a long period of time as medical knowledge accrues. As a result, nomenclature may not be revised and terms employed in common usage may not be defined.

This is particularly true in 'Parkinson's disease'. Synonyms include 'parkinsonism', 'idiopathic parkinsonism', 'parkinsonian syndrome', 'Lewy-body disease', 'paralysis agitans', and the original 'shaking palsy'. We also have 'post-encephalitic parkinsonism', 'arteriosclerotic parkinsonism' and, more recently, 'drug-induced parkinsonism'. Is a new term, *Parkinson's disease complex*, more helpful (Capildeo *et al.*, 1982)?

The use of terminology is not simply a question of semantics. It questions our present understanding of disease and disease processes. In order to study disease, we must first define the disease in question and then define the patient group that we wish to study.

In this chapter, 'Parkinson's disease' will be examined using these concepts. We begin by reviewing the original description of James Parkinson and then follow the growth of this eponymous disease with respect to the major clinical features in order to compare this with our present understanding. In this context, the relevance of the terms currently employed can be examined.

THE CONTRIBUTION OF JAMES PARKINSON

In his 'An Essay on the Shaking Palsy', Parkinson (1817) defines the 'shaking palsy' (paralysis agitans) as:

involuntary tremulous motion with lessened muscular power, in parts not in action and even when supported; with a propensity to bend the trunk forward, and to pass from a walking to running pace: the senses and intellects being uninjured.

He comments that:

the term shaking palsy has been vaguely employed by medical writers in general. By some it has been used to designate ordinary cases of palsy, in which some slight tremblings have occurred, whilst by others it has been applied to certain anomalous affections, not belonging to palsy.

With respect to tremor, he refers to the observations of Galen, Sylvius de la Boë, Sauvages and Juncker. Juncker divided tremor into 'active and passive', meaning those produced by 'terror or anger' as opposed to those dependent on a debilitating cause 'such as advanced age, palsy, etc.' Sylvius de la Boë (1614-72), a Leyden professor whose pupils included Willis, de Graaf, Stensen and Swammerdam, distinguished between tremors that are produced by attempts at voluntary motion and those that occur at rest. Parkinson (1817) quotes Sauvages (1763):

as distinguishing the latter of these species (tremor coactus) by observing that the tremulous parts leap, and as it were vibrate, even when supported: whilst every other tremor, he observes, ceases, when the voluntary exertion for moving the limb stops, or the part is supported, but returns when we will the limb to move; whence, he says, tremor is distinguished from every other kind of spasm.

Parkinson defines tremor and further states that:

Tremor can indeed only be considered as a symptom, although several species of it must be admitted. In the present instance the agitation produced by the peculiar species of tremor, which here occurs, is chosen to furnish the epithet by which this species of palsy, may be distinguished.

James Parkinson described six case histories (see table 20.1). All the cases were male, with ages ranging from 50 to 72 yearrs.

Since two cases were 'casually met with in the street' (Cases II and III), Case V was 'seen at a distance' and the 'particulars could not be obtained' and Case IV was lost to follow-up, it is a surprise that he was able to compile his observations on the natural history of the disease as he did, chiefly, it would appear, from Cases I and VI (see pp. 3 to 9 of the 'Essay'). It is unlikely that the editor of a modern journal would accept the case studies or even have them refereed! Since tremor is a salient feature according to Parkinson's definition, it is a surprise that one case history (Case V) is given where it is not a feature. However, he only saw this case at a distance. He does describe unilateral tremor and notes the process of the disease with tremor eventually developing on the other side.

Parkinson's observations on the gait patterns of his subjects are superb, painting memorable pictures with his pen. Case V is poignant, the poor man requiring his attendant to sway him backwards and forwards until he was able to start at a running pace, the attendant having to catch him after 20 paces. In all the cases except Case IV (lost to follow-up) there were characteristic disturbances of gait. The important observation, which many modern authors have failed to pick up, is that the person 'walks almost entirely on the forepart of the feet' (see Case II). Parkinson expands further on this in his general history.

But as the malady proceeds, even this temporary mitigation of suffering from the agitation of the limbs is denied. The propensity to lean forward becomes invincible, and the patient is thereby forced to step on the toes and forepart of the feet, whilst the upper part of the body is thrown so far forward as to render it difficult to avoid falling on the face. In some cases, when this state of the malady is attained, the patient can no longer exercise himself by walking in his usual manner, but is thrown on the toes and forepart of the feet; being at the same time, irresistibly impelled to take much quicker and shorter steps, and thereby to adopt unwillingly a running pace. In some cases it is found necessary entirely to substitute running for walking; since otherwise the patient, on proceeding only a few paces, would inevitably fall.

Yet 'the propensity to bend the trunk forwards, and to pass from a walking to a running pace' had been observed previously; Parkinson cites Gaubius and again Sauvages. The latter termed it *scelotyrbe festinans* (the origin of 'festinant gait' still currently used) which, he says, 'is a peculiar species of scelotyrbe, in which the patients, whilst wishing to walk in the ordinary mode, are forced to run'. Sauvages then confuses the issue by stating 'a similar affection of the speech, when the tongue outruns the mind, is termed volubility'!

'Walking on the forepart of the feet' appears to be Parkinson's own observation. Using an objective technique for measuring gait, polarised light goniometry (Capildeo *et al.*, 1981a), it has been possible to confirm this observation and in particular to demonstrate the loss of heel-strike in the parkinsonian subject which occurs after the forefoot is lowered to the ground. This is the reversal of normal gait when heel-strike occurs first followed by lowering of the forefoot. This observation has led to more appropriate physiotherapy techniques being employed (Flewitt *et al.*, 1981).

The contribution of James Parkinson can be defined using his own words (p. 27 of the 'Essay').

Having made the necessary inquiries respecting these two affections, tremor coaction of Sylvius de la Boë and of Sauvages, and scelotyrbe festinans of the latter nosologist which appear to be characteristic symptoms of this disease it becomes necessary, in the next place to endeavour to distinguish this disease from others which may bear a resemblance to it in some particular aspects.

In other words, he recognised that the two symptoms, the 'involuntary tremulous motion' and the characteristic gait disturbance, were the two cardinal features of this disease. There is no mention of rigidity or bradykinesia (although the latter is implied in the description of the natural history).

Table 20.1 Case histories from 'An Essay on the Shaking Palsy'.

	Patient description	Clinical features	Parkinson's comments
Case I	Male 'More than 50 years' Gardener	Slight trembling of left hand and arm' (steady decline)	'Life of remarkable temperance and sobriety' No 'Rheumatism, sudden seizure which could be referred to apoplexy or hemiplegia'
Case II	'Casually met with in the street' Male 62 years Attendant at magistrates' office	'All extremities were considerably agitated . . . speech much interrupted . . . body bowed and shaken . . . walked almost entirely on forepart of feet . . . fallen every step if not supported by stick'	'Suffered from disease 8–10 years' Gradual onset 'irregularities in his mode of living and particularly of indulgence in spiritous liquours' 'Since fully assurred of incurable nature, declined making any attempts for relief'
Case III	Also 'noticed casually in the street' Male About 65 years Athletic frame Formerly a sailor	'Agitation of limbs . . . head . . . whole body . . . too vehement to allow it to be designated as trembling Entirely unable to walk . . . body so bowed . . . head thrown so forward . . . obliged to go on a continued run . . . employed stick every 5 or 6 steps to force him into upright posture'	Patient attributed his complaint to several months in a Spanish prison Disease 'had continued so long, made such progress, as to afford little or no prospect of relief'
Case IV	Male 55 years	'Trembling of arms for 5 years' 'Inflammation over lower ribs on left side . . . termination in formation of matter beneath fascia'	'About a pint removed after making the necessary opening . . . discharged daily for 2–3 weeks' Recovered from inflammation and lost to follow-up 'by his removal to a distant part of the country'
Case V	Male 'Particulars . . . could not be obtained' 'Seen at a distance'	'. . . Supported by his attendant, standing before him . . . hand on each shoulder . . . swaying backward and forward . . . when giving the word, he would start in a running pace, the attendant sliding from before him and running forward . . . ready to receive him . . . after his having run about 20 paces'	'One of the characteristic symptoms of this malady, the inability for motion, except in a running pace, appeared to exist in an extraordinary degree'

Case VI Male 72 years	(Describes clinical course)	
	'... 11, 12 or more years ago ... weakness in left hand and arm, soon after trembling ... 3 years after the right arm in a similar manner: soon after the convulsive motions affected the whole body and began to interrupt the speech'	'Life of temperance' '20 years ago, lumbago'
	'Of late years ... constipation ... very strong cathartics'	(constipation improved ... 'perhaps owing to an increased secretion of mucus'
	'A year since, on waking at night lost the use of the right side ... tremor stopped' (on paralytic side)	Patient recovered from 'palsied state'. . . 'in a fortnight ... shaking returned'

So, with respect to terminology, we take Parkinson's name in vain when we talk of 'parkinsonian rigidity' (Walton, 1977) and 'parkinsonian facies', a term first attributed to Osler.

THE CONTRIBUTION OF JEAN-MARTIN CHARCOT

It was still necessary to separate 'Parkinson's disease' from other tremulous disorders and, until Charcot, multiple sclerosis and Parkinson's disease remained confused (Charcot, 1877, see p. 134). Today, more than 100 years later, Charcot's contribution to neurology (apart from numerous eponyms) remains sadly forgotten outside France (Capildeo, 1982). One reason was the controversy surrounding his later years when he tried to apply to the classification of hysteria the same methodology that proved so successful in defining diseases of the nervous system. Guillain's (1959) biography of Charcot was published in 1955 but not translated into English until 1959 by Pearce Bailey, former Director of the National Institutes of Health, Bethesda, Maryland.

Charcot noted that paralysis agitans 'assails persons already advanced in age, those especially who have passed their fortieth or fiftieth year'. He also commented that 'the symptoms of paralysis agitans are not all of the same value'. He talked of the march of paralysis agitans as '. . . slow and progressive. Its duration is long—sometimes it has gone on for thirty years'.

In an excellent description of the tremor, including samples of handwriting, he states that:

the head is always nearly quite respected at every stage of the disease, even in the most intense cases; and this is a character to which we shall, hereafter, give prominence, for the contrary is often observed in the cerebro-spinal form of disseminated sclerosis.

> Far from trembling, the muscles of the face are motionless, there is even a remarkable fixity of look, and the features present a permanent expression of mournfulness, sometimes of stolidness or stupidity. The nystagmus which so frequently figures in the symptomatology of disseminated sclerosis has no existence in paralysis agitans.

He also noted that:

> in some patients, the thumb moves over the fingers, as when a pencil or paper-ball is rolled between them; in others it is more complicated and resembled what takes place in crumbling a piece of bread.

In this 'Lecture', Charcot (1877) stated the following:

> We shall now point out a characteristic which we believe was overlooked by Parkinson as well as by most of his successors: we allude to the rigidity to be found at a certain stage of the disease, in the muscles of the extremities, of the body, and, for the most part, in those of the neck also. When this symptom declares itself, the patients complain of cramps, followed by stiffness, which at first transient, is afterwards more or less lasting, and is subject to exacerbations. Generally the flexor muscles are the first, as they are always the most intensely affected.

It was this muscular stiffness, Charcot maintained, that was responsible for the head and neck to be bent forward as if 'fixed in that position'. He also described the typical flexed position of the arms and hands 'held a little apart from the chest'. Charcot makes the important observation that rigidity may be an early feature.

> Gentlemen, there are cases, though these are rare indeed, in which muscular rigidity is a symptom of the early stage of the disease, and a really predominant one. I have recently observed an example which belongs to this category. The patient had scarcely noticed the tremor which, in fact, showed little intensity in his case, and was confined to one hand. He already displayed, however, in a high degree, the peculiar attitude of the body and its members, the difficulty of movement, and the characteristic gait.

There is an interesting footnote to this 'Lecture' (p. 144). A man of 50 years is described (another patient).

> attacked by 'Parkinson's disease'. . . having all the symptoms and especially the attitude. . . but the tremor was likewise deficient. Finally, Mr Gowers has communicated to M. Charcot a case, noted by him in the National Hospital for Epilepsy and Paralysis of London; the patient, a woman named Anne Phillips, exhibited all the symptoms of paralysis agitans, excepting the trembling, which is barely perceptible in her movements.

[My co-editor, Dr Leslie Findley, has been unsuccessful in obtaining this case record. It may be the same case as Gowers (1893) describes in his textbook (see p. 642, vol. II, 2nd edn).]

Slowness of movement was demonstrated by Charcot in some of the patients during the course of the 'Lecture' who recognised

the significant fact, that in such cases, there is rather retardation in the execution of movements than real enfeeblement of the motor powers. The patient is still able to accomplish most of the motor acts, in spite of the trembling, but goes about performing them with extreme slowness.

DISCUSSION

This historical review has dealt with the major features of this disease, the historical basis of which also seems to be the most poorly understood. The clinical application is still relevant today. For example, the problem in diagnosis of a patient presenting with either unilateral tremor, tremor with little rigidity, rigidity and bradykinesia without tremor—subjects discussed by the expert of today with his colleagues—were diagnostic problems well known to Charcot. But what to call the disease?

Gowers (1893) in his textbook (p. 636) comments that since the original description by Parkinson (1817):

it has been called 'Parkinson's disease' but the name which he gave to it of 'shaking palsy', is both apt and adequate as the designations of most diseases, and both it and its Latin form are firmly established.

He adds a footnote:

to the name 'paralysis agitans', it has been objected by Charcot that either the weakness or tremor is sometimes slight and occurs late; but the fact does not lessen the general applicability of the name, since in the majority of the cases both symptoms are conspicuous.

So Gower favoured Parkinson's original term 'shaking palsy'.

What of today's authors? In *Brain's Diseases of the Nervous System* (Walton, 1977) we find the 'whole' presented as 'the parkinsonian syndrome' defined as follows:

The Parkinsonian syndrome, named after James Parkinson, who first described paralysis agitans in 1817, is a disturbance of motor function characterized chiefly by slowing and enfeeblement of emotional and voluntary movement, muscular rigidity and tremor. Parkinsonism may be produced by a number of different pathological states and is usually ascribed to lesions involving the substantia nigra and its efferent pathways.

Yet, 'parkinsonian syndrome' is not a widely used term. There is no mention in this definition of the gait disorder, and bradykinesia, although implied, is not specified. In the text following the definition 'parkinsonism' is used and not 'parkinsonian syndrome'. Under 'forms of parkinsonism' we find 'paralysis agitans', 'parkinsonism following encephalitis lethargica' and 'arteriosclerotic parkinsonism', descriptions from previous decades. Also in the text (figure 105), a caption to a photograph states 'the characteristic posture of severe paralysis agitans (idiopathic parkinsonism)' but the term 'idiopathic parkinsonism' is not used elsewhere. Under 'muscular rigidity' we find the synonym 'parkinsonian rigidity' yet as we know Parkinson did not describe rigidity.

As Parkinson said 'the term shaking palsy has been vaguely employed by medical writers in general'; this could be paraphrased substituting 'parkinson's disease' for 'shaking palsy' and thereby making his comment pertinent for today.

Parkinson's disease is not a single disease entity. Post-encephalitic parkinsonism is a frequently quoted variant but the pathological, clinical and immunological findings indicate that it is quite distinct from so-called 'idiopathic parkinsonism' (Duvoisin and Yahr, 1965). In an update 50 years after the publication of his original paper in the journal *Brain*, Macdonald Critchley (1981) indicated that the term 'arteriosclerotic pseudo-parkinsonism' would have been more appropriate. Again the pathological and clinical findings are different to idiopathic parkinsonism. 'Paralysis agitans' as distinct from 'parkinsonian syndrome' is not a viable separation as suggested by Walton (1977).

Nowadays we consider two types of parkinsonism, namely idiopathic and drug-induced. As their names imply, the underlying aetiology is quite different as is the pathological and clinical substrate. 'Idiopathic parkinsonism' although generally used is not a satisfactory term: 'idiopathic', a convenient word used in medicine to denote ignorance of the underlying aetiology; and 'parkinsonism' can be defined differently according to each author. Are the clinical categories previously described purely different presentations of the same disease process, that is, do they have the same underlying neuropathological and neurochemical basis? Clinical impression would suggest that they may be different. It is difficult to explain unilateral tremor on the hypothesis of generalised depletion of dopamine in the brain. Why do some patients have severe tremor whilst in others with predominant rigidity and bradykinesia may tremor not be clinically obvious? The presence or absence of dementia further clouds the diagnosis. Although general opinion is against Parkinson's concept of 'the senses and intellects being uninjured', this has not been proven definitely. If dementia exists, is it of the Alzheimer-type, suggesting more widespread disturbances neurochemically than just dopamine depletion? In fact it is rather too simple to suggest that dopamine levels can change in the 'neurochemical cake' without disturbing other neurotransmitters in the brain. At the end of the day, we have to return to clinical description of our cases since, at present, we have no idea in an individual patient what neuropathological or neurochemical changes have occurred. For this reason, using the term 'Lewy-body disease' is inappropriate except within the framework of a pathological study. An indirect way of determining the neurochemical disturbance may be by monitoring the clinical response to therapeutic agents, particularly L-dopa. Within the group of patients with 'idiopathic' parkinsonism, response to L-dopa is not always predictable or consistent. However, a group of patients can be defined who respond to L-dopa alone, L-dopa in combination with a dopa decarboxylase inhibitor or a dopamine agonist. Patients who react badly to these drugs from the outset or who develop early side-effects or drug-related movement disorders have, presumably, a different neurochemical profile to the so-called 'responders'. These differences may be eventually defined and correlated with neuropathological and neurochemical changes.

There is enough clinical data to suggest that what is commonly called 'idiopathic parkinsonism' is in fact a heterogeneous group of diseases.

It is suggested that the term *Parkinson's disease complex* may be more appropriate than various terms previously employed. The term corresponds to the group of patients with so-called 'idiopathic parkinsonism'. However, the implications are different. 'Parkinson's disease' has been retained because of its 'time-honoured' image but the qualifying word 'complex' indicates that we are dealing with a heterogeneous patient group and serves as a constant reminder that we must define the patient or patient group from the outset; for example, 'this 70-year-old male patient has the following features of the Parkinson's disease complex. . .' or 'we describe the effects of a new therapeutic agent in 100 patients, all of whom had the following features of the Parkinson's disease complex. . .'. In this way a physician could easily compare this clinical description to the type of patient(s) he sees and therefore he would be able to consider the relevance of the quoted observations to his patient group. It is not enough to talk of a patient with 'idiopathic parkinsonism' or a group of patients with 'idiopathic parkinsonism'. Demographic details are important since a group of patients studied with 'idiopathic parkinsonism' with a stated age range of '25-70 years of age' is likely to be quite different from patients of 70 years and over.

We can define our patients using simple descriptions of the type used in our everyday clinical practice for the purposes of defining (clinically) homogeneous patient groups (Capildeo *et al.*, 1981b). This is essential for future neuroepidemiological studies, clinical studies and for interpreting the clinical correlates of neuropathological and neurochemical changes seen in the brain.

Our terminology indicates our current thinking, hence 'Parkinson's disease complex—restyling an old overcoat!'

REFERENCES

Capildeo, R. (1982). Charcot in the 80's. In Rose, F. C. and Bynum, W. F. (eds), *Historical Aspects of the Neurosciences*, Raven Press, New York, pp. 383-96.

Capildeo, R., Flewitt, B. and Rose, F. C. (1981a). The measurement of parkinsonian gait using polarised light goniometry. In Rose, F. C. and Capildeo, R. (eds), *Research Progress in Parkinson's Disease*, Pitman Medical, Tunbridge Wells, pp. 390-6.

Capildeo, R., Haberman, S. and Rose, F. C. (1981b). The classification of parkinsonism. In Rose, F. C. and Capildeo, R. (eds), *Research Progress in Parkinson's Disease*, Pitman Medical, Tunbridge Wells, pp. 17-24.

Capildeo, R., Wallace, M. G. and Rose, F. C. (1982). Dementia and Parkinsonism. *Br. J. Clin. Pract.*, 16, Suppl. 25-6.

Charcot, J. M. (1877). Lecture V on Paralysis Agitans. *Lectures on the Diseases of the Nervous System*, transl. George Sigerson, The New Sydenham Society, London.

Critchley, M. (1981). Arteriosclerotic pseudo-Parkinsonism. In Rose, F. C. and Capildeo, R. (eds), *Research Progress in Parkinson's Disease*, Pitman Medical, Tunbridge Wells, pp. 40–2.

Duvoisin, R. C. and Yahr, M. D. (1965). Encephalitis and parkinsonism. *Arch. Neurol.*, 12, 227–39.

Flewitt, B., Capildeo, R. and Rose, F. C. (1981). Physiotherapy and assessment in Parkinson's disease using the polarised light goniometer. In Rose, F. C. and Capildeo, R. (eds), *Research Progress in Parkinson's Disease*, Pitman Medical, Tunbridge Wells, pp. 404–13.

Gowers, W. R. (1893). *A Manual of Diseases of the Nervous System*, 2nd edn, J. & A. Churchill, London.

Guillain, G. (1959). *Jean-Martin Charcot: His Life—His Work*, transl. and ed. Pearce Bailey, Paul B. Hoeber, New York.

Parkinson, J. (1817). *An Essay on the Shaking Palsy*, Sherwood, Neely and Jones, London.

Walton, J. N. (1977). *Brain's Diseases of the Nervous System*, Oxford University Press, Oxford, pp. 579–95.

21
Tremor and rhythmical involuntary movements in Parkinson's disease

L. J. FINDLEY and M. A. GRESTY

INTRODUCTION

All behavioural types of tremor occur in Parkinson's disease (Findley *et al.*, 1981). The resting tremor that develops typically in the dependent limb is considered to be the hallmark of the disease. A separate postural tremor occurs as frequently as resting tremor but is a less conspicuous feature because it usually has a smaller amplitude. The cogwheel phenomenon is another disorder of movement occurring in this disease and consists of a periodic resistance to passive movement about a joint. The feature of periodicity would suggest that it has a mechanism with at least some features in common with tremogenic processes. A similar periodic resistance to movement develops when the joint is actively moved by the patient. This is universally termed an 'action tremor'. It is felt by the subject when he moves his limb and may be visibly present or be detected by the examiner if the limb at the region of the joint is palpated during the movement. An exacerbation of tremor at the termination of guided movement can occur in some parkinsonian patients, which is by definition an intention tremor. In approximately 10% of patients, and particularly those with a predominant postural tremor, it is possible to evoke a strong 'clonus-like' tremor in an affected limb by sustained passive tendon stretch (Denny-Brown, 1968).

It is proposed that the above, apparently diverse, phenomena can be attributed to the following mechanisms, summarised in table 21.1. One involves the inherent tendency to rhythmicity in diencephalic–cortical structures (see Llinás, this volume, chapter 10) and expresses itself as the typical resting tremor. The other tremulous phenomena are provoked by passive or active movement or the maintenance of posture, appear to occur in the presence of rigidity and, we will argue, have similar origins either to clonus or to enhanced physiological tremor.

RESTING TREMOR

Since Parkinson's 'Essay' (1817), there have been many accounts of the behavioural characteristics of the resting tremor (Denny-Brown, 1968; Selby, 1968;

295

Table 21.1 Tremulous phenomena in Parkinson's disease.

Classification	Frequency (Hz)	Mechanism
Rest tremor	4–5.5	rhythmical instability in thalamic neurones
Postural tremor of high amplitude, clonus, cogwheel phenomenon and action tremor, tremor of isometric stretch	~6	spinal mechanisms related to clonus(?)
Intermediate-frequency postural tremors	6.5–8.5	synchronisation from CNS(?)
High-frequency postural tremor and high-frequency cogwheel ('ripple')	9.5–11	long-term synchronisation involving stretch reflexes

Struppler *et al.*, 1978; Findley *et al.*, 1981). The resting tremor of Parkinson's disease affects primarily the distal upper limbs and more rarely the proximal upper limbs and the lower limbs. Involvement of the head and trunk is rarer. At onset the tremor is frequently either entirely unilateral or asymmetrical and may remain so throughout the natural history of the disorder. The tremor of an individual affected limb has a relatively stable frequency between 4 and 5.3 Hz. The frequency rarely varies through day or month by more than 0.3 Hz in any individual patient. The tremor typically attenuates or disappears prior to or with the onset of voluntary movement. Several seconds after the movement it may become re-established in posture with an identical frequency and similar waveform. The tremor in some severely affected patients does not seem to be markedly affected by movement.

The amplitude of resting tremor fluctuates widely and, to some extent, unpredictably, which has made it a difficult phenomenon to measure, particularly when attempting to assess the effect of tremolytic drugs. To date, methods of rating resting tremor have depended almost entirely upon a 'blind' clinical assessment or upon patients' self-assessment on rating scales (Webster, 1968; Gresty *et al.*, this volume, chapter 23). In some patients the tremor may have a peak acceleration, measured at the first interspace of the dorsum of the hand, of 1g (approximately 10 m s^{-2}, which is a peak amplitude of displacement of 1–1.5 cm). It is generally accepted that Parkinson's disease with predominant tremor, particularly when unilateral, is an indication for stereotaxis (see Andrew, this volume, chapter 25).

The rest tremor of Parkinson's disease results from reciprocal activation of antagonistic muscle groups (Rondot and Bathien, 1978). Within each agonist muscle group, individual muscles may contract in a sequential order during the activation cycle. This results in a complex waveform. The fundamental frequency of the waveform is determined by the cycle time for reciprocal activation. The complex shape of the waveform is determined by the timing of the individual muscle contributions and in the terminology of waveform analysis is referred to as 'harmonic distortion'. Fourier analysis of the rest tremor produces a spectrum with a fundamental frequency component and several harmonics (components at integer multiples of the fundamental frequency) (see figure 2.1, Gresty and Findley, this volume, chapter 2). These waveform characteristics are found almost exclusively in the rest tremor of Parkinson's disease and are features that can be helpful in the differential diagnosis of tremors, particularly in the elderly. Other tremors have waveforms that are more purely sinusoidal in shape. For the purposes of assessing the magnitude of rest tremor, the harmonic distortion of the waveform must be taken into account.

Although one may debate the precise origin of the tremor at rest, the most constant central pathological feature of parkinsonism with rest tremor is the degeneration of the nigro-striatal pathway with consequent depletion of dopamine in the striatum (Ehringer and Hornykiewicz, 1960). In contrast, typical rest tremor is rare in drug-induced parkinsonism and uncommon in the post-encephalitic types, where the nigro-striatal tract is not necessarily the prime focus or only site of pathological change. Degeneration of the nigro-striatal pathway removes the dopaminergic, inhibitory tonus on striatal neurones, which has secondary effects at the level of the pallidum and ventrolateral thalamus (Rondot and Bathien, 1978). Llinás (this volume, chapter 10) describes the oscillatory properties inherent in animal thalamic neurones investigated in studies *in vitro*. It is probable that this type of activity in thalamic neurones, evoked by a functional change in afferentation and relayed through the motor cortex, is the prime generator of the tremulous process. Hence the ventrolateral thalamus is the most appropriate and successful site for stereotaxic lesions aimed at abolishing tremor.

POSTURAL TREMOR

Symptomatic postural tremor occurs as frequently as the classical rest tremor although, when either is well developed, they tend to be mutually exclusive in terms of amplitude (Lance *et al.*, 1963; Findley *et al.*, 1981). Postural tremor is invariably distributed in the distal parts of the upper limbs. In any given limb it has a fixed frequency, which may be between 5.5 and 8 Hz; however, in our experience, postural tremors of large amplitude are invariably at a frequency of ~6 Hz. The maximal amplitude of postural tremor that we have recorded is only one-tenth that of maximal amplitudes of rest tremor observed. In contrast to the rest tremor, the waveform of postural tremor is sinusoidal and therefore gives a single peak, without harmonics, on a frequency spectrum (figure 21.1, upper traces). In appearance, the postural tremor of Parkinson's disease is similar to essential tremor, a characteristic that can be a source of difficulty in differential diagnosis (Salisachs and Findley, this volume, chapter 15).

Patients with a well developed postural tremor (~6 Hz) will show a marked action tremor and tremor at the termination of guided movement. These tremors have the same frequency as the postural tremor. On occasion a postural tremor

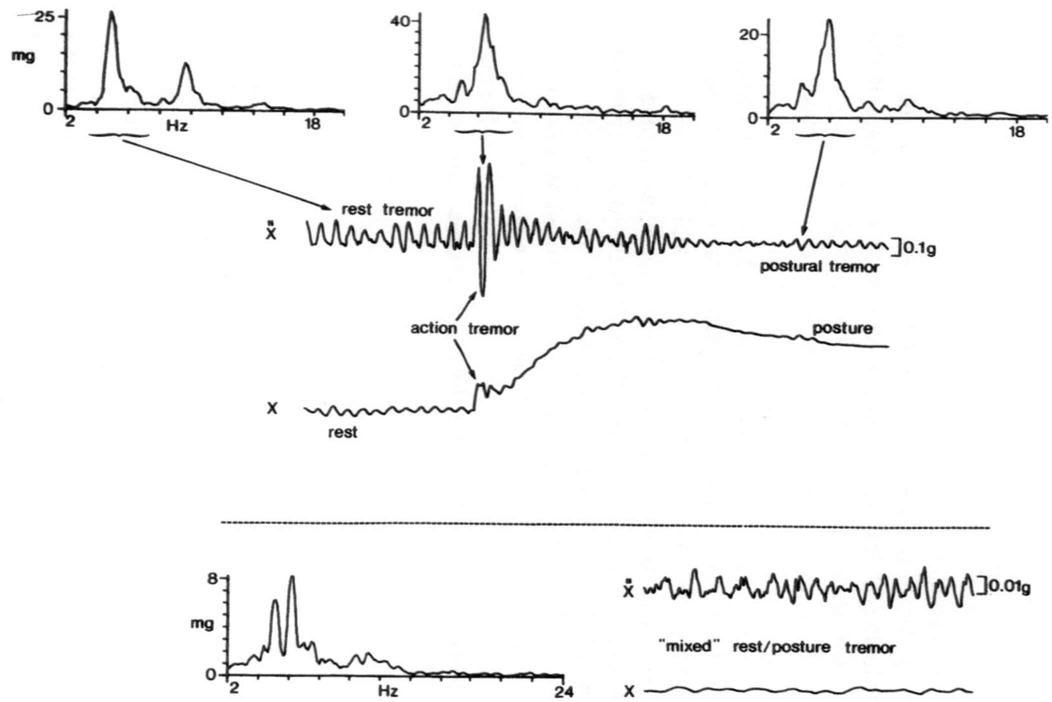

Figure 21.1 Recordings of time series and frequency spectra of acceleration $(\ddot{x})$ and displacement (x) of the hand (in the plane of extension/flexion) of a patient with postural and resting tremor associated with Parkinson's disease. Upper traces show the hand, first at rest, then lifting into posture. Lower traces show the hand maintained in posture with the resting and postural types of tremor vying for dominance, producing a spectrum with two harmonically unrelated peaks.

can transform into an action tremor when the limb is moved without their being any discontinuity, or change of frequency or waveform. Thus there is no reason to propose different origins for the postural and movement tremors.

In Lance *et al.'s* (1963) study, the action tremor developed on the basis of an unusual degree of grouping of muscle unit activity which was usually synchronous in all muscles involved, i.e. there was co-contraction of antagonistic muscles.

The majority of symptomatic postural tremors observed in our patients have had a frequency ~6 Hz. However, in agreement with Lance *et al.'s* observations, some patients do have symptomatic postural tremor at higher frequencies ranging upwards to 12 Hz. We would propose two possible origins for these higher-frequency postural tremors. Those in the frequency band of approximately 9.5–12 Hz are 'enhanced physiological tremor', which is tremor arising from long-term synchronisation between motor units determined by short-latency stretch reflexes (Allum, this volume, chapter 8). Symptomatic postural tremor at frequencies between approximately 6.5 and 9 Hz cannot be attributed to the stretch reflexes because the timings of the reflex loops are inappropriate. The likely mechanism that could generate tremor in these frequency bands is short-term synchronisation of motor units resulting from an unusual degree of synchronisation between descending facilitatory inputs to α-motoneurones. These types of higher-frequency postural tremor could either result from the pathophysiology of the disease or be a consequence of medication.

CONCURRENCE OF RESTING AND POSTURAL TREMORS

In some patients, at times, the normally regular postural tremor will change into an irregular tremor. The frequency spectrum of the irregular portion of the tremor record will have two peaks, one at a frequency in the range 4–5.5 Hz (i.e. comparable with the resting tremor), together with a higher-frequency peak at the frequency of the regular portion of the postural tremor record (i.e. 6 Hz or more) (figure 21.1, lower traces). The concurrence of the double peak in the spectrum suggests that the resting and postural tremors have separate mechanisms. Stronger proof that the resting and postural types of tremor arise from different mechanisms is that they can be shown by electromyography to run concurrently in the same muscle. This is illustrated in figure 21.2.

Lamarre and Dumont (1972) produced a model of parkinsonian resting tremor in monkeys with midbrain tegmentum lesions. When the same animal was injected intravenously with harmaline after a separate dentate or brachium conjunctivum lesion, a separate, predominantly postural, tremor at a higher frequency was produced. Electromyography showed that both tremor frequencies could be supported by the same muscle (see Lamarre, this volume, chapter 11). This model would seem to be a close parallel phenomenologically of tremors in patients with Parkinson's disease.

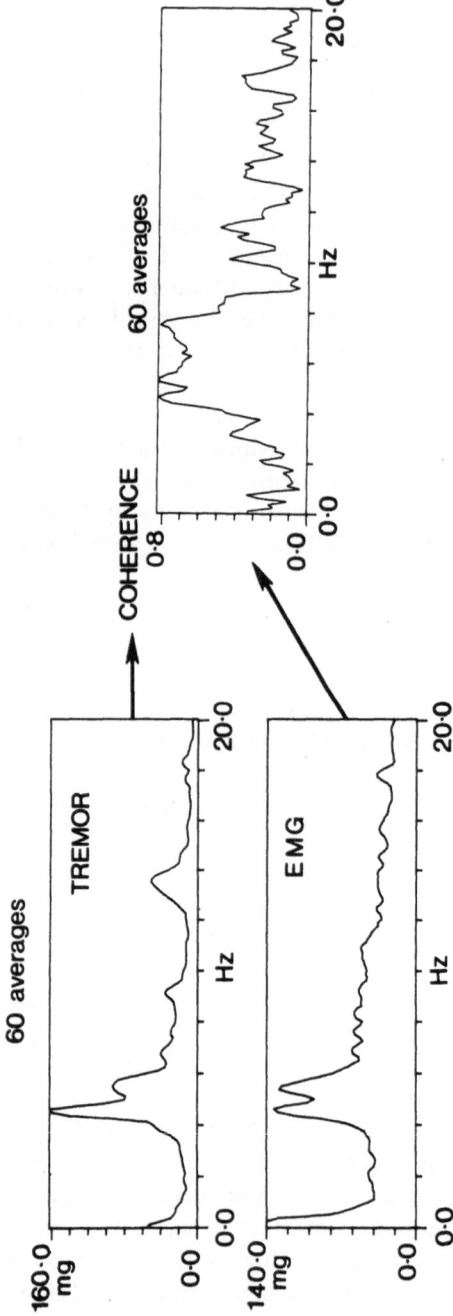

Figure 21.2 Averaged spectra derived from recordings of postural tremor of the hand and corresponding rectified EMG activity in a single extensor muscle during hand posture in a patient with Parkinson's disease. The tremor spectrum has two dominant peaks, one at 4.5 Hz and a second at 5.8 Hz of about half the amplitude. The spectrum of the rectified EMG has two similar peaks of comparable amplitude. The coherence calculated for the relationship between the EMG and tremor has a value of 0.9 at these frequencies. This value is highly significant for 60 averages and is evidence of a high correlation (implying causal relationship) between the EMG activity and overall limb tremor. The presence of a third peak of significance on the coherence function (at 7.7 Hz) indicates that there is a third frequency present that is common to both rectified EMG and tremor, although this is represented by low levels of magnitude on the individual spectra. This possibly represents a residual of some component of physiological tremor. (From Gresty and Findley (1984). In *7th Int. Symp. on Parkinson's Disease*. Reproduced by permission of Raven Press, New York.)

ACTION TREMOR AND THE COGWHEEL PHENOMENON

It has been shown that the postural and action tremors ~6 Hz have similar characteristics. Recordings of the action tremor and the cogwheel phenomenon show that, when well developed for several cycles, the cogwheel phenomenon is similar in terms of frequency and waveform to the action tremor. Thus both have the same frequency as postural tremor in the same limb. Furthermore, as the limb moves into posture, evoking the action tremor, the cycles of action tremor merge smoothly into postural tremor without discontinuity (figure 21.1, upper traces). Spectral analysis of samples of action tremor, the cogwheel phenomenon and postural tremor confirms that they are at the same frequency (figure 21.1, upper traces). These features suggest the hypothesis that the cogwheel phenomenon and action tremor are derived from the same processes as the postural tremor. When the 'cogwheel phenomenon' occurs in a different context, for example in essential tremor usually brought out as a positive 'Froment's sign', then it also has the same frequency and waveform as the postural tremor (Salisachs and Findley, this volume, chapter 15).

We have described rare patients notably without symptomatic postural tremor in whom the cogwheel phenomenon and action tremor occur at frequencies much higher than 6 Hz, that is around 10 Hz, and this we have called 'rippling' (Findley *et al.*, 1981). This is most likely to be a manifestation of 'enhanced physiological tremor' (*vide supra*) and can be found in the normal subject exhibiting stress or anxiety tremor.

INTERPRETATION

The clue as to the origin of the action and postural tremors may come from an unusual and neglected feature found in a small percentage of otherwise entirely typical parkinsonian patients; that is, the tremor produced by muscle stretch. This was first described by Denny-Brown (1968) and in our own series occurred in 15% of patients. The phenomenon is illustrated in figure 21.3. In pyramidal lesions the evocation of rhythmical involuntary movement (~6 Hz) by stretch is identified as clonus, whose mechanism, according to Dimitrijevic *et al.* (1980), is located in the spinal cord and seems to depend upon the pattern and degree of facilitation at that level. The hypothesis clearly presents itself that the tremor of Parkinson's disease produced by passive stretch may be closely related to clonus in the spastic patient. As there is a close resemblance between the tremor of stretch and the postural and action tremors of Parkinson's disease, the further hypothesis suggests itself that all these phenomena relate to a common mechanism. The part of this mechanism responsible for the generation of the rhythm of the movements is probably located in the spinal cord (Walshe, 1976; Dimitrijevic *et al.*, 1980).

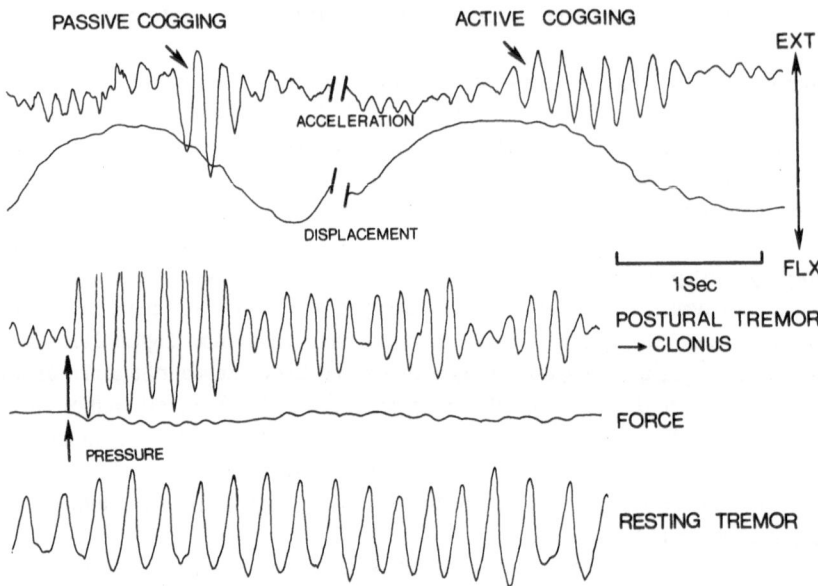

Figure 21.3 Recordings of cogwheeling, active cogwheeling (action tremor), resting tremor, postural tremor and clonus taken from a patient with idiopathic Parkinson's disease. The records were obtained in the same session within a few minutes of each other. The traces on the upper left show acceleration and displacement records of passive cogwheeling evoked at a frequency of 6 Hz. A few seconds later the patient moved his own hand in flexion and extension producing the active cogwheeling (upper right). The middle traces are accelerometric recordings of the hand tremor in posture, which goes into clonus as the patient presses down (hand extension) on a force platform. The arrows indicate the point at which he begins to press on the platform. The frequency of the clonus is 6 Hz. In the lowest trace the hand is at rest and develops a typical resting tremor at 4.3 Hz. A constant gain on the accelerometer traces is maintained throughout. (From Findley *et al.* (1981). *J. Neurol. Neurosurg. Psychiatr.*, **44**, 534–46. Reproduced by permission.)

RELATIONSHIP BETWEEN THE COGWHEEL PHENOMENA AND THE SHORT- AND LONG-LATENCY REFLEXES

Sudden perturbation of a limb produces a short-latency (M1) stretch reflex, which is normal in patients with Parkinson's disease (Lee and Tatton, 1978). When the subject is voluntarily opposing the perturbation, later EMG activity is recorded reflecting the longer-latency reflexes (M2 and M3). Lee and Tatton have shown that in parkinsonian patients with cogwheel rigidity the responses beginning at M2 and including M3 are up to five times larger than normal. In patients recorded without alteration in tone but with otherwise classical Parkinson's disease, the M2 and M3 components were normal. The enhancement of long-latency reflexes in

Parkinson's disease has been confirmed by more recent studies (Rothwell *et al.*, 1983; Berardelli *et al.*, 1983). However, the specificity of this finding to parkinsonian rigidity has been questioned (Evarts *et al.*, 1979). It is not clear whether repeated cycles of these long-latency reflexes evoked by continuation of stretch can occur, giving rise to a rhythmical interruption of movement with the properties of the cogwheel phenomenon. Lee and Tatton have argued that the motor cortex represents a potential site for interaction between the basal ganglia output and the proposed pathway for the M2 and M3 responses, which would be against a spinal location for the mechanism of the cogwheel phenomenon. However, Eklund *et al.* (1982) have shown that the entire M complex can be accounted for by peripheral/spinal mechanisms.

There is a reconciliation for these contrasting views as argued by ourselves and Llinás in this volume. The harmonious concordance of neural and muscular events in the body must require that short and long loop pathways (i.e. intraspinal or spinocerebral) have timing properties that would provide the correct conditions for the synchronisation of muscular events. Thus it is likely that the longer-latency reflexes (M3) traverse pathways that are both restricted to the spinal segment and project via central neuronal pathways.

REFERENCES

Berardelli, A., Sabra, A. F. and Hallett, M. (1983). Physiological mechanisms of rigidity in Parkinson's disease. *J. Neurol. Neurosurg. Psychiatr.*, **46**, 45-53.

Denny-Brown, D. (1968). Clinical symptomatology of disease of the basal ganglia. In Vinken, P. J. and Bruyn, G. W. (eds), *Handbook of Clinical Neurology*, vol. 6, *Diseases of Basal Ganglia*, North-Holland, Amsterdam, pp. 133-72.

Dimitrijevic, M. R., Nathan, P. W. and Sherwood, A. M. (1980). Clonus: the role of central mechanisms. *J. Neurol. Neurosurg. Psychiatr.*, **43**, 321-32.

Ehringer, H. and Hornykiewicz, O. (1960). Verteilung von Noradrenalin und Dopamine (3-hydroxytyramin) im Gehirn des Menschen und ihr Verhalten bei Erkrankungen des extrapyramidalen. *Syst. Wien Klin. Weitschr.*, **38**, 1236-9.

Eklund, G., Hagbarth, K. E., Hagglund, J. V. and Wallin, E. U. (1982). The late reflex responses to muscle stretch: the resonance hypothesis versus the long loop hypothesis. *J. Physiol.*, **326**, 79-90.

Evarts, E. V., Terävainen, H., Beuikert, B. E. and Calne, D. B. (1979). Pathophysiology of motor performance in Parkinson's disease. In Fuxe, I. K. and Calne, D. B. (eds), *Dopaminergic Ergot Derivatives and Motor Function*, Proc. Int. Symp., Wenner-Gren, Stockholm, 1978, Pergamon, Oxford, pp. 45-9.

Findley, L. J., Gresty, M. A. and Halmagyi, G. M. (1981). Tremor, the cogwheel phenomenon and clonus in Parkinson's disease. *J. Neurol. Neurosurg. Psychiatr.*, **44**, 534-46.

Gresty, M. A. and Findley, L. J. (1984). Postural and resting tremors in Parkinson's disease. In Hassler, R. G. (ed.), *Seventh International Symposium on Parkinson's Disease*, Raven Press, New York.

Lamarre, Y. and Dumont, M. (1972). In Goldsmith, E. I. and Moor-Jankowski, J. (eds), *Medical Primatology*, Karger, Basel, pp. 274-81.

Lance, J. W., Schwab, R. S. and Peterson, E. A. (1963). Action tremor and the cogwheel phenomenon in Parkinson's disease. *Brain*, **86**, 95-110.

Lee, R. G. and Tatton, W. G. (1978). Long loop reflexes in man: clinical applications. In Desmedt, J. E. (ed.), *Cerebral Motor Control in Man: Long Loop Mechanisms, Progress in Clinical Neurophysiology*, vol. 4, Karger, Basel, pp. 320-33.

Parkinson, J. (1817). *An Essay on the Shaking Palsy*, Whitingham Rowland, London.

Rondot, P., and Bathien, N. (1978). Pathophysiology of Parkinsonian tremor. In Desmedt, J. E. (ed.), *Physiological Tremor, Pathological Tremor and Clonus, Progress in Clinical Neurophysiology*, vol. 5, Karger, Basel, pp. 138-49.

Rothwell, J. C., Obeso, J. A., Traub, M. M. and Marsden, C. D. (1983). The behaviour of the long-latency stretch reflex in patients with Parkinson's disease. *J. Neurol. Neurosurg. Psychiatr.*, 46, 35-44.

Selby, G. (1968). Parkinson's disease. In Vinken, P. J. and Bruyn, G. W. (eds), *Handbook of Clinical Neurology*, vol. 6, *Diseases of Basal Ganglia*, North-Holland, Amsterdam, pp. 173-211.

Struppler, A., Erbel, F. and Velho, F. (1978). Overview on the pathophysiology of Parkinsonian and other pathological tremors. In Desmedt, J. E. (ed.), *Physiological Tremor, Pathological Tremor and Clonus, Progress in Clinical Neurophysiology*, vol. 5, Karger, Basel, pp. 114-28.

Walshe, F. M. R. (1976). Clonus: beats provoked by the application of a rhythmic force. *J. Neurol. Neurosurg. Psychiatr.*, 39, 266-74.

Webster, D. D. (1968). Critical analysis of the disability of Parkinson's disease. *Mod. Treat.*, 5, 257-82.

22
Neurochemical basis of parkinsonian tremor

P. JENNER and C. D. MARSDEN

INTRODUCTION

The major biochemical deficit in Parkinson's disease is a loss of cerebral dopamine pathways (Ehringer and Hornykiewicz, 1960; Hornykiewicz, 1963; Bernheimer *et al.*, 1973; Lloyd *et al.*, 1975a; Price *et al.*, 1978). The rest tremor characteristic of this disorder could be due to cerebral dopamine deficiency. The tremor often can be relieved by the administration of L-dopa or other dopamine agonist compounds. However, a proportion of patients (at least 20–30%) exhibit little or no tremor, despite the presence of marked akinesia and rigidity. Presuming that such patients have the characteristic severe dopamine deficiency of Parkinson's disease, for they exhibit obvious akinesia and rigidity, then it can be argued that neuronal loss in addition to that of dopamine systems may be of importance to the neurochemistry of tremor. Indeed, of all the cardinal symptoms of Parkinson's disease, tremor may be the most difficult to control with L-dopa therapy.

The object of the present chapter is to review the current evidence on the neurochemical changes associated with rest tremor in Parkinson's disease. First we will examine the data presently available on post-mortem studies in Parkinson's disease, and then we will review the neurochemical alterations occurring in some animal models of parkinsonian tremor. Our conclusion is that the neurochemical basis of parkinsonian tremor is not yet known.

EVIDENCE ON THE NEUROCHEMICAL BASIS OF PARKINSONIAN TREMOR FROM POST-MORTEM STUDIES

The major neurochemical deficit in Parkinson's disease is a profound loss of dopamine in all dopamine-containing areas of the brain (see Hornykiewicz, 1982). However, other neurones degenerate in this illness. Loss of cells in the nucleus locus coeruleus leads to a deficit of noradrenaline in various areas of the brain (Farley and Hornykiewicz, 1976) and there is also a decrease in cerebral 5-HT concentrations (Bernheimer *et al.*, 1961). In many patients, particularly those

305

Table 22.1 Loss of dopamine (DA) and homovanillic acid (HVA) in basal ganglia of parkinsonian patients with mild or marked akinesia, tremor and rigidity.

	Controls	Akinesia		Tremor		Rigidity	
		Mild	_Marked_	_Mild_	_Marked_	_Mild_	_Marked_
Caudate nucleus							
DA	2.64 ± 0.30	0.58 ± 0.12	0.22 ± 0.08*	0.53 ± 0.14	0.55 ± 0.11	0.74 ± 0.19	0.43 ± 0.11
HVA	3.23 ± 0.27	1.68 ± 0.25	0.59 ± 0.18*	1.68 ± 0.35	1.26 ± 0.20	1.69 ± 0.59	1.03 ± 0.16
Putamen							
DA	3.44 ± 0.29	0.44 ± 0.21	0.05 ± 0.02	0.65 ± 0.37	0.12 ± 0.07	0.31 ± 0.27	0.32 ± 0.19
HVA	4.29 ± 0.68	1.60 ± 0.39	0.83 ± 0.28	2.03 ± 0.55	1.07 ± 0.22*	1.68 ± 0.50	1.28 ± 0.34
Pallidum							
HVA	2.12 ± 0.27	1.30 ± 0.32	0.60 ± 0.17	1.71 ± 0.36	0.70 ± 0.12*	1.16 ± 0.51	0.94 ± 0.27

Concentration (µg/g wet weight of tissue)

Means ± 1 SEM are shown; $n = 4$–28.
*$p < 0.05$ compared to mildly affected group using Student's t test.
Adapted from Bernheimer et al. (1973).

exhibiting dementia, there is loss of cerebral choline acetyl transferase (Javoy-Agid *et al.*, 1981). Alterations in the activity of glutamic acid decarboxylase suggests changes in GABA function (Lloyd and Hornykiewicz, 1973; Lloyd *et al.*, 1975b), and recent studies have indicated changes in the brain concentrations of various peptides and in the numbers of enkephalin receptors (see for example Studler *et al.*, 1982; Rinne, 1982).

Most of these changes are thought to be subsidiary to the major loss of dopamine neurones and their contribution to the symptomatology of Parkinson's disease remains unknown. However, it is clear that a complex series of neuronal changes occur in the illness, so more than one neurochemical parameter may be involved in the pathophysiology of parkinsonian tremor.

Correlation of the extent of dopamine loss in the striatum (in brains from patients with Parkinson's disease taken at necropsy) with the severity of the symptoms in life has shown that akinesia, rigidity and tremor generally become manifest clinically only after striatal dopamine levels fall to about 70-80% of normal (Bernheimer *et al.*, 1973). The degree of akinesia correlates well with the degree of loss of dopamine, and of its metabolite homovanillic acid (HVA), in the caudate nucleus, and there are similar trends for the putamen and pallidum (table 22.1). No clear correlation between the degree of rigidity and the reduction in dopamine or HVA is evident, although there is a trend towards such a correlation in the caudate nucleus. The severity of tremor parallels the decrease of HVA in the pallidum, although a trend towards a decrease of both dopamine and HVA was observed in the putamen as well. There is no clear indication of a correlation between the degree of loss of dopamine in the caudate nucleus and the extent of tremor.

It is unfortunate that the degree of dopamine loss in other areas of the brain was not included in this study. In addition, measurement of changes in other neurotransmitters, particularly noradrenaline and 5-hydroxytryptamine (5-HT), might have revealed other contributions to the symptomatology of the disease. Indeed, there appears to have been only one attempt to correlate the symptomatology of Parkinson's disease with the extent of general monoamine loss (Fahn *et al.*, 1971). The comparison involved only two patients, one of whom exhibited no tremor whereas the other exhibited marked tremor. As can be seen in table 22.2, there was no correlation between tremor and the loss of dopamine or relative loss of noradrenaline or 5-HT.

No judgement can be made on two isolated cases, and further material is required. It is surprising that there has been no comprehensive attempt made to compare the neurochemical deficit in those patients exhibiting little or no tremor with those patients exhibiting marked tremor in such necropsy studies.

CEREBELLAR AND VENTROMEDIAL TEGMENTAL LESIONS IN MONKEYS

As reported in detail elsewhere in this volume, electrolytic or radiofrequency lesions placed in the ventromedial tegmentum in monkeys cause parkinsonism

Table 22.2 Correlation of symptoms of Parkinson's disease with monoamine deficiency in two patients.

Parameter	Severity of involvement	
	Patient DM	Patient SM
Tremor	0	++
Rigidity	+	+++
Akinesia	++	++++
Pathology (nigral cell loss)	+	++
Biochemical changes as percentage of normal values Reduced dopamine		
putamen	8	4
caudate	37–48	46–92
Reduced noradrenaline	51	30
Reduced 5-HT	15–49	21–91

Adapted from Fahn *et al.* (1971).

(Poirier, 1960; Poirier *et al.*, 1969; Pechadre *et al.*, 1976; Goldstein *et al.*, 1969a,b). Such animals exhibit hypokinesia and tremor (see Lamarre, this volume, chapter 11). In a typical animal, which had previously received incomplete lesions of the cerebellar dentate nuclei that did not cause motor impairment, subsequent bilateral tegmental lesions caused aphagia, profound akinesia, rigidity and postural tremor (Pechadre *et al.*, 1976). In this animal the lesion involved not only the ventromedial area of the upper midbrain, but also the caudal part of the hypothalamus and the medial part of the subthalamus (figure 22.1). There was an almost complete degeneration of the neurones of substantia nigra. More dorsally the lesions destroyed most of the parvocellular division of the red nucleus and interrupted corresponding cerebello-thalamic fibres. The magnocellular division of the red nucleus and corresponding rubral and tegmental descending pathways were spared.

Thus these lesions damage an area of midbrain to interrupt not only the ascending nigro-striatal dopamine pathway but also the cerebello-thalamic pathways, and the rubro-olivo-dentato-rubral loop.

Lesions of the ventral-medial tegmentum sparing substantia nigra, sometimes caused ballistic or choreic movements (Sourkes and Poirier, 1966). Lesions of the nigro-striatal pathway alone did not cause tremor but, if bilateral, they produced hypokinesia due to loss of dopamine-containing neurones (Pechadre *et al.*, 1976). Tremor only occurred if the lesion also had interrupted the ascending cerebello-thalamic and cerebello-rubral pathways.

This conclusion was supported by the neurochemical data obtained from these experiments (Sourkes and Poirier, 1966; Poirier *et al.*, 1966; Sourkes *et al.*, 1969). Lesions that only involved the nigro-striatal pathway led to a fall in dopamine but

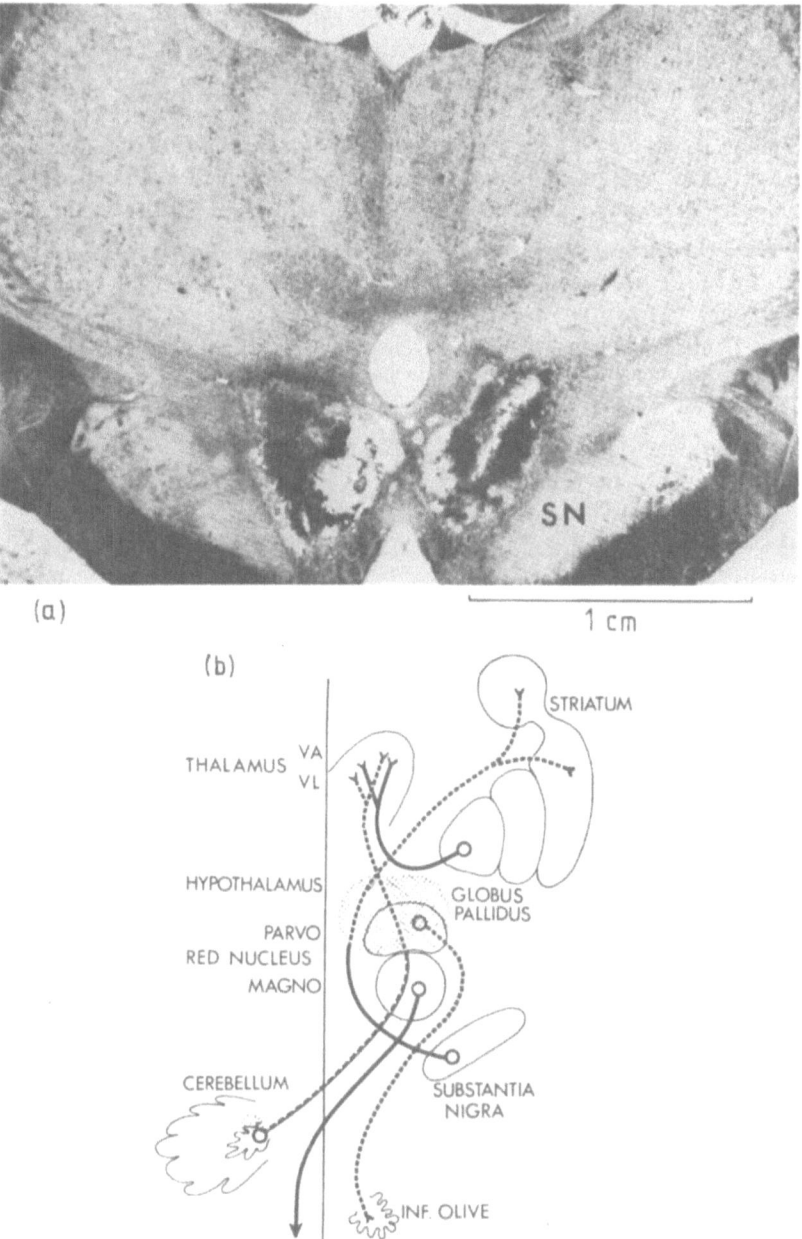

Figure 22.1 A typical lesion of the ventromedial tegmentum resulting in the production of sustained akinesia, rigidity and tremor. (a) Transverse section through upper brainstem to illustrate bilateral lesions involving the caudal hypothalamus, medial subthalamus and rostral midbrain. Section stained with basic fuchsin and fast blue (× 4 approx.). (b) Schematic drawing to illustrate the main neuronal features bilaterally involved in the same animal. They include the parvocellular division of the red nucleus and corresponding rubro-olivary fibres, the nigro-striatal pathway and cerebello-thalamic and cerebello-rubral ascending fibres. Taken from Pechadre *et al.* (1976).

not in 5-HT concentrations, and no tremor (table 22.3). In contrast, lesions involving more dorsal ventral-lateral areas of the tegmentum, but not the nigro-striatal pathway, caused a loss of 5-HT but no corresponding loss of dopamine and no tremor. It was only lesions of both areas that produced a fall in both dopamine and 5-HT, and resulted in tremor. The implication from these findings is that a combined loss of dopamine and 5-HT may be important for the production of parkinsonian tremor.

Table 22.3   Alterations in striatal dopamine (DA) and 5-HT concentrations produced by ventromedial tegmental lesions in monkey.

Lesioned area	Effect	Striatal concentration (µg/g wet weight of tissue)	
		DA	5-HT
None	—	3.56 ± 0.27	0.46 ± 0.06
Substantia nigra	Hypokinesia	0.30 ± 0.15*	0.5
Other tegmental areas	Choreiform and ballistic movements	5.95 ± 1.50*	0.20 ± 0.07*
Substantia nigra plus other tegmental areas	Tremor	0.28 ± 0.06*	0.04 ± 0.02*

Means ± 1 SEM are shown; n = 2–5.
*$p < 0.05$ compared to intact brain areas using Student's t test.
Adapted from Sourkes and Poirier (1966).

This argument has been strengthened by the findings of Goldstein and colleagues (Goldstein et al., 1969a,b). They showed that radiofrequency lesions of ventromedial tegmentum, which caused tremor, reduced the endogenous dopamine and 5-HT content of the ipsilateral striatum and reduced the synthesis of dopamine and 5-HT from labelled precursors. Such lesions also decreased tyrosine hydroxylase and dopa decarboxylase activity in striatum. Interestingly, a later study showed ventromedial tegmentum lesion to increase the staining intensity for acetylcholinesterase in globus pallidus (Nakatani et al., 1970), although the meaning of this change is not clear.

The primary importance of loss of dopamine-containing neurones in the induction of tremor has also been emphasised by the discovery that the dopamine agonists apomorphine (0.015–0.2 mg kg^{-1} i.m.) or piribedil (1.5–2.5 mg kg^{-1} i.m.) may reverse tremor in such animals (Pechadre et al., 1976). Surprisingly, L-dopa (30 mg kg^{-1} i.p.) produced no noticeable effect. There was no indication, however, that the dose of L-dopa was effective in elevating brain dopamine content and no attempt was made to utilise a peripheral decarboxylase inhibitor. It is of interest that Poirier et al. (1967) had previously demonstrated that lesions of the ventromedial tegmentum may drastically reduce the ability of L-dopa to increase striatal dopamine content.

There are a number of criticisms of the dopamine/5-HT hypothesis. Radio-frequency or electrolytic lesions of this area may damage many fibre pathways so that the loss of 5-HT in the striatum may only be coincidental. No specific lesions of the raphe nuclei have been carried out with nigro-striatal lesions to determine whether this combination results in tremor in primates. Control lesions of adjacent neuronal structures are also lacking. Administration of 5-hydroxytrypto-phan to the animals with ventromedial tegmental lesions did not prevent the tremor, suggesting that 5-HT may not be the critical component (Sourkes and Poirier, 1966; Poirier *et al.*, 1966). In conclusion, lesions of the ventromedial tegmentum in monkeys can produce a parkinsonian rest tremor, which can be reversed by dopamine agonist drugs. However, the model reveals little of the underlying biochemical pathology of tremor, apart from the requirement for neuronal loss in addition to that of dopaminergic pathways.

Similar conclusions can be reached from lesions placed more caudally to interrupt the rubro-olivo-cerebello-rubral loop (Larochelle *et al.*, 1970, 1971; Bedard *et al.*, 1970; Lamarre and Dumont, 1972; Lamarre, 1975; Poirier *et al.*, 1975) (figure 22.2). Such lesions do not damage the nigro-striatal tract and do not cause any loss of brain dopamine content. They do not produce spontaneous tremor. However, administration of dopamine antagonists to such animals elicits tremor. Thus, in animals with lesions of the dentate nucleus, tremor was induced by the administration of α-methyl-*p*-tyrosine, reserpine, and phenothiazine and butyrophenone neuroleptic drugs (Bedard *et al.*, 1970; Larochelle *et al.*, 1971). The tremor produced by such treatment could be suppressed by the administration of L-dopa, apomorphine or anticholinergic agents. Obviously some deficit other than simple loss of dopamine is required for the appearance of parkinsonian tremor in such animals, but dopamine deficit is required before whatever other mechanism is involved becomes of importance.

A further clue to the neurochemical basis of parkinsonian tremor may come from the actions of harmaline. In studies where monkeys received tegmental lesions, only 30% of animals developed tremor. The administration of harmaline to these animals exaggerated the tremor when present and induced tremor in those animals not exhibiting it (Poirier *et al.*, 1966; Battista *et al.*, 1970; Lamarre and Joffroy, 1970). In animals with lateral cerebellar lesions, the administration of harmaline initiated tremor (Larochelle *et al.*, 1970; Lamarre and Dumont, 1972). Harmaline did not produce parkinsonian rest tremor in normal monkeys but induced a fine generalised rest tremor (Poirier *et al.*, 1966). These two forms of tremor appear to depend on different neuronal mechanisms. The parkinsonian-like tremor is generated at the thalamo-cortical level (Lamarre and Joffroy, 1970), while the generalised tremor is generated from the olivo-cerebellar system (Lamarre *et al.*, 1971, de Montigny and Lamarre, 1973; Llinás and Volkind, 1973). In lesioned animals, following curarisation of the animal or deafferentation of the trembling limb by section of the dorsal roots (C_2-T_4) to prevent peripheral feedback, rhythmic unit activity at the frequency of the experimental parkinsonian tremor was recorded in thalamic regions following harmaline administration. In contrast, in the unlesioned but decerebrate cat, harmaline induced sustained rhythmic activity in the olivo-cerebello-bulbar system.

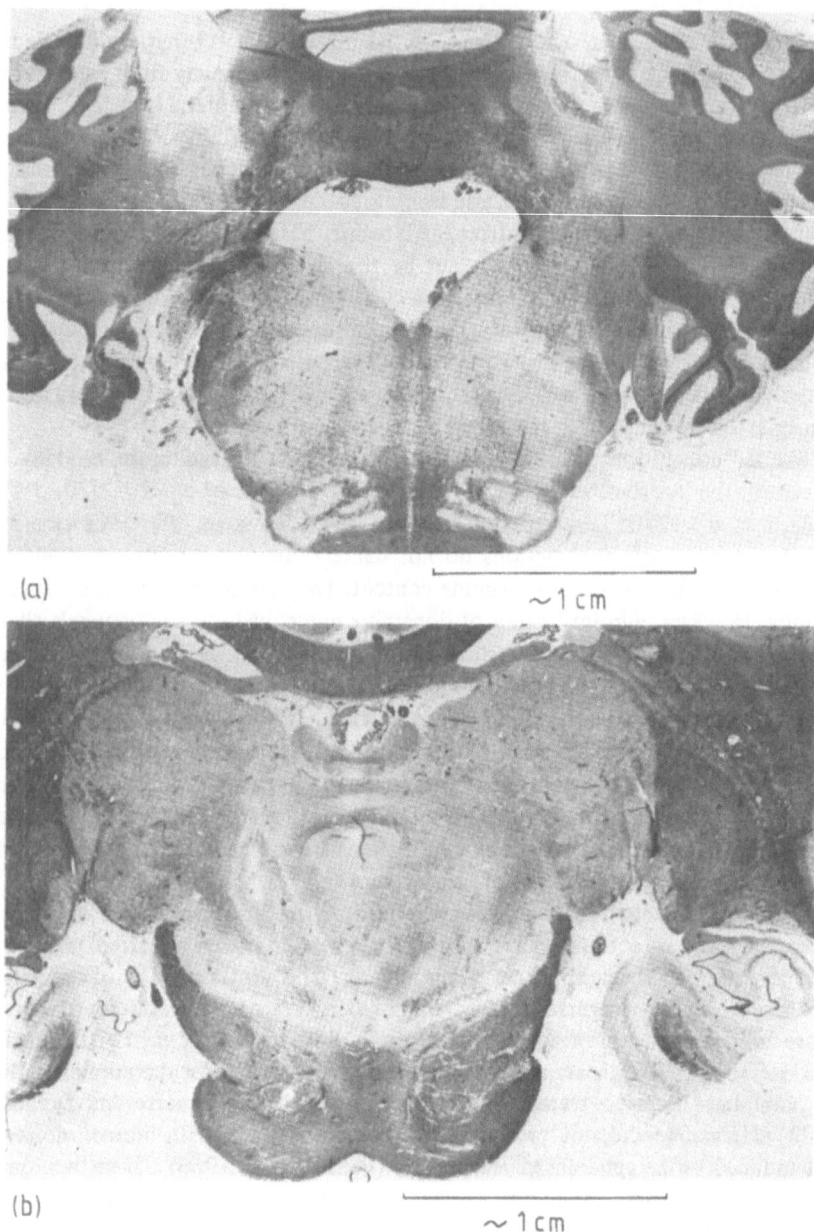

(a)

~1 cm

(b)

~1 cm

Figure 22.2 Typical lesions placed in the brainstem to interrupt the rubro-olivo-cerebello-rubral loop, which did not result in the production of tremor. (a) Transverse section through the cerebellum and medulla of a monkey showing a bilateral lesion involving the lateral cerebellar nuclei. (b) Transverse section through the lower midbrain of a monkey showing a unilateral lesion in the area of the red nucleus that extends to the dorsal part of the tegmental area. Note that the nigral cells are intact. Sections stained with basic fuchsin and fast blue (× 3.5 approx.). Taken from Larochelle *et al.* (1971).

Surprisingly, the mechanism by which harmaline induces tremor is unclear. The drug is a weak monoamine oxidase inhibitor, causing increases in brain 5-HT and dopamine concentrations (Udenfriend *et al.*, 1958), and may also possess direct 5-HT agonist actions (see Pinder, this volume, chapter 34). While such mechanisms may be important in the olivo-cerebellar actions of harmaline, they would appear not to explain the exaggeration of parkinsonian-like tremor, which is associated with reduced monoamine content of the brain. Indeed, other potent monoamine oxidase inhibitors such as tranylcypromine are without effect (Sourkes and Poirier, 1966).

There has been no detailed neurochemical analysis of the deficits that occur in these primate models of parkinsonian tremor. One of the limiting factors in such studies is the small number of animals that can be employed. There appears, however, to have been little attempt to determine whether similar lesions in rodents, in which more detailed neurochemical studies might be undertaken, will result in tremor.

TREMOR PRODUCED BY CHOLINERGIC MANIPULATION OF THE STRIATUM

The conclusion from the data discussed above must be that little is known about the neurochemical changes that contribute to the production of parkinsonian tremor, other than the basic requirement for loss of striatal dopamine.

The beneficial effects of anticholinergic drugs in the treatment of Parkinson's disease gave rise to the idea that there is an inherent dopaminergic–cholinergic balance within the striatum which is disrupted by the disease. This idea is supported by a large body of experimental evidence from animals, which has demonstrated the reciprocal relationship between striatal dopamine and acetylcholine function (Stadler *et al.*, 1973; Butcher, 1977).

The focal injection of cholinergic drugs into striatum of the cat can also induce a rest tremor (Baker *et al.*, 1976). Such tremor can be produced by cholinergic agonists such as carbachol (Connor *et al.*, 1966a), and by the injection of cholinesterase inhibitors such as physostigmine, to increase inherent cholinergic tone (Lalley *et al.*, 1970) (table 22.4). Present evidence suggests that acetylcholine receptors found within striatum are mainly muscarinic. Indeed Connor and coworkers produced much data to suggest that intrastriatal administration of muscarinic agonists and antagonists was effective in altering tremor (Connor *et al.*, 1966a,b; Baker *et al.*, 1969; Lalley *et al.*, 1970). However, there is dispute over the role played by nicotinic drugs, since peripheral administration of nicotine certainly evokes tremor as in man, mouse and rabbit (see for example Silvette *et al.*, 1962). The ability of cholinergic agonists to induce tremor on focal injection into striatum supports the general idea that disruption of normal dopaminergic–cholinergic balance is responsible for parkinsonian tremor, as suggested two decades ago by McGeer *et al.* (1961) and Barbeau (1962). However, there are a number of reasons for questioning this view.

Table 22.4 Cholinergic drugs inducing tremor and anticholinergic drugs inhibiting carbachol-induced tremor on intracaudate injection in the cat.

(a) Cholinergic agonists and cholinergic inhibitors

Cause tremor	Inactive
Carbachol	Nicotine
Bethanechol	
Methacholine	
Acetylcholine	
Oxotremorine	
Arecoline	
Physostigmine	
DFP	

(b) Cholinergic antagonists and acetylcholine synthesis inhibitors

Inhibit carbachol tremor	Inactive
Scopolamine	Hexamethonium
Atropine	Tetraethylammonium
Biperiden	Decamethonium
Benztropine	Dihydro-β-erythroidine
Hemicholinium-3	d-Tubocurarine

Adapted from Baker *et al.* (1976).

Simply decreasing dopamine function in striatum does not induce tremor, so it is difficult to see why intrastriatal injection of cholinergic compounds causes tremor by altering dopaminergic–cholinergic balance. This may, of course, simply reflect the differing pathophysiological basis of tremor in the cat and monkey. In addition, the injection of cholinergic agents into other areas of basal ganglia, such as into the globus pallidus and substantia nigra, can also produce tremor (George *et al.*, 1964; Cox and Potkonjak, 1969). So this effect is not a specific striatal phenomenon.

The results of pharmacological manipulation of striatal cholinergic tremor by catecholamines is also somewhat surprising. The action of catecholamines focally injected into the striatum to inhibit tremor induced by pilocarpine ranks in the order expected for stimulation of a β-receptor (Connor *et al.*, 1967; Lalley *et al.*, 1970). Isoprenaline was far more potent that dopamine in causing inhibition (table 22.5). Also, while β-receptor antagonists inhibited this catecholamine action, phentolamine and chlorpromazine were without effect. Recently, it was observed that striatal β-adrenoceptor stimulation by (–)-isoprenaline increased the spontaneous release of dopamine both *in vitro* and *in vivo* (Reisine *et al.*, 1982). This effect was antagonised by the β-blockers propranolol and practolol.

Experiments utilising cholinergic drugs have also provided some evidence for involvement of monoamines other than dopamine in the mechanism of tremor. In a recent study of tremorine-induced tremor and rigidity in the rat (Dickenson and Slater, 1982), lesions of the locus coeruleus reducing brain noradrenaline concentration decreased the ability of tremorine to induce tremor and rigidity, but

Table 22.5 The effect of intracaudate administration of catecholamines and related agents on carbachol-induced tremor
and the effect of adrenergic blocking agents on the
antagonistic action of adrenaline.

Drug	Dose abolishing carbachol tremor (µg/g)
Isoprenaline	7.8 ± 0.7
Adrenaline	10.3 ± 1.0
Noradrenaline	51.5 ± 3.2
Dopamine	99.7 ± 6.8
Ephedrine	> 150
Methylamphetamine	> 150

Drug	Dose preventing adrenaline suppression of carbachol tremor (µg/g)
Propranolol	25
Dichloroisoprenaline	25
Phentolamine	> 200
Chlorpromazine	> 200

Adapted from Connor *et al.* (1967).

lesions of the raphe nuclei were without effect on tremor, although they did
reduce rigidity. This evidence, in contrast to that from humans and monkeys,
suggests that noradrenaline rather than 5-HT may be involved in tremor mechanisms.

CONCLUSIONS

This review of the sparse literature presently available reveals that little is known
of the detailed neurochemical changes that occur in parkinsonian tremor. Perhaps
most surprising is the lack of post-mortem studies of the underlying alteration in
brain transmitter content. Parkinson's disease is sufficiently prevalent to allow a
comparison of tissue from those patients exhibiting gross tremor to those with
little or no tremor in order to detect neurochemical changes. Present neurochemical techniques are such that subtle alterations in both pre- or postsynaptic
events might be detected. It is probable that the uncertainty as to which brain
area or which transmitter substance might be involved in parkinsonian tremor has
prevented a detailed analysis of post-mortem tissue.

The lesions of the ventromedial tegmentum in monkeys have shed some light
on those pathways that appear initially involved in the production of a parkinsonian tremor. However, the neurochemical studies in these animals were carried
out approximately 15 years ago at a time when only few neurotransmitter substances had been identified. It is not surprising, therefore, that the information on
transmitter change in these animals was limited. The critical requirement for a loss

or disruption of brain dopamine function was recognised, as was the need for some other neurochemical change that allowed the manifestation of tremor. At the present time there is only weak evidence to implicate either 5-HT or noradrenaline. The possible role played by these substances appears even less likely when considering that there is little evidence from clinical studies to suggest any marked benefit of drugs altering brain 5-HT or noradrenaline function in the treatment of the tremor of Parkinson's disease (Jenner and Marsden, 1982). In the light of present knowledge it would seem important to determine the transmitter substances utilised by the cerebello-thalamic fibres and the rubro-olivo-dentato-rubral loop. The former would seem of particular relevance since a thalamic oscillator appears important in producing a parkinsonian-like tremor in monkeys with a cerebellar lesion treated with harmaline. Measurement of these neurotransmitters in lesioned monkeys, or in post-mortem brain tissue from parkinsonian patients, might reveal the critical neurochemical imbalance resulting in tremor production.

The production of tremor by alteration of striatal cholinergic function in the cat is somewhat difficult to reconcile with the studies in monkeys. Perhaps species differences in the mechanism of tremor production occur. This raises the important issue of whether tremor produced in the cat can be equated to that in the monkey, or indeed in man. Presently there is not sufficient evidence to make a detailed judgement on the anatomical or neurochemical basis of tremor production in different species. Certainly, in each case, a parkinsonian-like rest tremor is produced. Compared to the rest tremor of Parkinson's disease, which occurs at a frequency of 5–6 Hz, the tremor in cats induced by cholinergic agents is dissimilar, occurring at 19–23 Hz, whereas in monkeys with ventromedial tegmental lesions tremor occurs at 4–6 Hz. This might suggest that the primate model, as would be expected, more closely mimics what occurs in man.

Although the lesioned monkey appears to represent a good model for parkinsonian rest tremor, it is inconceivable that the extensive neurochemical investigation required could be carried out in this species. At the present time there appears to have been no attempt to determine whether similar lesions in rodents can induce rest tremor which sufficiently resembles that occurring in man to provide a viable neurochemical test bed.

On the basis of present studies we can only conclude that the neurochemical basis of parkinsonian tremor is unknown.

ACKNOWLEDGEMENTS

This work was supported by the Parkinson's Disease Society, the Medical Research Council, the Wellcome Trust and the Research Funds of the Bethlem Royal Hospital and Maudsley Hospital and King's College Hospital.

REFERENCES

Baker, W. W., Connor, J. D., Rossi, G. V. and Lalley, P. M. (1969). In Barbeau, A. and Brunette, J. R. (eds), *Progress in Neurogenetics*, vol. 1, Excerpta Medica, Amsterdam, pp. 390-408.

Baker, W. W., Lalley, P. M., Connor, J. D. and Rossi, G. V. (1976). Neuropharmacologic analysis of cholinergic tremor mechanisms in the caudate nucleus. *Pharmacol. Ther. C: Clin. Pharmacol. Ther.*, 1, 459-73.

Barbeau, A. (1962). The pathogenesis of Parkinson's disease: a new hypothesis. *Can. Med. Assoc. J.*, 87, 802-7.

Battista, A. F., Nakatani, S., Goldstein, M. and Anagnoste, G. (1970). Effect of harmaline in monkeys with central nervous system lesions. *Exp. Neurol.*, 28, 513-24.

Bedard, P., Larochelle, L., Poirier, L. J. and Sourkes, T. L. (1970). Reversible effect of L-dopa on tremor and catatonia induced by α-methyl-*p*-tyrosine. *J. Physiol. Pharmacol.*, 48, 82-4.

Bernheimer, H., Birkmayer, W. and Hornykiewicz, O. (1961). Verteilung des 5-Hydroxytryptamines (Serotonin) im Gehirn des Menschen und sein Verhalten bei Patienten mit Parkinson-Syndrom. *Klin. Wochenschr.*, 39, 1056-9.

Bernheimer, H., Birkmayer, W., Hornykiewicz, O., Jellinger, K. and Seitelberger, F. (1973). Brain dopamine and the syndromes of Parkinson and Huntington: clinical, morphological and neurochemical correlations. *J. Neurol. Sci.*, 20, 415-55.

Butcher, L. L. (1977). Nature and mechanism of cholinergic–monoaminergic interaction in the brain. *Life Sci.*, 21, 1207-26.

Connor, J. D., Rossi, G. V. and Baker, W. W. (1966a). Characteristics of tremor in cats following injections of cabachol into the caudate nucleus. *Exp. Neurol.*, 14, 371-82.

Connor, J. D., Rossi, G. V. and Baker, W. W. (1966b). Analysis of the tremor induced by injection of cholinergic agents into the caudate nucleus. *Int. J. Neuropharmacol.*, 5, 207-16.

Connor, J. D., Rossi, G. V. and Baker, W. W. (1967). Antagonism of intracaudate cerebral tremor by local injection of catecholamines. *J. Pharmacol. Exp. Ther.*, 155, 545-51.

Cox, B. and Potkonjak, D. (1969). An investigation of the tremorgenic effects of oxotremorine and tremorine after stereotaxic injection into rat brain. *Int. J. Neuropharmacol.*, 8, 291-7.

de Montigny, C. and Lamarre, Y. (1973). Rhythmic activity induced by harmaline in the olivo-cerebello-bulbar system of the cat. *Brain Res.*, 53, 81-95.

Dickenson, S. L. and Slater, P. (1982). Effect of lesioning dopamine noradrenaline and 5-hydroxytryptamine pathways on tremorine-induced tremor and rigidity. *Neuropharmacology*, 21, 787-94.

Ehringer, H. and Hornykiewicz, O. (1960). Verteilung von Noradrenalin und Dopamine (3-Hydroxytyramin) im Gehirn des Menschen und ihr Verhalten bei Erkrankungen des extrapyramidalen. *Syst. Wien Klin. Weitschr.*, 38, 1236-9.

Fahn, S., Libsch, L. R. and Cutler, R. W. (1971). Monoamines in the human neostriatum: topographic distribution in normals and in Parkinson's disease and their role in akinesia, rigidity, chorea and tremor. *J. Neurol. Sci.*, 14, 427-55.

Farley, I. J. and Hornykiewicz, O. (1976). Noradrenaline in subcortical brain regions of patients with Parkinson's disease and control subjects. In Birkmayer, W. and Hornykiewicz, O. (eds), *Advances in Parkinsonism*, Editiones Roche, Basle, pp. 178-85.

George, R., Haslett, W. L. and Jenden, D. J. (1964). A cholinergic mechanism in the brainstem reticular formation: induction of paradoxical sleep. *Int. J. Neuropharmacol.*, **3**, 541–52.

Goldstein, M., Anagnoste, B., Battista, A. F., Owen, W. S. and Nakatani, S. (1969a). Studies of amines in the striatum in monkeys with nigral lesions. *J. Neurochem.*, **16**, 645–53.

Goldstein, M., Battista, A. F., Anagnoste, B. and Nakatani, S. (1969b). Tremor production and striatal amines in monkeys. In Gillingham, F. G. and Donaldson, I. M. L. (eds), *Third Symposium on Parkinson's Disease*, Livingstone, Edinburgh, pp. 37–40.

Hornykiewicz, O. (1963). Die topische Lokalisation und das Verhalten von Noradrenalin und Dopamin (3-Hydroxytyramin) in der Substantia nigra des normalen und Parkinsonkranker Menschen. *Syst. Wien. Klin. Weitschr.*, **75**, 309–12.

Hornykiewicz, O. (1982). Brain neurotransmitter changes in Parkinson's disease. In Marsden, C. D. and Fahn, S. (eds), *Movement Disorders*, Butterworth Scientific, London, pp. 41–58.

Javoy-Agid, F., Ploska, A. and Agid, Y. (1981). Microtopography of TH, GAD and CAT in the substantia nigra and ventral tegmental area of control and parkinsonian brain. *J. Neurochem.*, **37**, 1218–27.

Jenner, P. and Marsden, C. D. (1982). Noradrenaline and 5-hydroxytryptamine modulation of brain dopamine function: implications for the treatment of Parkinson's disease. *Br. J. Clin. Pharmacol.*, **15**, Suppl. 2, 277S–905.

Lalley, P. M., Rossi, G. V. and Baker, W. W. (1970). Analysis of local cholinergic tremor mechanisms following selective neurochemical lesions. *Exp. Neurol.*, **27**, 258–75.

Lamarre, Y. (1975). Tremorgenergic mechanisms in primates. *Adv. Neurol.*, **10**, 23–34.

Lamarre, Y. and Dumont, M. (1972). Activity of cerebellar and lower brain stem neurons in monkeys with harmaline-induced tremor. In Goldsmith, E. I. and Moor-Jankowski, J. (eds), *Medical Primatology*, Karger, Basel, pp. 274–81. 274–81.

Lamarre, Y. and Joffroy, A. J. (1970). Thalamic unit activity in monkey with experimental tremor. In Barbeau, A. and McDowell, F. H. (eds), *L-Dopa and Parkinsonism*, Davis, Philadelphia, pp. 163–70.

Lamarre, Y., de Montigny, C., Dumont, M. and Weiss, M. (1971). Harmaline-induced rhythmic activity of cerebellar and lower brain stem neurons. *Brain Res.*, **32**, 246–50.

Larochelle, L., Bedard, P., Boucher, R. and Poirier, L. J. (1970). The rubro-olivo-cerebello-rubral loop and postural tremor in the monkey. *J. Neurol. Sci.*, **11**, 53–64.

Larochelle, L., Bedard, P., Poirier, L. J. and Sourkes, T. L. (1971). Correlative neuroanatomical and neuropharmacological study of tremor and catatonia in the monkey. *Neuropharmacology*, **10**, 273–88.

Llinás, R. and Volkind, R. A. (1973). The olivo-cerebellar system: functional properties as revealed by harmaline-induced tremor. *Exp. Brain Res.*, **18**, 69–87.

Lloyd, K. G., Davidson, L. and Hornykiewicz, O. (1975a). The neurochemistry of Parkinson's disease: effect of L-DOPA therapy. *J. Pharmacol. Exp. Ther.*, **195**, 453–64.

Lloyd, K. G. and Hornykiewicz, O. (1973). L-glutamic acid decarboxylase in Parkinson's disease: effect of L-DOPA therapy. *Nature*, **243**, 521–3.

Lloyd, K. G., Mohler, H., Hertz, P. H. and Bartholini, G. (1975b). Distribution of choline acetyltransferase and glutamic acid decarboxylase within the substantia nigra and other brain regions from control and parkinsonian patients. *J. Neurochem.*, **25**, 789–95.

McGeer, P. L., Boulding, J. E., Gibson, W. W. and Foulkes, R. G. (1961). Drug-induced extrapyramidal reactions. *J. Am. Med. Assoc.*, **177**, 665–70.

Nakatani, S., Battista, A. F. and Goldstein, M. (1970). Acetylcholinesterase content in the basal ganglia in monkeys with tegmental lesions. *Trans. Am. Neurol. Assoc.*, **95**, 292–5.

Pechadre, J. C., Larochelle, L. and Poirier, L. J. (1976). Parkinsonian akinesia, rigidity and tremor in the monkey: histopathological and neuropharmacological study. *J. Neurol. Sci.*, **28**, 147–57.

Poirier, L. J. (1960). Experimental and histological study of midbrain dyskinesias. *J. Neurophysiol.*, **23**, 534–51.

Poirier, L. J., Bouvier, G., Bedard, P., Boucher, R., Larochelle, L., Olivier, A. and Singh, P. (1969). Essai sur les circuits neuronaux impliqués dans le tremblement postural et l'hypokinesie. *Rev. Neurol.*, **120**, 15–40.

Poirier, L. J., Pechadre, J. C., Larochelle, L., Dankova, J. and Boucher, R. (1975). Stereotaxic lesions and movement disorders in monkeys. *Adv. Neurol.*, **10**, 5–22.

Poirier, L. J., Singh, P., Sourkes, T. L. and Boucher, R. (1967). Effect of amine precursors on the concentration of striatal dopamine and serotonin in cats with and without unilateral brain stem lesions. *Brain Res.*, **6**, 654–66.

Poirier, L. J., Sourkes, T. L., Bouvier, G., Boucher, R. and Carabin, S. (1966). Striatal amines, experimental tremor and the effect of harmaline in the monkey. *Brain*, **89**, 37–55.

Price, K. S., Farley, I. J. and Hornykiewicz, O. (1978). Neurochemistry of Parkinson's disease: relation between striatal and limbic dopamine. *Adv. Biochem. Psychopharmacol.*, **19**, 293–300.

Reisine, T. D., Chesselet, M. F., Lubetski, C., Cheramy, A. and Glowinski, J. (1982). A role for striatal β-adrenergic receptors in the regulation of dopamine release. *Brain Res.*, **241**, 123–30.

Rinne, U. K. (1982). Brain neurotransmitter receptors in Parkinson's disease. In Marsden, C. D. and Fahn, S. (eds), *Movement Disorders*, Butterworth Scientific, London, pp. 59–74.

Silvette, H., Hoff, E. C., Larseon, P. S. and Haag, H. B. (1962). The actions of nicotine on central neuron system functions. *Pharmacol. Rev.*, **14**, 137–73.

Sourkes, T. L. and Poirier, L. J. (1966). Neurochemical basis of tremor and other disorders of movement. *Can. Med. Assoc. J.*, **94**, 53–60.

Sourkes, T. L., Poirier, L. J. and Singh, P. (1969). In Gillingham, F. G. and Donaldson, I. M. L. (eds), *Third Symposium on Parkinson's Disease*, Livingstone, Edinburgh, pp. 54–60.

Stadler, H., Lloyd, K. G., Gadea-Ciria, M. and Bartholini, G. (1973). Enhanced striatal acetylcholine release by chlorpromazine and its reversal by apomorphine. *Brain Res.*, **55**, 476–80.

Studler, J. M., Javoy-Agid, F., Cesselin, F., Legrand, J. C. and Agid, Y. (1982). CCK-8-Immunoreactivity distribution in human brain: selective decrease in the substantia nigra from parkinsonian patients. *Brain Res.*, **243**, 176–9.

Udenfriend, S., Withrop, B., Redfield, B. G. and Weissback, H. (1958). Studies with reversible inhibitors of monoamine oxidase: harmaline and related compounds. *Biochem. Pharmacol.*, **1**, 160–5.

23
Assessment of resting tremor in Parkinson's disease

M. A. GRESTY, ROSALEEN McCARTHY and L. J. FINDLEY

INTRODUCTION

Of the three cardinal features of Parkinson's disease, rigidity, bradykinesia and tremor, it is the tremor at rest that responds least predictably to drug therapy (Boshes, 1976). The evaluation of response to drug treatment is further complicated by the difficulties encountered when attempting objective assessments of tremor magnitude. The problems of assessing the resting tremor arise because its amplitude is subject to sudden and extreme fluctuations. These fluctuations can be the result of circadian variations, alterations in anxiety level, external stresses such as those produced by difficult tasks and, of course, fluctuations in the 'availability' of dopaminergic agents at receptor sites. Although these factors undoubtedly contribute to the variability in the amplitude of rest tremor, the commonest observed fluctuation, i.e. the abrupt change in amplitude seen in the apparently unstimulated patient, appears to be unrelated to any of the above factors. It is such fluctuations, of unknown origin, that make the assessment of this tremor particularly difficult.

Parkinsonian tremor, at rest, is one of the most common symptomatic tremors encountered in clinical practice, and thus it is hardly necessary to stress the need for some method for its assessment, particularly in terms of response to anti-parkinsonian drugs. As yet there is no convenient, objective method of assessing parkinsonian resting tremor. Current methods consist of monitoring long epochs in an uncontrolled environment (Ackmann *et al.*, 1977) or, more commonly, of making assessments on clinical rating scales, either by patient self-assessment, assessment by a companion or 'blind' evaluation by a clinician (Webster, 1968).

In this chapter we present an evaluation of a method of assessing resting tremor in Parkinson's disease. The objective is to provide a reliable method of assessing disability and response to tremolytic anti-parkinsonian drugs.

IDEAL REQUIREMENTS FOR ASSESSMENT

Ideally, any method of assessing tremor should fulfil certain requirements. The

321

method should be quick, so that it may be readily implemented in the clinic, involve a minimal number of assessment sessions and use apparatus that is easily available. Of utmost importance, the method should indicate the highest levels of tremor that the patient is likely to experience given the stage of his disease and the level of effective medication. Thus the method should reveal the maximum magnitudes of tremor resulting from attentional demand or stress. Assuming that the patient's status does not alter, one would expect the maximum levels of tremor to be reproducible on successive assessments. If the method could reveal maximum levels of tremor by provocative tasks, this would circumvent the problems of spontaneous fluctuations and provide a reliable baseline against which response to drugs may be evaluated. In order that it may be implemented in the clinic, the procedure should be relatively insensitive to minor variations in the timing of the test and be flexible enough to allow for the intellectual abilities of the individual patient. Broadly speaking there are two possible approaches, now outlined.

Long-term monitoring

Typically this involves devices that attach to the tremulous limb and record continuously or sample epochs of tremor. Analysis can be on- or off-line and involves digital filtering to restrict the recording to the frequency band of the tremor and to eliminate artefacts from stray movements with a frequency content outside the passband of the system. This 'carpet bombing' method has severe drawbacks, for there is no control over the particular situations experienced by the individual during any particular session and the recordings are heavily contaminated by movement artefacts derived from whatever the patient happens to be doing. However, this is the only method of detecting the maximum levels of tremor that the patient experiences in his own environment or the proportion of time that he is tremulous.

Assessment of short epochs of behaviour under controlled conditions

We opted to explore the use of a paradigm in which tremor would be assessed whilst the patient performed various tasks stressing particular dimensions of psychological function. We hoped that such a design would control the patient's arousal and produce more constant and reproducible tremor levels. A previous attempt to control tremor levels by tasks such as mental arithmetic has been described by Terävainen and Calne (1980). However, they gave no evaluation of the effectiveness of their procedure.

EXPERIMENTAL DESIGN

Each patient was assessed 'before' (or 'off') and 'on' drug therapy. Under each of these regimens, two assessments were given, one in the morning and the second in the afternoon at approximately the same times for all patients (10.30 h and 14.00 h) and at the same time after medication. In each assessment the patients were given a series of four standard tasks selected in order to emphasise particular dimensions of attentional demand. Each lasted approximately 1 min, during which tremor was recorded. Hence 16 samples of tremor were obtained in an assessment. The total time for an assessment was less than 40 min. Some patients were assessed on several different days under each regimen.

Throughout the tasks the patient sat comfortably in a carver chair with fore-arms resting in a standardised position. Tremor of the most symptomatic hand was recorded using a miniature piezoresistive accelerometer mounted on the limb with its sensitive axis oriented in the direction of greatest excursion.

The tremor signals were measured on-line using a spectral analyser, which computed an average spectrum derived by fast Fourier transformation from 100 overlapping 10.24 s samples of tremor. A velocity spectrum was calculated from the acceleration spectrum, and tremor magnitude during the assessment was estimated as the mean sum of velocity-squared frequency components in the frequency band 1.5 to 32 Hz with a resolution of 0.15 Hz. The resulting measurement is an estimate of the average kinetic energy dissipated by the tremor and has the powerful property of partially compensating for variations in harmonic distortion exhibited by resting tremor (Gresty and Findley, this volume, chapter 2).

Task characteristics

In pilot experiments we explored a variety of tasks and the following were selected because they were the most successful in inducing reproducible levels of tremor over repeated testing.

'Stroop' task

The patient was presented with a large matrix of words which spelt the names of common colours (red, yellow, green, blue). Each word was printed in coloured ink but the colour of the ink and the printed names did not correspond. The patient's task was to name the colour of the inks in which each word was written but to ignore the written word (Stroop, 1935). Successful performance requires an intellectual effort due to demands made on selective attention in a conflict situation. The conflict arises because reading is a more overlearned response than colour naming, and thus the patient has to inhibit the dominant tendency to say the word.

Colour naming task

The patient was required to name the colours (red, yellow, blue, green) of a set of rectangles presented in a matrix. This task ensures consistent levels of alertness, and sustained attention without involving response conflict.

Number matrix task

The patient was given one of a variety of tasks graded according to ability (e.g. summing columns of numbers or summing repetitions of the same digit). Such tasks involve the use of a variety of cognitive processes and ensure sustained attention and mental effort.

'Control condition'

The patient was told to relax and to do nothing.

The tasks were presented using 35 mm slide projection onto a tangent screen. The order of presentation of tasks was in a latin square design to control for practice, fatigue effects and adaptation to the situation. For all tasks the patients were instructed to take their time and to be accurate. Their performance was monitored and only achievement above the 95% correct level was accepted. The matrix task was modified if the patient failed to achieve this criterion.

Patients

Ten patients were the subject of this pilot study. These were classified as follows:

Six patients were first assessed when they were recently diagnosed, untreated cases with rest tremor as a dominant feature (frequency range 4–5.4 Hz). The patients had a range of duration of symptoms from six months to 1 year and none had received any previous dopaminergic medication. Each was assessed in the untreated condition in both the morning and afternoon of the same day and further assessments were made when treatment had started.

The remaining four patients had an established history of Parkinson's disease with a duration of symptoms up to five years. They had been, and were, taking dopaminergic medication at the time of assessment. In none of these patients was tremor satisfactorily controlled. Patients on medication were receiving either L-dopa with decarboxylase inhibitor (Sinemet) or bromocriptine (Parlodel). One patient showed best response to a combination of both types of dopaminergic therapy given concurrently.

RESULTS

Generally speaking, two broad patterns of results were found. In patients who were assessed before starting treatment, tasks enhanced tremor to magnitudes above control levels and there were consistent proportional relationships between tremor under all conditions. In patients receiving medication, tasks enhanced tremor generally above control levels; however, tremor magnitude under control conditions fluctuated unpredictably.

The results were analysed in detail with a view to estimating the reliability of the assessment procedure in provoking reproducible, statistically stable levels of tremor.

Test–retest reliability

This measure gives an indication of the ability of the various tasks to elicit comparable levels of tremor on repeated assessments. It was estimated using the Spearman rho (ρ) correlation coefficient on a sample of seven patients including the six untreated and one poorly controlled patient whose level of medication was constant, morning (a.m.) and afternoon (p.m.). The correlation coefficients between rank order of tremor magnitude a.m. and rank order of tremor magnitude p.m. are shown in table 23.1. The high correlation coefficients for enhanced

Table 23.1   Correlation coefficients (see text).

	ρ	p
Control	0.89	< 0.05
Colour patch	1.0	< 0.01
Stroop	0.86	$= 0.5$
Arithmetic	0.66	> 0.5

tremor under colour patch and Stroop tasks indicate that on repeated assessments the ordering of patients on these tasks in terms of magnitude of tremor does not change. In contrast the ordering of patients in terms of magnitude of tremor under the arithmetic task was not maintained on repeated assessment.

Differences between tasks in their ability to provoke tremor

For both the treated and the untreated patients, these were estimated using the Friedman analysis of variance on the means of two samples (a.m. and p.m.). For the untreated patients, the mean level of tremor on the first two samples (a.m. and p.m.) was used and for nine treated patients the first assessment was used in the analyses. There was a significant difference between the tasks in their ability to provoke tremor in both groups—untreated group: $F = 13.2$, $n = 6$, $K = 3$, $p < 0.001$; treated group: $F = 61.2$, $n = 9$, $K = 3$, $p < 0.001$. Arithmetic was not included in either of these analyses because of some patients' inability to attain criterion.

Pairwise contrasts between control and colour patch naming and control versus Stroop task were significant, showing that both of these tasks enhanced tremor above control levels. There were no significant differences between Stroop and colour patch naming in their ability to enhance tremor. Supplementary pairwise contrasts showed that arithmetic enhanced tremor magnitude above control levels but its enhancing effect was significantly weaker than that of the Stroop and colour patch tasks.

The ability of the various tasks to enhance tremor was found to be in the following order:

$$\text{control} < \text{arithmetic} < \text{colour patch} = \text{Stroop}$$

Inter-test relationships

Arithmetic was not included because of reduced n, due to inability of some subjects to attain criterion on the test. The tremor magnitude for these three conditions under which the patients were able to perform to a 95% criterion were intercorrelated in order to obtain an indication of task interrelationships. The relevant correlation matrices for treated ($n = 10$) and untreated ($n = 6$) patients are shown in table 23.2.

A demonstration of the consistency of this method of assessing rest tremor is provided by the results derived from one patient (figure 23.1) who was assessed repeatedly, at similar times of day, over a period of approximately nine months.

Table 23.2   Correlation matrices (see text).

(a)   Untreated patients

	Control	Colour patch	Stroop
Control	–	0.95	0.95
Colour patch		–	0.89
Stroop			–

(b)   Treated patients

	Control	Colour patch	Stroop
Control	–	< 0.5	< 0.5
Colour patch		–	0.98
Stroop			–

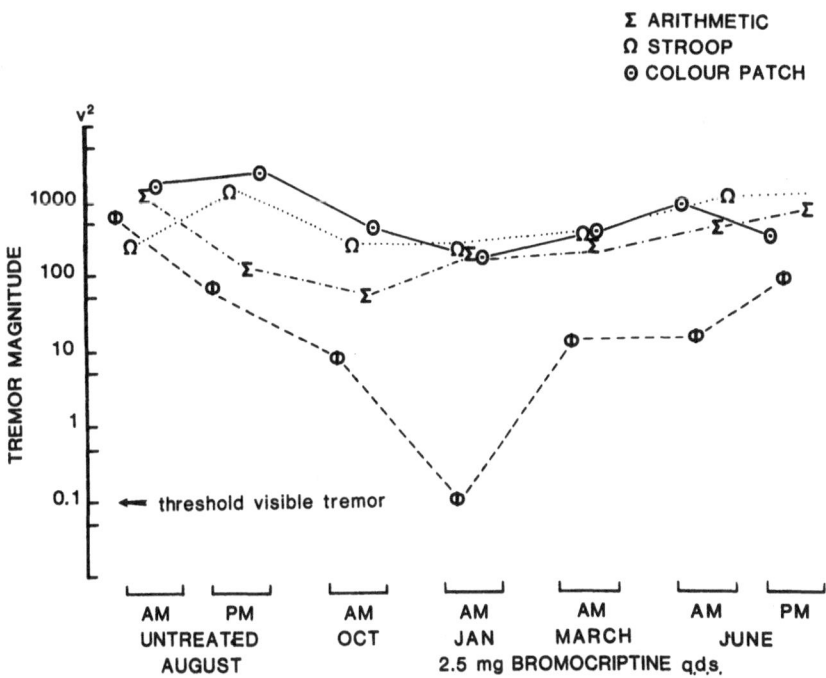

Figure 23.1   Results obtained on repeated assessments of tremor magnitude in a 55-year-old man with 18 months history of Parkinson's disease with predominant right-sided tremor. The axis is scaled on a log scale of velocity squared (units 9.81 m s^{-1}) and the abscissa indicates repeated assessments on different dates, a.m. and p.m. Low and unchanging doses of bromocriptine were introduced from January, and were ineffective in reducing the tremor on clinical assessment and by objective measurement.

The magnitudes of tremor recorded under Stroop and colour patch naming conditions were consistently the highest observed and varied by less than one decade in an observed total range of five decades. In contrast, under the control condition, tremor magnitude varied more than 3.5 decades. Tremor magnitudes recorded under the arithmetic task varied by more than one decade.

DISCUSSION

These results indicate that certain conditions, which control the patients' behaviour by presenting selected tasks in an appropriate experimental design, reliably produce high levels of tremor magnitude in parkinsonian patients with symptomatic tremor. Patients' own reports consistently confirmed that the highest levels of tremor obtained under task in our assessment protocol reliably indicated the maximum levels they experienced in their 'ordinary lives'. This type of paradigm would seem to be suitable both for the assessment of the range of fluctuation of tremor magnitude under various stresses and for monitoring effects of medication.

The results revealed that the type of task used to stress the subjects could be of vital importance in controlling behaviour such that high and consistent levels of tremor were provoked. In this respect it is interesting to note that mental arithmetic tasks, which have been used previously by other authors, were not reliable in provoking either high or consistent levels of tremor magnitude (see table 23.1). An additional problem with mental arithmetic is that some patients were unable to perform consistently to the same criteria from one session to another, which also detracts from test–retest reliability. This observation was particularly true for patients receiving dopaminergic drugs. Thus it would seem that mental arithmetic is a poor choice of task for the control of behaviour in patients with Parkinson's disease.

There were differences between the responses of previously untreated patients with early Parkinson's disease and those of patients who were on or who subsequently received treatment. The significance of the correlation matrices for the treated and untreated patients is as follows: In untreated patients, tremor under task can be reliably predicted from the 'baseline' tremor recordings taken under the control condition. In treated patients who were 'partially' controlled, the magnitude of tremor observed in response to tasks was independent of the tremor under the control condition. It would seem, therefore, that different factors are involved in the provocation of tremor in new or untreated patients as opposed to the patients on medication. In untreated patients the high correlations between tremor magnitude measured under control and task conditions could indicate that simple common factor as the primary determinant of the tremogenic properties of these conditions. In contrast, in the patients taking medication, the lack of correlation between the behaviour of tremor under control and under task conditions implies that Stroop and colour patch naming are tapping an independent factor from the control condition.

A surprising finding was that colour patch naming was extremely effective in provoking reliable and high magnitudes of tremor. This means that such a task, which has simple criteria that are easy to attain for all patients and easy to score, can be first choice for controlling patients' behaviour during tremor assessment. The simplicity of the colour patch naming task and its effectiveness in provoking tremor have the obvious implication that it could be used routinely in the clinic to indicate the maximum levels of tremor that the patient is likely to experience.

CONCLUSIONS

This study shows that, by controlling patients' behaviour with tremor-enhancing tasks in an appropriate experimental design, one can make reliable assessments of the upper ranges of magnitude of rest tremor that the patient normally experiences. Intellectual difficulty is not a necessary characteristic of tremor-enhancing tasks, as shown by the fact that mental arithmetic enhanced tremor weakly in comparison with colour patch naming. There are differences between untreated and treated patients in the ability of tasks to enhance tremor, which demonstrates that drugs can change the factors involved in its provocation.

REFERENCES

Ackmann, J. J., Sances, A., Larson, S. J. and Baker, J. B. (1977). Quantitative evaluation of long term Parkinson tremor. *IEEE Trans. Biomed. Eng.*, BME-24, 49–56.

Boshes, B. (1976). Further insights into Parkinsonian tremor. In Birkmeyer, W. and Hornykiewicz, O. (eds), *Advances in Parkinsonism*, Roche, Basel, pp. 303–18.

Stroop, J. R. (1935). Studies of interference in serial verbal reactions. *J. Exp. Psychol.*, 18, 643–62.

Teräväinen, H. and Calne, D. (1980). Quantitative assessment of Parkinsonian defects. In Rinner, Klinger and Stamm (eds), *Parkinson's Disease*, Elsevier/ North-Holland, Amsterdam, pp. 145–64.

Webster, D. D. (1968). Critical analysis of the disability in Parkinson's disease. *Mod. Treat.*, 5, 257–82.

24
Medical treatment of tremor in Parkinson's disease

J. A. OBESO and J. M. MARTÍNEZ LAGE

INTRODUCTION

In a retrospective analysis of clinical trials on the effectiveness of treatment of tremor in Parkinson's disease, one encounters some difficulties with methodology, which makes interpretation of results very difficult. One of the problems is that in most reported studies the cardinal symptoms of Parkinson's disease had not been analysed separately with respect to the effect of treatment. Another crucial point concerns the evaluation of tremor for, although we now know that there are different forms of tremulous movement in Parkinson's disease (Findley et al., 1981), reports have only devoted attention to the slow 4–5 Hz 'resting' tremor, little work having been published on the clinical importance of postural and action tremor in Parkinson's disease and their possible modification by treatment. Thus, we shall limit this review mainly to the impact of drug therapy on resting tremor in patients usually classified as or above grade II of Hoehn and Yahr's (1967) scale.

EARLY TREATMENTS (1892–1963)

Anticholinergics

Charcot initiated the pharmacological treatment of Parkinson's disease, introducing hyoscine (scopolamine) in 1892. Hyoscine, atropine and stramonium were the generally accepted treatment for Parkinson's disease for many years, until favourable reports on the use of some belladonna alkaloid extracted from white wine (Price and Merrit, 1941; Fabing and Zeligs, 1941) prompted an intensive search for synthetic compounds. The least toxic and most efficient among the initial synthetic anticholinergics was caramiphen hydrochloride (Parpanit), which produced fewer side-effects, such as confusion, nightmares, psychosis and pupil dilation, than atropine or scopolamine (Grunthal, 1946). In a model research study of its time, Schwab and Leigh (1949) found a mean 25% improvement in

62% of 50 parkinsonian patients treated with Parpanit alone. These authors were not favourably impressed with the action of Parpanit on tremor, although about half of the patients experienced a reduction in shaking. Subsequently, in 1947, benzhexol (Artane) was introduced for the treatment of Parkinson's disease. Doshay and Constable (1949) reported improvement in 89 of 117 patients (76%), and Corbin (1949) also obtained benefit in 77% of the patients treated with this drug. Rigidity was felt in general to improve most frequently (75% of the patients); however, tremor was reduced in about 50% of the cases. The chemical congeners cycrimine (Pagitane), procyclidine (Kemadrin) and biperiden (Akineton) were available soon after Artane (Schwab and Chafetz, 1955; Zier and Doshay, 1957; England and Schwab, 1959). Overall, these drugs provided only a moderate improvement in akinesia and rigidity and usually only slight reduction of tremor. It should not be forgotten that these small and variable improvements can be very significant in individual patients.

Antihistaminics

This group of drugs became 'fashionable' in the drug therapy for Parkinson's disease in the 1940s. Diphenhydramine (Benadryl), phenindamine tartrate (Thephorin) and benztropine (Cogentin), this last compound combining atropine and antihistaminic effects, were generally accepted as being efficacious (McGavack et al., 1947; Budnitz, 1948; Ryan and Wood, 1949). In an extensive study, Effron and Denker (1950) obtained the best therapeutic results with a combination of Artane, Cogentin and hyoscine. Amelioration of tremor, however, was achieved in only 25% of patients.

The role of anticholinergic and antihistaminic drugs in the treatment of Parkinson's disease has clearly been eclipsed by the introduction of levodopa (L-dopa). However, it is well recognised now that in a number of patients tremor may be significantly improved with anticholinergics and antihistaminics for a long period of time, thus allowing delay in the introduction of levodopa therapy. This applies particularly to a subgroup of patients who have a very slowly progressive form of the disease, usually confined to one side of the body, and with tremor as the main complaint (Scott and Brody, 1971).

DOPAMINERGIC AGONISTS (1963–1983)

Levodopa

Soon after the introduction of levodopa for the treatment of Parkinson's disease, it became recognised that tremor was usually the least responsive of the major cardinal signs. There is no doubt, however, that tremor in some patients may be markedly improved by levodopa, as shown by the data in table 24.1, even though it is generally agreed that akinesia and rigidity usually respond more spectacularly.

Table 24.1 Average overall improvement in cardinal symptoms (%) after oral levodopa therapy.

	No. patients	*Rigidity*	*Akinesia*	*Tremor*
Levodopa alone				
Keenan (1970)	360	57	62	61
Levodopa + benserazide				
Miller and Wiener (1974)	17	90	71	71
Rinne *et al.* (1972)	30	68	68	79
Levodopa + carbidopa				
Ohmoto and Kiskisawa				
(1975)	14	70*	67*	43*
Agnoli *et al.* (1974)	28	76	72	65
Martínez Lage *et al.*				
(1974)	32	62	58	60

*Maximum improvement only.

The reasons for such special 'selective' sensitivity of certain symptoms and signs in Parkinson's disease to drug therapy are unknown, but a better understanding of the pathophysiology and biochemistry underlying tremor, rigidity and brady-kinesia may allow us to give a more rational therapy according to the individual patient's symptom profile.

Interestingly, we have observed that tremor may be indeed facilitated or triggered off by 'low' levodopa stimulation in some patients. We first noticed such a phenomenon in patients with diphasic dyskinesias (Muenter *et al.*, 1977). In these cases, dyskinetic movements in the form of chorea, ballism or dystonia herald the beginning and end of the action of each dosage of levodopa (figure 24.1a). However, a period of tremor may actually precede and follow dyskinesias (figure 24.1b). This tremor, which mainly affects the upper limbs, disappears or wanes during the peak 'on' or 'off' states. Otherwise, when present, the tremor has all the typical features of resting parkinsonian tremor. On the other hand, we have studied a few patients with rigidity and bradykinesia as main symptoms during the 'off' phases who will show resting tremor for a few minutes before any therapeutic response is obvious. Dyskinesias are not observed as an accompanying feature. Tremor may appear in many of these patients with a 'one-phase pattern' (figure 24.1c), a phenomenon also frequently observed in patients with typical diphasic dyskinesias (Marsden *et al.*, 1982).

Ergot alkaloid derivatives

Several ergot alkaloid derivatives (*ergolines*) have recently been introduced as a complement to or substitute for levodopa therapy. The rationale behind this is to avoid the long-term side-effects of levodopa therapy, particularly the 'on'-'off' phenomena.

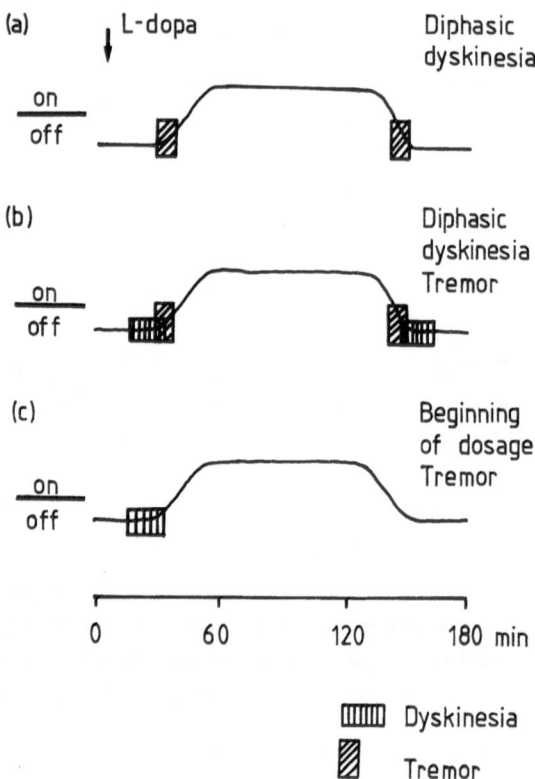

Figure 24.1 (a) Schematic representation of diphasic dyskinesias. Ballistic movements, dystonia or chorea occur only at the onset and end of action of dose. (b) Resting tremor affecting upper and lower limbs may precede and follow typical diphasic dyskinesia in some patients. Usually, the severity of dyskinesias is such that tremor receives little attention. (c) Unilateral or generalised resting tremor may precede the beneficial effect of levodopa in some patients who do not show tremor during the 'on'–'off' states.

The effect of *bromocriptine* on parkinsonian tremor is summarised in table 24.2. Even though data available for analysis are limited, it seems that the tremolytic effect of bromocriptine is maximum when given in low dosages (less than 30 mg per day).

Lergotrile was the next ergoline to be introduced. In the initial studies the four cardinal features of Parkinson's disease were reduced significantly when this drug was added to levodopa (Lieberman *et al.*, 1975a). However, lergotrile has had to be abandoned as an anti-parkinsonian drug because of the unacceptably high incidence of adverse effects that it provoked.

Pergolide and *lisuride*, two newer semisynthetic ergot alkaloid derivatives, have recently been introduced for Parkinson's disease. Both drugs have proved useful in reducing oscillations in motor capability, prolonging 'on' periods and decreasing

Table 24.2 Effect of bromocriptine on resting tremor.

Reference	N	Mean daily dosage (mg)	Significant improvement
Lieberman *et al.* (1976)	11	26.7	no
Parkes *et al.* (1976)	20	25.9	no
Kartzinel *et al.* (1976)	20	34	yes (50%)
Kartzinel and Calne (1976)	20	75	no
Rinne and Marttila (1978)	24	30	yes (46%)
Rascol *et al.* (1979)	12	20–75	? (32%)
Teychenne *et al.* (1982)	22	13	yes (48%)

early-morning akinesia, but neither one relieves tremor more effectively than previously available drugs (Lieberman *et al.*, 1981; Gopinathan *et al.*, 1981; Le Witt *et al.*, 1982). However, a dramatic reduction of tremor has been reported in a few patients (Parkes *et al.*, 1981; Lang *et al.*, 1982), and that is also our impression in a small number of patients with very severe tremor unresponsive to standard therapy.

Piribedil

Piribedil (pyrimidyl piperinyl piperazine) was introduced by Carrodi, Fuxe and Ungersted (1971). This drug was found to be effective in relieving tremor in monkeys (Goldstein *et al.*, 1973) and was subsequently used as an oral agent in the treatment of Parkinson's disease. Tremor was the main sign ameliorated by Piribedil (Rondot *et al.*, 1975; Feigenson *et al.*, 1976), but the proportion of patients obtaining a significant improvement was no greater than with levodopa therapy (Lieberman *et al.*, 1975b). Possible reasons for the relative failure of oral against intravenous Piribedil could be related to the higher serum levels that were able to be achieved intravenously or because the active agent may have been a metabolite of Piribedil that could not reach a sufficient intracerebral concentration after oral administration (Lieberman *et al.*, 1975b). The effectiveness of Piribedil in relieving tremor was limited by its strong tendency to induce dyskinesias. The use of this drug may deserve reconsideration for the occasional patient with severe tremor, who is not responding to any other medication.

A controlled trial studying the change of postural and action tremor after different drug treatments and the effect of beta-blockers on the three types of tremors of Parkinson's disease has not yet been carried out. Such an undertaking could provide objective data on the actual value of certain drugs that, like propranolol, are sometimes employed to treat tremor in Parkinson's disease in a very empirical manner.

CONCLUSION

The effect of treatment on resting tremor in Parkinson's disease cannot be assessed in isolation, i.e. it is necessary to consider tremor in relation to the degree of akinesia and rigidity. Almost every anti-parkinsonian drug will have some effect on tremor, but it is not possible to select a particular therapeutic regimen on the basis of tremolytic effect alone.

It can fairly be stated that patients with unilateral tremor as the predominant symptom should be considered for surgical treatment, i.e. thalamotomy (see Andrew, this volume, chapter 25). This will remain so until more predictably effective drugs with high therapeutic indices and selectivity, and without long-term adverse effects, are developed.

REFERENCES

Agnoli, A., Casacchia, M., Fazio, C., Ruggieri, S., Zamponi, A., Mancini, G., Muratorio, A. and Perro, R. (1974). Comparison between the therapeutic effects of L-dopa and L-Dopa plus Dopa decarboxylase inhibitors in Parkinson's disease. In Yahr, M. (ed.), *Current Concepts in the Treatment of Parkinsonism*, Raven Press, New York, pp. 87–94.

Budnitz, J. (1948). The use of Benadryl in Parkinson's disease: a preliminary report of 8 cases. *New Engl. J. Med.*, **238**, 874–5.

Carrodi, H., Fuxe, J. and Ungerstedt, U. (1971). Evidence for a new type of dopamine receptor stimulating agent. *J. Pharm. Pharmacol.*, **23**, 989–91.

Corbin, K. B. (1949). Trihexyphenidyl: evaluation of a new agent in treatment of parkinsonism. *J. Am. Med. Assoc.*, **141**, 377–82.

Doshay, L. J. and Constable, K. (1949). Artane therapy for Parkinsonism: preliminary study of results of 117 cases. *J. Am. Med. Assoc.*, **140**, 1317–22.

Effron, A. S. and Denker, P. G. (1950). A clinical evaluation of certain antihistamine and antispasmodic drugs in Parkinson's disease. *J. Am. Med. Assoc.*, **144**, 5–8.

England, A. C. and Schwab, R. S. (1959). Management of Parkinson's disease. *Arch. Intern. Med.*, **104**, 439–68.

Fabing, H. D. and Zeligs, M. A. (1941). Treatment of the post-encephalitic parkinsonism syndrome with desiccated white wine extract of V.S.P. belladonna root. *J. Am. Med. Assoc.*, **117**, 332–4.

Feigenson, J. S., Sweet, R. D. and McDowell, F. H. (1976). Piribedil: its synergistic effect in multidrug regimens for parkinsonism. *Neurology*, **26**, 430–3.

Findley, L. J., Gresty, M. A. and Halmagyi, G. M. (1981). Tremor, the cogwheel phenomenon and clonus in Parkinson's disease. *J. Neurol. Neurosurg. Psychiatr.*, **44**, 534–46.

Goldstein, M., Battista, A. F. and Ohmoto, A. F. (1973). Tremor and involuntary movements in monkeys: effect of L-Dopa and of a dopamine receptor stimulating agent. *Science*, **179**, 816–17.

Gopinathan, G., Terävainen, H., Dambrosia, J. M., *et al.* (1981). Lisuride in parkinsonism. *Neurology*, **31**, 371–6.

Grunthal, E. (1946). Ueber Parpanit einen neuen, extrapyramidalmotorische Störungen beeinflussenden. *Stoff Schwiz. Med. Wochenschr.*, **76**, 1286–9.

Hoehn, M. M. and Yahr, M. D. (1967). Parkinsonism: onset, progression and mortality. *Neurology*, **17**, 427–42.

Kartzinel, R. and Calne, D. B. (1976). Studies with bromocriptine. Part I. 'On-off' phenomena. *Neurology*, 26, 508-10.

Kartzinel, R., Teychenne, P., Gillespie, M. M., *et al.* (1976). Bromocriptine and levodopa (with or without carbidopa) in Parkinsonism. *Lancet*, 2, 272-5.

Keenan, R. E. (1970). The Eaton collaborative study of levodopa therapy in parkinsonism: a summary. *Neurology*, 20, 46-52.

Lang, A. E., Quinn, N., Brincat, S., Marsden, C. D. and Parkes, J. (1982). Pergolide in late-stage Parkinson's disease. *Ann. Neurol.*, 12, 243-7.

Le Witt, P. A., Gopinathan, G., Ward, C. D., *et al.* (1982). Lisuride versus bromo-criptine treatment in Parkinson's disease: a double-blind study. *Neurology (NY)*, 32, 69-72.

Lieberman, A. N., Goldstein, M., Leibowitz, M., *et al.* (1981). Treatment of advanced Parkinson's disease with pergolide. *Neurology (NY)*, 31, 675-82.

Lieberman, A. N., Myamoto, T. and Battista, A. (1975a). Studies on the anti-parkinsonian efficacy of lergotrile. *Neurology*, 25, 459-62.

Lieberman, A. N., Shopsin, B., Le Brun, Y., *et al.* (1975b). Studies on Piribedil in parkinsonism. In Calne, D. B., Chase, T. N. and Barbeau, A. (eds), *Advances in Neurology*, vol. 9, Raven Press, New York, pp. 399-407.

Lieberman, A., Zolfaghari, M., Boal, D., *et al.* (1976). The antiparkinsonian efficacy of bromocriptine. *Neurology*, 26, 405-9.

McGavack, T. H., Elias, H. and Boyd, L. J. (1947). Some pharmacological and clinical experiences with dimethylaminoethyl benzhydryl ether hydrochloride (Benadryl). *Am. J. Med. Sci.*, 213, 418-34.

Marsden, C. D., Parkes, J. D. and Quinn, N. (1982). Fluctuations of disability in Parkinson's disease. Clinical aspects. In Marsden, C. D. and Fahn, S. (eds), *Movement Disorders*, Butterworth, London, pp. 96-124.

Martínez Lage, J. M., Marti Masso, J. F., Carrera, N., *et al.* (1974). A single-blind comparative study with the combination of carbidopa and L-Dopa in Parkinson's disease treatment. In Yahr, M. (ed.), *Current Concepts in the Treatment of Parkinsonism*, Raven Press, New York, pp. 3-11.

Miller, E. M. and Wiener, L. (1974). Ro 4-4602 and levodopa in the treatment of Parkinsonism. *Neurology*, 24, 482.

Muenter, M. D., Sharpless, N. S., Tyce, G. M., *et al.* (1977). Patterns of dystonia (I-D-I' and D-I-D') in response to L-Dopa therapy for Parkinson's disease. *Mayo Clin. Proc.*, 52, 163-74.

Ohmoto, T. and Kiskisawa, H. (1975). L-Dopa therapy combined with peripheral decarboxylase inhibitor (MIC-486) in Parkinsonism. *Folia Psychiatr. Neurol. Jpn.*, 29, 1-13.

Parkes, J. D., Marsden, C. D., Donaldson, I., *et al.* (1976). Bromocriptine treat-ment in Parkinson's disease. *J. Neurol. Neurosurg. Psychiatr.*, 39, 184-93.

Parkes, J. D., Schachter, M., Marsden, C. D., *et al.* (1981). Lisuride in Parkin-sonism. *Ann. Neurol.*, 9, 48-52.

Price, J. C. and Merrit, H. H. (1941). The treatment of Parkinsonism: result obtained with wine of Bulgarian belladonna alkaloid of V.S.P. belladonna. *J. Am. Med. Assoc.*, 117, 335-7.

Rascol, A., Guiraud, B., Montastruc, J. L., *et al.* (1979). Long-term treatment of Parkinson's disease with bromocriptine. *J. Neurol. Neurosurg. Psychiatr.*, 42, 143-50.

Rinne, U. K. and Marttila, R. (1978). Brain dopamine receptor stimulation and the relief of Parkinsonism: relationship between bromocriptine and levodopa. *Ann. Neurol.*, 4, 263-7.

Rinne, U. K., Sonninen, V. and Siirtola, T. (1972). Treatment of Parkinson's disease with L-Dopa and decarboxylase inhibitor. *Z. Neurol.*, 202, 1-20.

Rondot, P., Bathien, N. and Ribadeau-Dumas, J. L. (1975). Indications of Piribedil in L-Dopa treated parkinsonians. In Calne, D. B., Chase, T. N. and Barbeau, A. (eds), *Advances in Neurology*, vol. 9, Raven Press, New York, pp. 373-81.

Ryan, G. M. S. and Wood, J. S. (1949). Benadryl in the treatment of Parkinsonism: results in 40 cases. *Lancet*, 1, 258-9.

Schwab, R. S., and Chafetz, M. E. (1955). Kemadrin in the treatment of Parkinsonism. *Neurology*, 5, 273-7.

Schwab, R. and Leigh, D. (1949). Parpanit in the treatment of Parkinson's disease. *J. Am. Med. Assoc.*, 139, 629-34.

Scott, M. R. and Brody, J. A. (1971). Benign early onset of Parkinson's disease: a syndrome distinct from classic postencephalitic parkinsonism. *Neurology*, 21, 366-8.

Teychenne, P. F., Bergsrud, D., Anis Racy, P. A.-C., *et al.* (1982) Bromocriptine: low-dose therapy in Parkinson's disease. *Neurology (NY)*, 32, 577-83.

Zier, A. and Doshay, L. J. (1957). Procyclidine hydrochloride (Kemadrin). Treatment of Parkinsonism: result in 108 patients. *Neurology*, 7, 485-9.

25
Surgical treatment of tremor

JOHN ANDREW

HISTORICAL BACKGROUND

Parkinson (1817) reported that a patient with the 'shaking palsy' lost the tremor on the side of the body affected by a hemiplegic stroke. This observation has led neurosurgeons in the present century to perform partial interruptions of the pyramidal and extrapyramidal pathways in an attempt to relieve parkinsonian tremor and rigidity, as well as other movement disorders and other forms of tremor, without causing permanent hemiplegia.

Removal of the motor or premotor cortex usually resulted in spastic hemiplegia, and such operations are no longer practised (Bucy and Case, 1939; Klemme, 1940). Partial section of the anterior limb of the internal capsule through the lateral ventricle did not permanently relieve the tremor (Meyers, 1940, 1942), but the same author reported greater success by dividing the pallido-fugal pathways in the ansa lenticularis and fascicularis. Crossed pyramidal tract section (Putnam, 1940) at the level of the second cervical segment usually gave good relief of tremor, with mild persisting weakness. More lasting relief, with a greater risk of increased weakness, was obtained if the whole of the lateral columns on the affected side were sectioned sufficiently to cause some disturbance of pain appreciation in the opposite leg (Oliver, 1949). Cerebral pedunculotomy (Walker, 1949), when the outer three-fifths of the peduncle were divided under direct vision, was also successful for tremor and was followed by remarkably little permanent weakness.

The next important milestone in the surgical treatment of parkinsonian tremor was during an operation for pedunculotomy when the anterior choroidal artery was injured and ligàted; the peduncle was left unsectioned. The tremor and rigidity were relieved without undesired sequelae (Cooper, 1953). This operation was then performed on a number of occasions, but the results were unpredictable, and other surgeons reported hemiplegia as a complication. The anterior choroidal artery does not irrigate the same field in all subjects, but the medial part of the lentiform nucleus (globus pallidus crus 1 and 2), the ansa lenticularis and neighbouring portion of the anterior limb of the internal capsule receive their blood supply from this vessel.

THE ADVENT OF STEREOTAXIC SURGERY

Surgical attention was now centred on the globus pallidus and the pallido-fugal pathways. Blind division of the ansa lenticularis was performed through a frontal craniotomy on one side under local anaesthetic. The frontal lobe was elevated and the loop divided above the optic tract. This was a formidable procedure, although often successful. Stereotaxic methods were then developed to reach the same target for cases of parkinsonism, and the method was developed by various workers (e.g. Guiot and Gillingham, Cooper, Riechert, Narabayashi, and Spiegel and Wycis).

The principles of stereotaxic surgery are to relate the surgical target to nearby structures that can be visualised radiographically, and then to direct an electrode, or a probe, to the target with minimal possible damage (stereotaxis, from Greek, *stereos* = solid, *taxis* = arrangement). In the early days, when the surgical techniques were less well developed and lesions were sometimes made in the thalamus and not in the globus pallidus, the more posterior the lesion the better the result for the tremor. An attempt was made to identify a named thalamic nuclear parcellation as the ideal target site, but there were difficulties. First, there are the two systems of nomenclature: the American (Walker, 1938) and the German (Hassler, 1959). From the original descriptions, the boundaries of the current popular target—ventralis oralis posterior (Vop) and ventralis intermedius (Vim) in the Hassler terminology, or ventralis lateris (VL) in that of Walker—do not exactly correspond. Secondly, there is a variability in distances of the thalamic nuclear boundaries between the midline and radiological reference points in the third ventricle. Atlases of the thalamus and basal ganglia were published where serial slices through the brain were placed in a template so that the various structures could be related in distance to the midline, and to the reference points, such as the anterior and posterior commissures (AC, PC) and the interventricular foramen (IVF), and the reference planes (Spiegel and Wycis, 1952; Talairach *et al.*, 1957; Schaltenbrand and Bailey, 1959). A more detailed variability study of the nuclear boundaries, with a model of an average thalamus, was prepared by examining slices of 1 mm thickness in the coronal plane through 26 thalamuses (Andrew and Watkins, 1969). Perhaps because of the problems of localisation, temporary reversible lesions were made, using an inflatable balloon, or a cryoprobe to lower the temperature and suppress the ambient neuronal activity; if the tremor ceased by either method, then a permanent lesion was made using, in the first group, an alcoholic paste, or in the second, by freezing (Cooper and Bravo, 1958; Cooper *et al.*, 1965).

THE CURRENT 'TARGET' USED IN THE ALLEVIATION OF TREMOR

In an attempt to find a 'physiological' target, microelectrode recording of spontaneous and evoked cell activity was introduced (Albe-Fessard *et al.*, 1962; Jasper and Bertrand, 1966). They noted spontaneous tremor rhythm firing from Vim. The posterior border of this is the anterior limit of the sensory relay nuclei, ventralis caudalis externus (Vce) and ventralis caudalis internus (Vci). Spontaneous rhythmic firing, synchronous with the tremor, may be seen and heard with an audiovisual display system, and the tremor itself recorded with an accelerometer through the same system (figure 25.1). At this site, the firing is not

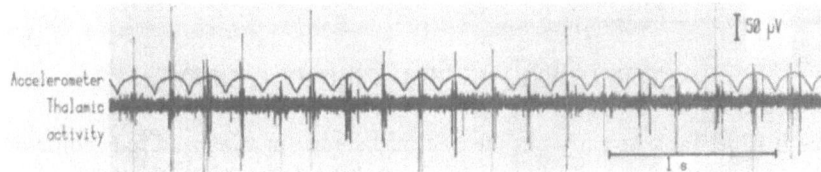

Figure 25.1 Visual display of thalamic cell bursts believed to be in Vim, and the tremor recorded by accelerometer.

thought to be responsive to the tremor, since it may be heard a few seconds before a still arm begins to shake, and to cease a few seconds after the arm becomes still again. The Vim receives afferents from muscle spindles in its lateral part, and vestibular pathways in its medial. It projects to the sensorimotor cortex. Anterior to Vim is the Vop which is thought to correspond to VL of Walker. This nucleus receives input from the cerebellar dentate nucleus, which has passed through the red nucleus first and then to the motor cortex (Hassler *et al.*, 1979). Whether the tremor rhythm firing, and therefore the tremor, is generated in the Vim (tremor pacemaker), where it is usually recorded, or whether it is transmitted through that zone from elsewhere, and presumably on its way to the motor cortex which triggers the tremor, is not known. Rhythmic firing recorded from the sensory relay nuclei, more posteriorly in Vce, is thought to be responsive to, and not initiating, tremor. The paucity of post-mortem material reflects the low mortality, but denies us anatomical confirmation. When passive muscle stretch responses have been recorded near the Vim-Vce border, a small thermo-coagulative lesion, up to 30 cmm (Ohye *et al.*, 1981) is sufficient to suppress tremor, although a larger lesion is required for a coarser tremor. That this target is Vim has been disputed (Hassler *et al.*, 1979) since, from his post-mortem material of successfully treated tremor cases, it was found that there may have been no destruction in Vim. It is suggested that the tremor bursts have been recorded from cerebellar pathways in the fields of Forel passing to Vop and that a lesion at either of these sites may presumably be effective. Whether this tremor firing comes from a tremogenic zone, as suggested by the French school, or is simply responsive to tremor activity, as suggested by the German, one thing is clear: in those cases of tremor where firing is recorded anterior to the sensory relay nuclei, a small lesion at that site, to include the muscle stretch responsive zone—never more than 1-2 mm posterior—is usually effective in abolishing tremor. Whether the tremor firing is in Vop, Vim or the fields of Forel, or dorsal tegmental area (HI), may be therapeutically unimportant. It is known that the posterior border of Vim has a 4 mm scatter in the sagittal plane behind the interventricular foramen (IVF), and a slightly greater scatter in relation to the mid-commissural point used by most stereotaxic surgeons as the reference point; and that the inferior borders of Vim and Vce have at least a 2 mm scatter in the first standard deviation (Andrew and Watkins, 1969, pp. 46, 39). Without post-mortem examination, the precise site of tremor firing and muscle stretch responses, as well as the lesion, can never be known.

STEREOTAXIC METHOD USED BY ANDREW

Since it is desirable to carry out the electrical studies in a well and fully conscious patient, the technique of Oliver (1967) has been followed, with modifications by E. S. Watkins (1961, personal communication). Staged operations are performed. At the first, under general anaesthesia, a large burr hole is made about 3 cm from the midline, immediately anterior to the fronto-parietal suture, on the side opposite that being treated. The base of a metal cup (figure 25.3a) is pegged into the outer table over the burr hole. The stereotaxic frame is attached to the head, and the patient sat up. Myodil (Iodophenylate), 6 ml, is injected into the lateral ventricle and it fills the third ventricle. Lateral and frontal X-rays are taken to relate the anterior and posterior commissures (AC, PC), and the interventricular foramen of Munro (IVF) and the midline (figure 25.2), to grids attached to the frame. A multiperforated sphere is then fixed into the metal cup (figure 25.3a), aligned so that a probe passing through its central hole will reach a point in the thalamus 14 mm posterior to the IVF on the IVF–PC plane (x plane), the IVF being the only reference point used for measurement. Many surgeons prefer to use the AC–PC as the x plane, and the mid-commissural point as the reference point. We prefer the IVF as a single reference point and IVF–PC as the x plane, since the variability of the distance from this reference point to the borders of thalamic nuclei is less (Andrew and Watkins, 1969, pp. 9–23). Further X-rays are taken in the lateral and frontal views with a check probe to the target point, and the first stage completed. It often happens that the mere passage of the electrode probe for the check X-rays is sufficient to abolish the tremor for one or two days. If alignment is not exact, the neighbouring perforations in the sphere allow the target zone to be reached with accuracy.

A few days later, when the patient has fully recovered, under local anaesthesia and without sedation, the target zone is explored by microelectrode recording and electrical stimulation.

The recording electrode is monopolar (figure 25.3c), encased within a 1.6 mm diameter stainless-steel tube. The active element is a 0.05 mm diameter PTFE tungsten wire passed through the tube. The tip of the wire is electrochemically etched. The casing is the indifferent element for recording. The tungsten wire tip tapers over a distance of 1 mm from 5 μm to 10 μm. The exposed conical tip is 50 μm in length, ending in a hemisphere of 5 μm radius (Howe *et al.*, 1983). The proximal end of the electrode is connected to a switching box (Medelec SP 268) and to a standard EMG machine (Medelec MS6) (Fowler *et al.*, 1984).

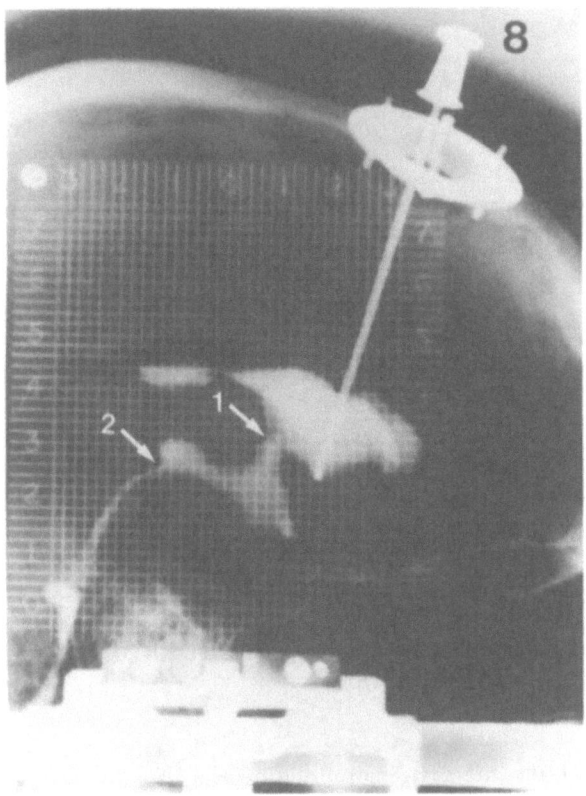

Figure 25.2 Lateral radiograph of skull, showing cup for electrode guide, cannula in frontal horn, and myodil in frontal horn, third ventricle and aqueduct; the IVF and PC are easily related to the graticule. Arrows: 1, interventricular foramen of Munro; 2, posterior commissure.

The accelerometer is attached to the trembling limb and connected through a pre-amplifier to the Medelec, and the tremor displayed on a second channel.

As the electrode advances through the Vim, it is usually possible to record the tremor visually and audibly in cases of parkinsonism, benign essential tremor, and sometimes in multiple sclerosis. At each advance of 1 mm, or sometimes less, the joints are passively stretched and evoked responses listened for. These are usually not heard until the tremor firing zone has been passed through. The background cell firing increases in amplitude, or microvoltage, on the passage of the electrode posteriorly, reaching its maximum in the posterior part of the sensory relay nuclei, Vce or Vci, where tactile sensory responses are evoked. Different patterns and voltages of background cell activity have been described for the zones of the thalamus likely to be traversed, as well as for the fields of Forel and the red nucleus.

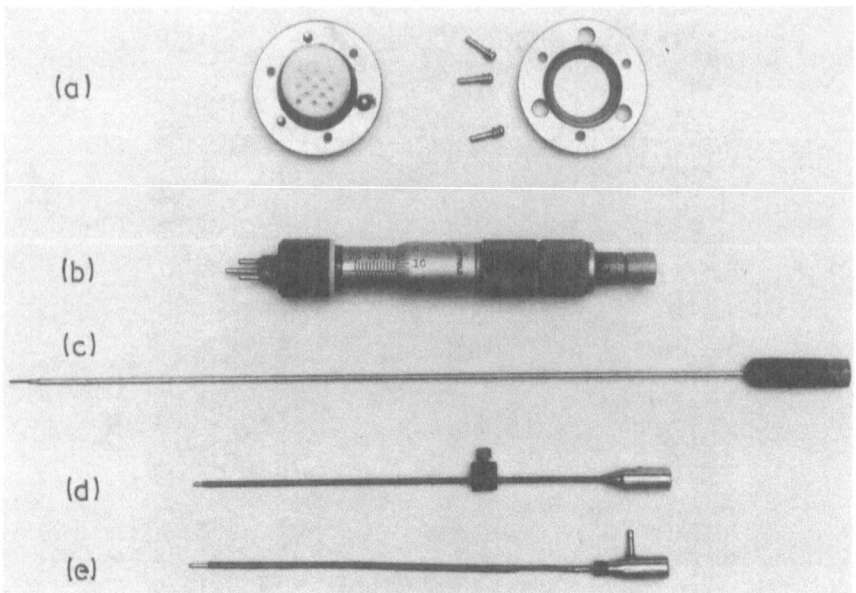

Figure 25.3 (a) Metal cup and cap; Teflon sphere and pegs. (b) Micrometer screw for propelling recording electrode. (c) Recording electrode. (d) Stimulating electrode. (e) Lesion-making electrode.

Stimulation at the site of tremor firing or evoked muscle stretch responses is then carried out with a different electrode, which is unipolar, has a bared tip of 1 mm, and is 1.5 mm in diameter (figure 25.3d). A current of 0.1-2.0 V is used, 50-100 Hz. When—as rarely happens—there has been no rhythmic tremor firing or evoked sensory responses, stimulation at the estimated target site may be the only physiological guide for the lesion. When a small current, 0.5 V or less, causes paraesthesia in the opposite arm or leg or side of the face, it is presumed that the needle tip is too posterior in the Vce or Vci, or near the medial lemniscus, and a lesion there may cause permanent paraesthesia, principally in the corner of the mouth and periphery of the upper limb. A larger current of 1.0 V or more causing paraesthesia usually means the correct site has been reached. Stimulation may also aggravate or suppress the tremor, again a favourable sign for target localisation. If a small current of 0.5 V results in a myoclonic jerk, then the needle tip is too close to the internal capsule. The multiperforated sphere allows a fairly wide zone of exploration, since the perforations are 3 mm apart in the sagittal and coronal planes, and, provided the distances advanced by the electrode are known, then its point can be related to the reference point, the midline and the x or IVF-PC plane by simple geometric calculation.

The ideal target is one that straddles the zones from which spontaneous tremor rhythm firing has been recorded, and muscle stretch responses from the trembling arm evoked. Also, if the tremor is markedly modified by the stimulus at a given point, then this is usually a favourable site for a lesion. A special electrode (figure 25.3e) is used for this. It has a bared tip of 6 mm and is hollowed out for the insertion of a thermocouple to record the temperature at the electrode tip. A radiofrequency current is used to raise the temperature at the electrode tip to 67°C for 150 s, producing a coagulum the shape of an oblate spheroid. If the tremor does not abate, the lesion may be lengthened, or a further coagulation made parallel with, above, or to one side of the first. The guide is left in place for a few days so that a further lesion can be made if the tremor returns. It is usually possible to make a single lesion in cases of parkinsonism, which will be effective if physiological identification of the target has been carried out. Intervals of a few days for further lesions are allowed for. The presumed site and shape of the lesion are represented in figure 25.4. The CT scan appearance of a recent and successful lesion is shown in figure 25.5.

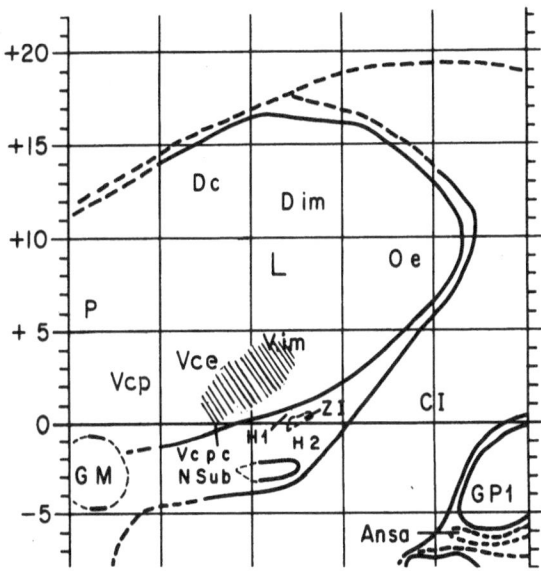

Figure 25.4 Sagittal section through an average thalamus at 14 mm from midline. Hatched area = presumed lesion. Dc, dorsalis caudalis; Dim, dorsalis intermedius; Oe, oralis externus; L, lateral mass of thalamus; Vim, ventralis intermedius; Vce, ventralis caudalis externus; Vcp, ventralis caudalis portae; CI, internal capsule; Vcpc, ventralis caudalis parvocellularis; GP1, globus pallidus crus 1; H1, H2, dorsal and ventral tegmental areas; ZI, zona incerta; NSub, subthalamic nucleus of Luys; P, pulvinar; and GM, medial geniculate.

Although time-consuming, microelectrode recording of evoked sensory responses does offer, in addition, a unique opportunity to study some of the processes in the normal human thalamus. For example, in the sensory relay nuclei (Vce, Vci), cell units responsive to both sides of the mouth area, one side of the mouth and the hand on the same side, or to both lower limbs, have been found.

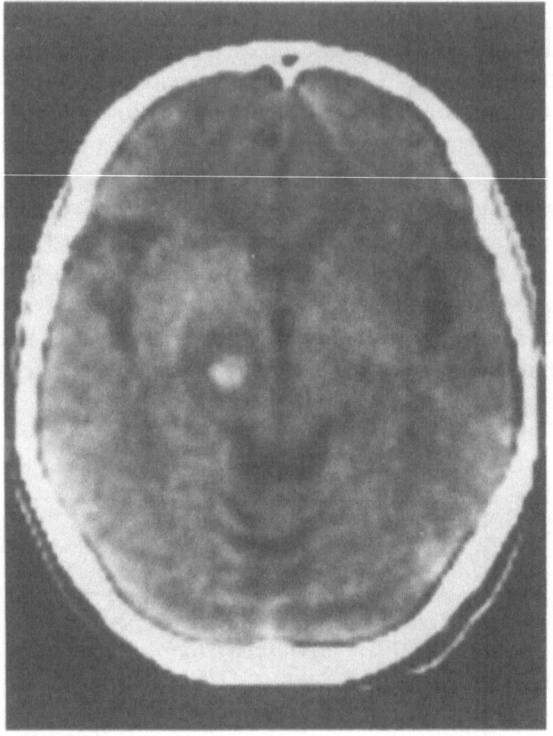

Figure 25.5 Stereotaxic lesion at 10 days post-operation, appearing as a small haemorrhagic infarct with some surrounding oedema.

This suggests a feedback system for integrated movements in such activities as chewing, feeding oneself (hand to mouth) and walking (Andrew and Rudolf, 1972, 1973).

TYPES OF TREMOR FOR WHICH STEREOTAXIS IS MOST USEFUL

Parkinsonism

The tremor of parkinsonism was the first to be treated, and it is of interest that the target for its alleviation is the same as that now used for tremor in other conditions which will be described. Usually the size of lesion required is substantially less in parkinsonism.

After the initial enthusiasm subsided, and after many operations had been performed only because of the lack of any effective alternative, the indications for surgery became clear. These included tremor and rigidity, particularly when predominantly unilateral. It was first found, however (Gillingham *et al.*, 1964), that, with carefully performed stereotaxis, if a smaller lesion had been made by other surgeons effectively, then an operation could be performed on the opposite side with safety, provided there was an interval of at least a number of weeks between the two procedures. The earlier large lesion produced by the inflatable balloon, followed by injection of chemicals, if performed on the second side could be disastrous. It was the use of microelectrode recording that permitted the making of smaller lesions and reduced the side-effects of operation on one side, allowing safer bilateral surgery. However, vegetative disturbances, akinesia or weakness, and impairment of balance, were often made worse by surgery, even when performed on one side. The patients with these problems are most likely to be benefited by L-dopa. When this drug became generally available 15 years ago, and particularly when carbidopa was added, the number of operations fell considerably and, in fact, there are very few of the younger surgeons today who are acquainted with stereotaxic surgery.

Unfortunately, Sinemet (L-dopa plus carbidopa) does not help the tremor as much as it does the rigidity and akinesia and, furthermore, it has undesirable side-effects, particularly when administered for a long time. These included the 'on'-'off' phenomenon, the need for frequent administration of small doses, and loss of effectiveness, as well as unpleasant oro-facial and limb dystonia. This has only recently been appreciated, so that patients are once again being referred for surgery, particularly when the proper indications exist. The time to perform the operation is considered to be when the tremor and rigidity are beginning seriously to interfere with the patient's professional or domestic life and work. It has been the experience of the author to treat patients whose tremor has persisted to a disabling degree for a number of years, in spite of long-term L-dopa administration, and then, when an operation has finally been suggested and performed, to see the tremor disappear following a successful lesion. It may be argued that when the tremor predominates, and particularly if it is unilateral, and provided that the general health of the patient is good, then an operation should be considered early rather than late, and Sinemet should be withheld until the other symptoms, which are not amenable to surgery, develop as the disease progresses. Following operation, the tremor is permanently relieved in 80–90% of cases (Ohye *et al.*, 1981), and there is a relapse rate of about 10% in the hands of the author, when there is some return of tremor, but rarely to the same extent as before the operation. The mortality rate should be less than 1% but the complication of hemiplegia is about 2% and more likely to occur in elderly hypertensives. The relief of rigidity may suggest some slight weakness which passes after one or two weeks.

Benign essential tremor

The results of thalamotomy in these cases are usually very good (Ohye *et al.*, 1981). They report 15 successfully treated patients, all requiring small lesions and with no late relapse. In the author's experience of 10 patients so treated, one developed hemiplegia which largely recovered, and one patient still had a persisting tremor. In three other cases, the tremor was much improved, and in the rest it almost completely disappeared, and certainly the functional use of the affected arm in these eight patients was considerably improved to the extent that it was possible to hold and drink a glass of water without spilling. Occasional myoclonic jerks were seen.

Now that beta-blockers are sometimes effective in this group, it is hoped that pharmacological development will render surgery unnecessary.

Tremor following head injury

Nine patients with post-traumatic tremor were successfully treated by operation, the tremor and associated involuntary myoclonic jerks being largely abolished, much increasing the use of the affected arm. In none of these had drugs given any benefit. Eight cases have recently been reported (Andrew *et al.*, 1982). They had all suffered severe closed head injuries and were under the age of 23 years at the time of the accident; older people would probably not have survived. They were the victims of road traffic accidents; with the improved primary care of such cases, it is likely that more such causes of tremor will be seen in the future. The tremor is both postural and kinetic, resting tremor usually being less pronounced. All the patients reported had shown ocular-motor disturbances after the injury, and in six the tremor appeared as they recovered from an initial hemiplegia. They also showed some cerebellar ataxia. The clinical findings supported the view that the causative lesion was located in the midbrain close to the red nucleus and brachium conjunctivum, and in one patient the CT scan showed a recent upper midbrain lesion (Holmes, 1904; Kremer *et al.*, 1947). Surgical complications included a worsening, usually temporary, of any dysarthria or ataxia of gait; if these are pronounced, then operation is now considered inadvisable, since their deterioration caused a severe handicap in two patients, outweighing the benefit from relief of tremor. In that series, the shortest interval between accident and surgery was three years. Since some of the patients were still growing, this was considered to be an excessive delay; every effort should be made to encourage independent and integrated use of the affected limb into everyday life, and this can only be achieved by abolition of the tremor by pharmacological means (which to date has been disappointing) or by surgical means.

Multiple sclerosis

There have been some remarkable improvements of tremor in these patients following thalamotomy. The tremor resembles that seen in the elderly with head injuries and, presumably, the causative lesion is situated in the same locality in the cerebral peduncle. As in the post-traumatic cases, drugs seem to have little influence. The chances of failure and of severe complications, including hemiplegia, worsened ataxia and exacerbation of the disease, present a formidable risk. This is particularly so in patients in whom these disabilities are already pronounced, and who are deteriorating. There are unfortunately few patients suitable for surgery, and in these the neurological condition should have been static for some considerable time. Pressures from the referring physician, and a sympathy for the patient in his terrible plight, may lead the surgeon to perform ill-advised operations, bringing this treatment into disrepute and depriving the few who could benefit. It is always explained to the patient and family that operation is very likely to help the tremor, on the one hand, but that there is a risk that there may be a temporary hemiparesis, and the other symptoms of the disease may be worse, particularly of gait and balance. Any pre-existing ataxia in the arm, for which the operation has been performed, will still be present after the thalamotomy, and ataxia, if severe, would be a contra-indication to an operation for tremor, since improved function would be only slight. When the disease has been static for two or three years, these post-operative complications described have not occurred. Even so, the operation is performed under steroid cover, 80 units ACTH daily being given for a 10 day period, starting immediately prior to the first stage, and then being reduced after 10 days. It is inadvisable to operate on the opposite side if the first side is successful, since the risk of pseudo-bulbar palsy and disturbances of gait and balance would be very great indeed. The author has operated on nine patients, and in three the results were very worth while; two died shortly after, and in four there was only slight benefit. It was from this group that the contra-indications to thalamotomy were learnt.

Other causes of tremor

These are rare, and include cerebrovascular accident as a cause, and writing tremor (Ohye *et al.*, 1981). They may both be associated with hemidystonia or focal dystonia respectively, which may also be improved surgically, although a larger lesion will usually be required.

THE FUTURE OF SURGICAL TREATMENT FOR TREMOR

Until fresh advances are made in pharmacology of the neurotransmitters involved in the different forms of tremor discussed, there will continue to be a place for surgical treatment. The methods described are invasive and destructive. To avoid the amount of invasion, stereotaxic radiosurgery has been suggested, but this would not allow adequate target localisation by cell recording, stimulation, or a reversible lesion. To avoid destruction of normal brain, a chronic electrode implanted under the thalamus near the nucleus of Luys and substantia nigra area, which stimulates the area when triggered by active movement of the affected limb, has been reported (Brice and McLellan, 1980). This was specifically designed for victims of multiple sclerosis. It will be interesting to follow any development of this project.

ACKNOWLEDGEMENTS

The author wishes to thank Dr H. Townsend, Dr N. de M. Rudolf and Dr. C. J. Fowler for their help with the microelectrical recordings over a period of nearly 20 years, as well as the Department of Clinical Measurement and Dr A. J. Hewer, at the Middlesex Hospital, London.

REFERENCES

Albe-Fessard, D., Arfel, G., Guiot, G., Hardy, J., Vourc'h, G., Hertzog, E., Aleonard, P. and Derome, P. (1962). Dérivations d'activités spontanées et evoquées dans les structures cérébrales de l'homme. *Rev. Neurol.*, **106**, 89–105.

Andrew, J., Fowler, C. J. and Harrison, M. J. G. (1982). Tremor after head injury and its treatment by stereotaxic surgery. *J. Neurol. Neurosurg. Psychiatr.*, **45**, 815–19.

Andrew, J. and Rudolf, N. de M. (1972). Micro-electrode recordings in the human thalamus during stereotaxic surgery. In Nicholson, J. P. (ed.), *Interdisciplinary Investigation of the Brain*, Plenum Press, London and New York.

Andrew, J. and Rudolf, N. de M. (1973). Somatic representation in the human thalamus. *J. Neurol. Neurosurg. Psychiatr.*, **36**, 154.

Andrew, J. and Watkins, E. S. (1969). *A Stereotaxic Atlas of the Human Thalamus and Adjacent Structures*, Williams and Wilkins, Baltimore.

Brice, J. and McLellan, L. (1980). Suppression of intention tremor by contingent deep brain stimulation. *Lancet*, **1**, 1221–2.

Bucy, P. C. and Case, J. T. (1939). Tremor: physiologic mechanism and abolition by surgical means. *Neurol. Psychiatr. (Chic.)*, **41**, 721–46.

Cooper, I. S. (1953). Ligation of anterior choroidal artery for involuntary movements—parkinsonism. *Psychiatr. Q.*, **27**, 317–19.

Cooper, I. S. and Bravo, G. J. (1958). Chemopallidectomy and chemothalamotomy. *J. Neurosurg.*, **15**, 244.

Cooper, I. S., Giono, G. and Terry, R. (1965). The cryogenic lesion. *Confin. Neurol.*, **26**, 161–77.

Fowler, C. J., Howe, N., Andrew, J. and Harrison, M. J. G. (1984). In preparation.

Gillingham, F. J., Kalyanaraman, S. and Donaldson, A. A. (1964). Bilateral stereotaxic lesions in the management of parkinsonism and the dyskinesias. *Br. Med. J.*, **5410**, 656–9.

Hassler, R. (1959). Anatomy of the thalamus. In Schaltenbrand, G. and Bailey, P. (eds), *Introduction to Stereotaxis, with an Atlas of the Human Brain*, Thieme, Stuttgart, pp. 230–90.

Hassler, R., Mundiger, F. and Riechert, T. (1979). *Stereotaxis in Parkinson's Syndrome*, Springer-Verlag, Berlin, Heidelberg and New York, pp. 201–4.

Holmes, G. (1904). On certain tremors in organic cerebral lesions. *Brain*, **27**, 327–75.

Howe, N. and Baldwin, A. and Fowler, C. J. (1983). In preparation.

Jasper, H. H. and Bertrand, G. (1966). Thalamic units involved in somate sensation in voluntary and involuntary movements in man. In Purpura, D. P. and Yahr, M. D. (eds), *The Thalamus*, Columbia University Press, New York, pp. 365–90.

Klemme, R. (1940). Surgical treatment of dystonia, paralysis agitans and athetosis. *Arch. Neurol. Psychiatr. (Chic.)*, **44**, 926.

Kremer, M., Ritchie Russell, W. and Smyth, G. E. (1947). A mid-brain syndrome following head injury. *J. Neurol. Neurosurg. Psychiatr.*, **10**, 49–60.

Meyers, R. (1940). Surgical procedure for post-encephalitic tremor with notes on the physiology of premotor fibres. *Arch. Neurol. Psychiatr. (Chic.)*, **44**, 455.

Meyers, R. (1942). Surgical interruption of the pallidofugal fibres. Its effect on the syndrome of paralysis agitans and technical considerations in its application. *NY State J. Med.*, **42**, 317-25.

Ohye, C., Hirai, T., Miyazaki, M., Shibazaki, T. and Nakajima, H. (1981). Vim thalamotomy for the treatment of various kinds of tremor. *Appl. Neurophysiol.*, **45**, 275-80.

Oliver, L. C. (1949). Surgery in Parkinson's disease. Division of lateral pyramidal tract for tremor: report on 48 operations. *Lancet*, **1**, 910-13.

Oliver, L. C. (1967). *Parkinson's Disease*, Heinemann Medical, London.

Parkinson, J. (1817). *An Essay on the Shaking Palsy*, Sherwood, Neely and Jones, London.

Putnam, T. J. (1940). Treatment of unilateral paralysis agitans by section of the lateral pyramidal tract. *Arch. Neurol. Psychiatr. (Chic.)*, **44**, 950-76.

Schaltenbrand, G. and Bailey, P. (1959). *Introduction to Stereotaxis, with an Atlas of the Human Brain*, Thieme, Stuttgart.

Spiegel, E. A. and Wycis, H. T. (1952). *Stereoencephalotomy*, Grune & Stratton, New York.

Talairach, J., David, M., Tournoux, P., Corredor, H. and Kvasina, T. (1957). *Atlas d'Anatomie Stéréotaxique*, Masson, Paris.

Walker, A. E. (1938). *The Primate Thalamus*, Chicago University Press, Chicago.

Walker, A. E. (1949). Cerebral pedunculotomy for the relief of involuntary movements. *Acta Psychiatr. Scand.*, **24**, 723-6.

SECTION 5
CEREBELLAR TREMOR

26
Cerebellar tremor: clinical aspects

STANLEY FAHN

There is perhaps no symptom in neurology whose anatomical basis or the physiology of whose production is less understood than those involuntary movements which, though varying in their character and accompanying conditions, are collectively known as tremors.

Holmes (1904)

HISTORICAL ASPECTS

When Parkinson (1817) described the entity 'the shaking palsy', which now bears the name of Parkinson's disease, he pointed out that clinicians had long distinguished between tremor while the body is at rest, which he called 'palpitation of the limbs'*, and tremor produced by attempts at voluntary motion, which he called simply 'tremor'. Although Parkinson described the disease in patients who had only tremor at rest, for a great many years thereafter the presence of any type of tremor commonly led to the condition being diagnosed as 'paralysis agitans' (Parkinson's disease). In Romberg's (1853) textbook, tremors are ascribed only to paralysis agitans, mercurial poisoning, alcoholism, fever, and to senile tremor; there is no mention of the cerebellum. Recognition that intention tremor was related to multiple sclerosis awaited the definitive description of that entity by Charcot (1868). There was disagreement initially as to whether tremor in multiple sclerosis is manifested only when voluntary movements are performed (see Hammond, 1871), but Charcot (1879) clearly differentiated the rest tremor of parkinsonism from the intention and action tremors of multiple sclerosis.

Benedikt (1889) was one of the first to localise action tremor. He described a patient who had a right oculomotor paralysis and a left-sided tremor that increased with voluntary activity. A tuberculoma was found in the right cerebral peduncle, as predicted by him. Benedikt postulated that action tremor is caused by lesions in the midbrain. Holmes (1904) described nine cases of tremor caused by midbrain lesions; two of the cases were verified by autopsy findings. The

*Called *Palmos* by Galen and *Tremor coactus* by de la Boë, according to Parkinson (1817).

355

patients had both an action-type (and sometimes intention) tremor and a rest tremor, as well as some signs of parkinsonism. Holmes emphasised that the intention (and action) tremor was due to involvement of the superior cerebellar peduncle or of the red nucleus. Today, we could assign the parkinsonian symptoms, including the tremor at rest, to destruction of monoaminergic fibres ascending through this region of the midbrain. To support his deduction that the action tremor in his patients was due to a lesion of the superior cerebellar peduncle, Holmes cited the studies of Ferrier and Turner (1894), who produced action tremor in monkeys with ablative lesions of the ipsilateral superior cerebellar peduncle. He also cited the case report of Sander (1898) describing intention tremor associated with a tumour of the ipsilateral cerebellar hemisphere that destroyed the dentate nucleus and superior cerebellar peduncle, and also the report of Touche (1900).

Holmes (1917) studied the effect of acute cerebellar injuries from gunshot wounds acquired during World War I. He recognised that action tremor did not develop acutely, but became more prominent in later stages. Holmes also recognised the existence of postural tremor in patients with cerebellar injuries. He referred to this as 'deviation from the line of movement' and attributed the oscillating swaying of the elevated and unsupported limbs as being due to hypotonia of the muscles that normally fix the proximal joints of the limbs. Although Holmes referred to this postural tremor as static tremor, he clearly indicated in this paper that he was not defining static tremor as rest tremor. He 'never observed tremor while the limbs and body were at rest and fully supported but it often appears during the maintènance of posture that requires muscular contractions'. Holmes noted that action tremor requires the activity of agonist and antagonist muscles, and that in postural tremor the role of the antagonist is to counteract the force of gravity. Holmes also commented about this type of postural tremor involving the head and body when the patient is sitting and standing, respectively. He felt this was 'due to irregular and discontinuous contractions of muscles that should maintain the attitude'. Today, we refer to this head and body tremor as titubation.

In his Croonian Lectures delineating the clinical symptoms of cerebellar disease, Holmes (1922) pointed out that there are three types of tremor associated with cerebellar lesions: postural, intention and rest. However, he then described rest tremor as being associated with midbrain lesions, rather than cerebellar lesions per se. He also continued to use the term 'static tremor' for our current definition of postural tremor. In his last major paper on cerebellar symptomatology, Holmes (1939) discussed recent observations by other investigators and did not review tremor in any detail.

In more recent developments, Cooper (1960a) showed that ventrolateral thalamotomy can relieve contralateral intention tremor. Most recently, Gilman et al. (1981) published a major scholarly review of cerebellar disorders and presented data on the incidence of symptoms in 162 patients with focal cerebellar lesions.

CLINICAL FEATURES

Symptomatology

In addition to tremor, which is discussed in greater detail below, there are a host of other symptoms associated with cerebellar pathology in humans. Holmes (1917, 1922, 1939) was a most careful observer of the results of cerebellar lesions, and he analysed his findings to list a specific set of symptoms that occur with cerebellar pathology. This list includes muscle hypotonia, which in turn leads to abnormal postural attitudes, alteration of associated movements, pendular tendon reflexes, postural tremor and the rebound phenomenon. The most prominent cerebellar symptoms are those associated with voluntary locomotor activity due to faulty agonism, antagonism, synergy and fixation. These include dysmetria, decomposition of movement into its component parts, slower rate of movement, lack of 'check', incoordination of movement, dysdiadochokinesia, poor equilibrium with wide-based station and gait, ataxic gait and intention tremor. Phonation and particularly articulation of speech are affected to produce a slurred-type of dysarthria. With involvement of the vestibular system, nystagmus may occur. I use the term 'ataxia of the limbs' (limb ataxia) to indicate a combination of dysmetria, lack of check, asynergia and decomposition of movement. I find that many clinicians fail to distinguish between limb ataxia and intention tremor, and tend to use the term 'intention tremor' to refer to both types of phenomena. Since they can usually be differentiated if attention is paid to doing so, and because their pathophysiology and anatomical localisations (and probably their future pharmacotherapy) are most likely different, I believe we should be precise and distinguish between these two phenomena.

Tremor

Definitions

Tremor, defined by Holmes (1904) as involuntary oscillations of any part of the body around any plane, can be divided into four major phenomenological categories.

Rest tremor refers to tremor that is present when the affected body part is in repose and supported against gravity so that there are no normally required muscle contractions.

Postural tremor refers to tremor that is present when the affected body part is not in voluntary locomotor activity except to maintain it in a posture against the force of gravity. Common examples of such postural activity are sustaining the arms horizontally in front of the body and keeping the head erect and the body erect. Postural tremor can be considered as a special form of action tremor.

Action tremor refers to tremor present during voluntary locomotor activity, such as when moving a limb, when pouring liquid from a cup and when writing.

Intention tremor refers to an exaggeration of action tremor when the limb is reaching for a target, and is most pronounced on approaching the destination.

This classification is useful because placing tremor in the appropriate category is the first step to diagnosis (Marshall, 1968; Fahn, 1972; Jankovic and Fahn, 1980). Moreover, these descriptive adjectives, similarly defined, are also applied to categorise other abnormal involuntary movements, such as myoclonus and dystonia. Such consistency in movement disorder terminology is highly desirable.

One problem in discussing tremor is that different terminologies for the same type of tremor have been used by different authors. This creates confusion, and one must be careful to interpret the results of a study according to the definitions given by the author and not necessarily by the definitions that the reader may have assumed. Commonly used terms in the literature are static, kinetic, ataxic and terminal tremors.

Static tremor has been used to refer to rest tremor (Marshall, 1968; Fahn, 1972; Griffith, 1973) and also to postural tremor (Holmes, 1917, 1922; Gilman *et al.*, 1981). Some authors have confused Holmes's use of static tremor as meaning rest tremor (Carpenter, 1961). Since the term 'static' can cause such confusion, it is best avoided.

Kinetic tremor has been used to refer to both action tremor and intention tremor (Gilman *et al.*, 1981).

Ataxic tremor has been used to refer to a combination of limb ataxia and intention tremor (Holmes, 1917; Carpenter, 1961).

Terminal tremor refers to tremor that develops as the limb is approaching the target.

In contrast, intention tremor has come to mean tremor that is present also during the entire voluntary locomotor activity but is exaggerated as the target is approached. Gilman *et al.* (1981) do not like the term 'intention', claiming that its meaning is ambiguous and could 'be used in reference to tremors on contemplating, initiating, performing, or completing a movement'. However, the term is so commonly used that its meaning is usually unambiguous and it has constantly been defined as in the above paragraph.

Intention tremor

Intention tremor is the most classic form of cerebellar tremor. But, in all probability, it is secondary to a lesion of the main neocerebellar outflow pathway, the dentate nucleus and its fibre bundle, the superior cerebellar peduncle (Holmes, 1904, 1917, 1922), rather than to a lesion of the cerebellar cortex. Animal studies support this concept (Ferrier and Turner, 1894; Botterell and Fulton, 1938; Carrea and Mettler, 1947; Peterson *et al.*, 1949; Carpenter, 1961). Since there are few clinicopathological studies of patients available to confirm or deny this concept, it is useful to mention the case of a patient with postural, action and intention tremors of both arms, in whom there are kinematographic recordings of the tremor and a pathological study of the post-mortem brain. This patient had demyelinating plaques in both superior cerebellar peduncles secondary to multiple sclerosis. There were also plaques in the middle cerebellar peduncle and in the cerebellar white matter, but not in the cerebellar cortex. This demonstration is compatible with, but does not prove, the concept that a lesion of the superior cerebellar peduncle may be essential for the pathogenesis of intention tremor.

The severity of the intention tremor influences the amplitude of the tremor, the timing of its appearance during the locomotor activity and whether it is distal or proximal. When mild, the tremor appears only when the limb is approaching the target, and it tends to affect only the distal musculature. The more severe the tremor, the sooner it appears with action, even when the limb is still far from the target. In other words, it now also becomes an action tremor, but the amplitude still intensifies as the target is approached. This is the most common appearance of intention tremor. In this form, milder tremors will tend to be located distally in the limb, and more severe tremors tend to involve the proximal muscles as well. The amplitude of intention tremor ranges from barely perceptible distal oscillations as the finger approaches the target to gross, ballistic-type oscillations proximally with the slightest of active movements. In its most severe form, intention tremor occurs with any degree of locomotor activity, including posture holding. When the tremor is even moderately severe and present with posture holding, the arms may oscillate about the shoulder joints, producing a characteristic proximal postural tremor, known as 'wing-beating'. The legs can also be involved in intention tremor, including wing-beating. Although some authors refer to intention tremor as being proximal (Gilman *et al.*, 1981), it can also be distal. Most authors cite a frequency of about 3 Hz for intention tremor.

As discussed above, intention tremor, although commonly referred to as a 'cerebellar' tremor, is probably due to a lesion of the cerebellar outflow pathway, i.e. the dentate nucleus and its fibre bundle, the superior cerebellar peduncle. Lesions of this pathway, as distal from the cerebellum as the red nucleus (Carpenter, 1961), will produce an intention tremor ipsilateral to the side of the 'involved' cerebellum. Thus, with a lesion of the red nucleus involving the fibres of the superior cerebellar peduncle passing through this area, the tremor is contralateral to the side of the lesion since the superior cerebellar peduncle has already decussated. Lesions in this area of the midbrain will frequently also involve the ascending dopaminergic nigro-striatal pathway and produce a contralateral rest tremor as well as the intention tremor. This combination of tremors is referred to as 'midbrain' or 'rubral' tremor. The most common disorder to cause intention tremor is multiple sclerosis. Wilson's disease, although far less common, can also produce such a tremor. Essential tremor can sometimes be difficult to differentiate from intention tremor since, although primarily a distal tremor with posture holding that does not usually increase during action, it usually intensifies somewhat as the hand approaches a target. Thus, there is an intention tremor component to essential tremor. The presence of any cerebellar or other neurological findings on examination can be helpful in classifying the tremor as intention tremor rather than as essential tremor. Contrariwise, if tremor is the only finding, then essential tremor or even enhanced physiological tremor must be seriously considered.

Postural tremor

The second type of cerebellar tremor is a postural tremor due to compensation of drifting of hypotonic muscles (Holmes, 1917, 1922). This produces a very slow oscillation of the outstretched arms about the shoulder joints. This tremor tends to develop as the patient maintains the arms in the outstretched posture. The tremor is explained in terms of alternate contraction of certain groups of muscles and their antagonists. Brain (1940) stated it clearly:

> The hypotonic fixators fail to maintain the posture of the unsupported limb, with the result that the voluntarily contracting antagonists pull the limb out of the desired alignment. The appropriate fixators for this new position fail to maintain it, owing to their lack of tone, with the result that the old agonists, which for the moment have become the new antagonists, by their contractions pull the limb into its previous position. Consequently the limb oscillates around the point it should occupy. This kind of tremor may develop in any part of the body, when that part has to be maintained in the absence of support in any new position against gravity.

This type of tremor of the axial muscles affects the head and trunk when the patient is erect; it is known as titubation. Truncal titubation develops when the patient is standing, and head titubation can also occur when the patient is sitting as well. Although titubation has been considered by Holmes (1917) to be a postural tremor due to hypotonic muscles, resulting in muscular contraction to maintain the postural attitude, it seems reasonable to consider that it may also be a more 'active' tremor and may be due to active rhythmical contractions of the axial musculature. Mauritz et al. (1981) suggested that delayed and enhanced long-loop reflexes, which they observed in seven patients with anterior lobe cortical cerebellar atrophy, may be responsible for truncal antero-posterior sway.

Other tremors

Griffith (1973) described five patients with cerebellar disease who also had persistent or transient rest tremors. Four of the patients had space-occupying lesions, and it is possible that there were pressure effects on the midbrain to produce the rest tremor. One of these four patients was autopsied; although the midbrain was structurally normal, no chemical studies were carried out to determine if the nigro-striatal dopaminergic pathway was involved. Not enough information was obtained on the fifth patient to be able to reach any conclusion about her. It is impossible to reach any decision as to what the mechanism is for the observed rest tremor in these patients, but the data are not adequate to implicate pure cerebellar pathology as the sole explanation.

Silfverskiold (1977) described a 3 Hz 'kicking' tremor of the leg in alcoholic cerebellar degeneration. The leg is held up against gravity, flexed at the hip and knee. If the leg was held in a slightly abducted posture, a 3 Hz synchronous coarse adduction tremor in the thighs also appeared.

TREATMENT

Treatment of intention tremor is far from satisfactory. Adding weights to the limbs can reduce the severity of the tremor (Chase *et al.*, 1965; Hewer *et al.*, 1972), but this approach was of therapeutic benefit in only 36% of 50 patients studied by Hewer *et al.* (1972).

Cooper (1960a) showed that ventrolateral thalamotomy can relieve the contra-lateral intention tremor. This has been confirmed by a number of other reports (Cooper, 1960b, 1965; Broager and Fog, 1962; Krayenbuhl and Yasargil, 1962, Laitinen, 1965; Fox and Kurtzke, 1966 Samra *et al.*, 1970).

Rascol *et al.* (1981) reported that 5-hydroxytryptophan, the precursor of serotonin, can reduce cerebellar symptoms, including intention tremor. Details are meagre. Their study has not yet been replicated and it awaits confirmation.

Recently, Sabra *et al.* (1982) reported that isoniazid (800 to 1200 mg daily) reduced severe intention tremor in all four patients with multiple sclerosis to whom it was administered. These workers postulate that the improvement may be due to increased cerebral GABA content with isoniazid treatment. This study also needs confirmation.

An effective pharmacotherapeutic approach to treating cerebellar tremor is clearly needed.

REFERENCES

Benedikt, M. (1889). Tremblement avec paralysie croisée du moteur oculaire commun. *Bull. Med.*, **3**, 547-8; English translation published in Wolf, J. K. (1971). *The Classical Brain Stem Syndromes*, C. C. Thomas, Springfield, IL, pp. 103-9.

Botterell, E. H. and Fulton, J. F. (1938). Functional localization in the cerebellum of primates. III. Lesion of hemispheres (neocerebellum). *J. Comp. Neurol.*, **69**, 63-87.

Brain, W. R. (1940). *Recent Advances in Neurology*, Blakiston, Philadelphia, p. 141.

Broager, B. and Fog, T. (1962). Thalamotomy for the relief of intention tremor in multiple sclerosis. *Acta Neurol. Scand.*, **38**, Suppl. 3, 143-56.

Carpenter, M. B. (1961). Brain stem and infratentorial neuraxis in experimental dyskinesia. *Arch. Neurol.*, **5**, 504-24.

Carrea, R. M. E. and Mettler, F. A. (1947). Physiologic consequences following extensive removals of the cerebellar cortex and deep cerebellar nuclei and effect of secondary cerebral ablations in the primate. *J. Comp. Neurol.*, **87**, 169-288.

362   S. Fahn

Charcot, J. M. (1868). *Gaz. Hop. Civ. Milit.*, 41, as cited by Wilson, S. A. K. (1940). *Neurology*, vol. 1, Williams & Wilkins, Baltimore, p. 148.
Charcot, J. M. (1879). *Clinical Lectures on Diseases of the Nervous System*, vol. I, 2nd edn, transl. Sigerson, G., Henry C. Lea, Philadelphia.
Chase, R. A., Cullen, J. K. Jr, Sullivan, S. A. and Ommaya, A. K. (1965). Modification of intention tremor in man. *Nature*, 206, 485–7.
Cooper, I. S. (1960a). Neurosurgical relief of intention tremor due to cerebellar disease and multiple sclerosis. *Arch. Phys. Med.*, 41, 1–4.
Cooper, I. S. (1960b). Neurosurgical alleviation of intention tremor of multiple sclerosis and cerebellar disease. *New Engl. J. Med.*, 263, 441–4.
Cooper, I. S. (1965). Clinical and physiologic implications of thalamic surgery for disorders of sensory communication: II. Intention tremor, dystonia, Wilson's disease and torticollis. *J. Neurol. Sci.*, 2, 520–33.
Fahn, S. (1972). Differential diagnosis of tremors. *Med. Clin. N. Am.*, 56, 1363–75.
Ferrier, D. and Turner, W. A. (1894). A record of experiments illustrative of the symptomatology and degenerations following lesions of the cerebellum and its peduncles and related structures in the monkey. *Phil. Trans. R. Soc. B.*, 185, 719–78.
Fox, J. L. and Kurtzke, J. F. (1966). Trauma-induced intention tremor relieved by stereotaxic thalamotomy. *Arch. Neurol.*, 15, 247–51.
Gilman, S., Bloedel, J. R. and Lechtenberg, R. (1981). *Disorders of the Cerebellum*, Davis, Philadelphia.
Griffith, H. (1973). Static (resting) cerebellar tremor. *Proc. R. Soc. Med.*, 66, 36–7.
Hammond, W. A. (1871). *A Treatise on Diseases of the Nervous System*. Appleton, New York.
Hewer, R. L., Cooper, R. and Morgan, M. H. (1972). An investigation into the value of treating intention tremor by weighting the affected limb. *Brain*, 95, 579–90.
Holmes, G. (1904). On certain tremors in organic cerebral lesions. *Brain*, 27, 327–75.
Holmes, G. (1917). The symptoms of acute cerebellar injuries from gunshot wounds. *Brain*, 40, 461–535.
Holmes, G. (1922). The Croonian Lectures on the clinical symptoms of cerebellar disease and their interpretation. *Lancet*, 1, 1177–82.
Holmes, G. (1939). The cerebellum in man. *Brain*, 62, 1–30.
Jankovic, J. and Fahn, S. (1980). Physiologic and pathologic tremors. Diagnosis, mechanism, and management. *Ann. Intern. Med.*, 93, 460–5.
Krayenbuhl, H. and Yasargil, M. G. (1962). Relief of intention tremor due to multiple sclerosis by stereotaxic thalamotomy. *Confin. Neurol.*, 22, 368–74.
Laitinen, L. (1965). Stereotaxic treatment of hereditary tremor. *Acta Neurol. Scand.*, 41, 74–9.
Marshall, J. (1968). Tremor, In Vinken, P. J. and Bruyn, G. W. (eds), *Handbook of Clinical Neurology*, vol. 6, North-Holland, Amsterdam, pp. 809–25.
Mauritz, K. H., Schmitt, C. and Dichgans, J. (1981). Delayed and enhanced long latency reflexes as the possible cause of postural tremor in late cerebellar atrophy. *Brain*, 104, 97–116.
Parkinson, J. (1817). *An Essay on the Shaking Palsy*, Sherwood, Neely and Jones, London.
Peterson, E. W., Magoun, H. W., McCulloch, W. S. and Lindsley, D. B. (1949). Production of postural tremor. *J. Neurophysiol.*, 12, 371–84.
Rascol, A., Clanet, M., Montastruc, J. L., Delage, W. and Guiraud-Chaumeil, B. (1981). L5H Tryptophan in the cerebellar syndrome treatment. *Biomedicine*, 35, 112–13.

Romberg, M. H. (1853). *A Manual on the Nervous Diseases of Man*, vol. II, transl. Sieveking, E. H., Sydenham Society, London.

Sabra, A. F., Hallett, M., Sudarsky, L. and Mullally, W. (1982). Treatment of action tremor in multiple sclerosis with isoniazid. *Neurology*, 32, A113.

Samra, K., Waltz, J. M., Riklan, M., Koslow, M. and Cooper, I. S. (1970). Relief of intention tremor by thalamic surgery. *J. Neurol. Neurosurg. Psychiatr.*, 33, 7–15.

Sander, M. (1898). Ein pathologisch-anatomischer Beitrag sur Functin des Klein-hirns. *Dtsch Z. Nervenheil.*, 12, 363–83.

Silfverskiold, B. P. (1977). A 3/sec leg tremor in a 'cerebellar' syndrome. *Acta Neurol. Scand.*, 55, 385–93.

Touche, R. (1900). Deux cas de remollissement du cervelet (pseudosclerose en plaques cérébelleuses. Chorée cérébelleuse). *Rev. Neurol. (Paris)*, 8, 149–152.

27
Motor control in cerebellar tremor

P. RONDOT and N. BATHIEN

INTRODUCTION

Cerebellar lesions can provoke two main types of tremors (Rondot *et al.*, 1979), kinetic and postural:

Kinetic tremor is the most common. It is characterised by a succession of discontinuous contractions, occurring when the hand is directed towards an object, in the finger-to-nose test for example, provoking a jerky movement without altering its direction. 'Instead of being continuous, tonic as in normal states, it is discontinuous, clonic, epileptoid' (Thomas and Durupt, 1914). Often, oscillations perpendicular to the direction of movement also occur, which are provoked by the rhythmical contraction of the proximal muscles of the shoulder. These oscillations next to the target provoke an intention tremor. Where this tremor is particularly intense, it appears from the beginning of the movement and gives a 'clonic' aspect to the contractions, which can simulate myoclonus. We have proposed to call it *hyperkinetic tremor* (Rondot *et al.*, 1972); it is common in multiple sclerosis.

Postural tremor can also be found occasionally, particularly when the amplitude of the kinetic tremor is large: the finger that is maintained level with the target at the end of a movement can only be kept so with tremor.

There is a very particular spontaneous rhythmical activity that follows lesions to the dentate nucleus; it can be localised to the velo-laryngo-pharyngeal muscles, and is called *palatal myoclonus*. This activity can occasionally spread to the muscles of the limbs, 'myoclonies squelettiques' of French authors. The term 'myoclonus' is probably a misnomer because the activity has the characteristics of tremor (Rondot and Ben Hamida, 1968). This activity is also observed in cases of tegmental bundle lesions. Owing to its particular characteristics, it will not be discussed further here.

METHODOLOGY

We have studied cerebellar tremor in seven cases of cerebellar atrophy, three cases of cerebellar hemisphere tumours and 10 cases of multiple sclerosis. It is most typical with cerebellar atrophy, in the absence of additional lesions to the posterior columns and pyramidal tracts.

This study has been carried out by recording with a potentiometer and an accelerometer the displacement and acceleration of the flexion and extension movements of the forearm during the gesture of bringing the forefinger to the nose. In 14 cases, the device used by Conrad *et al.* (1974) with monkeys was adapted to human beings (Bathien *et al.*, 1984): the patient was sitting down with the elbow in a fixed position and the forearm lying in a splint that was mobile around the axis of the elbow. The patient was asked to move his forefinger, from an intermediary position, between two target positions, illuminated at random and requiring a movement either of flexion or of extension of the forearm (figure 27.1). In certain cases, these movements were carried out before and after applying 100 Hz vibrations to the tendon of the triceps by means of a Heiwa-Denshi vibrator. The displacement obtained was up to 2 mm.

In cases of cerebellar hemisyndrome, the other side was recorded as a control.

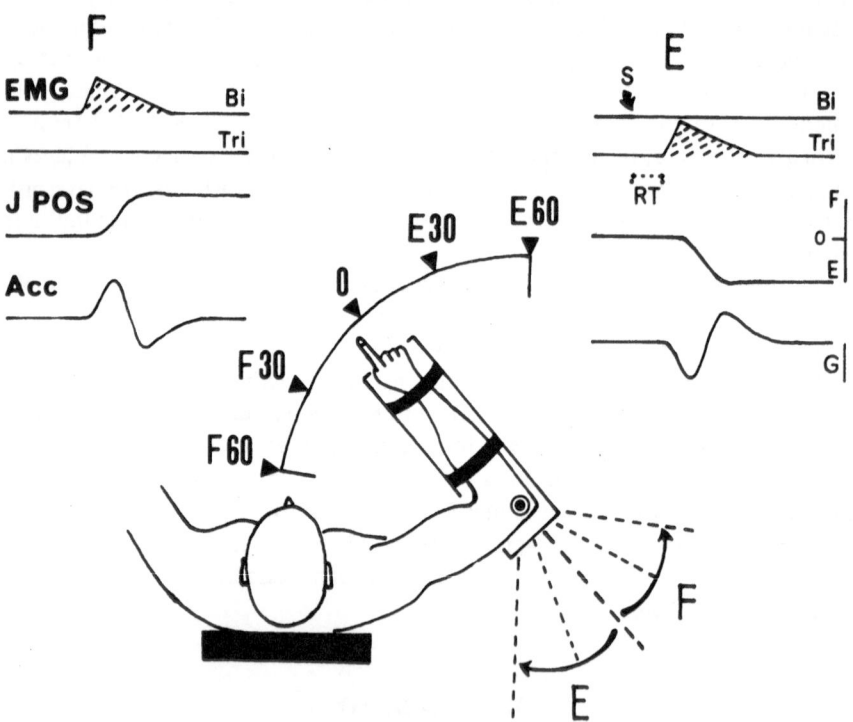

Figure 27.1 Flexion and extension movements at the elbow joint between two targets indicated on the screen by coloured lights.

RESULTS

In order to study the disorder of motor control in cerebellar tremor, it is necessary to observe it throughout the sequence of movement, i.e. the beginning of the movement, its development, its end, and maintenance of posture will be considered successively.

The beginning of the movement

The beginning of the movement is characterised by a longer reaction time than that of the healthy side. This delay is from 60 to 80 ms for the biceps and triceps muscles (cf. table 27.1). The application of vibrations does not modify this result.

Table 27.1 Changes in reaction times in a patient with a unilateral cerebellar syndrome. Reaction time was measured from the warning visual signal to the onset of the EMG activity in the agonist muscle. Triceps was recorded during extension and biceps during flexion. Values are mean ± SEM. The *p* values are two-tailed significance levels of the comparison of reaction time in affected side against control side.

Type of movement	*Reaction time (ms)*		p value
	Control side	*Affected side*	
Extension, $n = 15$	171.89 ± 9.07	253.53 ± 15.18	$p < 0.001$
Flexion	178.16 ± 10.92	238.53 ± 15.55	$0.04 < p < 0.01$

The movement

The EMG activity, instead of being tonic progressive, is registered as relatively short wide bursts which occurred earlier in the course of the movement with more severe cerebellar syndrome. These bursts were recorded in the agonist at a frequency of 3-7 Hz. The antagonist was also frequently the site of a simultaneous burst of activity (figure 27.2). Sometimes only the agonist presented this type of activity; sometimes, more rarely, the burst alternated from agonist to antagonist. In the same patient, a synchronisation of agonist-antagonist activities with slow movements and an alternation with rapid movements was observed.

The bursts appeared earlier during movement when its acceleration was greater (figure 27.3).

The proximal muscles of the upper limb were often the site of activity, even though the elbow was supported. This activity, more intense than in the normal patient, predominated in the deltoid and infra-spinatus muscles during extension and in the pectoralis major during flexion. When the activity of the agonist was rhythmical, this rhythm spreads to the proximal muscles of the limb (figure 27.3), provoking large vertical oscillations when the elbow was not supported.

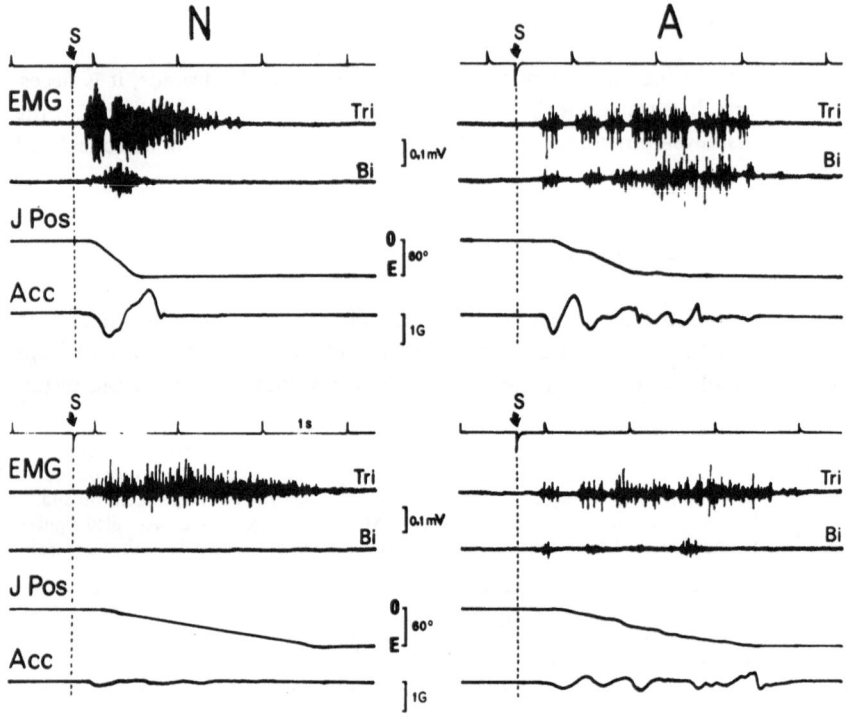

Figure 27.2 Extension movements of the elbow in a patient with unilateral cerebellar deficit. Traces are (from the top downwards): timescale with marker of visual signal (S); triceps EMG (Tri); biceps EMG (Bi); position of the elbow (J Pos); and accelerometric recording of the movement (Acc). Samples of 60° movements with an initial peak acceleration of 1.0g and 0.1g are compared. (N = normal side; A = affected side.) Note the bursting activity from the affected side.

When vibrations of 100 Hz frequency were applied to the tendons of the biceps or triceps muscles, a decrease, often even the disappearance, of the rhythmical bursts occurred (figure 27.4) and regularised the movement.

It should be noted that the movement of the cerebellar patient, like that of the normal subject (figure 27.2), began with a burst of activity of a phasic aspect recorded on the agonist. However, in the case of the cerebellar subject, contrary to what is observed in the normal patient, the activity that followed this first starting burst was also fragmented in bursts, which appeared clinically as a kinetic tremor (figure 27.2). In the normal patient, or on the normal side, the activity that follows the first and only burst appears continuous and tonic. It was very difficult for the cerebellar patient to accomplish a slow movement with small acceleration.

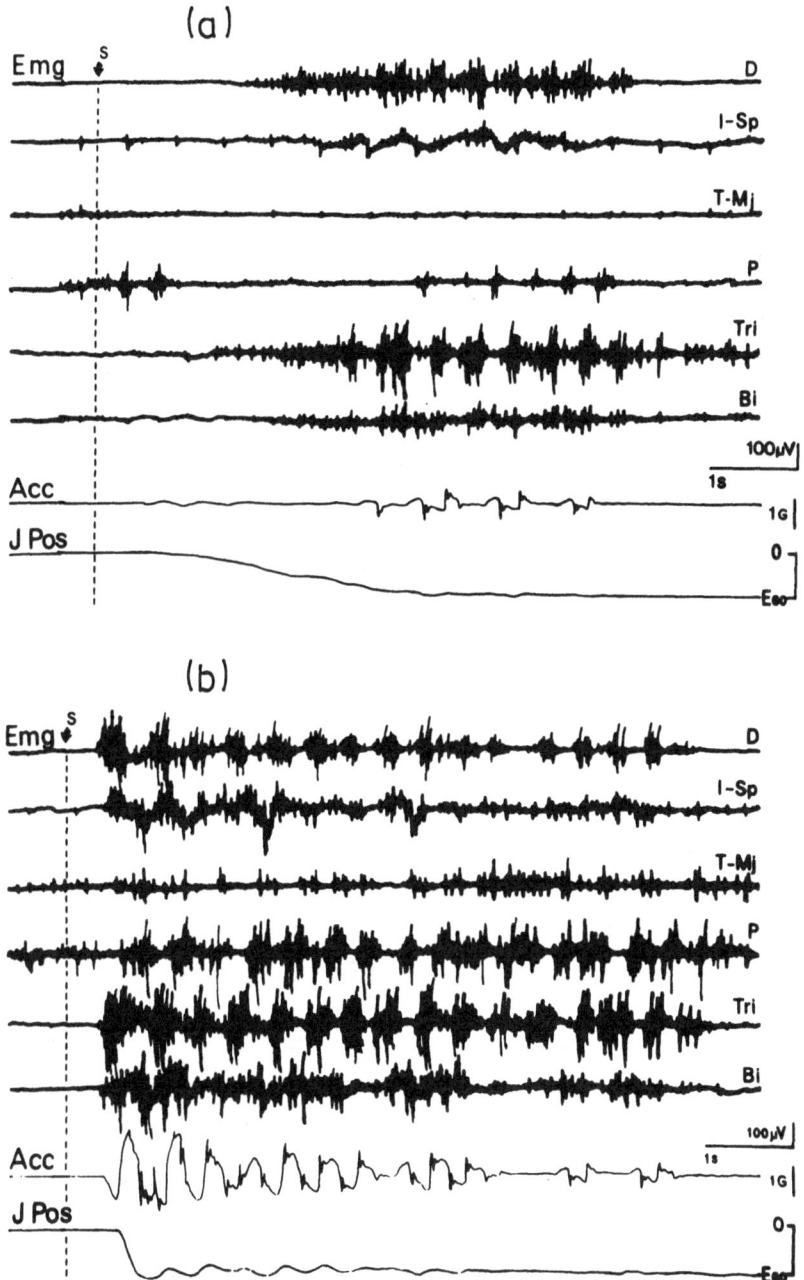

Figure 27.3 Cerebellar tremor initiated by extension movements of the elbow. Traces are (from the top downwards): EMG of the shoulder muscles (D = deltoid, I-Sp = infra-spinatus, T-Mj = teres major, P = pectoralis) and the arm muscles (Tri = triceps, Bi = biceps); accelerometric recording (Acc); and position of the elbow (J Pos). Note the number of bursts according to the level of acceleration and the bursting activity in proximal muscles.

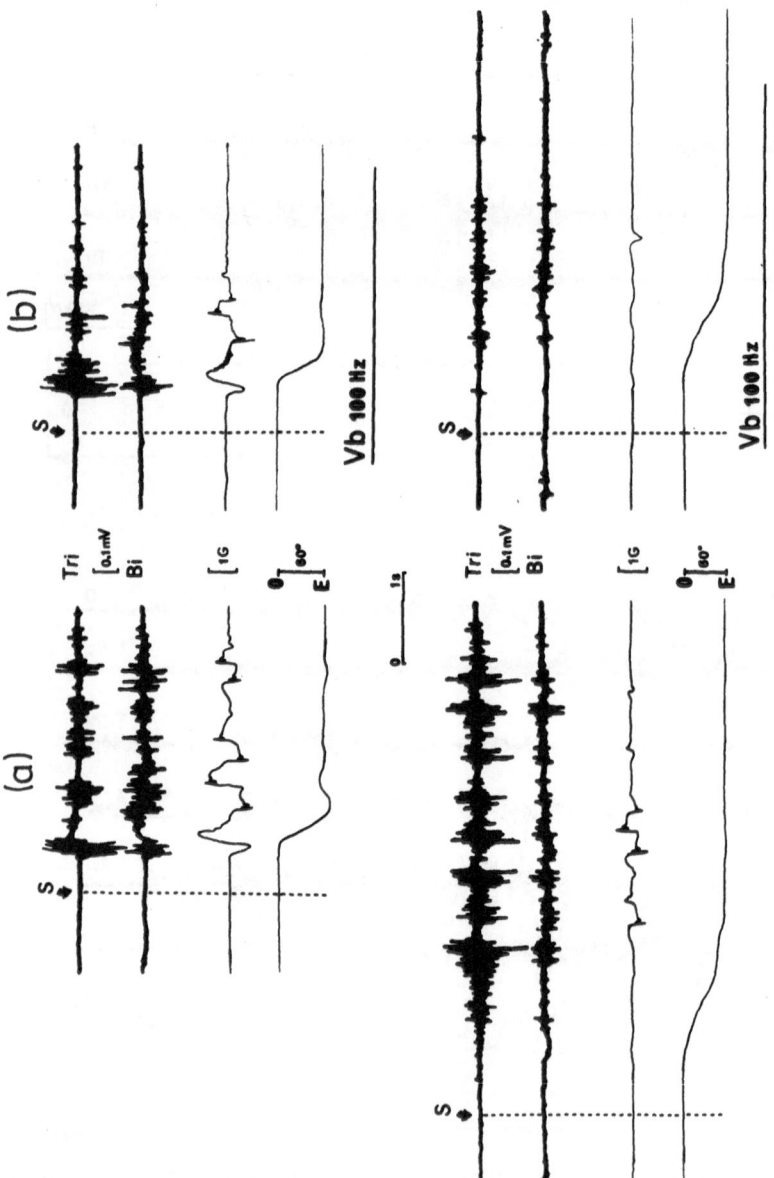

Figure 27.4 Extension movements of the elbow in a patient (a) before and (b) during vibrations applied to the tendon of the triceps.

The end of the movement

This was characterised by accentuation of the rhythmical oscillations, particularly in the hyperkinetic tremor (figure 27.5). When the tremor did not appear during the movement, one or more oscillations, which were sometimes only visible on the accelerometric recording, were evident at the end of it. The completion of movement is inaccurate and delayed, resulting in overshooting of the target followed by one or more adjustments. At the end of the movement, a rhythmical activity of variable frequency, 4 to 8 Hz, occasionally persisted in certain groups of muscles, often at a distance from the agonists (figure 27.4). The rhythmical bursts were not separated from each other by the phase of silence that is characteristic of parkinsonian tremor (Rondot and Bathien, 1976). The activity often lasted several seconds, whereas on other occasions it persisted for as long as muscular contraction was maintained to hold a fixed posture (figure 27.6). In this case the tremor often, but not always, resulted from activity alternating from agonist to antagonist.

DISCUSSION

The first anomaly observed during this study was the increase in reaction time for the initiation of movement. Holmes (1917, 1922) has already pointed out this anomaly, which Thomas (1937) called dyschronometry. In unilateral cerebellar syndrome, when a patient is asked to bring both forefingers simultaneously to the nose, a delay is noted for the forefinger on the cerebellar side. This delay at the beginning of movement does not account for the onset of the cerebellar tremor. However, such a delay in the antagonist muscle is the cause of the oscillations at the end of the movement, in that because the contraction of the antagonist is delayed it is unable efficiently to slow down the movement at the target. It should be noted that hypotonia cannot be held responsible for this delay in contraction. Indeed, if the muscular tonus is increased with the vibratory tonic reflex (Matthews, 1966), the subsequent delay is not shortened. This increase in reaction time may thus be attributed to a central effect. This effect may be due either to a decrease in tonic precentral discharge levels, or to the fact that the movement command that reached the cerebellum as a specific signal has been relayed too late to spinal motor neurones via thalamus and motor cortex. Meyer-Lohmann *et al.*'s (1977) experimental study is in favour of this last hypothesis, which is not contradicted by our observations.

In kinetic tremor, the oscillations at the end of movement (see above) must be distinguished from the oscillations that appear during the course of movement. These oscillations may be due to various causes. They may depend on a central mechanism that could act as either a thalamic or a cortical pacemaker, sending impulses to the spinal cord after having been liberated of the inhibiting cerebellar influences, or, in the absence of a pacemaker, following a mechanism similar to

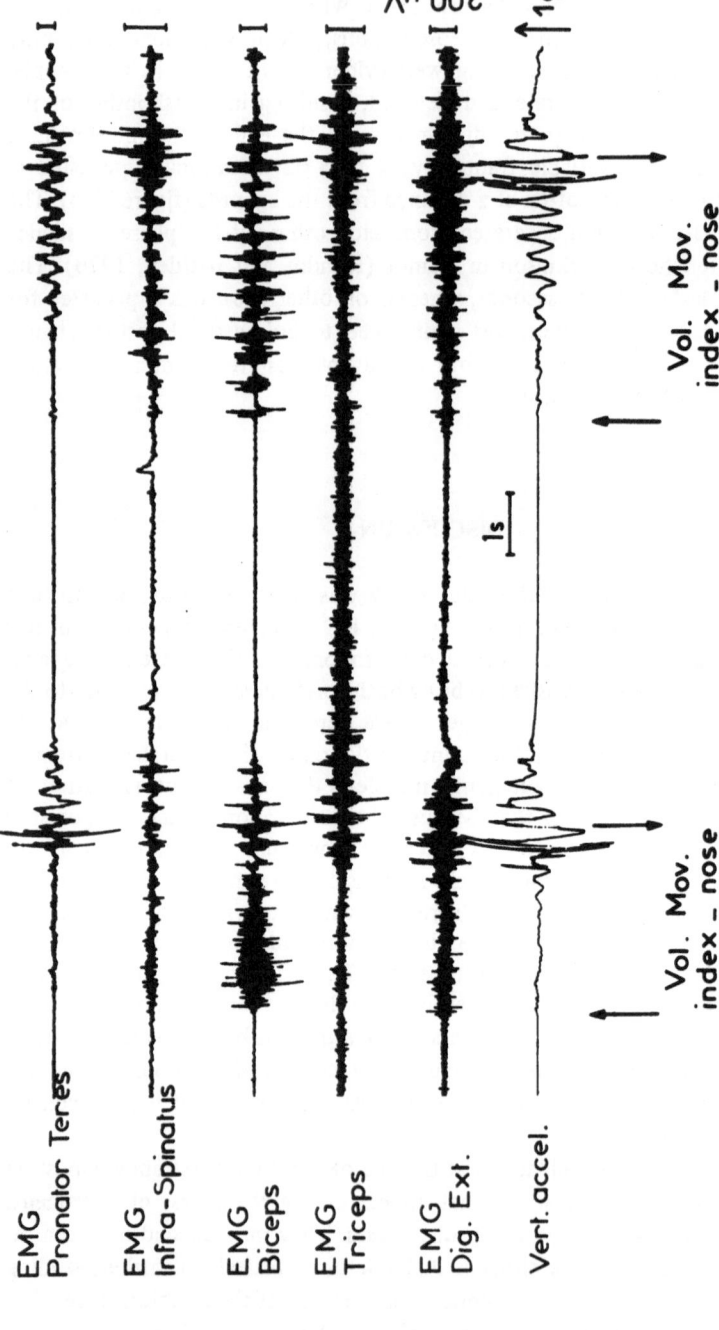

Figure 27.5 Hyperkinetic tremor, EMG activity in pronator teres, infra-spinatus, biceps, triceps and digitorum extensor; and accelerometric recording of the movement (vert. accel.). Note accentuation of the rhythmical oscillations at the end of the flexion movement.

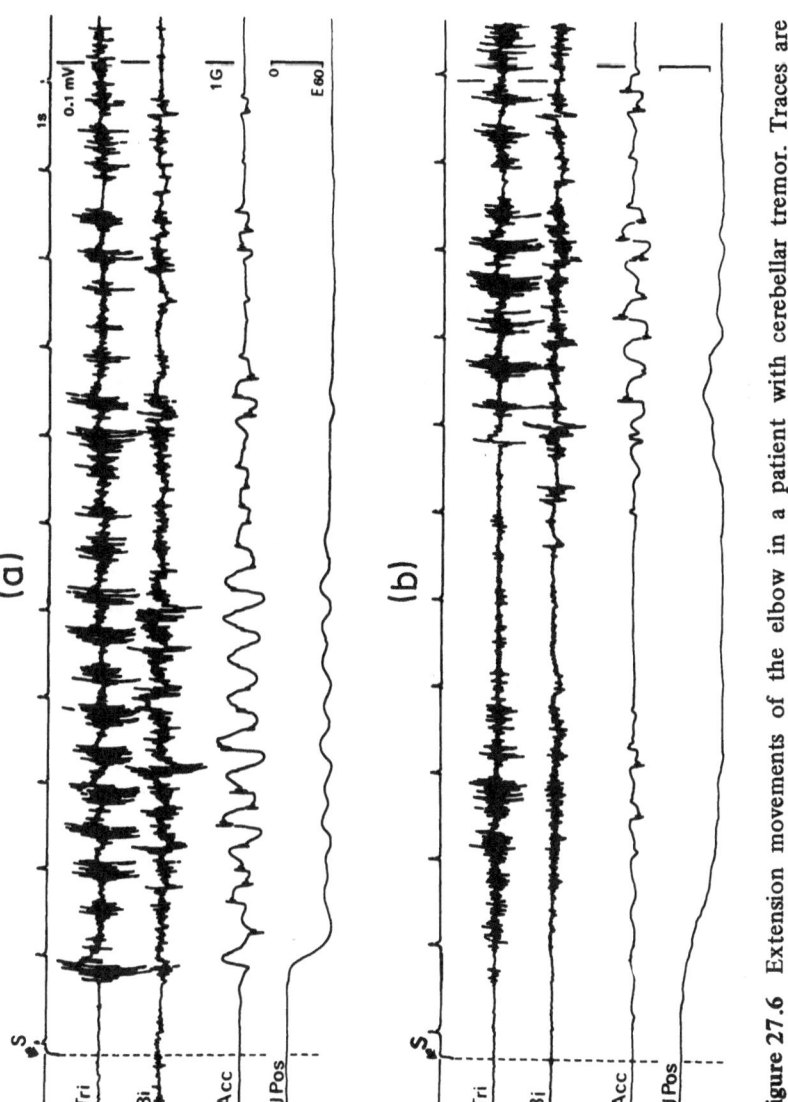

Figure 27.6 Extension movements of the elbow in a patient with cerebellar tremor. Traces are (from the top downwards): timescale with marker (S); triceps EMG (Tri); biceps EMG (Bi); accelerometric recording (Acc); and elbow position (J Pos). (a) The bursting activity in the agonist muscle continues during the holding phase of the rapid movement. (b) In this case a postural tremor is also recorded following the rhythmical activity initiated by a slow movement.

that which conditions the 'clonic' bursts of an epileptic fit. A peripheral mechanism can also be considered in which the cerebellar tremor is comparable to a clonus that maintains itself under cover of an exaggeration of the myotatic reflex.

The observations made in man can be compared to the results of experimental investigations. Recently Vilis and Hore (1980), by cooling the dentate nucleus of the cerebellum in the monkey, provoked a kinetic and sometimes a postural tremor analogous to that noted in man. They observed that during movement correction, after a torque pulse perturbation, the excitatory second cortical response (related to the activity of the muscle that caused the return movement) was delayed and the correction could be due to both segmental and suprasegmental reflexes. For these authors, activation of the antagonist, which must permit the limb to return to its original position, did not happen at the right time and was replaced by a reflex activity. The latter nevertheless occurred with much delay, and lasted too long to allow a correctly adjusted movement to the target, thus inducing oscillations. This hypothesis could explain why these oscillations occur earlier during the course of a movement if it is executed more rapidly. Indeed, the stretch reflex is facilitated by the speed of the stretching.

Nevertheless, several factors argue against the exaggeration of a segmental or plurisegmental reflex as the determining cause in cerebellar kinetic tremor. This tremor is most often observed in voluntary movement executed towards a target. It is not conditioned by the length of the movement but by the approach to the target. If the movement is small, there will be fewer oscillations, but they will begin earlier than oscillations that appear when the movement is greater, though of equal speed and acceleration. According to the hypothesis of a segmental or suprasegmental reflex activation of the antagonist, one should be led to presume that this reflex could be modulated according to the distance to be covered; such modulation has not been proven to this day.

Furthermore, Meyer-Lohmann *et al.* (1977) have shown that the more the dentate nucleus is cooled, the greater is the magnitude of the cerebellar tremor. The paradoxical conclusion should be that the more intense the cerebellar syndrome, the lower the threshold of the myotatic reflex becomes. However, it is known that cerebellectomy provokes a depression of the fusimotor system (Gilman, 1972). In fact, cooling of the dentate nucleus caused the disappearance of the discharges in the precentral neurones observed during extension of the forearm, and these neurones are predominantly related to flexion (Meyer-Lohmann *et al.*, 1975). If the activity recorded during extension before cooling is related to the stretching of the extensor, far from increasing, this activity disappeared after cooling.

It should also be mentioned that on the EMG recordings the agonist and antagonist muscles are activated either simultaneously or alternately. Thus activation may not only be due to the stretching of the antagonist. We have observed that the application of vibrations to the agonist and antagonist muscles diminishes the amplitude of the oscillations and sometimes stops them. These vibrations provoke a tonic vibratory reflex in the muscle by increasing large muscle spindle primary afferent discharges (Hagbarth and Eklund, 1968). By facilitating the myotatic reflex, they should also increase the amplitude of the oscillations, whereas the opposite is observed. Thus the oscillations observed during the movement may not be accounted for by exaggeration of the myotatic reflex.

The pathophysiology of cerebellar tremor may not be limited to the modification of a segmental or suprasegmental reflex, as is clonus. The pathophysiology must take into account several factors. Cerebellar tremor is most obvious in voluntary movement. It is conditioned by the target to be reached or the goal to be achieved, and is influenced by several parameters. Before movement is initiated, the distance between hand and target is evaluated visually. During movement, the location of the hand in relation to the target relies on sight and proprioceptive input arising from various muscle and joint receptors. These data enable movement to be slowed at the appropriate time to reach the target accurately. The cerebellum has to integrate visual and proprioceptive data to establish a temporal programme of activation for the antagonist muscle. When cerebellar dysfunction occurs, it is no longer possible to establish this programme, which leads to a delayed substitution under the guidance of visual control. This defect in the movement programme is the primary factor accounting for the oscillations at the end of movement.

A second factor may be of equal importance in explaining the origin of cerebellar tremor. We have mentioned the difficulty encountered by the cerebellar patient in executing a slow movement. This corresponds to the phasic characteristic of electrical activity, which is grouped in bursts of varying length from the beginning of movement. Miller and Freund (1980) have also observed that, in cerebellar dyssynergia in humans, abrupt movements are executed with excessive speed. The grouping of bursts of electrical activity noted on the EMG during movements executed by cerebellar patients can be correlated to experimental data obtained by recording the precentral unit activity, which, after cooling of the dentate nucleus, 'was far less finely structured and appeared more as a dense burst' (Meyer-Lohmann *et al.*, 1977). The two peaks of activity recorded before cooling had melted into one, thus changing from multimodal to unimodal firing.

CONCLUSION

The absence of tonic activity explains the major difficulty encountered by the cerebellar patient in adjusting a movement that remains brusque at the beginning and at the end of its course. Normally, the cerebellum must act either as a filter protecting the cortex and motor system from excessively intense discharges and/or as a programmer establishing the temporal sequence of the movement whilst modulating the level of cortical activation to adjust the acceleration of the guided movement in relation to the target. It may be assisted in this function by proprioceptive inputs received at the cortical level during movement. When these proprioceptive inputs are lacking, cerebellar tremor becomes more intense. This is observed during multiple sclerosis, where it becomes a 'hyperkinetic tremor'.

The cerebellar patient is unable to modulate his activity, particularly to adapt the acceleration of the movement to bring it to the target. Thus the resulting movement is delayed, brusque and clonic—hence, cerebellar kinetic tremor.

REFERENCES

Bathien, N., Toma, S. and Rondot, P. (1984). Tremor and bursting EMG pattern in movement performance of patients with cerebellar deficit. *EEG Clin. Neurophysiol.*, in press.

Conrad, B., Matsunami, K., Meyer-Lohmann, J., Wiesendanger, M. and Brooks, V. B. (1974). Cortical load compensation during voluntary elbow movements. *Brain Res.*, **71**, 507-14.

Gilman, S. (1972). The nature of cerebellar dyssynergia. In Williams, D. (ed.), *Modern Trends in Neurology*, Butterworths, London, pp. 60-79.

Hagbarth, K. E. and Eklund, G. (1968). The effects of muscle vibration in spasticity, rigidity and cerebellar disorders. *J. Neurol. Neurosurg. Psychiatr.*, **31**, 207-13.

Holmes, G. (1917). The symptoms of acute cerebellar injuries due to gunshot wounds. *Brain*, **40**, 461-535.

Holmes, G. (1922). The Croonian lectures on the clinical symptoms of cerebellar disease and their interpretation. *Lancet*, **202**, 1231-7.

Matthews, P. B. C. (1966). The reflex excitation of the soleus muscle of the decerebrate cat caused by vibration applied to its tendon. *J. Physiol. (Lond.)*, **184**, 450-72.

Meyer-Lohmann, J., Conrad, B., Matsunami, K. and Brooks, V. B. (1975). Effects of dentate cooling on precentral unit activity following torque pulse injections into elbow movements. *Brain Res.*, **94**, 237-51.

Meyer-Lohmann, J., Hore, J. and Brooks, V. B. (1977). Cerebellar participation in generation of prompt arm movements. *J. Neurophysiol.*, **40**, 1038-50.

Miller, R. G. and Freund, H. J. (1980). Cerebellar dyssynergia in humans: a quantitative analysis. *Ann. Neurol.*, **8**, 574-9.

Rondot, P. and Bathien, N. (1976). Peripheral factors modulating parkinsonian tremor. In Birkmayer, W. and Hornykiewicz, O. (eds), *Advances in Parkinsonism*, Roche, Basel, pp. 269-76.

Rondot, P., Bathien, N. and Toma, S. (1979). In Massion, J. and Sasaki, K. (eds), *Cerebro-cerebellar interactions*, Elsevier/North-Holland Biomedical Press, Amsterdam, New York and Oxford, pp. 203-30.

Rondot, P. and Ben Hamida, M. (1968). Myoclonies du voile et myoclonies squelettiques. Etude clinique et anatomique. *Rev. Neurol.*, **119**, 59-83.

Rondot, P., Said, G. and Ferrey, G. (1972). Les hyperkinesies volitionnelles. Etude electrologique. Classification. *Rev. Neurol.*, **126**, 415-26.

Thomas, A. (1937). La dyschronométrie cérébelleuse. Réflexe antagonists, équilibre actif. Réactions d'équilibration. *Presse Méd.*, **45**, 1643-6.

Thomas, A. and Durupt, A. (1914). *Localisations Cérébelleuses*, Vigot, Paris, pp. 151-5.

Vilis, T. and Hore, J. (1980). Central neural mechanisms contributing to cerebellar tremor produced by limb perturbation. *J. Neurophysiol.*, **43**, 279-91.

28
Treatment of cerebellar tremor

N. J. LEGG

INTRODUCTION

The disorders of movement produced by cerebellar disease are complex (Holmes, 1939). They include dysmetria, dysdiadochokinesis and decomposition of movement as well as intention tremor. The combination is disabling, and clinical descriptions of patients with cerebellar disorders often do not distinguish between the various modalities, but content themselves with describing the whole disability as cerebellar ataxia. Observations of improvement with treatment often use the same approach, assessing the patient's competence on a number of motor tasks and recording the performance in terms of the time taken to complete them. This is a valid means of assessing function, for it uses as a yardstick tasks similar to those that the patient has to carry out from day to day. It is not helpful, however, to an understanding of the pharmacology of an individual item such as tremor (see Fahn, this volume, chapter 5). Thus a review of the treatment of cerebellar tremor cannot be strictly that: it is a review of the treatment of cerebellar disorders, in which tremor plays a prominent but not a solo role.

To begin with, mention should be made of those cerebellar syndromes that are due to a treatable cause. These include acute intoxication with alcohol and other sedative drugs; possibly chronic alcohol toxicity and hypothyroidism; certainly chronic phenytoin toxicity; and certain tumours. Severe ataxia in such cases can completely disappear when the underlying disease is treated, even when this is a malignant tumour remote from the cerebellum, suggesting that perhaps some currently untreatable cerebellar diseases might also benefit symptomatically if the right pharmacological key could be found.

SYMPTOMATIC TREATMENT

Symptomatic treatment of cerebellar ataxia has been tried for some years, using mechanical damping devices to begin with. Holmes (1939) observed that holding a heavy bar improved alternating pronation and supination movements almost to normal in a patient with cerebellar disease, and Hewer et al. (1972) showed that intention tremor could be reduced by lead weights strapped to the wrist.

This method has not found widespread support, perhaps because there are critical loads above which the effect is reversed (Hewer *et al.*, 1972) and because the effects of loading flexors and extensors may be quite different (Chase *et al.*, 1965). An analogous technique is the application of viscous damping to the limbs (Rosen *et al.*, 1979). This has proved too cumbersome to be convenient, but viscous damping of certain items of equipment, of value for particular tasks, can be useful and such devices are under evaluation at present (A. W. S. Brown, 1983, personal communication).

DRUG TREATMENT

Physostigmine

Drug treatment has been tried extensively over the years, but no success was reported until the late 1970s, when Kark *et al.* (1977) showed improvement in response to physostigmine, an anticholinesterase that passes the blood-brain barrier. The rationale for this therapy at that stage was its influence in other movement disorders, such as Huntington's chorea (Klawans and Rubovits, 1972), parkinsonism (Duvoisin, 1967) and chorea (Tarsy *et al.*, 1974), in which its effects were thought to be due to enhanced cholinergic activity. An abnormality of pyruvate oxidation had already been shown in some cases of Friedreich's ataxia (Kark *et al.*, 1974; Barbeau *et al.*, 1976), but the suggestion that this might be related to a relative deficiency of brain acetylcholine had not yet been made (Barbeau, 1978). The trial of physostigmine used both intravenous and oral administration to patients with Friedreich's ataxia, olivo-ponto-cerebellar atrophy, cerebellar cortical atrophy, combined cerebral and cerebellar cortical atrophy, and Ramsay-Hunt syndrome. Neurological examinations were recorded on videotape and assessed on a semiquantitative scale. Forty minutes after physostigmine 1 mg i.v., scores improved by 35%, and a similar improvement was recorded in long-term studies on patients taking oral tablets in doses of up to 1 mg two-hourly. However, clinical benefit could not be detected without the use of videotapes, and most patients could not distinguish between the effects of physostigmine tablets and placebo.

Choline

Choline, either free as the chloride or bound to phospholipid as in lecithin, is the rate-limiting substrate for acetylcholine synthesis, and its oral administration raises brain choline and acetylcholine levels (Cohen and Wurtman, 1976). It had been shown to improve patients with chronic tardive dyskinesia (Davis *et al.*, 1975; Growdon *et al.*, 1977) and Huntington's chorea (Davis *et al.*, 1976). Barbeau (1978) reviewed the uses of choline and lecithin (phosphatidylcholine) in neuro-logical diseases, and suggested a relation between abnormal pyruvate metabolism and a deficiency of brain acetylcholine in Friedreich's ataxia. He reported that 12 patients with various cerebellar degenerations had been treated with lecithin, in doses of up to 24 g daily, and that improvement had averaged 30% after two months.

In the same year I reported the case of a 62-year-old man with late-onset idiopathic cerebellar degeneration, present for six years (Legg, 1978). At that stage he could walk only with a stick, on a wide base, and could not stand with his feet together. His writing was very poor and he showed titubation. He was treated with choline chloride, 1 g four times daily, and the improvement, which began on the second day of treatment, was dramatic. He could walk without a stick even over rough surfaces, could perform Romberg's test and tandem standing, and could hop on either foot. Titubation improved, the time taken for tests of manual dexterity was reduced by 50% or more, and his writing and drawing were much better. Drawings of helices, made with the wrist unsupported, recorded a tremor before treatment which was almost abolished by the choline. This therapeutic effect was reduced by propantheline 15 mg four times a day and abolished by 15 mg six times a day. No benefit was obtained from physostigmine 6 mg daily. Lecithin had the same effect as choline, but he preferred the latter. He has remained on choline ever since, and the benefit has been maintained. One pair of objective measurements (accelerometric) of his tremor on and off treatment failed to show any difference, suggesting that much of the improvement may have been in dysmetria.

A subsequent report described a further 13 patients with various cerebellar diseases, including degenerations, multiple sclerosis, vascular disease and trauma, who had been treated with choline chloride in doses up to 20 g a day without deriving any benefit (Legg, 1979). These observations were purely clinical, incorporating writing and drawing tasks and timed tests of motor function but without any videotape analysis. Negative results were also reported by Philcox and Kies (1979) in six patients with a dominantly inherited cerebellar ataxia of late onset characterised mostly by gait disturbance.

Sehested *et al*. (1980) described a double-blind crossover study in six patients with cerebellar ataxia, given choline chloride 5 g daily for four days. No improvement was noted on clinical assessment or videotape study. The treatment period in this study was rather short for establishing lack of any therapeutic effect. Lawrence *et al*. (1980) did a double-blind study on 14 patients with idiopathic cerebellar degeneration, Friedreich's ataxia, mixed cerebral and cerebellar signs or alcoholic cerebellar disease. Observations were made clinically, with the assistance of an ataxiometer, and scores were allotted for hand function, walking time and ataxia. Only one patient improved significantly, a man of 53 with a five-year history of progressive imbalance, dysarthria and poor handwriting. Walking speed was substantially reduced by choline 4 g daily or 150 mg kg^{-1} daily, but not until treatment had been going on for a few days. Hand function also improved, but not the ataxiometer score. His imporvement corresponded to a plasma choline level that would produce a 55% increase in cerebellar acetylcholine concentration in the rat (Eckernas and Aquilonius, 1977).

A further controlled trial was reported by Livingstone *et al.* (1981). Twenty patients were studied, suffering from Friedreich's ataxia, mixed corticospinal and cerebellar signs, or idiopathic cerebellar ataxia. They received 6 g or 12 g choline daily for six weeks. The assessment was by clinical examination using an ataxia score for each limb, a questionnaire to indicate functional disability, and videotape recordings of motor function that were scored blind by three independent clinicians. Ten patients showed mild but significant improvement in upper-limb coordination and two experienced improvement in gait and lower-limb coordination. The 12 g of choline a day appeared more effective than did 6 g per day, but produced more side-effects as well. The improvement was only modest: no patient regained independence and no chair-bound patients became able to walk. However, one became able to feed himself and another became able to put a key in a lock and to fill in a football pools coupon. Insofar as the abnormalities revealed by drawing tests can be separated into tremor and dysmetria, it appears from the published achievements of one patient that both were improved.

Thus the beneficial effects of choline seem to be confined to one or two patients. Nothing stands out to identify them at present, and although there are also a few unpublished cases who have benefited (e.g. C. B. Wynn-Parry, 1980, personal communication), the total number who have been successfully or usefully improved is very small.

Baclofen and sodium valproate

Owing to this lack of success with choline, a preliminary attempt was made (Legg, 1979) to improve cerebellar deficits by modifying GABA activity, since GABA is known to be an important neurotransmitter in the cerebellum. Thirteen patients were treated with baclofen, a GABA analogue, or with sodium valproate, which at least at high doses can increase brain GABA levels, or with both drugs together. No patient improved, and several deteriorated, both subjectively and objectively. One patient was also treated with isoniazid, but without any effect.

Isoniazid

Isoniazid was at that time being investigated for its effects in Huntington's chorea, in which brain GABA levels were known to be reduced (Perry *et al.*, 1973; Bird and Iversen, 1974). Imidazole, a GABA agonist, had proved clinically ineffective (Shoulson *et al.*, 1975). Preliminary observations on isoniazid suggested only a possibility of clinical benefit (Perry *et al.*, 1979) but established that CSF GABA levels could be elevated three-fold by isoniazid 300 mg t.d.s. (Manyam *et al.*, 1981; Perry *et al.*, 1982). Sabra *et al.* (1982) first described the use of isoniazid in subjects with cerebellar disorders. These were four patients with multiple sclerosis and a gross action tremor, similar if not identical to rubral tremor. Treatment with isoniazid, 800 to 1200 mg daily, produced significant improvement in all four patients, enabling them to carry on their normal daily activities with greater ease. One patient was intolerant of the drug and developed abnormal liver function, so treatment had to be stopped. The improvement in these patients was confined to this specific tremor, at 2.5-3.0 Hz and with an average EMG burst duration of 200-250 ms. In two patients it was observed that dysmetria was not altered, and in one of these it became the dominant disability after the tremor had been ameliorated.

So far no extension of this study has been published. We do not yet know, for instance, how many patients with a similar tremor have been treated without benefit, and there are no data on the effect of isoniazid on other components of cerebellar disease. I have used isoniazid at 300 mg t.d.s. in five patients with multiple sclerosis or cerebellar degeneration, with moderate ataxia of the upper limbs and of gait but without the 'rubral' type of tremor described by Sabra *et al.*, and have seen no benefit. If the effect of isoniazid is indeed confined solely to this one form of cerebellar tremor, however, it will still be a very significant advance in management for what is otherwise a very disabling movement disorder.

Valproic acid

While still on the subject of GABA activity and its modification, mention should be made of the case of Somerville *et al.* (1982), who obtained marked clinical benefit from valproic acid in a case of dyssynergia cerebellaris myoclonica. The benefit was essentially to the myoclonus, which improved so much on a dose of 250 mg t.d.s. that the patient became able to walk, eat, write and partially dress herself, all of which had previously been impossible. There may well be similarities of pharmacological abnormality between this type of abnormal movement and the rubral tremor that was improved in Sabra's patients and is usually due to multiple sclerosis.

L-5-Hydroxytryptophan

One report describes beneficial effects from L-5-hydroxytryptophan, a precursor of serotonin, in cerebellar syndromes (Rascol *et al.*, 1981). The rationale was the known effectiveness of this preparation in other movement disorders such as post-anoxic action myoclonus. The trial was uncontrolled, and was carried out in 24 patients, 14 suffering from multiple sclerosis, four with spinocerebellar degenerations and six with miscellaneous cerebellar diseases. The dose of drug was not specified. Twelve patients were improved, but the benefit was transient in some. Benefit seems to have been obtained in some patients with severe intention tremor of 'rubral' type. No other reports have so far appeared about this mode of treatment. There is a single description of improvement with propranolol in two brothers with familial ataxia (Braham *et al.*, 1979).

SURGERY

Surgical treatment of tremor is dealt with elsewhere in this volume by Andrew (chapter 25). A variant on surgery was described by Brice and McLellan (1980), who treated severe intention tremor in five patients with multiple sclerosis by means of contingent deep-brain stimulation. Electrodes were implanted between the thalamus and midbrain on each side, and square-wave stimuli with a pulse width of 500 μs, a frequency of 50–150 Hz and currents of up to 2 mA were employed. There were some clinical changes at the time of electrode placement, including improvement in some signs and exacerbations of others, ascribed to the trauma of multiple electrode insertions. Subsequently stimulation improved intention tremor in three patients, one of whom was then treated by thalamotomy. Permanent electrodes were implanted in the other two, and the most effective stimulus parameters were established by trial and error. Stimulation was then maintained via bilateral implanted radio receivers and external transmitters, which were triggered by EMG signals from the appropriate deltoid muscle, thus confining stimulation to times when the arm was being used. Both these patients obtained substantial improvement in control of their upper limbs, becoming able to carry out simple personal tasks such as feeding and dressing which had previously been impossible. The effectiveness of treatment had been maintained for some six months at the time of publication, and it continued for some eighteen months in all (McLellan, personal communication). The remaining two patients derived no benefit.

BIOFEEDBACK

The final method of treatment to be described is that of electromyographic (EMG) biofeedback, reported by Davis and Lee (1980). This was based on methods developed for rehabilitation of hemiplegia (Brudny *et al.*, 1974; Basmajian *et al.*, 1975) and other motor disorders, which were modified to provide a visual feedback representing activity in an agonist/antagonist pair of muscles. Three patients were treated, one with multiple sclerosis and two with spinocerebellar degenerations. All three subjects improved in the regularity and accuracy of alternating flexion and extension movements at the wrist. In two of them this appeared to be due to reduced coactivation of opposing muscles. After four feedback sessions, each of 15 min, one patient could maintain the improved performance even without the feedback in operation. The specificity of the feedback effect was assessed in one subject by offering distorted feedback some of the time. Although this had some beneficial effect, presumably via increased attention or motivation, the improvement with true feedback was very much greater. So far this limited study is the only one published about the use of this method.

CONCLUSIONS

What is the present status of therapy for cerebellar ataxia and its various components? So far we have perhaps a few pointers, but no real guidelines and certainly no indications. It seems clear that only very few patients can be helped by enhancing cholinergic activity, and those who can will probably be suffering from cerebellar degeneration rather than multiple sclerosis. Choline chloride or lecithin achieve this effect much better than physostigmine. A trial of two weeks on choline chloride, up to 10 g daily, should be enough to determine whether this approach is worth while. Patients with a severe intention tremor of rubral type, who will usually be suffering from multiple sclerosis, can be offered a trial of treatment with isoniazid 300 mg t.d.s., in combination with pyridoxine 100 mg daily and a careful watch for hepatic side-effects.

Both of these drug treatments are readily available and easy to organise. Rubral tremor is so disabling that patients unresponsive to isoniazid may be considered for deep-brain stimulation or thalamotomy. However, the former is still at an experimental stage, and both techniques demand specialised neuro-surgical expertise.

All other treatments are purely experimental. L-Tryptophan is expensive and not easy to obtain, but it clearly needs full assessment in a properly conducted trial. EMG biofeedback likewise merits further appraisal, and is not essentially a difficult method to set up. There seems to be no place for isoniazid in most cerebellar syndromes, but the evidence against it is only anecdotal and needs firming up.

The treatments described here have mostly been tried on the basis of clinical analogy and inspiration rather than on an understanding of abnormal cerebellar physiology. The abnormality of pyruvate metabolism in some cases of Friedreich's ataxia appeared to provide a rationale for the use of drugs to enhance cholinergic activity (Barbeau, 1978), but in the event improvement with choline chloride has not been confined to Friedreich's form of ataxia (Legg, 1978; Livingstone *et al.*, 1981) and no data have been published to indicate whether responders do in fact have abnormal pyruvate metabolism. Furthermore, there is no direct information about the level of acetylcholine synthesis or activity in cerebellar disease.

It now appears unlikely that a common pharmacological deficit will be found to underlie all, or even most, cases of cerebellar ataxia: the analogy with Parkinson's disease (Barbeau, 1978) was a hope that has been dashed by experience. Cerebellar movement disorders are probably associated with dysfunction in several neuro-transmitter systems, and the extent to which each one is affected may well differ profoundly from one disease to another, even though the clinical manifestations are similar.

Recent research has illustrated these variations, but has not yet provided an overall guide to them or to their therapeutic implications. A reduction in CSF GABA levels, for example, has been reported in cases of olivo-ponto-cerebellar and late cortical cerebellar atrophy but not in hereditary cerebellar ataxia (Ogawa *et al.*, 1982). Noradrenergic function varies in different forms of hereditary cerebellar ataxia in mice (Muramoto *et al.*, 1982). The role of acetylcholine even in normal cerebellar function is still under review (Woodward *et al.*, 1982; Crepel and Dhanjal, 1982). Diazepam is thought to enhance GABA activity and might therefore be expected to alleviate cerebellar disorders, but it can itself produce an ataxia of cerebellar type, and its effects on spontaneous and induced firing in Purkinje cells differ from species to species (Mariani and Delahaye-Bouchaud, 1978).

These data should become clearer and fit into some generalised scheme in due course, but there is no guarantee that this will lead to a rational programme of treatment for patients with cerebellar disorders. It would be quite wrong, therefore, to sit back and wait for a rationale before trying out new therapeutic regimes, and it is much more appropriate to adopt an experimental approach to the management of individual cases. In the present state of play the clinical scientist is in as strong a position as anyone to make crucial observations.

REFERENCES

Barbeau, A. (1978). Emerging treatments: replacement therapy with choline or lecithin in neurological diseases. *Can. J. Neurol. Sci.*, **5**, 157–60.

Barbeau, A., Butterworth, R. F., Ngo, T., Breton, G., Melancon, S., Shapcott, D., Geoffroy, G. and Lernieux, B. (1976). Pyruvate metabolism in Friedreich's ataxia. *Can. J. Neurol. Sci.*, **3**, 379–88.

Basmajian, J. V., Kukula, C. G., Nabrayan, M. G. and Takebe, K. (1975). Biofeedback treatment of footdrop after stroke compared with standard rehabilitation technique: effects on voluntary control and strength. *Arch. Phys. Med. Rehabil.*, **56**, 231–6.

Bird, E. D. and Iversen, L. L. (1974). Post-mortem measurement of glutamic acid decarboxylase, choline acetyltransferase and dopamine in basal ganglia. *Brain*, **97**, 457–72.

Braham, J., Sadeh, M., Turgman, J. and Sarova-Pinchas, I. (1979). Beneficial effect of propranolol in familial ataxia. *Ann. Neurol.*, **5**, 207.

Brice, J. and McLellan, L. (1980). Suppression of intention tremor by contingent deep-brain stimulation. *Lancet*, **1**, 1221–2.

Brudny, J., Korein, J., Levidow, L., Grynbaum, B. B., Lieberman, A. and Friedmann, L. W. (1974). Sensory feedback therapy as a modality of treatment in central nervous system disorders of voluntary movements. *Neurology*, **24**, 925–32.

Chase, R. A., Cullen, J. K., Sullivan, S. A. and Ommaya, A. K. (1965). Modification of intention tremor in man. *Nature*, **206**, 485–7.

Cohen, E. L. and Wurtman, R. J. (1976). Brain acetylcholine: control by dietary choline. *Science*, **191**, 561–2.

Crepel, F. and Dhanjal, S. S. (1982). Cholinergic mechanisms. Neurotransmission in the cerebellum of the rat. An *in vitro* study. *Brain Res.*, **244**, 59–68.

Davis, A. E. and Lee, R. G. (1980). EMG biofeedback in patients with motor disorders: an aid for coordinating activity in antagonistic muscle groups. *Can. J. Neurol. Sci.*, **7**, 199–206.

Davis, K. L., Berger, P. A. and Hollister, L. E. (1975). Choline for chronic tardive dyskinesia. *New Engl. J. Med.*, **293**, 152.

Davis, K. L., Hollister, L. E., Barchas, J. D. and Berger, P. A. (1976). Choline in tardive dyskinesia and Huntington's disease. *Life Sci.*, **19**, 1507–16.

Duvoisin, R. C. (1967). Cholinergic–anticholinergic antagonism in parkinsonism. *Arch. Neurol.*, **17**, 124–6.

Eckernas, S. A. and Aquilonius, S. M. (1977). A simple radio-enzymatic procedure for the determination of choline and acetylcholine in the brain regions of rats sacrificed by microwave irradiation. *Acta Physiol. Scand.*, **100**, 446–51.

Growdon, J. H., Hirsch, M. J., Wurtman, R. J. and Wiener, W. (1977). Oral choline administration to patients with tardive dyskinesia. *New Engl. J. Med.*, **297**, 524–7.

Hewer, R. L., Cooper, R. and Morgan, M. H. (1972). An investigation into the value of treating intention tremor by weighting the affected limb. *Brain*, **95**, 579–90.

Holmes, G. (1939). The cerebellum of man. *Brain*, **62**, 1–30.

Kark, R. A. P., Blass, J. P. and Engel, W. K. (1974). Pyruvate metabolism in neuromuscular diseases. Evidence of a genetic defect in two families with the syndrome of Friedreich's ataxia. *Neurology (Minneap.)*, **24**, 964–71.

Kark, R. A. P., Blass, J. P. and Spence, M. A. (1977). Physostigmine in familial ataxias. *Neurology*, **27**, 70–2.

Klawans, H. C. and Rubovits, R. (1972). Central cholinergic–anticholinergic antagonism in Huntington's chorea. *Neurology (Minneap.)*, **22**, 107–16.

Lawrence, C. M., Millac, P., Stout, G. S. and Ward, J. W. (1980). The use of choline chloride in ataxic disorders. *J. Neurol. Neurosurg. Psychiatr.*, **43**, 452–54.

Legg, N. J. (1978). Oral choline in cerebellar ataxia. *Br. Med. J.*, **2**, 1403–4.

Legg, N. J. (1979). Oral choline in cerebellar ataxia. *Br. Med. J.*, **2**, 133.

Livingstone, I. R., Mastaglia, F. L., Pennington, R. J. T. and Skilbeck, C. (1981). Choline chloride in the treatment of cerebellar and spinocerebellar ataxia. *J. Neurol. Sci.*, **50**, 161–74.

Manyam, B. V., Katz, L., Hare, T. A., Kaniefski, K. and Tremblay, R. D. (1981). Isoniazid-induced elevation of CSF GABA levels and effects on chorea in Huntington's disease. *Ann. Neurol.*, **10**, 35–7.

Mariani, J. and Delahaye-Bouchaud, N. (1978). Effect of diazepam on the spontaneous and harmaline-induced electrical activity of Purkinje cells in the cerebellum of the rat and rabbit. *Neuropharmacology*, **17**, 45–51.

Muramoto, O., Ando, K. and Kanazawa, I. (1982). Central noradrenaline metabolism in cerebellar ataxic mice. *Brain Res.*, **237**, 387–95.

Ogawa, N., Kuroda, H., Ota, Z., Yamamoto, M. and Otsuki, S. (1982). Cerebrospinal fluid γ-aminobutyric acid variations in cerebellar ataxia. *Lancet*, **2**, 215.

Perry, T. L., Hansen, S. and Khoster, M. (1973). Huntington's chorea: deficiency of γ-aminobutyric acid in brain. *New Engl. J. Med.*, **288**, 337–42.

Perry, T. L., Wright, J. M., Hansen, S. and MacLeod, P. M. (1979). Isoniazid therapy of Huntington's disease. *Neurology*, **29**, 370–5.

Perry, T. L., Wright, J. M., Hansen, S., Thomas, S. M. B., Allan, B. M., Baird, P. A. and Diewold, P. A. (1982). A double-blind clinical trial of isoniazid in Huntington's disease. *Neurology*, **32**, 354–8.

Philcox, D. V. and Kies, B. (1979). Choline in hereditary ataxia. *Brain*, **98**, 309.

Rascol, A., Clanet, M., Montastruc, J. L., Delage, W. and Guiraud-Chaumeil, B. (1981). L5H tryptophan in the cerebellar syndrome treatment. *Biomedicine*, **35**, 112–13.

Rosen, M. J., Dunfee, D. E. and Adelstein, B. D. (1979). Suppression of abnormal intention tremor by application of viscous damping. *Proc. 4th Congr. Int. Soc. Electrophysiology and Kinesthesiology*, Boston.

Sabra, A. F., Hallett, M., Sudarsky, L. and Mullally, W. (1982). Treatment of action tremor in multiple sclerosis with isoniazid. *Neurology*, 32, 912–13.

Sehested, P., Lund, H. I. and Kristensen, O. (1980). Oral choline in cerebellar ataxia. *Acta Neurol. Scand.*, 62, 124–6.

Shoulson, I., Chase, T. N., Roberts, E. and van Balgooy, J. N. A. (1975). Huntington's disease—treatment with cinidazole-4-acetic acid. *New Engl. J. Med.*, 293, 504–5.

Somerville, E. R. and Olanow, C. W. (1982). Valproic acid. Treatment of myoclonus in dyssynergia cerebellaris myoclonica. *Arch. Neurol.*, 39, 527–8.

Tarsy, D., Leopold, N. and Sax, D. S. (1974). Physostigmine in choreiform movement disorders. *Neurology (Minneap.)*, 24, 28–33.

Woodward, W. R., Blank, N. K. and Seil, F. J. (1982). Choline acetyltransferase activity in mouse cerebellar cultures. *Brain Res.*, 241, 323–7.

SECTION 6
TREMORS IN PERIPHERAL NEUROPATHY

29
Tremor associated with peripheral neuropathy

B. T. SHAHANI

INTRODUCTION

There are a variety of movement disorders that are seen in association with peripheral neuropathies (Shahani and Young, 1976a,b). Sensory ataxia, which gets worse with the eyes closed, can usually be easily distinguished from 'cerebellar' ataxia, which is most prominent in the terminal part of the movement, producing slow, large-amplitude oscillations of the limb in different directions in three-dimensional space. 'Contraction fasciculations', which are seen in patients with chronic denervation and reinnervation, are due to pathology of motoneurones and/or their axons. They can be easily identified clinically through weakness in the affected muscles and by electromyography (EMG), where there is evidence of prolonged duration and large-amplitude motor unit potentials recorded with conventional needle EMG. In addition to these movement disorders, there are specific types of action tremors seen in association with different types of peripheral neuropathies. The purpose of this chapter is to discuss some of these clinical entities with emphasis on the underlying pathophysiological mechanisms responsible for them.

PHYSIOLOGICAL TREMOR IN PERIPHERAL NEUROPATHIES

Physiological tremor, which can be demonstrated in all normal individuals, can also be seen in patients with different types of peripheral neuropathies. Both the frequency (8–12 Hz) and other physiological features, such as continuous EMG activity (appearance of full voluntary 'recruitment pattern') recorded with surface EMG electrodes, remain unchanged. However, factors such as stressful situation, injection of beta-adrenergic stimulating agents (isoproterenol), fatigue, etc., which produce enhancement of physiological tremor in normal subjects (by producing grouping of the discharges of motor units around the ongoing optimal tremor frequency), fail to do so in patients with severe sensory peripheral neuropathy.

389

In a patient with severe pansensory neuropathy we had previously reported severe involvement of all sensory fibres with preservation of the function of α motor axons (Adams *et al.*, 1973). This 40-year-old man had a familial disorder characterised by a chronic progressive sensory neuropathy with autonomic dysfunction with virtually complete sparing of motor fibres. He had gradual neurological deterioration at least from age 18 with complete loss of all sensory modalities, greatest in the extremities but also very severe over trunk, neck and face. There was areflexia and wide-based 'ataxic' gait. The patient's sister had a similar disorder with severe sensory loss and ataxic gait; she died at age 29 following a fracture and consequent osteomyelitis. Detailed electrophysiological studies including EMG with concentric needle electrodes, conventional motor and sensory nerve conduction and late response studies, 'silent period' and unloading responses and *in vitro* sural nerve conduction studies were performed. There was no evidence of active or chronic denervation on needle EMG examination. The maximum motor conduction velocity measurements were normal in all nerves tested (median nerve $53 \, \mathrm{m \, s^{-1}}$ with terminal latency of 2.8 ms, ulnar nerve $69 \, \mathrm{m \, s^{-1}}$ with terminal latency of 2.7 ms, peroneal nerve $47 \, \mathrm{m \, s^{-1}}$ with terminal latency of 6 ms). F responses recorded from intrinsic hand muscles had minimal latency of 26 ms, suggesting that nerve conduction was normal even in proximal segments on α motor axons. Sensory nerve action potentials could not be recorded from median or ulnar nerves. The proprioceptive silent periods could not be recorded from intrinsic hand muscle and unloading reflexes were absent in the biceps muscle in the upper extremity. *In vitro* sural nerve conduction studies showed absence of α, δ and C peaks. Electron microscope studies showed disappearance of all myelinated axons with relative sparing of Schwann cells. A few non-myelinated fibres were seen within Schwann cells. There were no onion bulbs and no amyloid deposits. Further studies were performed on this patient to analyse control of voluntary movement and movement disorders in the 'deafferented' subject. A low-amplitude physiological tremor with frequency of 10–12 Hz and continuous EMG activity in antagonistic muscles was present when the arms were held outstretched. However, it was impossible to produce *enhanced* physiological tremor in this patient. Neither anxiety nor holding a 2–3 kg weight for several minutes produced any increase in the amplitude of the tremor or synchronisation of motor unit potentials. It is clear from these studies that servo-loop and muscle spindles are essential for producing enhanced physiological tremor, as shown by studies of Hagbarth and Young (see Young, this volume, chapter 7). Studies of ballistic and ramp movements during a visual matching task had shown that the triphasic EMG pattern seen in normal subjects was also present in this patient during the ballistic movements (Hallett *et al.*, 1975). Further studies have shown many times that the triphasic EMG pattern is followed by discrete bursts of EMG activity in both agonist and antagonist muscles. These studies suggest that post-ballistic movement oscillations do not require an intact stretch reflex arc and may be related to some central oscillatory mechanism. When the arms are held outstretched holding a 2–3 kg weight for 3–5 min, the patient, instead of developing enhanced physiological tremor, develops slow (2–3 Hz) oscillations of the entire arm due to movements at proximal joints. These slow oscillations have a regular rhythm and must also be related to central oscillatory mechanisms.

In patients with a subclinical peripheral neuropathy in whom the function of the stretch reflex arc is preserved, both the enhanced physiological tremor and enhanced essential tremor can be demonstrated. It is well known that the amplitude of action tremor in chronic alcoholic subjects is significantly larger than that found in normal subjects. We have demonstrated that there are at least two distinct types of tremor (physiological and essential) that are exaggerated, most probably due to a peripheral mechanism involving peripheral tremogenic beta-adrenergic receptors (Marsden *et al.*, 1967; Young *et al.*, 1975), because of sympathetic overactivity during alcohol withdrawal. This exaggeration of different types of tremor is present as long as the neuropathy is mild and the function of the stretch reflex arc is preserved. In *severe* alcoholic and other types of neuropathies with loss of tonic and phasic stretch reflexes, enhancement of tremors is not seen; however, underlying physiological and essential tremors are still present.

In a recent study Said *et al.* (1982) reported the occurrence of tremor in 14 patients with acquired peripheral neuropathies of different origin and in patients with motor neurone disease. Sensory changes, aetiology and course of neuropathy varied in different patients and no unique pattern of histopathology could be demonstrated with detailed morphological studies. All patients showed electrophysiological evidence of denervation, and minimal weakness was the only clinical finding common to all patients. The tremor frequency in different limbs ranged from 4 to 12 Hz. These authors claim that 'benign essential tremor may be considered as enhanced physiological tremor and the tremor of peripheral neuropathy has the same electrophysiological characteristics as essential tremor. Both are often irregular and present the same range of frequencies.' On the basis of their findings the authors conclude that 'in patients with neuropathy we believe that the tremor is due to enhancement of physiologic tremor by minimal weakness and possibly by impairment of the stretch reflex, both of which increase central drive.' These observations and interpretations obviously do not agree with the modern concepts of the pathophysiological mechanisms of the familial essential tremor or the physiological mechanisms of enhanced physiological tremor, which require the preservation of the stretch reflex arc.

NEUROPATHIC TREMOR

In a small group of patients with acquired, chronic, relapsing–remitting polyneuropathies, a type of action tremor has been described (Adams *et al.*, 1972; Shahani *et al.*, 1973a). This 'neuropathic tremor' is most prominent in distal muscles and is most severe during a certain stage of the disease. Surface EMG recordings from a pair of antagonistic muscles and accelerometric tracings show an irregular tremor with bursts of EMG activity which are synchronous or alternating with no definite fixed pattern as seen with some other types of tremor. The rate of this tremor is 6–8 Hz. With the improvement in neuropathy, there is reduction in the amplitude of the tremor. Detailed electrophysiological studies including motor and sensory conduction, late response studies and recording of proprioceptive 'silent period' suggest that this tremor is produced by selective involvement of large sensory fibres. The maximum motor conduction velocity in many of these patients with neuropathic tremor is extremely slow, suggesting segmental demyelination as the primary pathological process underlying the neuropathy. However, severity of the neuropathic tremor is related more to the presence or absence of proprioceptive silent period rather than to slowing of nerve conduction. When the silent period is absent, the tremor is more marked, and a significant improvement is seen when the silent period is present. These studies suggest that the neuropathic tremor is produced by selective affection of large sensory fibres, including those responsible for proprioceptive input from muscle spindles. We have not seen this type of tremor in patients who had deafferentation procedures for intractable pain (with absent proprioceptive silent periods) and in patients with amyloid neuropathy with selective involvement of small sensory fibres but preservation of tendon jerks and proprioceptive silent period.

TREMOR WITH CHARCOT-MARIE-TOOTH DISEASE

Charcot-Marie-Tooth (CMT) disease is a familial peripheral neuropathy that affects both motor and sensory nerve fibres. Based on detailed clinical, electrophysiological and morphological studies, Dyck and Lambert (1968) divided patients with CMT into two genetically determined diseases. In one group of patients (called 'hypertrophic' type) there was morphological evidence of segmental demyelination and remyelination with onion bulb formation; the other group, which was designated 'neuronal' type, did not show any evidence of segmental demyelination. There are patients who present clinically as peroneal muscular atrophy in limbs without involvement of sensory fibres. This group is designated as hereditary distal spinal muscular atrophy (Dyck and Lambert, 1968; Harding and Thomas, 1980).

The patients with peroneal muscular atrophy (CMT disease) who have additional involvement of sensory fibres have been classified as hereditary motor and sensory neuropathy (HMSN). Based on the estimation of maximum motor conduction velocity in the median nerve, the HMSN is divided into two subgroups: (a) type I with marked slowing of motor nerve conduction velocity (less than $38\,\mathrm{m\,s^{-1}}$) and (b) type II in which nerve conduction velocity is only mildly affected. Although many investigators consider type I and type II HMSN as two genetically different forms of the disease (Dyck and Lambert, 1968; Harding and Thomas, 1980), Salisachs et al. (1982) are of the opinion that motor conduction velocity studies in the median nerve should not be used as a means of 'genetic' classification of CMT disease.

A movement disorder with features of familial essential tremor and plantar ulcers of the feet was described by Dyck and Lambert (1968) in the hypertrophic (type I) variety of CMT disease but not in the neuronal (type II) type. According to Salisachs (1976) and Salisachs *et al.* (1982) clinical features including features of essential tremor and plantar ulcers can be seen in both types and he is of the opinion that CMT disease should not be divided into two categories. In a series of reports (Salisachs, 1976, 1981; Salisachs *et al.*, 1979, 1982) it was shown that essential tremor can be present in patients with CMT disease with or without significant slowing of nerve conduction. It was concluded that CMT disease and essential tremor are not the result of association of two separate dominant characteristics which are generally inherited as mendelian dominant traits. Salisachs (1976) concluded that 'in spite of the diversity of the clinical manifestations of the peripheral neuropathy, the semiologically different types of essential tremor and the electrophysiological data, it is concluded that patients who develop peripheral neuropathy on a familial basis and who exhibit clinical features of similar character, suffer from a common type of pathological disorder.' Although Salisachs and his colleagues have made some important observations on the association of movement disorders with CMT disease, these studies suffer from the lack of detailed electrophysiological and pharmacological analysis of the movement disorders present in this patient population.

The neuropathic tremor described above should be differentiated from the action tremor seen in some patients with CMT disease (Shahani *et al.*, 1973b). It has been suggested by some authors (Yudell *et al.*, 1965) that a combination of action tremor and CMT disease in the same patient constitutes the syndrome described by Roussy and Levy (1926). However, detailed electrophysiological studies including physiological and pharmacological analysis of tremor in our laboratory have shown that the familial–essential tremor is seen in certain kinships with CMT disease. Some members in the family have only the essential tremor or the neuropathy, while some have a combination of both. In patients who have both neuropathy and tremor, there is marked slowing of nerve conduction, suggesting segmental demyelination. Because of a severe neuropathy there is involvement of both phasic (with absent tendon jerks and H reflexes) and tonic stretch reflexes (with decreased resistance to passive movement, absent tonic vibration reflex and silent periods). However, the tremor has characteristic features of familial–essential tremor with synchronous bursts of EMG activity in antagonistic muscle groups and a rate of 6–8 Hz. Unlike neuropathic tremor, which does not respond to beta-adrenergic blocking agents, this tremor responds well to treatment with oral propranolol. Our findings and observations on these patients suggest that: (1) the stretch reflex arc is not necessary for the production of familial–essential tremor but is necessary for 'enhanced' essential tremor; and (2) the response to treatment with propranolol in patients with familial–essential tremor is due to its effects on central rather than peripheral mechanisms.

MOVEMENT DISORDERS IN GUILLAIN-BARRÉ-STROHL SYNDROME

Diagnosis of Guillain-Barré-Strohl (GBS) syndrome is usually made on the basis of characteristic history, physical examination and laboratory findings of increased

CSF protein with low cell count. Many authors claim that, during the early phases of the disease, electrophysiological studies do not show any abnormality. However, detailed electrophysiological studies performed in our laboratory suggest that both studies early during the course of the disease and sequential studies carried out thereafter are helpful in diagnosis and monitoring of GBS syndrome. Moreover, we believe that electrophysiological studies, which are the most sensitive laboratory tests (abnormal prior to elevation of CSF proteins), are also helpful in elucidating underlying physiological mechanisms responsible for a variety of movement disorders seen in some patients with GBS syndrome. Both morphological and physiological studies have shown that 'blockage' of impulses is the most prominent feature during early phases of the disease. This results in decreased persistence or absence of late responses (F responses and H reflex) and reduction in the amplitude of compound muscle action potentials. Studies (using collision techniques) performed in our laboratory for evaluation of the function of different diameter α motor axons have shown selective involvement of smaller-diameter motor nerve fibres. Subsequently, when segmental demyelination takes place, there is marked slowing of nerve conduction (greater than 40% of normal values) and prolonged latencies of late responses.

A variety of movement disorders including spontaneous discharges of single motor units producing fasciculations, facial myokymia, neuropathic tremor and ataxis of the 'sensory' and 'cerebellar' type may be seen in GBS syndrome at different stages of the illness. Out of 48 consecutive adult patients with GBS syndrome, facial or limb myokymia was present in eight, which is approximately 17% of the patient population (Mateer *et al.*, 1983). Electrophysiological studies showed some slowing of motor conduction and abnormalities or absence of sensory nerve action potentials. In all muscles of patients with myokymia, the bursts of EMG activity occurred at 3–8 Hz with intervals that were relatively stable for each motor unit potential. The bursts appeared as singlets, doublets, triplets or multiplets. Within a burst, inter-spike intervals ranged from 6 to 40 ms. Blocking of the terminal spike potential occurred when the preceding interval was prolonged (Brick *et al.*, 1982). The authors suggested that myokymia was caused by ectopically generated potentials in the segmentally demyelinated nerves and that the tetanic bursts were produced by a 'multiplier effect' as seen in dystrophic mice with demyelinated axons (Rasminsky, 1978, 1980).

The neuropathic tremor seen in some patients with GBS syndrome at a certain stage during the course of recovery has typical features of this tremor described above. In most patients this tremor disappears as the neuropathy improves.

Since the original description by Fisher (1956), there have been a number of reports of a variant of GBS syndrome with ophthalmoplegia, areflexia and ataxia. As the movement disorder has features of 'cerebellar' rather than 'sensory' ataxia, we have performed detailed clinical and electrophysiological studies (Shahani and Ropper, 1982; Ropper and Shahani, 1983) in some of these patients. By recording proprioceptive silent periods from different muscles (proximal and distal) and by careful clinical evaluation of joint position sense in different joints, we find that ataxia clinically indistinguishable from cerebellar ataxia is present only when there is differential involvement of proprioceptive input coming from muscle spindles versus joint position sense receptors. When both joint position sense and muscle spindle afferents are equally involved, as may be the case in most patients with GBS syndrome, ataxia is not seen. It is suggested that mismatching of information from these two different sensory systems responsible for monitoring limb position in the central nervous system may result in ataxia. When the neuropathy is severe, with loss of the function of all sensory fibres, the movement disorder has features of 'sensory' ataxia, which gets worse with eyes closed and can be corrected when the eyes are open. In the light of our findings, it is important to note that in a recent study McCloskey *et al.* (1983) have shown that pulling or vibrating the exposed tendons of normal, awake subjects can give sensations of joint movements, even when the joints concerned are not moved.

MOVEMENT DISORDERS IN REFSUM'S DISEASE

Refsum's disease is a recessively inherited neurological disorder, the cardinal features of which are chronic progressive peripheral neuropathy, retinitis pigmentosa and excess of phytanic acid in various tissues of the body. In addition 'cerebellar' ataxia is considered to be one of the major features of this disorder. Detailed clinical, electrophysiological and biochemical studies were performed on three patients with Refsum's disease in our laboratory. We found that electrophysiological and clinical findings of neuropathy may range from a severe demyelinating neuropathy with secondary axonal degeneration in some to no evidence of neuropathy in others even when the most sophisticated electrophysiological techniques (including late response studies and collision techniques) for detection of peripheral nerve pathology are used (Domingue *et al.*, 1982). It is our view that the movement disorders associated with Refsum's disease should be carefully re-evaluated using modern electrophysiological techniques in order to understand the pathophysiological mechanisms responsible for 'cerebellar ataxia' in these patients.

MOVEMENT DISORDERS PRODUCED BY PERIPHERAL NERVE ENTRAPMENT SYNDROMES

In recent years we have seen a number of musicians (including pianists, violinists, drummers and a sitar player) in whom a lesion of the peripheral nervous system in the form of entrapment syndrome (even mild) results in lack of coordinated activity of the whole hand and a 'flexion dystonia' of digits 4 and 5 on clinical examination. Some of these patients have a carpal tunnel syndrome—a lesion that is not directly related to the control of digits 4 and 5. Others may have injury to any other peripheral nerve or one of its branches. In most patients peripheral nerve injuries involve branches of the median, ulnar or radial nerves; however, we have seen patients with involvement of a branch of a proximal nerve, such as axillary nerve, resulting in incoordination of voluntary movements of the upper extremity. In some patients we have analysed the movement disorder by surface EMG recordings from several muscles of the arm during appropriate tasks for different types of musicians and athletes. In addition to surface EMG recordings, behaviour of single motor units was studied using special needle EMG recording electrodes. Detailed studies showed that the size principle of recruitment (Henneman *et al.*, 1976) was well preserved in individual muscles studied by this technique. In some instances joint interval histograms were plotted for single motor unit recordings from different muscles of musicians, and even these were completely normal. Although each muscle studied individually was normal, patients were unable to produce coordinated movements necessary for playing a musical instrument. In order to produce the fine coordinated movements required for playing musical instruments, there is a need for proper integration of signals not only from suprasegmental structures but also from reflex and sensory inputs at the segmental level. Any lesion that may produce the slightest abnormality of any of these inputs results in the loss of fine coordinated movements essential for playing a musical instrument. Although the whole hand is affected, the abnormality is most prominent in digits 4 and 5, which are most vulnerable from the point of view of motor control. In many of these patients, early detection and treatment of the entrapment syndrome results in significant improvement of function. In others, in whom the process has lasted for longer periods of time, resulting in changes in the central motor programmes, there is a need for retraining with physiological techniques such as EMG audiovisual feedback in addition to treating the primary cause.

CONCLUSIONS

It is clear that different lesions of the peripheral nervous system, depending upon the degree and site of involvement of specific peripheral nerve fibres, can produce different types of movement disorders. The qualities of different types of sensory inputs, their interpretation and the way in which they are incorporated in a particular movement determine the type of movement disorder produced by specific lesions of peripheral nerve fibres. It is essential to recognise the importance of manifold sources of afferent activity that play upon different levels of the central nervous system to produce functionally integrated responses and it is not necessary to explain every movement disorder, such as tremors and 'cerebellar' type of ataxia, on the basis of lesions of the central nervous system.

REFERENCES

Adams, R. D., Shahani, B. T. and Young, R. R. (1972). Tremor in association with polyneuropathy. *Trans. Am. Neurol. Assoc.*, **97**, 44-8.

Adams, R. D., Shahani, B. T. and Young, R. R. (1973). A severe pansensory poly-neuropathy. *Trans. Am. Neurol. Assoc.*, **98**, 67–9.

Brick, J. F., Gutmann, L. and McComas, C. F. (1982). Calcium effect on genera-tion and amplification of myokymic discharges. *Neurology*, **32**, 618–22.

Domingue, J. N., Shahani, B. T. and Kolodny, E. (1982). Electrophysiologic studies in Refsum's disease. *Trans. Am. Neurol. Assoc.*, **106**, 173–4.

Dyck, P. J. and Lambert, E. H. (1968). Lower motor and primary sensory neuron diseases with peroneal muscular atrophy. Part 1. Neurologic, genetic and electrophysiologic findings in hereditary polyneuropathies. *Arch. Neurol.*, **18**, 603–18.

Fisher, C. M. (1956). An unusual variant of acute idiopathic polyneuritis (syn-drome of ophthalmoplegia, ataxia and areflexia). *New Engl. J. Med.*, **225**, 57–75.

Hallett, M., Shahani, B. T. and Young, R. R. (1975). EMG analysis of stereotyped voluntary movements in man. *J. Neurol. Neurosurg. Psychiatr.*, **38**, 1154–62.

Harding, A. E. and Thomas, P. K. (1980). The clinical features of hereditary motor and sensory neuropathy. Types I and II. *Brain*, **103**, 259–80.

Henneman, E., Shahani, B. T. and Young, R. R. (1976). Voluntary control of human motor units. In Shahani, M. (ed.), *The Motor System: Neurophysio-logy and Muscle Mechanisms*, Elsevier, Amsterdam, 73–8.

McCloskey, D. I., Cross, M. J., Honner, R. and Potter, E. K. (1983). Sensory effects of pulling or vibrating exposed tendons in man. *Brain*, **106**, 21–37.

Marsden, C. D., Foley, T. H., Owen, D. A. L. and McAllister, R. G. (1967). Peripheral beta-adrenergic receptors concerned with tremor. *Clin. Sci.*, **33**, 53–65.

Mateer, J. E., Gutmann, L. and McComas, C. F. (1983). Myokymia in Guillain-Barré syndrome. *Neurology*, **33**, 374–6.

Rasminsky, M. (1978). Ectopic generation of impulses and cross-talk in spinal nerve roots of 'dystrophic' mice. *Ann. Neurol.*, **3**, No. 4, 351–7.

Rasminsky, M. (1980). Ephaptic transmission between single nerve fibres in the spinal nerve roots of dystrophic mice. *J. Physiol. (Lond.)*, **305**, 151–69.

Ropper, A. H. and Shahani, B. T. (1983). Proposed mechanisms of ataxia in Fisher syndrome. *Arch. Neurol.*, **40**, No. 9, 537–8.

Roussy, G. and Levy, G. (1926). Sept cas d'une maladie familiale particulière. Troubles de la marche, pieds bots et aréflexie tendineuse generalisée avec acces-soirement maladresse des mains. *Rev. Neurol.*, **2**, 427–50.

Said, G., Bathien, N. and Cesaro, P. (1982). Peripheral neuropathies and tremor. *Neurology*, **32**, 480–5.

Salisachs, P. (1976). Charcot–Marie–Tooth disease associated with 'essential tremor'. *J. Neurol. Sci.*, **28**, 17–40.

Salisachs, P. (1981). Unusual presentation of Charcot–Marie–Tooth disease — incoordination with absent or minimal wasting. *J. Neurol. Sci.*, **50**, 175–80.

Salisachs, P., Codina, A., Gimenez-Roldan, S. and Zarranz, J. J. (1979). Charcot-Marie–Tooth disease associated with 'essential tremor' and normal and/or slightly diminished motor conduction velocity. *Eur. Neurol.*, **18**, 49–58.

Salisachs, P., Findley, L. J., Codina, A. and Martinez-Lage, J. M. (1982). Should Charcot–Marie–Tooth disease be genetically subgrouped on motor conduction velocity? *J. Neurol. Neurosurg. Psychiatr.*, **45**, 182–4.

Shahani, B. T. and Ropper, A. (1982). Mechanisms of ataxia in Fisher syndrome. *Ann. Neurol.*, **12**, 77.

Shahani, B. T. and Young, R. R. (1976a). A review of physiological and pharma-cological studies of human tremor. In Shahani, M. (ed.), *The Motor System—Neurophysiology and Muscle of Human Tremor*, Elsevier, Amsterdam, pp. 307–13.

Shahani, B. T. and Young, R. R. (1976b). Physiological and pharmacological aids in the differential diagnosis of tremor. *J. Neurol. Neurosurg. Psychiatr.*, **39**, 772–83.

Shahani, B. T., Young, R. R. and Adams, R. D. (1973a). Neuropathic tremor. *EEG Clin. Neurophysiol.*, **34**, 800.

Shahani, B. T., Young, R. R. and Adams, R. D. (1973b). The tremor in the Roussy–Levy syndrome. *Neurol.*, **23**, 425–6.

Young, R. R., Growdon, J. H. and Shahani, B. T. (1975). Beta-adrenergic mechanisms in action tremor. *New Engl. J. Med.*, **293**, 950–3.

Yudell, A., Dyck, P. J. and Lambert, E. H. (1965). A kinship with the Rousey–Levy syndrome. *Arch. Neurol. (Chic.)*, **13**, 432–40.

30
Tremor in peripheral neuropathy

I. S. SMITH, P. FURNESS and P. K. THOMAS

INTRODUCTION

Tremor is an unusual symptom in peripheral neuropathy, but it has been described in a significant proportion of patients with chronic relapsing inflammatory neuropathy, hereditary motor and sensory neuropathy (HMSN) and benign IgM paraproteinaemic neuropathy. It has also been reported in a few cases of neuropathy caused by diabetes, uraemia or porphyria (Ridley, 1969; Said *et al.*, 1982) and is sometimes found in the recovery stages of the Guillain-Barré-Strohl syndrome. Tremor should be distinguished from other movement disorders found in neuropathies, such as sensory ataxia, choreiform movements or pseudoathetosis.

In this chapter, the word 'tremor' is used in the clinical sense to mean an abnormal rhythmic movement of part of the body which can be seen on examination. The exception to this is when reference is made to physiological tremor, which is usually not detectable clinically.

CHRONIC RELAPSING INFLAMMATORY NEUROPATHY

This neuropathy probably has an autoimmune pathogenesis. During a relapse, there may be severe generalised weakness with some sensory loss. Nerve conduction velocities are reduced and peripheral nerves show extensive segmental demyelination and sometimes focal accumulations of inflammatory cells. Some, but not all, cases are benefited by corticosteroids.

There have been several reports of cases of chronic relapsing inflammatory neuropathy with tremor. One such case, described by Thomas *et al.* (1969), developed a coarse intention tremor in both arms during the fourth relapse of the neuropathy. Motor conduction velocity was reduced to 13 m s^{-1}. Case 2 of Matthews *et al.* (1970) had tremor in the hands which came on two years after the onset of the neuropathy. It was evident when the arms were outstretched and was almost regular, at about 6 Hz. The patient also had a rest tremor that was identical to the 'pill-rolling' tremor of Parkinson's disease. No rigidity was found in the arms. The tremor persisted during a remission when the weakness had completely resolved, but disappeared during the next similar remission only to reappear during a subsequent relapse. The cases of Shahani and Young (1978) also showed this tendency for tremor to appear during a relapse and to improve when the neuropathy remitted. Their motor conduction velocities were markedly reduced. These authors emphasised that, unlike essential tremor, this was an irregular tremor and it did not respond to propranolol. It was seen in the outstretched arms, most prominent distally, and was accentuated by performing discrete movements. The frequency found in their patients was around 6–8 Hz. Similar observations were made by Dalakas and Engel (1981) who reported a series of 25 cases, six of whom had tremor. Motor conduction velocities ranged from 17 to 28 m s^{-1}. They described a postural tremor in the distal muscles of the arms which was irregular and also present during action. It usually appeared in the second or third relapse of the disease and resolved as the neuropathy improved. The tremor was not related to the severity of weakness or proprioceptive loss, nor to corticosteroid therapy, which can cause mild tremor in high dosage. Propranolol did not affect the tremor in one patient.

The above descriptions of tremor in chronic relapsing inflammatory neuropathy show certain fairly consistent features. Tremor appears some time after the onset of the neuropathy. It is an irregular tremor which is present during movement and maintenance of posture. Relapse and remission of the neuropathy may be accompanied by similar changes in the tremor, although it is not specifically related to the degree of weakness or sensory loss. Treatment with propranolol is ineffective.

HEREDITARY MOTOR AND SENSORY NEUROPATHY

Hereditary motor and sensory neuropathy (HMSN) types I and II comprise the majority of cases diagnosed clinically as Charcot-Marit-Tooth disease (see Shahani, this volume, chapter 29). A small proportion, without sensory involvement, represents hereditary distal spinal muscular atrophy. These are all chronic genetically determined disorders. HMSN type I is characterised by markedly reduced nerve conduction velocity and extensive segmental demyelination in nerve biopsies; type II, by contrast, shows normal or modestly reduced conduction velocity and considerably less evidence of demyelination in biopsies.

Tremor is more commonly found in HMSN type I but also occurs in type II (Dyck, 1975; Harding and Thomas, 1980). Cases of HMSN with pronounced tremor constitute the Roussy-Lévy syndrome. The tremor is regular and is seen in the hands when the arms are outstretched. It is not greatly exaggerated by movement and may respond to propranolol. In many ways, it resembles benign essential tremor.

PARAPROTEINAEMIC NEUROPATHY

Chronic demyelinating neuropathy with benign IgM paraproteinaemia is a condition that has been described in recent years (for references see Smith *et al.*,

1983). It is a chronic neuropathy that is mixed sensorimotor in type. Motor conduction velocities are markedly reduced. Nerve biopsies have shown changes compatible with a predominantly demyelinating neuropathy. Immunological investigations suggest that this is an autoimmune disease. Antibody specific for human peripheral myelin has been found in the sera of these patients. Nerve biopsies studied by direct immunofluorescence showed the presence of IgM antibody on surviving myelin sheaths.

Ten of the 12 patients reported by Smith *et al.* (1983) had tremor. The other two patients were severely ataxic. Tremor was present at rest in three of these cases, two having tremor in the thumb. The other case had rest tremor which resembled the 'pill-rolling' tremor of Parkinson's disease, although he had no other features of the disease. All cases had tremor in the hands with the arms outstretched. It was irregular in that the amplitude would vary considerably over a short period. Also different antagonistic muscle groups would be involved at different times to produce a compound tremor that could vary in character almost continuously. The tremor was enhanced by movement, particularly during the terminal part of the action. Tremor in these cases varied from being a very mild disorder to one that was extremely disabling. The muscles responsible for the tremor were generally not weak and joint position sense was often normal or only slightly impaired, even in some of the cases with severe tremor. The tremor did not respond to propranolol nor to anti-parkinsonian drugs.

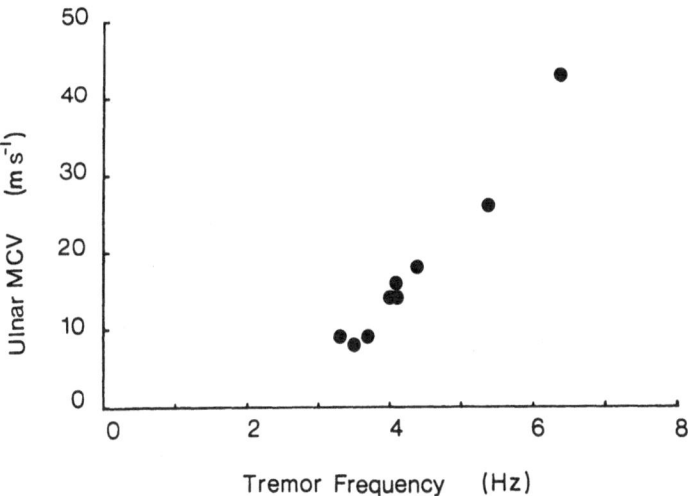

Figure 30.1 Relationship between tremor frequency in the thumb and motor conduction velocity in the ulnar nerve in the forearm for nine cases of para-proteinaemic neuropathy. The tremor recording was obtained while pressing on a strain gauge under isometric conditions and exerting a force of between approx. 2.5 N and 5 N.

Preliminary observations on the frequency of tremor in the thumb have been made on nine cases using a strain gauge (Smith and Furness, unpublished observations). The mean tremor frequency in these cases varied from 3.3 to 6.4 Hz. Motor conduction velocity in the forearm segment of the ulnar nerve was measured in each of the nine cases using standard methods. When the frequency of tremor in the thumb was plotted against this velocity, there was a direct relationship, as shown in figure 30.1, although observations on more cases are required for confirmation. There was no clear relationship between velocity and amplitude of tremor.

MECHANISMS OF TREMOR IN NEUROPATHY

The causes of tremor in peripheral neuropathy are not known but several possible mechanisms have been put forward. It is not at present clear whether any one explanation might apply to all forms of neuropathic tremor.

Delay in the stretch reflex arc

Since many cases of neuropathy with tremor have reduced motor conduction velocities, the possibility has been considered that the tremor may be related to increased conduction time in peripheral servomotor loops (Adams *et al.*, 1972; Thomas, 1975). Physiological tremor is in part related to delay in the stretch reflex arc (Hammond *et al.*, 1956; Halliday and Redfearn, 1956). It may be that increasing this delay could give rise to a pathological tremor. However, this does not explain why only some patients with neuropathy and slowing of conduction have tremor. Dalakas and Engel (1981) have studied tremor in chronic relapsing inflammatory neuropathy and found no significant difference between the conduction velocities of those with and those without tremor. Many cases of HMSN type I, who have markedly reduced conduction velocities, do not have tremor and, conversely, some cases of HMSN type II, with normal or slightly reduced conduction velocities, do have tremor. These observations show that slowing of nerve conduction is neither a sufficient nor a necessary condition for the production of tremor. A similar conclusion was reached by Adams *et al.* (1972) and Thomas (1975).

Selective loss of sensory nerve fibres

Shahani and Young (1978) have proposed that an imbalance in the sensory input to the motor neurone pool, caused by loss of function in proprioceptive fibres from muscles, could produce tremor in neuropathy (see Shahani, this volume, chapter 29).

Muscle weakness

Said *et al.* (1982) looked at a heterogeneous group of patients with neuropathy and tremor. Most were diabetic or uraemic but there were single cases of alcoholic, vasculitic and amyloid neuropathy. The only consistent finding on examination was mild weakness in the tremulous limb. Tremor frequency was not related to conduction velocity. No common abnormality was found on morphological study of peripheral nerve biopsy specimens. They concluded that the tremor was physiological tremor, which was enhanced by minimal muscle weakness and possibly by impairment of the stretch reflex. Again, this did not explain why most cases with neuropathic weakness do not have tremor.

Associated essential tremor

The resemblance of the tremor in HMSN to benign essential tremor led Dyck and his coworkers to consider the possibility that the association between tremor and this neuropathy is due to a combination of the dominant gene for HMSN and that for essential tremor (Dyck, 1975). The results of their genetic studies were not compatible with this hypothesis.

Central origin

Dyck, in the discussion following the paper by Adams *et al.* (1972), noted that several of his cases of chronic relapsing inflammatory neuropathy with tremor had pathological changes in the central nervous system. It was implied that the tremor may have been caused by an associated abnormality in the central nervous system. This might explain why only some patients with neuropathy have tremor. If there were no central abnormality, then tremor would not be present. It may be that this central disorder could generate the frequency of tremor seen in the limbs by means of an oscillating neuronal mechanism, as has been proposed for Parkinson's disease.

The presence of a central disorder would seem reasonable as the clinical observations on the paraproteinaemic cases suggested that the tremor and the neuropathy were separate processes. Tremor often appeared and progressed over a time when the neuropathy was static. Cases with very similar neuropathies in terms of weakness and sensory loss could have a mild tremor or else a very severe and extremely disabling one. The muscles responsible for the tremor were usually not weak and it did not appear to be related to proprioceptive loss. The presence of tremor was not correlated with motor conduction velocity, as has been found in HMSN and chronic relapsing inflammatory neuropathy. The tremor had some of the features of 'central' tremors such as those found in Parkinson's disease and cerebellar disorders. It often resembled essential tremor, which may well be central in origin.

However, if the tremors in the paraproteinaemic cases were due to a central abnormality, a relationship between frequency and nerve conduction would not be compatible with it being generated by a central oscillating mechanism, since the frequency seen in the limbs would not be affected by slowing of peripheral nerve conduction. The time interval between the arrival of nerve impulses at a muscle would not be altered by the speed at which they were conducted along the nerve fibres.

Combined central and peripheral origin

The preliminary observations on cases of paraproteinaemic neuropathy described here suggest that there is a correlation between tremor frequency and motor conduction velocity. This raises the possibility of a causal relationship, although it is also possible that both are related to the severity of the underlying disease process. The correlation would be compatible with the tremor being caused by increased delay in the stretch reflex arc. However, there is also evidence to suggest that tremor is central in origin. The apparent discrepancy between these two conclusions may be resolved by the hypothesis that tremor is the resultant of two separate processes, one taking place centrally and the other peripherally. It seems possible that an abnormality in the central nervous system is the primary cause of the tremor, since there is no clear relationship between any single aspect of the neuropathy and the presence of tremor, but when tremor does appear its frequency may be determined by the degree of slowing of conduction in the peripheral nervous system. If the tremor frequency is related to increased delay in the stretch reflex arc, it may be that a central abnormality has interfered with the central control of this reflex. On this view, the tremor is due to effects of the disease on physiological tremor which has been increased in amplitude by a central disorder and reduced in frequency by slowing of peripheral nerve conduction.

The above hypothesis may be supported by the results of Marsden and Meadows (unpublished observations) (reported by Marsden, 1978) who showed that, in seven patients with chronic relapsing inflammatory neuropathy and slow conduction, the tremor frequencies were slower and the amplitudes smaller than those of normal physiological tremor. In three of their cases who recovered, the conduction velocities increased from a mean of 27 to 45 m s^{-1} and tremor peak frequency increased from 7.0 to 8.7 Hz. If these figures are plotted on a graph of velocity against frequency, the slope is similar to that seen for the present results (see figure 30.1), although the plot would be shifted by between 1.5 and 2 Hz to the right.

This hypothesis implies that the stretch reflex is still intact. There have been no published studies on the stretch reflex in paraproteinaemic neuropathy, but it may be relevant to consider two patients in the series reported by Smith *et al.* (1983) who did not have tremor. They were very ataxic and had the most severe loss of sensation in the whole of that series. The absence of tremor may have been related to the functional state of the stretch reflex, which could have been markedly impaired by muscle deafferentation. These cases are perhaps analogous to the three severely deafferented tabetic patients described by Halliday and Redfearn (1958), who did not have the normal physiological tremor peak of 9 Hz. The other less severely affected tabetic patients all had normal or increased tremor peaks. It was concluded that absence of the peak in the former was consistent with the stretch reflex arc having been disrupted.

CONCLUSIONS

Clinical observations on tremor in a group of patients with peripheral neuropathy and IgM paraproteinaemia suggest that the tremor may be due to a disorder of the central nervous system. The relationship between tremor frequency and nerve conduction velocity may mean that this central abnormality allows an increased oscillation in a peripheral servo-loop system to take place. It is also possible that this relationship is determined by some underlying factor such as the severity of the disease process. It is at present uncertain how far these conclusions could apply to other types of neuropathic tremor.

REFERENCES

Adams, R. D., Shahani, B. T., and Young, R. R. (1972). Tremor in association with polyneuropathy. *Trans. Am. Neurol. Assoc.*, 97, 44–8.

Dalakas, M. C. and Engel, W. K. (1981). Chronic relapsing (dysimmune) polyneuropathy: pathogenesis and treatment. *Ann. Neurol.*, 9, Suppl., 134–5.

Dyck, P. J. (1975). Inherited neuronal degeneration and atrophy affecting peripheral motor, sensory and autonomic neurons. In Dyck, P. J., Thomas, P. K. and Lambert, E. H. (eds), *Peripheral Neuropathy*, W. B. Saunders, Philadelphia, pp. 825–67.

Halliday, A. M. and Redfearn, J. W. T. (1956). An analysis of the frequencies of finger tremor in healthy subjects. *J. Physiol. (Lond.)*, 134, 600–11.

Halliday, A. M. and Redfearn, J. W. T. (1958). Finger tremor in tabetic patients and its bearing on the mechanism producing the rhythm of finger tremor. *J. Neurol. Neurosurg. Psychiatr.*, 21, 101–8.

Hammond, P. H., Merton, P. A. and Sutton, G. G. (1956). Nervous gradation of muscular contraction. *Br. Med. Bull.*, 12, 214–18.

Harding, A. E. and Thomas, P. K. (1980). Autosomal recessive forms of hereditary motor and sensory neuropathy. *J. Neurol. Neurosurg. Psychiatr.*, 43, 669–78.

Marsden, C. D. (1978). The mechanisms of physiological tremor and their significance for pathological tremors. In Desmedt, J. E. (ed.), *Progress in Clinical Neurophysiology*, vol. 5, Karger, Basel, pp. 1–16.

Matthews, W. B., Howell, D. A. and Hughes, R. C. (1970). Relapsing corticosteroid-dependent polyneuritis. *J. Neurol. Neurosurg. Psychiatr.*, 33, 330–7.

Ridley, A. (1969). The neuropathy of acute intermittent porphyria. *Q. J. Med.*, 38, 307–33.

Said, G., Bathien, N. and Cesaro, P. (1982). Peripheral neuropathies and tremor. *Neurol. (Minneap.)*, 32, 480–5.

Shahani, B. T. and Young, R. R. (1978). Action tremors: a clinical neurophysiological review. In Desmedt, J. E. (ed.), *Progress in Clinical Neurophysiology*, vol. 5, Karger, Basel, pp. 129–37.

Smith, I. S., Kahn, S. N., Lacey, B. W., King, R. H. M., Eames, R. A., Whybrew, D. J. and Thomas, P. K. (1983). Chronic demyelinating neuropathy associated with benign IgM paraproteinaemia. *Brain*, **106**, 169-95.

Thomas, P. K. (1975). Clinical features and differential diagnosis. In Dyck, P. J., Thomas, P. K. and Lambert, E. H. (eds), *Peripheral Neuropathy*, W. B. Saunders, Philadelphia, pp. 495-512.

Thomas, P. K., Lascelles, R. G., Hallpike, J. F. and Hewer, R. L. (1969). Recurrent and chronic relapsing Guillain-Barré polyneuritis. *Brain*, **92**, 589-606.

SECTION 7
TREMULOUS AND TREMOR-LIKE
MOVEMENTS OF THE EYES

31
Mechanisms of ocular oscillations

DAVID S. ZEE and LANCE M. OPTICAN

INTRODUCTION

Ocular oscillations are of many types and usually reflect instability in one of the four major subclasses of eye movements: saccadic, pursuit, vestibular, or vergence. Since the systems that generate eye movements receive afferent (e.g. visual) and probably internal ('efference copy') feedback about their performance, one can analyse ocular motor performance using control systems theory (Robinson, 1981b). Feedback systems are susceptible to instability and oscillations. An increase in the gain (output/input ratio) or in the phase (or delay from input to output) may lead to instability. Recent experimental research has emphasised several physiological mechanisms that may underlie some types of instability and oscillation that occur in the ocular motor system.

These physiological mechanisms can be divided into two categories: inhibitory gating functions and adaptive control of modifiable gain elements. The purpose of an inhibitory gate is to keep an inherently unstable system off when it is not needed. This prevents unwanted oscillations. Modifiable gain elements allow the performance of a neurological control system to be adjusted to meet best the needs of the organism. This is accomplished by an adaptive control system that monitors ocular motor performance and makes the appropriate changes to ensure that eye movements remain accurate. Using these concepts we will analyse several different types of ocular oscillations.

INHIBITORY GATING MECHANISMS

Malfunction of an inhibitory gate is exemplified by ocular oscillations that consist of back-to-back, to-and-fro saccades without an intersaccadic interval (Zee and Robinson, 1979a). These include microsaccadic oscillations and voluntary nystagmus (which occur in normal individuals) and opsoclonus and ocular flutter (which occur in patients with neurological disease) (figure 31.1). This group of oscillations is to be distinguished from macrosaccadic oscillations, which consist of to-and-fro saccades (about the position of a target), separated by an intersaccadic interval.

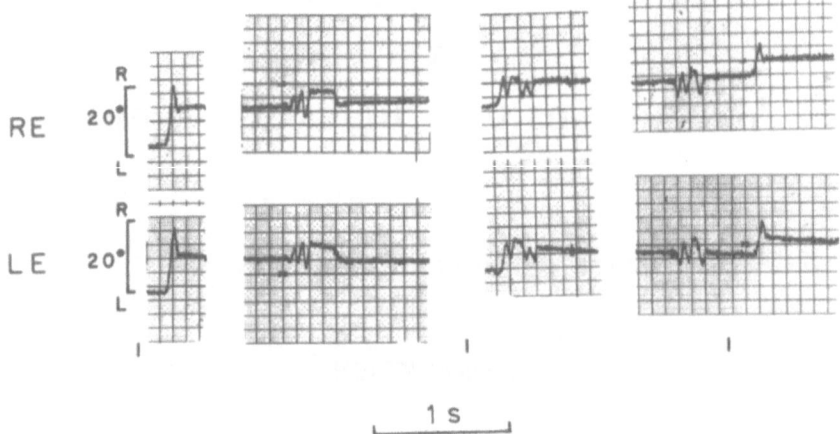

RE   20°

LE   20°

1 s

Figure 31.1 Spontaneous and post-saccadic horizontal saccadic oscillations (ocular flutter). Vertical bars indicate a target jump. Note the bursts of back-to-back, to-and-fro saccades without an intersaccadic interval. (From Zee and Robinson (1979a). *Ann. Neurol.,* **5**, 405–14. Reproduced by permission of Little, Brown & Co.)

This disorder reflects an increase in saccadic system gain and an abnormality of the adaptive control of saccade size (see below).

Before considering the specific nature of these different types of saccadic oscillations, it will be useful to review ideas of how saccades are generated normally (Robinson, 1981a; Leigh and Zee, 1982). Saccades are created by a pulse-step (phasic–tonic) change in motor innervation. The saccadic pulse is an eye velocity command that generates the high-frequency burst of innervation seen during the saccade. It moves the eye rapidly from one position to another against orbital viscous forces. The saccadic step is an eye position command that generates the appropriate level of innervation at the end of the saccade to hold the eye in its new position against orbital elastic restoring forces. For saccades to be both rapid and accurate the saccadic pulse must be of the appropriate height and size, respectively. For the eye to stop abruptly at the end of the saccade, to allow steady fixation, the saccadic step must be sustained and its size must be appropriately matched to that of the saccadic pulse.

It is generally thought that the immediate premotor commands for the pulse change in innervation are created by a neural circuit in the brainstem called the *saccadic pulse generator* (figure 31.2). This network is made up of a number of cell types including so-called *saccadic burst cells.* These neurones are normally silent but burst at a high discharge rate immediately preceding, and time-locked to, the high-frequency burst of neural activity that occurs in ocular motor neurones during a saccade. Burst cells for horizontal saccades are located in the pontine

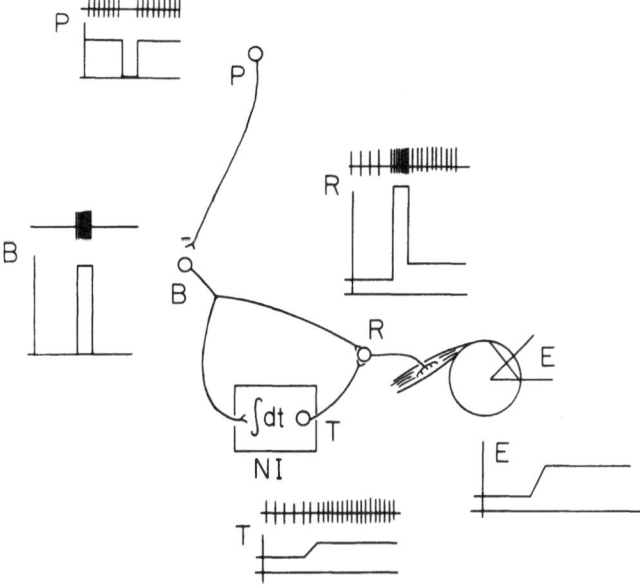

Figure 31.2 Relationship between pause (P) cells, burst (B) cells and tonic (T) cells. Pause cells act as an inhibitory gate and prevent extraneous burst cell activity except when a saccade is called for. Then pause cells cease discharging. The neural integrator (NI) integrates the saccadic pulse to produce the step that is seen on tonic neurones. The pulse and step combine to produce the innervational change (R) that produces the saccadic eye movement (E). (From Zee (1982). In Lessell and van Dalen (eds), *Neuro-Ophthalmology*. Reproduced by permission of Excerpta Medica.)

reticular formation; for vertical saccades, in the mesencephalic reticular formation.

The step of innervation is thought to be created by a central gaze-holding network, or neural integrator, that integrates (in the mathematical sense) the saccadic eye velocity command (pulse) to produce the appropriate position-coded information (step) for the ocular motor neurones. Another set of cells located in the brainstem reticular formation, *tonic neurones*, could provide such neural commands.

Exactly how the central nervous system creates a neural pulse of the appropriate height and duration for a given saccade is not known. One hypothesis, however, suggests that the duration of the burst cell discharge is controlled by an internal negative feedback loop that continuously compares desired eye position (based on the position of the target) and actual eye position (based on monitoring of efferent commands) (Zee and Robinson, 1979a; Zee *et al.*, 1976). In this hypothesis, the burst cells are continuously driven by an internal position error signal (the difference between desired and actual eye position). When this position error signal becomes zero, the burst cell discharge ceases and the saccade is over. The high gain of the burst cell discharge rate–position error relationship and the delay in the internal feedback loop make the saccadic pulse generator unstable.

Another class of cells, *pause neurones*, are clustered near the pontine midline and also change their discharge rate in relationship to saccades. Pause cells cease discharging (pause) immediately preceding, and time-locked to, the burst of neural activity that occurs during saccades; otherwise they discharge at a constant rate. When the pause cells are experimentally stimulated electrically in the monkey, the animal is unable to make saccades in any direction although other types of movements such as vestibular slow phases can still be elicited. In fact, if the pause cells are stimulated during a saccade, the eye movement is stopped in flight. These findings suggest that the pause cells tonically inhibit the burst cells, acting as a gate to prevent extraneous burst cell activity that might lead to saccadic oscillations (figure 31.2).

Two phenomena that have been described in normal human beings, namely *voluntary nystagmus* and *microsaccadic oscillations*, may reflect the inherent instability of the normal saccadic pulse generator. Voluntary nystagmus has been shown to consist of a series of back-to-back, to-and-fro saccadic eye movements (Shults *et al.*, 1977). Perhaps some individuals have learned to generate voluntary nystagmus by inhibiting their pause cells, which in turn would permit their burst neurones to oscillate. The brief period of small-amplitude oscillations that occurs after a very small saccade (microsaccadic oscillations) can be explained if one assumes that when pause cells shut off—for any sized saccade—they do not resume discharging again until a minimum period of time has elapsed, perhaps 30–40 ms. In this period, while the pause cells are silent, small-amplitude saccadic oscillations could occur.

Patients with certain neurological disorders may also show oscillations that consist of back-to-back, to-and-fro saccades without an intersaccadic interval. If these movements are restricted to the horizontal plane, they are called *ocular flutter*. If they are multidirectional, they are called *opsoclonus*. A disorder of the way that burst neurones are inhibited by pause cells could be the cause. Ocular flutter, in fact, appears to be an exaggerated form of voluntary nystagmus or microsaccadic oscillations with a slightly larger amplitude and corresponding lower frequency of oscillation. Opsoclonus may be an example of saccadic oscillations in which there is loss of inhibition to both the horizontal and vertical pulse generators.

It is conceivable that a mechanism similar to pause cell gating of saccadic burst neurones also exists for the circuits that generate pursuit eye movements. The pursuit system, with a delay in its visual feedback loop and a high (open-loop) gain necessary for accurate closed-loop tracking, could easily become unstable and show oscillations. In fact, normal individuals may show oscillations during smooth tracking. These oscillations would be deleterious during attempted fixation, so perhaps a gating mechanism for smooth pursuit exists. Of course, there must be some visual mechanism to assist ocular stabilisation during attempted fixation. This may or may not be the smooth pursuit system.

DISORDERED OR INAPPROPRIATE ADAPTIVE CONTROL

This may also be an important mechanism contributing to ocular oscillations. In the past decade, a major focus of ocular motor research has been upon the adaptive processes by which the brain 'repairs' itself in the face of disease and trauma as well as upon the changes accompanying normal development and ageing (Robinson, 1975; Ito, 1982). The inferior olive and cerebellum, in particular, appear to be involved in adaptive ocular motor control, with the cerebellum being likened to a 'repair shop' for ocular motor dysmetria of all types. The dorsal vermis and underlying fastigial nuclei function in the control of the size of the saccadic pulse (so that saccade size is appropriate) (Optican and Robinson, 1980). The flocculus functions in the control of the saccadic pulse-step match (so that the eye stops abruptly at the end of the saccade) as well as in control of the gain, phase and direction of the vestibulo-ocular reflex (so that images remain stationary on the retina during head movements) (Optican *et al.*, 1980; Schultheis and Robinson, 1981). These adaptive mechanisms respond to dysmetria slowly, over hours or days.

These considerations emphasise the concept that ocular motor disorders reflect the 'pure' effects of a lesion only when a patient is examined *immediately* after a neurological insult. Otherwise, one also observes the effects of attempted compensation. The adaptive repair mechanisms themselves must have adequate inputs to determine whether or not repair is needed, intact mechanisms for elaborating appropriate corrective adjustments, and access to the intrinsic structures and pathways that create and carry ocular motor commands. Furthermore, lesions within the adaptive networks in themselves could either create ocular motor abnormalities and/or possibly lead to a reversion to a previous state of 'disrepair'. The resulting ocular motor abnormalities would then reflect the organism's prior history of disease, trauma and natural development and ageing. For example, in the monkey, the effects of ablation of the flocculus upon vestibular ocular reflex (VOR) gain or the saccadic pulse-step match are idiosyncratic from animal to animal (Zee *et al.*, 1981). This variability may reflect a 'default' to an inherent state of ocular motor dysmetria.

Another form of saccadic oscillation, *macrosaccadic oscillations*, is an example of an inappropriately high gain. Macrosaccadic oscillations are sequences of *hypermetric saccades* separated by an intersaccadic interval of several hundred milliseconds. Each saccade takes the eye beyond the position of the target, preventing foveal fixation. Macrosaccadic oscillations are frequently a sign of lesions within the cerebellum and especially the dorsal vermis and underlying fastigial nuclei (Selhorst *et al.*, 1976) (figure 31.3). Experimentally, large lesions in this region lead to an enduring saccadic hypermetria (Optican and Robinson, 1980). The lesion therefore causes an increase in saccadic system gain (saccade size-retinal error relationship) as well as an inability to adjust the size of the saccadic pulse appropriately to produce accurate saccades. Thus, macrosaccadic oscillations are to be distinguished from ocular flutter and opsoclonus. The former, a series of discrete hypermetric saccades, reflects instability of the entire saccadic tracking

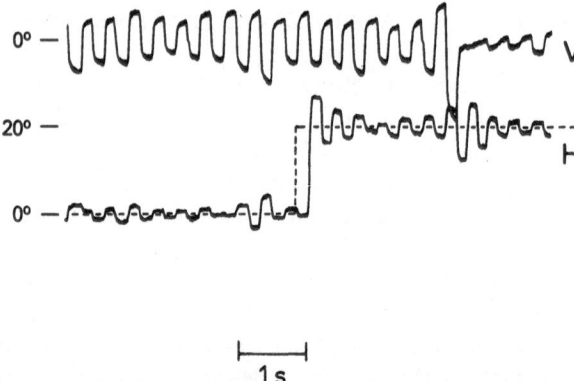

Figure 31.3 Macrosaccadic oscillations in a monkey after total cerebellectomy. The broken line indicates the target position. Note the oscillations in both the horizontal and vertical planes.

system. The latter, continuous saccadic oscillations, reflects instability of the intrinsic brainstem neurones that generate the saccadic pulse.

The manner in which high gains that are the result of an adaptive (or maladaptive) process can lead to macrosaccadic oscillations is well exemplified in the response of some patients with ocular myasthenia gravis who have no cerebellar or central nervous system dysfunction at all. If a myasthenic patient with a severe degree of ophthalmoparesis is given an anticholinesterase inhibitor to relieve the neuromuscular blockade, the patient's saccades may suddenly become much larger. When the patient is then required to fixate a target, the eyes may oscillate about the position of the target because the patient cannot make a saccade small enough to acquire the target (Zee and Robinson, 1979b). The reason is, of course, that the anticholinesterase inhibitor, by relieving the eye muscle weakness, unmasks the increased saccadic innervation that had been programmed by the central nervous system to overcome the peripheral muscle weakness. Now, for a given retinal error (the distance between the peripheral retinal location of the image of a target and the fovea), saccadic innervation is too large. This increase in saccadic system gain creates saccadic dysmetria (overshoot) and, when the gain is 2.0 or greater, sustained macrosaccadic oscillations occur.

A similar phenomenon can be demonstrated in patients with ophthalmoparesis in one eye who, for reasons of better acuity or ocular dominance, habitually view out of that paretic eye (Kommerell et al., 1976). Appropriate adaptation occurs to increase innervation (to both eyes because of Herring's law of equal innervation) for a given visual stimulus and so to overcome the effects of the muscle weakness. When such patients are transiently forced (by occluding the paretic eye) to view with their normally mobile eye, saccades become inappropriately large, creating saccadic overshoot. If the degree of paresis is marked, and is for saccades in both directions, then macrosaccadic oscillations may appear.

We have recently examined a patient with chronic, unilateral abducens nerve palsy and studied the effects of chronic viewing with the paretic eye on pursuit responses (Optican *et al.*, 1982). We found that pursuit system innervation (gain) increased when the patient viewed monocularly with the good eye. He had smooth pendular oscillations of the eyes (occurring at a frequency of about 3 Hz) during both attempted tracking and even occasionally during attempted steady fixation (figure 31.4). In other words, pendular oscillations were induced by an 'adaptive'

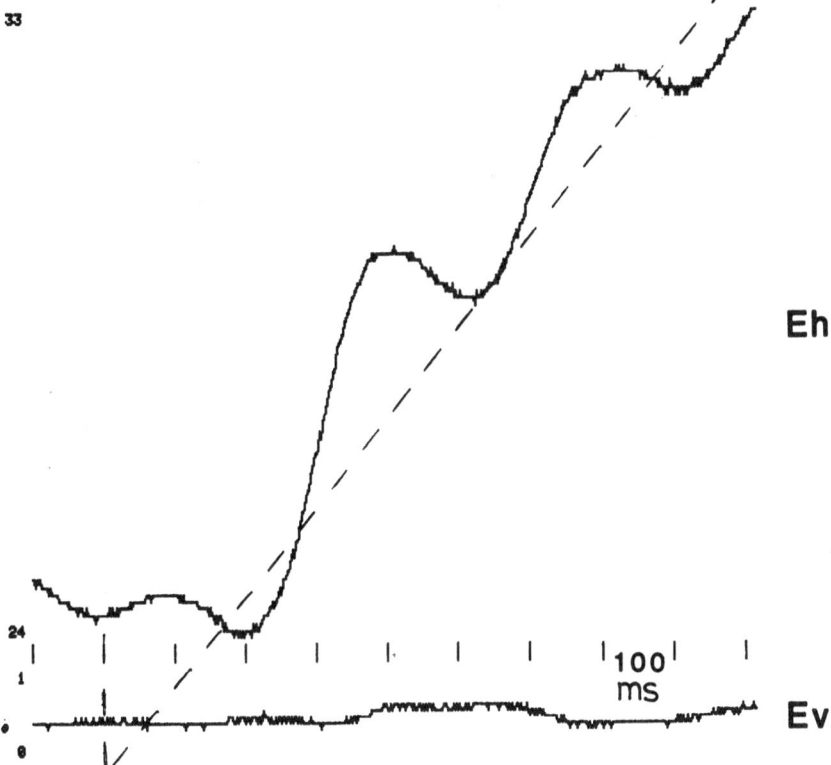

Figure 31.4 Pendular oscillations of the left eye in a patient with a right lateral rectus palsy who had been habitually viewing with the right eye. This record is with the left eye viewing. The broken line approximates the target position. Note slight oscillation even before the target begins moving.

increase in pursuit system gain. This finding suggests that pathological pendular oscillations can arise from an inappropriately increased pursuit system gain. In fact, increased pursuit system gain has also been hypothesised as one of the mechanisms underlying congenital nystagmus (Dell'Osso, 1982). Another potential cause of pursuit system oscillations is an increase in the delay necessary for visual feedback—perhaps due to prolonged transmission time in demyelinated axons.

Another ocular motor oscillation, *periodic alternating nystagmus* (PAN), also reflects (mal)adaptive ocular motor control (Leigh *et al.*, 1981). PAN consists of a horizontal jerk nystagmus that alternates direction every few minutes. PAN has been reported in a variety of circumstances but is especially common with acquired neurological lesions in the region of the caudal cerebellum and dorsal medulla. Sometimes this nystagmus is present only in darkness and it has been reported in blind patients with no other evidence of neurological disease.

A clue to the genesis of this oscillation was provided by Kornhuber (1959), who followed the course of a patient, who eventually developed PAN, for a number of years. Originally she showed an exaggeration of a vestibular response— the reversal phase of post-rotatory nystagmus—shown by normal individuals. This reversal phase, also called secondary nystagmus or post-postrotatory nystagmus, occurs during or on stopping a sustained rotational stimulus (velocity step). After the primary vestibular reaction has died away, a weak secondary response develops with slow phases in the opposite direction. This reversal phase has been attributed to a vestibular adaptation or repair process that would act to null persistent unidirectional nystagmus. (The reversal phase of optokinetic after-nystagmus has been thought to be a related phenomenon.) Kornhuber reported that his patient, prior to developing PAN, showed not one but several reversals of post-rotatory nystagmus before it died out. The period of this damped oscillation was similar to that of the fully formed PAN that she subsequently developed. Thus one can speculate that PAN is an exaggerated form of a normal adaptive process. We developed a hypothetical explanation for PAN using this idea.

We postulated that PAN arises from three factors. The first is an instability in the brainstem neural networks that generate the slow phases of vestibular and optokinetic nystagmus. The instability is due to an *inappropriately high gain within a postulated positive feedback loop in the vestibular-optokinetic system*. (The function of this feedback loop is both to increase the vestibular ocular reflex time constant and to produce optokinetic after-nystagmus. These responses ensure better image stabilisation both during and after sustained head movements.) Secondly, the development of PAN depends upon the appropriate *action of an adaptive network* that acts to null prolonged, inappropriate nystagmus. Thirdly, PAN persists because of an *inability to use visual information* (retinal image slip) for both immediate visual suppression of inappropriate nystagmus as well as for the long-term adaptive adjustment of the gain within the brainstem vestibular-optokinetic pathways.

Why does the gain of the brainstem positive feedback loop increase? One possibility is a loss of inhibition in vestibular pathways, possibly due to interruption of the vestibular commissure. In fact, many patients with PAN have lesions in the dorsal medulla which might be expected to interrupt the vestibular commissure. In the monkey, PAN has been created by a lesion that included the dorsal medulla (Burde *et al.*, 1975). Most patients and the experimental animal with PAN, however, also had a vestibulo-cerebellar lesion. This might account for both the inability to suppress the nystagmus in the light as well as the inability to adjust the gain of the positive feedback loop appropriately in the brainstem vestibular-optokinetic pathway. Interestingly PAN can be stopped pharmacologically with baclofen (Halmagyi *et al.*, 1980), a presumed GABA-ergic agent, which may act to augment transmission either in cerebellar Purkinje cell projections to the vestibular nuclei or in vestibular commissural pathways. Both pathways are thought to be inhibitory in nature and use GABA as a neurotransmitter.

One might ask why some blind patients, without other evidence of neurological disease, also show PAN. Such patients may have an inherently high gain within the positive feedback loop in their vestibular-optokinetic pathway that is normally' adjusted downwards by the cerebellum. When visual feedback is lost, however, the cerebellum does not have a way of knowing whether or not the feedback loop gain is appropriate. Thus a patient's performance may revert back to a 'default value' that, in particular cases, might be too high. In fact, PAN in blind patients is often relieved when vision is restored (Cross *et al.*, 1982). Whether this is simply the result of restoration of smooth pursuit function with the ability to suppress unwanted nystagmus or whether there is an adaptive adjustment in brainstem pathways to eliminate the periodic alternating nystagmus completely is not yet known. Interestingly, other types of ocular oscillations also make their appearance when patients or experimental animals become blind (Leigh and Zee, 1980; Zee *et al.*, 1982). Raising experimental animals in darkness or in continuous stroboscopic illumination (the latter does not permit smooth retinal image slip) may also lead to development of ocular oscillations (Conway *et al.*, 1981; Harris and Cynader, 1981; Melvill Jones *et al.*, 1981).

There are a number of additional types of ocular oscillations, not discussed here, that probably have mechanisms different from those that we have suggested (for example, see Ell *et al.*, this volume, chapter 32). Nevertheless, loss of an inhibitory gating mechanism and high gains associated with inappropriate adaptation to ocular motor dysmetria may play an important role in the genesis of many types of ocular oscillations.

CONCLUSIONS

We have proposed two types of mechanism, namely failure of inhibitory gating and abnormal feedback characteristics, that can reasonably account for several types of involuntary ocular oscillations occurring in neurological disease. It is appropriate, elegant and heuristic to couch these theoretical mechanisms in the conceptual framework of control systems theory, which gives us an understanding of how oscillatory processes can arise in neural control networks. Current neurophysiological evidence shows that many theoretical aspects of the control systems models have identifiable physiological realisations. Conversely, neurological data can provide insights into the nature of the systems involved in ocular motor control.

ACKNOWLEDGEMENTS

Vendetta Matthews provided editorial assistance. This research was supported by National Institutes of Health Grants EY01849 and EY00158.

REFERENCES

Burde, R. M., Stroud, M. H., Roper-Hall, G., Wirth, F. P. and O'Leary, J. L. (1975). Ocular motor dysfunction in total and hemicerebellectomized monkeys. *Br. J. Ophthalmol.*, **59**, 560–5.

Conway, J. L., Timberlake, G. T. and Skavenski, A. A. (1981). Oculomotor changes in cats reared without experiencing continuous retinal image motion. *Exp. Brain Res.*, **43**, 229–32.

Cross, S. A., Smith, J. L. and Norton, E. W. D. (1982). Periodic alternating nystagmus clearing after vitrectomy. *J. Clin. Neuro-ophthalmol.*, **2**, 5–11.

Dell'Osso, L. F. (1982). In Lennerstrand, G., Zee, D. S. and Keller, E. L. (eds), *Functional Basis of Ocular Motility Disorders*, Pergamon Press, Oxford, pp. 129–38.

Halmagyi, G. M., Rudge, P., Gresty, M. A., Leigh, R. J. and Zee, D. S. (1980). Treatment of periodic alternating nystagmus. *Ann. Neurol.*, **8**, 609–11.

Harris, L. R. and Cynader, M. (1981). The eye movements of the dark-reared cat. *Exp. Brain Res.*, **44**, 41–56.

Ito, M. (1982). Cerebellar control of the vestibulo-ocular reflex—around the flocculus hypothesis. *Annu. Rev. Neurosci.*, **5**, 275–96.

Kommerell, G., Olivier, D. and Theopold, H. (1976). Adaptive programming of phasic and tonic components in saccadic eye movements. Investigations in patients with abducens palsy. *Invest. Ophthalmol.*, **15**, 657–60.

Kornhuber, H. H. (1959). Der periodisch alternierende Nystagmus (Nystagmus alternans) und die Enthemmung des vestibularen Systems. *Arch. Ohren Nasen Kehlkopfheilkd.*, **174**, 182–209.

Leigh, R. J., Robinson, D. A. and Zee, D. S. (1981). A hypothetical explanation for periodic alternating nystagmus: instability in the optokinetic-vestibular system. *Ann. NY Acad. Sci.*, **374**, 619–35.

Leigh, R. J. and Zee, D. S. (1980). Eye movements of the blind. *Invest. Ophthalmol.*, **19**, 328–31.

Leigh, R. J. and Zee, D. S. (1982). *The Neurology of Eye Movements*, F. A. Davis, Philadelphia.

Melvill Jones, G., Mandl, G., Cynader, M. and Outerbridge, J. S. (1981). Eye oscillations in strobe reared cats. *Brain Res.*, **209**, 47–60.

Optican, L. M., Chu, F. C., Hays, A. V., Reingold, D. B. and Zee, D. S. (1982). Adaptive changes of oculomotor performance in abducens nerve palsy. *Soc. Neurosci. Abstr.*, **8**, 418.

Optican, L. M. and Robinson, D. A. (1980). Cerebellar dependent adaptive control of the primate saccadic system. *J. Neurophysiol.*, **44**, 1058–76.

Optican, L. M., Zee, D. S., Miles, F. A. and Lisberger, S. G. (1980). Oculomotor deficits in monkeys with floccular lesions. *Soc. Neurosci. Abstr.*, **6**, 474.

Robinson, D. A. (1975). How the oculomotor system repairs itself. *Invest. Ophthalmol.*, **14**, 413–15.

Robinson, D. A. (1981a). In Brooks, V. B. (ed.), *Handbook of Physiology*, vol. 2, part II, American Physiological Society, Washington, pp. 1275–320.

Robinson, D. A. (1981b). The use of control systems analysis in the neurophysiology of eye movements. *Annu. Rev. Neurosci.*, 4, 463–503.

Schultheis, L. W. and Robinson, D. A. (1981). Directional plasticity of the vestibulo-ocular reflex in the cat. *Ann. NY Acad. Sci.*, 374, 504–12.

Selhorst, J. B., Stark, L., Ochs, A. L. and Hoyt, W. F. (1976). Disorders in cerebellar oculomotor control. II. Macrosaccadic oscillations, an oculographic, control system and clinico-anatomic analysis. *Brain*, 99, 509–22.

Shults, W. T., Stark, L., Hoyt, W. F. and Ochs, A. L. (1977). Normal saccadic structure of voluntary nystagmus. *Arch. Ophthalmol.*, 95, 1399–404.

Zee, D. S. (1982). Ocular motor control. In Lessell, S. and van Dalen, J. T. W. (eds), *Neuro-Ophthalmology*, vol. 1, Excerpta Medica, Amsterdam, chap. 10, p. 131.

Zee, D. S., Optican, L. M., Cook, J. D., Robinson, D. A. and Engel, W. K. (1976). Slow saccades in spinocerebellar degeneration. *Arch. Neurol.*, 33, 243–51.

Zee, D. S. and Robinson, D. A. (1979a). A hypothetical explanation of saccadic oscillations. *Ann. Neurol.*, 5, 405–14.

Zee, D. S. and Robinson, D. A. (1979b). In Thompson, H. S. (ed.), *Topics in Neuro-Ophthalmology*, Williams and Wilkins, Baltimore, pp. 266–85.

Zee, D. S., Tusa, R. J., Optican, L. M. and Gucer, G. (1982). Effects of bilateral occipital lobe lesions on eye movements in primates: preliminary observations. *Soc. Neurosci. Abstr.*, 8, 291.

Zee, D. S., Yamazaki, A., Butler, P. H. and Gucer, G. (1981). Effects of ablation of flocculus and paraflocculus on eye movements in primate. *J. Neurophysiol.*, 46, 878–98.

32
Pendular nystagmus (ocular myoclonus) and related somatic tremors: their pharmacological modification and treatment

JONATHAN J. ELL, LESLIE J. FINDLEY and MICHAEL A. GRESTY

INTRODUCTION

Pendular nystagmus can be defined as an involuntary oscillation of the eye or eyes. When it occurs in conjunction with other body movements, it is often termed ocular myoclonus. In previous reports (Gresty *et al.*, 1982; Ell *et al.*, 1982) we have outlined in detail the essential characteristics of acquired pendular nystagmus. Approximately 30% of our patients and those reviewed from the literature had associated body tremors. Our analyses led us to the conclusion that the eye and body movements were causally related. Subsequent attempts at pharmacological modification of these movements have confirmed this conclusion.

PENDULAR NYSTAGMUS

The types of waveforms encountered are given in figure 32.1. It is noteworthy that the nystagmus can be monocular or binocular. In the case of a binocular pendular nystagmus, the eyes may move conjugately or disconjugately, i.e. the trajectories of motion of the two eyes may differ. An electro-oculographic trace illustrating disconjugate nystagmus is shown in figure 32.2. However, wave analysis of such a nystagmus shows that the two eyes move with a fixed and constant phase relationship. Coherence measurements (made using a spectrum analyser) indicate, furthermore, a high degree of synchronisation between the eyes.

Of our patients, approximately 50% had multiple sclerosis and 30% had brain-stem angioma (localised to the midbrain) or cerebrovascular disease. The commonly associated oculomotor abnormalities were:

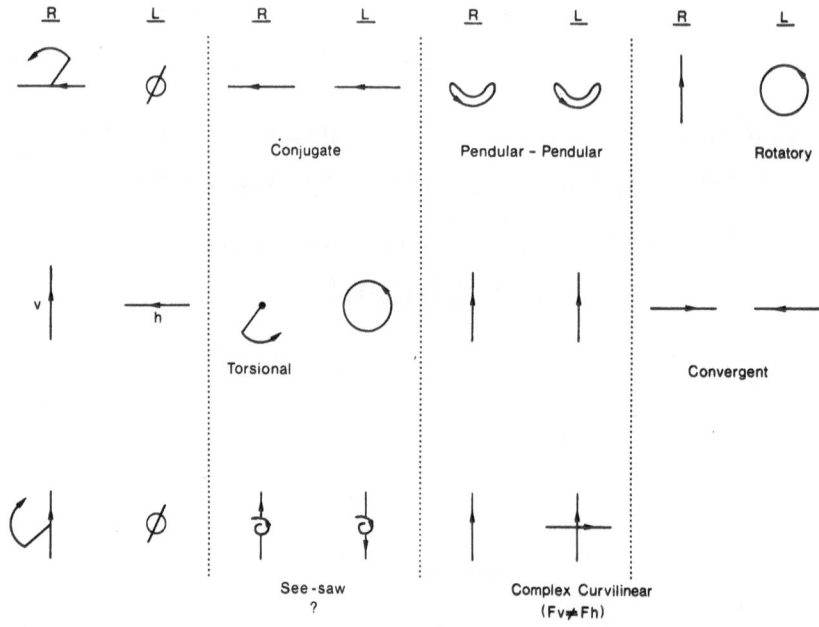

Figure 32.1 Trajectories of the eye/eyes encountered in our cases of acquired pendular nystagmus. The term 'complex curvilinear' refers to cases of monocular nystagmus in whom the frequencies of oscillation in the vertical and horizontal planes differ, producing an irregular 'hysteresis loop' trajectory.

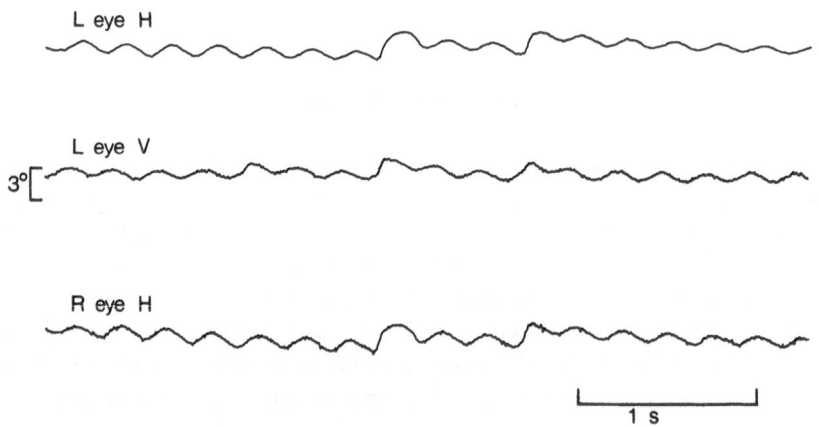

Figure 32.2 Disconjugate pendular nystagmus. The right eye oscillates in the horizontal plane, the left eye follows a circular trajectory (rotatory nystagmus). Recordings made by DC-coupled electro-oculography.

convergence failure	90%,
internuclear ophthalmoplegia	66%,
skew deviation	15%,
strabismus	5%.

Significantly the major oculomotor systems of saccades, optokinetic response, vestibulo-ocular reflex and pursuit could all be intact in the presence of pendular nystagmus.

RELATED SOMATIC TREMORS

In the 30% of our patients with associated somatic tremors, a high degree of correlation between the frequency of eye oscillation and tremor frequency was found. In some of our patients with the syndrome of 'oculo-palatal-laryngeal-pharyngeal-diaphragmatic myoclonus', spectral analysis of the various movements showed a high degree of correlation and suggested that they were causally related (as assessed by coherence values). An example of this is shown in figure 32.3. In some of our patients such a high degree of synchronisation between eye and body movements was not present. We consider that in this latter instance use of the term 'ocular myoclonus' is not really justified as it implies that the eye and limb 'tremors' share a unitary mechanism.

MECHANISM OF PENDULAR NYSTAGMUS AND CERTAIN SOMATIC TREMORS

Aschoff *et al.* (1974) postulated that acquired pendular nystagmus in multiple sclerosis represented a failure of the position-holding function of the cerebellar nuclei and was thus a direct indication of cerebellar disease. The hypothesis cannot explain the existence of monocular pendular nystagmus as cerebellar stimulation studies to date have revealed binocular projections (Ron and Robinson, 1973). We have proposed that, in some instances at least, the nystagmus arises from spontaneous oscillation in deafferented neurones proximal to the oculomotor nuclei. The frequency characteristics of the nystagmus make it unlikely to arise from activity within a feedback loop. Furthermore, the neuronal circuits involved with somatic and ocular movements are so dissimilar that it is improbable that such closely interrelated tremors could arise from disorders involving the respective primary pathways. Tahmoush *et al.* (1972), from a polygraphic study of oculo-palatal myoclonus with associated tremor of the extremities, suggested that the abnormal ocular, branchial and limb movements shared a common pathophysiological mechanism. Drawing upon the post-mortem examination findings of Guillain *et al.* (1933) and others, they proposed that the site of the rhythmic discharge responsible for the myoclonus was the inferior olivary nucleus. Llinás

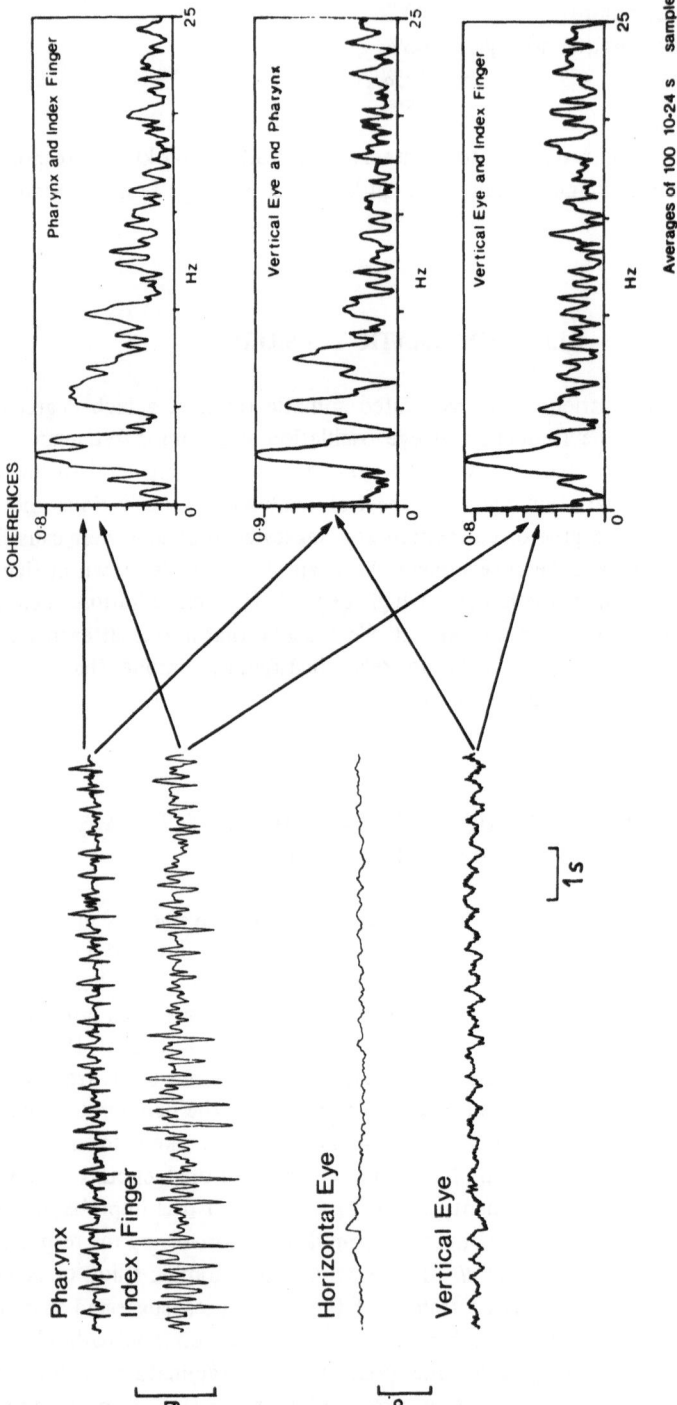

Figure 32.3 Recordings of myoclonus in the pharynx, finger and eyes in a patient with the syndrome of oculo-palatal myoclonus. Somatic tremors measured with piezoresistive accelerometers (magnitude in milli-g, r.m.s.). Coherences on the right indicate a high degree of synchronisation between the various involuntary movements.

and Yarom (1980) have cultured cells from the inferior olivary nucleus in the monkey which have spontaneous rhythmical activity that is Ca^{2+} mediated.

We share this view of a common rhythm generator and suggest that the occurrence of tremor in various body parts is dependent upon additional access of abnormal spontaneous neuronal oscillatory activity to appropriate circuits. Thus from a pathophysiological point of view, more than one 'lesion' is required to produce ocular and somatic tremors.

PHARMACOLOGICAL MODIFICATION OF PENDULAR NYSTAGMUS AND ASSOCIATED TREMORS

In the past, many attempts have been made to suppress pharmacologically both somatic tremors and pendular nystagmus with agents such as L-dopa, tetrabenazine, clonazepam and baclofen. Acquired pendular nystagmus often results in considerable visual handicap. Apart from constant oscillopsia, patients suffer difficulty with maintenance of target fixation under conditions of movement, reading difficulty secondary to impaired generation of normometric scanning steps and difficulty with viewing motion pictures. The physical handicaps resulting from low-frequency, large-amplitude postural and intention tremor are often of devastating severity.

Following on from the hypothesis of a common rhythm generator and neuronal membrane instability, we investigated the effects of the cardiac glycoside, ouabaine, upon pendular nystagmus. This drug alters cellular trans-membrane potentials through inhibition of the sodium pump. The results of a 250 μg i.v. injection of ouabaine given to a patient with multiple sclerosis who had a pendular nystagmus are shown in figure 32.4. Following administration, the amplitude of the nystagmus rose from its usual maximum level of $2.5°$ to a maximum of $5°$ after 5 min. The amplitude then declined to baseline level after 13 min. This response parallels the known pharmacokinetics of ouabaine in humans. An injection of normal saline given as a control had no effect. This exacerbation of pendular nystagmus following intravenous ouabaine has been confirmed in five other patients, all of whom had multiple sclerosis. However, in a single patient, a 62-year-old male with oculo-palatal-labial-laryngeal-diaphragmatic myoclonus developing after a brainstem stroke, a 250 μg i.v. injection of ouabaine completely abolished the involuntary movements for 7 min. A subsequent one-month trial of oral digoxin 0.25 mg per day showed no discernible effect.

Charcot's observations on the effects of the administration of certain plant alkaloids upon involuntary movements (Ordenstein, 1868) led us to examine the effects of hyoscine upon pendular nystagmus. From trials with several patients, it was clear that an intravenous dose of 400 μg resulted in complete suppression of their nystagmus. However, at this dosage they all experienced an unacceptable level of drowsiness. Not only did this make the use of hyoscine alone impracticable in clinical practice but also made interpretation of the positive response difficult as pendular nystagmus usually diminishes during periods of somnolence of any cause.

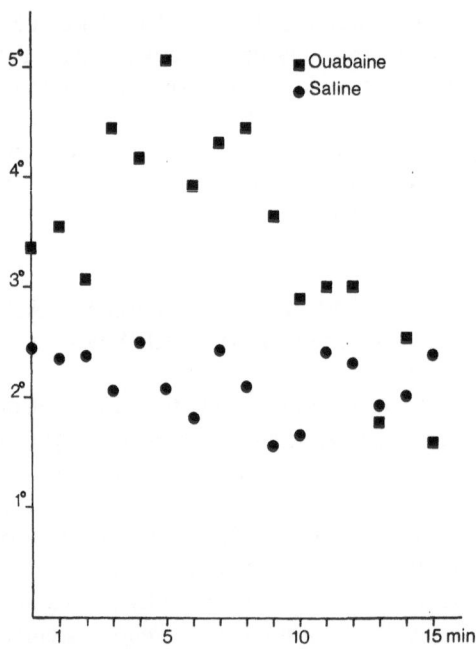

Figure 32.4 Effects of ouabaine upon the amplitude (in degrees peak) of pendular nystagmus. Also indicated is the saline control study.

The next drug investigated was the local anaesthetic, lignocaine hydrochloride. Intravenous administration of 100 mg over 5 min caused subsequent suppression of nystagmus for 3 min. No drowsiness was induced. In fact, the drug has an alerting effect. The effect of lignocaine 100 mg followed by hyoscine 200 µg i.v. upon a rotatory pendular nystagmus in a patient with multiple sclerosis is shown in figure 32.5. In this instance the nystagmus was suppressed (and visual acuity improved by two lines on the Snellen chart) for an hour.

Also illustrated in figure 32.5 is the effect of these two drugs in combination upon an associated postural tremor of the upper limbs in the same patient. Suppression of the tremor also continued for an hour. We have since confirmed these observations in eight patients (all with multiple sclerosis). The durations of suppression in these patients ranged from 1 to 12 h.

Hyoscine is readily absorbed, intact and active, by the gastrointestinal tract; however, lignocaine is not. Recently, a derivative of lignocaine, tocainide hydrochloride, has become available which is suitable for oral administration. We have investigated the effects of a combination of tocainide 2400 mg/day (six 400 mg doses) and hyoscine 600 µg b.d. in a 32-year-old woman with multiple sclerosis and a severe 4.5 Hz postural and intention tremor of the upper and lower limbs. Before this treatment was begun, it was confirmed that both her nystagmus and tremor were abolished or suppressed following intravenous lignocaine and hyoscine.

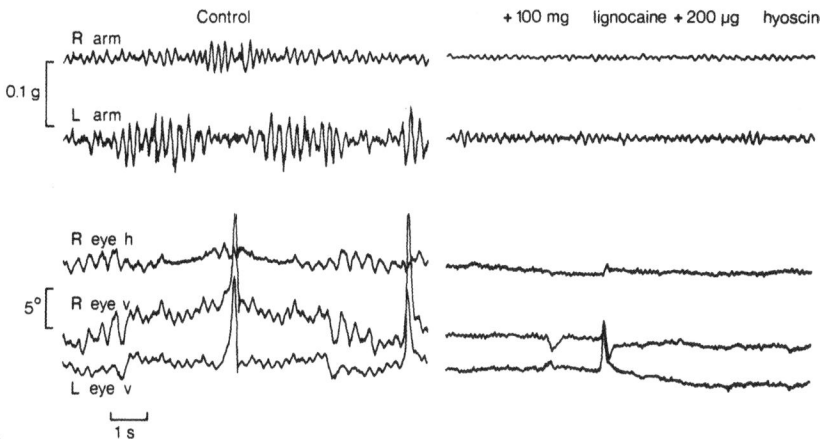

Figure 32.5 Effects of acute intravenous administration of lignocaine 100 mg and hyoscine 200 µg upon disconjugate pendular nystagmus and postural tremor in a patient with multiple sclerosis. Upper traces on left show tremor recordings, and lower traces show electro-oculograms (pre-drugs). Traces on right show suppression of tremor and nystagmus (post-drugs).

Treatment with tocainide and hyoscine was continued for two weeks until what we considered to be an optimum response was attained. The oral regime failed to suppress the pendular nystagmus. The effects of oral and intravenous therapies upon the postural tremor are shown in figure 32.6. Tremor magnitude as measured in milli-*g*, root mean square (r.m.s.), was reduced nearly 100-fold. As a result, she was able to walk unassisted and to write (albeit with difficulty) for the first time in three years. No untoward side-effects, apart from some dryness of the mouth, were encountered.

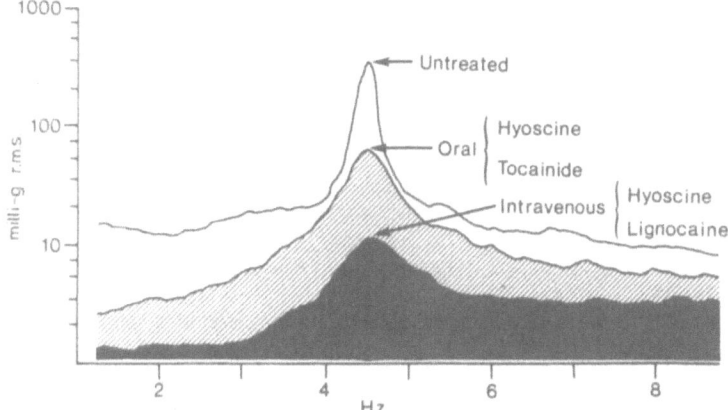

Figure 32.6 Effects of acute intravenous administration of lignocaine 100 mg and hyoscine 200 µg upon 4.5 Hz postural tremor of the upper limbs in a patient with multiple sclerosis (black area). Open area represents baseline recordings. Hatched area shows tremor magnitude at two weeks after commencing tocainide 2400 mg/day and hyoscine 1200 µg/day.

CONCLUSIONS

In general, it would appear that intravenous administration of hyoscine and lignocaine can abolish or suppress both acquired pendular nystagmus and low-frequency postural tremor. These two drugs have their actions upon cellular membranes. In the knowledge that other drugs that act through modification of chemical neurotransmission have little effect on such involuntary movements, we consider that our results provide firm evidence for the hypothesis of a common rhythm generator and neuronal membrane instability being the underlying causes of these movements. It must be stressed, however, that patients with pendular nystagmus and associated tremors are relatively rare. Such patients are all too frequently severely disabled, not only by their nystagmus and tremor but also by additional neurological deficits. From our experience, it is not possible to assess accurately the response to long-term oral therapy in severely disabled patients. We would suggest that treatment with oral tocainide and hyoscine be restricted to those patients with pendular nystagmus and associated tremor in the absence of any other significant neurological signs or disabilities.

REFERENCES

Aschoff, J. C., Conrad, B. and Kornhuber, H. H. (1974). Acquired pendular nystagmus with oscillopsia in multiple sclerosis: a sign of cerebellar nuclei disease. *J. Neurol. Neurosurg. Psychiatr.*, 37, 570-7.

Ell, J. J., Gresty, M. A., Chambers, B. R. and Findley, L. J. (1982). Acquired pendular nystagmus: characteristics, pathophysiology and pharmacological modification. In Roucoux, A. (ed.), *Physiological and Pathological Aspects of Eye Movements*, Proceedings of the Workshop Sponsored by the European Communities, Chateau Pont d'Oye, Belgium, Pergamon Press, Oxford, in press. Oxford, in press.

Gresty, M. A., Ell, J. J. and Findley, L. J. (1982). Acquired pendular nystagmus: its characteristics, localising value and pathophysiology. *J. Neurol. Neurosurg Psychiatr.*, 45, 431-9.

Guillain, G., Thurel, R. and Bertrand, I. (1933). Examen anatomo-pathologique d'un cas de myoclonies vélo-pharyngo-oculo-diaphragmatiques associées à des myoclonies squelettiques synchrones. *Rev. Neurol. (Paris)*, 2, 801-12.

Llinás, R. R. and Yarom, Y. (1980). Electrophysiological properties of mammalian inferior olivary cells *in vitro*. In Courville, J., de Montigny, C. and Lamarre, Y. (eds), *The Olivary Nucleus, Anatomy and Physiology*, Raven Press, New York, pp. 379-88.

Ordenstein, L. (1868). *Sur la Paralysie Agitante à la Sclerose en Plaques Generalisée*, Delahaye, Paris.

Ron, S. and Robinson, D. A. (1973). Eye movements evoked by cerebellar stimulation in the alert monkey. *J. Neurophysiol.*, 36, 1004-22.

Tahmoush, A. J., Brooks, J. E. and Keltner, J. L. (1972). Palatal myoclonus associated with abnormal ocular and extremity movements: a polygraphic study. *Arch. Neurol.*, 27, 431-40.

SECTION 8
DIVERSE TREMULOUS STATES

33
Atypical tremors, rare tremors and unclassified tremors

STANLEY FAHN

INTRODUCTION

Tremors have been conveniently classified according to their clinical appearance, as to whether they are present at rest, with posture holding, with action, or on approaching a target (Fahn, this volume, chapter 26). Within each of these categories are tremors of different aetiologies. Electrophysiological, pharmacological and pathological correlates of each tremor are being obtained to bring about a better understanding of the pathophysiology and treatment, as well as to aid in diagnosis and classification. Despite the convenience of our current classification scheme, there remain a number of unusual and undiagnosed types of tremor. In fact, from practical experience of seeing patients with a variety of movement disorders, I find that the disorders of tremor are probably filled with more patients undiagnosed in terms of aetiology and not fitting into previously established descriptions than any other category of movement disorder. In this chapter tremors that are atypical, rare and even unclassified at present in terms of diagnosis will be described.

Atypical tremors include dystonic tremor, spasmus nutans, rhythmical myoclonus and proximal parkinsonian tremor. Rare, but recognised, tremors, include primary writing tremor, hysterical tremor and hereditary chin quivering. Unclassified tremors to be described include paroxysmal tremor and tremor associated with naphthalene intoxication. It should be noted that the tremors presented here are only a fragment of a much larger number of unusual tremors that could be described. It will serve merely as an example of the broad spectrum of this problem.

ATYPICAL TREMORS

Dystonic tremors

Dystonic tremors are those oscillations seen as part of dystonic movements. Rhythmical group action potentials occur in dystonia (Yanagisawa and Goto,

431

1971), and these are manifested as tremors. Dystonic tremors are not the only type of tremor seen in patients with torsion dystonia. Many patients as well as members of the family have an associated essential tremor (Zeman *et al.*, 1960; Yanagisawa *et al.*, 1972; Bundey *et al.*, 1975; Couch, 1976). Perhaps the most common form of dystonic tremor is that seen in patients with spasmodic torticollis. Nuchal tremor is seen in many of these patients. Case 1 demonstrates that this tremor is seen when the patient attempts to resist the pulling of the tonically contracting muscles. This feature of the dystonic patient attempting to overcome and resist the contractions of the dystonic musculature appears to be a basic phenomenon giving rise to dystonic tremor. By asking the patient not to resist, but to relax and allow the contractions to occur, the tremor can disappear. Case 2 illustrates that a large-amplitude dystonic action tremor can also occur in a limb. This tremor is present only when the arm is in specific postures or actions, and disappears when the arm is allowed to be in a posture that does not resist the direction of the actively pulling muscles.

Case 1

A 53-year-old man had classical spasmodic torticollis so that his head was turned with the chin directed to the right shoulder. When his head was allowed to remain in this posture, no nuchal tremor was seen. When the patient attempted to straighten his head, a horizontal tremor of the neck began and persisted as long as the head was held straight, i.e. a resistance against the direction of the pulling of the dystonic contractions.

Case 2

An Ashkenazic Jewish man developed involuntary movements at the age of seven while writing with the right hand. Handwriting was switched to the left hand at the age of nine. At the age of 19, the left leg twisted when he walked. Examination at the age of 24 revealed dystonic movements of both arms and the left leg, but only with action and not at rest. The extended right arm tended to pronate involuntarily. When the patient attempted to keep that arm straight, a coarse pronation–supination tremor of that hand developed. It was maximum when the arm was supinated, and it disappeared when he allowed the arm to remain in a hyperpronated posture. On finger-to-nose manoeuvre, the right arm developed a coarse tremor as the finger approached the nose. However, if the patient allowed the right arm to be hyperabducted at the shoulder, no tremor developed during the finger-to-nose manoeuvre. These variations with posture distinguish dystonic tremors from the action tremor of essential tremor and enhanced physiological tremor.

Rhythmical and oscillatory myoclonus

It is frequently debated whether the rhythmical movements of so-called palatal myoclonus and ocular myoclonus are actually tremors or myoclonus. The fact that they may persist during sleep and that sychronous contractions may occur elsewhere in the body (Tahmoush *et al.*, 1972) strongly indicate that these indeed represent myoclonus rather than tremor. Their response to 5-hydroxytryptophan (Magnussen *et al.*, 1977; Williams *et al.*, 1978) supports this concept. The question arises whether other segmental rhythmical contractions are to be considered as rhythmical myoclonus or as a tremor. Case 3 describes a patient with rhythmical 2 Hz 'tremor' of the neck and arms that was eventually diagnosed as rhythmical segmental myoclonus on the basis that EMG recordings showed that the muscular contractions were firing synchronously in all affected muscles (Fahn and Singh, 1980).

Case 3

A 27-year-old left-handed man had infantile right hemiplegia secondary to a left hemisphere porencephalic cyst from a birth injury. He had a lifelong history of right hemiparesis, right hemianaesthesia, right homonymous hemianopia, and pendular and jerk nystagmus. Childhood seizures were controlled with phenytoin, 400 mg per day, and phenobarbital, 180 mg per day, which he has continued to take. At the age of 15, a rhythmical 'tremor' of the right shoulder developed and responded to trihexyphenidyl, which was eventually discontinued. At the age of 19, the 'tremor' returned. There was no response to trihexyphenidyl, diazepam or perphenazine. At the age of 23, a ventriculo-peritoneal shunt to drain the porencephalic cyst was carried out in an attempt to treat the 'tremor'. The 'tremor' disappeared for a few days, then returned. Meningitis led to the removal of the shunt catheter. The 'tremor' then spread to the neck. The following medications were tried without success: reserpine, tetrabenazine, clonazepam, diazepam, perphenazine, haloperidol and trihexyphenidyl. At the age of 27, the 'tremor' spread to involve the left shoulder also.

Examination at the age of 27 revealed simultaneous rhythmical contractions of the neck and both shoulders and proximal arms at a rate of 2 Hz. The head moved in a flexion–extension direction. The arms moved in an anterior–posterior direction when sitting or lying, but in an abduction–adduction direction when standing. All movements occurred simultaneously and symmetrically. There was no palatal or ocular myoclonus. The movements were not present during sleep. EMG recordings utilising surface electrodes revealed synchronous contractions of all muscles involved. Plasma levels of phenytoin and phenobarbital were within normal range. Treatment with 5-hydroxytryptophan (5-HTP) and carbidopa completely eliminated the involuntary movements. He continues to receive 67 mg per day of 5-HTP and 200 mg per day of carbidopa. When the drugs were discontinued on three occasions, the movements returned.

Oscillating myoclonus can also be mistaken for tremor. In contrast to rhythmical myoclonus, which is always segmental and continuous, oscillating myoclonus can be either segmental or generalised and it is transient (Fahn and Singh, 1981). It tends to be induced by specific stimuli, and after a brief period it fades away. Cases 4 and 5 demonstrate two examples of oscillating myoclonus.

Case 4

An Ashkenazic Jewish man was in good health until 1973 (aged 16) when he noticed jerky movements of the left arm while trying to drink water. These movements then occurred with anxiety and with other voluntary motor activity. Trials of valproate, haloperidol, levodopa and hypnosis were of no benefit. Over the next two years the jerky movements spread to involve the head, right arm, trunk and both legs. In April 1977 (aged 20) he underwent a right ventrolateral cryothalamotomy in Moscow, which relieved the abnormal involuntary movements for only a few hours. The symptoms have remained stable over the next $5\frac{1}{2}$ years, during which time he has emigrated to the USA. The movement disorder interfered with his ability to continue school and to work. He reported that he could have up to 2 h freedom from the involuntary movements when he is engrossed in mental activity. Heavy alcohol ingestion was also reported to reduce the movements.

There was no history of head trauma, encephalitis or exposure to toxins. He had been an excellent student and planned to enroll in medical school until the movement disorder developed and forced him to leave school. There was no family history of neurological disease. Examinations of both parents, the only sibling and a nephew were normal.

The patient was first seen in 1980. Neurological examination revealed sudden bursts of rapid oscillating movements which then faded and disappeared after several seconds. They could be brought on by stress, anxiety, painful stimuli and occasionally with loud noise or by talking. Attempting to 'hold still' would bring on the movements, and, in fact, this manoeuvre was the most reliable method to induce them. The involuntary jerky movements involved the head, trunk and all limbs; the arms were more severely affected than the legs, the left side was more involved than the right side, and the proximal muscles more than the distal muscles. Voluntary ballistic movements rarely induced them, but sometimes they would occur with slower ramp movements. Writing would usually cause the jerky movements to appear in most parts of the body, but not in the arm doing the writing. The general neurological examination was otherwise normal, including testing for cerebellar function. Computed tomography of the head (CT scan), electroencephalography (EEG), somatosensory evoked responses, and examination of the cerebrospinal fluid (CSF) were all normal, as were routine laboratory studies.

Electromyographic examination (EMG) using surface electrodes and a 20-channel EEG machine was carried out and revealed synchronised contractions in various muscles during the bursts of oscillatory movements. Clonazepam was slightly effective at a dosage of 16 mg per day, but this benefit was subsequently lost. There was no benefit from sodium valproate, either alone or together with clonazepam. Cyproheptadine, carbamazepine, propranolol, carbidopa/levodopa, carbidopa/5-hydroxytryptophan, pemoline, methylphenidate, reserpine and tetra-benazine were not effective. Baclofen, at a dosage of 60 mg per day, reduced the jerky movements a moderate amount, but this effect was eventually lost.

Case 5

A 45-year-old man previously in good health developed a mild action tremor of both arms. In 1971, at the age of 54, he noticed oscillatory movements of his head and trunk when he moved or changed position. This problem continued, and he lost his job as a supermarket manager. These movements worsened, and movements of his trunk occurred while driving, such as when he moved the right leg to apply the brakes. The oscillatory movements of the trunk would last for a few seconds, then gradually dampen and disappear. Drinking alcohol reduced both the oscillatory truncal movements and the tremor of the hands. His mother and a maternal aunt had a similar tremor of the hands.

The patient was first seen in 1978 (aged 60). Neurological examination revealed two types of abnormal involuntary movements. There was a mild-amplitude postural tremor of the hands that worsened with action and intention movements of the arms. The most obvious difficulty, however, was the presence of sudden bursts of rapid oscillating movements of the trunk and head which then faded and disappeared after several seconds. They were induced when he shifted his body, such as when arising from a sitting position, when leaning to one side, or when changing his posture during the act of sitting or lying. CT scan, EEG and CSF analysis were normal. Because of the oscillating movements, the initial diagnosis was an unusual action tremor of the trunk. Treatment with propranolol was of no benefit. Subsequently, after Case 4 was encountered, a diagnosis of action myo-clonus of the trunk was considered, and he was treated with clonazepam. At a dosage of 1 mg t.i.d., there was virtually complete relief of the movements. There has been no relapse after two years of treatment.

Proximal tremor in parkinsonism

Occasionally, proximal, rather than distal, tremor at rest of the arms is encoun-tered in patients with parkinsonism. This is an atypical location of a common tremor. This has given rise to consideration of other diagnoses. Cases 6 and 7 describe two patients; the first had a good response to levodopa/carbidopa and the second to ethopropazine and amantadine.

Case 6

A 76-year-old woman had tremor of the arms of two years duration. Six months later she noted tremor of her trunk and legs as well. Later she noted tremor of her voice. The arm tremor continued to worsen. Examination revealed marked-amplitude tremor at rest, most pronounced in the proximal muscles of both arms. The tremor became more severe on maintenance of posture but diminished on initiation of arm movement. There was mild rigidity. Rapid alternating movements were slow, gait was slow and shuffling, and she had postural instability. Trials of alcohol (1 oz 95%) and propranolol (240 mg per day) were without benefit. Carbidopa/levodopa (25–250 mg q.i.d.). produced considerable lessening of the tremor. The addition of ethopropazine (100 mg per day) markedly reduced the tremor.

Case 7

A 47-year-old man noted tremor of the right arm associated with stress five years previously. The tremor was present much of the time $3\frac{1}{2}$ years later. At that time tremor developed in the right leg. Examination revealed tremor at rest in both the proximal and distal muscles of the right arm and right leg, which disappeared on initiation of movement of those limbs. There was mild facial hypomimia, slight difficulty with rapid alternating movements, and reduced arm swing, all on the right side. Treatment with ethopropazine and amantadine markedly diminished the tremor.

RARE TREMORS

In the category of rare tremors, I place those conditions that have been reported in the literature, but are encountered rarely and may not even be recognised widely by neurologists. I will describe three types within this category: primary writing tremor, hereditary chin quivering and hysterical tremor.

Primary writing tremor

This condition was first described by Rothwell *et al.* (1979) in one boy beginning at the age of 12. Short bursts of shaking developed when trying to write or utilise the right forearm in any motor act involving pronation. If he wrote with the wrist held rigid and with movements only at the shoulder and elbow, no tremor was elicited. From this description, one could not be certain whether the tremor was due to action dystonia, in which dystonic tremor developed at a certain posture of the forearm. Klawans *et al.* (1982) reported six patients with tremor during handwriting and other activities involving pronation of the wrist. Three patients also had mild postural tremor, and three had mild intention tremor. Propranolol and levodopa were ineffective, while anticholinergic drugs ameliorated the tremor. From the above cases, one still cannot be certain whether primary writing tremor is a unique entity, a 'forme fruste' of action dystonia, or a mild case (variant) of essential tremor. Case 8 describes a woman with tremor during handwriting (only with the right hand), but very mild intention tremor was seen as well. Perhaps this patient fits the description of primary writing tremor, but perhaps it represents a variant of essential tremor. She declined to participate in drug trials.

Case 8

A 41-year-old woman had noted that for 20 years the left hand would shake when writing. The symptom worsened gradually over the years, and she had switched to writing with the right hand four years previously. In the last few months, she noticed that there was shaking of the left hand when bringing a spoonful of soup to her mouth. She had no difficulty writing on a blackboard. There is no family history of tremor. Examination revealed tremor of the left hand when writing. There was no tremor at rest, with outstretched arms, with winged posture of the arms, or with finger-to-nose testing. When writing, there was predominantly pronation–supination tremor. There was no 'tightening' of any muscles in the hand, forearm, or arm when writing.

Hysterical tremor

Tremor as the result of a conversion reaction has been recognised, but it is rarely encountered. Anecdotal reports indicate that the tremor is most pronounced when attention is paid to it, and that it may disappear when attention of the patient is diverted to another subject (Campbell, 1979). To be certain that the tremor is due to a conversion reaction, remission must occur either spontaneously, with psychotherapy, with supportive physiotherapy, or with placebo. I have seen both action and rest tremors as hysterical manifestations. Each type will be described.

Case 9

A 16-year-old boy in good health suddenly developed tremor of the right arm. Examination revealed a coarse tremor of the right arm, more pronounced in the distal rather than proximal muscles. It was present at rest, with posture holding and with action. It had a frequency of about 4 Hz. It did not lessen with action. However, it virtually disappeared when the right hand was engaged in careful motor activity, such as writing, tying shoe-laces, and approaching the target on the finger-to-nose manoeuvre. The direction of the tremor changed to that of least resistance. For example, when the palm was resting on his thigh, the tremor was side-to-side. When the hand was off his lap, the tremor was in a flexion–extension direction. There were no signs of parkinsonism other than decreased right arm swing when he walked. He had 'la belle indifférence'. Psychotherapy was initiated. Approximately four months later, he disclosed to the therapist that he was being bullied at school. The tremor suddenly disappeared, and he is now normal.

Case 10

A woman who worked in a state disability claims office was well until 1976 (aged 23), when she experienced a severe headache lasting several days. After a couple of days, she noted that her head was shaking involuntarily from side to side as if she was constantly saying 'no'. She was admitted to hospital; skull X-rays, EEG and CSF were were reported to be normal. Within a few days in hospital the tremor of the head disappeared spontaneously. In the following months, she had several episodes of head tremor. Initially, these episodes were intermittent, occurring several times a day. But soon the tremor became continuous, lasting several weeks. The head tremor returned in August 1977, and she was hospitalised elsewhere two months later. CSF, EEG and a CT scan of the head were normal. She underwent psychotherapy without improvement. She was then tried on many different drugs, including phenytoin, haloperidol, Sinemet, carbamazepine, pimozide, primidone and propranolol.

In January 1979, while on a ski trip, she suddenly developed severe tremor of the right hand which was noted to be between 3 and 4 Hz in a supination–pronation direction. The right arm and leg were noted to be slightly flexed and rigid. The head tremor was still present. She was admitted to another hospital in April 1979. CSF, EEG, CT scan and brain scan were normal. Because of the increased tone in the right limbs, a diagnosis of dystonia was made. Her neurologist placed her on trihexyphenidyl and when he saw her again in July 1979 the tremors had disappeared. By the end of 1979 dystonic posturing of the right arm and some dragging of the right foot were noticed. She began to complain of pain in many joints of the right limbs. Trials of clonazepam and baclofen were ineffective.

When I first examined her in December 1979, she had a slow horizontal head tremor at a rate of 2.5 Hz when she was sitting and 0.87 Hz when lying supine. No dystonic movements or postures were noted at that time. There was no palatal myoclonus. She was admitted to the Neurological Institute in January 1981, and some dragging of the right leg was present on admission. Somatosensory and brainstem auditory evoked potentials were normal. EMG recordings of both sternomastoid muscles revealed synchronous contractions in both. When the head was held firmly, then the upper trunk had the tremor. The tremor never ceased except during sleep. Suddenly in the hospital, the patient developed a pronation–supination tremor of the right hand at 3–3.5 Hz. The hand also developed a flexed posture and increased tone. The thumb had flexed into the palm. She had difficulty opening the clenched right fist. She was placed on trihexyphenidyl in increasing dosages daily. Over the next few days, she complained of tightness and dull aching pain in her thighs, back, shoulder and arm. Quinine provided partial relief. However, dystonic posturing with increased muscle tone of the right leg and foot developed. The foot was held in an equinovarus posture, and she walked on the lateral edge of the foot with her trunk bent forward and to the right. All this time she continued to have a 1.5 Hz tremor of the head and the 3 Hz tremor of the right hand. A psychiatric evaluation suggested some reactive depression, but no evidence for a conversion reaction. As the dosage of trihexyphenidyl was being increased, trials of Sinemet, carbamazepine, baclofen and 5-hydroxytryptophan were undertaken without benefit. At a dosage of trihexyphenidyl 50 mg per day the tremors subsided and the patient was discharged. Posturing of the right arm and leg slowly lessened.

In June 1981 she began to have painful spasms and 'paralysis' of her legs, and was admitted to the Neurological Institute. In spite of the inability to move her legs, the patient was calm and had 'la belle indifference'. The legs were in a frog position, flexed at the knees and slightly abducted at the thighs. At rest there was no increased tone. She was unable to move the legs despite attempts to do so accompanied by loud breathing sounds of effort. Passive manipulation of the legs was met by increased muscular resistance. After a few minutes of forcefully applied pressure trying to overcome the muscular resistance, the antagonistic muscles suddenly relaxed and the examined leg would drop to the bed with normal tonus. Tendon reflexes, plantar reflexes and sensation were intact. In view of the current situation, it was clear that the patient had a conversion reaction. She was treated with encouragement, physiotherapy and gradually switching placebo for trihexyphenidyl. The patient slowly improved, and she was discharged within one month after admission walking normally She was kept on placebo medication.

Attempts to treat with psychotherapy were unsuccessful due to lack of insight. The patient joined the local dystonia society chapter and became an active member. Once, some members commented that she looked as if she did not have dystonia. Shortly afterwards, she developed flexion of the left knee when walking. Despite outpatient physiotherapy and increased dosage of placebo, tremor of the right hand and equinovarus posturing of the right foot returned. She was readmitted to the Neurological Institute in September 1982. Shortly after admission, adduction-abduction tremor of both thighs also developed at a rate of 2.5 Hz. She continued to have 3.3 Hz tremor of the right hand. An intramuscular injection of saline (thought by the patient to be ACTH) relieved the thigh tremor. The psychiatrist and I confronted her with the diagnosis of a conversion reaction for all her symptoms. The patient was initially distressed and angry. However, with considerable attention and care, we dealt with her emotions daily, and gradually the symptoms began to fade. When she awakened one morning, she noticed that the right hand tremor had disappeared. She was discharged and treated with continuing psychotherapy. In October 1982, she had only mild equinovarus posturing of the right foot and was able to return to work.

Hereditary chin tremor

Autosomal dominantly transmitted quivering of the chin has been reported in several families (see Goldsmith, 1927; Laurance *et al.*, 1968). I have seen two patients with this condition, a father and his infant son. It causes no disability.

Cases 11 and 12

A 30-year-old black man had quivering of his chin all his life. He came for an evaluation, along with his eight-month old son who was noted to have a similar condition. Examination revealed low-amplitude, rapid tremor of the mentalis muscle in each of them. In the man, it was present most of the time. In his son, it would come and go. It would last less than a minute and then be absent for a minute or longer.

UNDIAGNOSED TREMORS

There are a number of patients with tremors that have not yet been categorised. In most of these cases, no known aetiological factor has been elucidated, and these patients are usually labelled as postural or action tremors of unknown aetiology. I will describe two patients with tremors that have not previously been described in the literature. Case 13 has paroxysmal tremor associated with paroxysmal ataxia, and Case 14 had a severe intention tremor that appears to have been induced by naphthalene intoxication.

Paroxysmal tremor and ataxia

Case 13

An 81-year-old woman noticed a tremor of the right hand that first interfered with writing and other delicate work in 1966. After that she had insidious development of unsteadiness of gait and falling. She was admitted to the Neurological Institute in 1970. Examination at that time revealed rest tremor in both hands that worsened with action and intention. There was also some ataxia of gait and dysmetria of both arms, right greater than left. There was no cogwheel rigidity, bradykinesia, masked facies or other stigmata of parkinsonism. At that time the differential diagnosis was between parkinsonism and cerebellar disease. She was given a trial of levodopa, but developed severe palpitations and discontinued it. Numerous medications were tried without benefit: diazepam, tricyclic antidepressants, propranolol, perphenazine/amitriptyline, trihexyphenidyl and amantadine. A trial of Sinemet in 1978 was also without benefit. There was a gradual progression of gait difficulty with increased falling.

While being followed in clinic, it was noticed that on some visits no tremor was seen, and on other visits the tremor was very pronounced. In 1978, she developed tremor of both legs. Examination in September 1978 revealed non-synchronous tremor in all extremities at a frequency of around 6 Hz, decreased tone, postural instability and a normal gait. At the time of her next clinic visit, her gait was wide-based and ataxic. I examined her in 1980 and obtained a history that she would develop episodes of sudden onset of tremor at rest of both legs, tremor of the voice, increased dysmetria of the arms and ataxia of gait. Just as suddenly, these increased symptoms would disappear. The episodes of transient worsening would appear several times a day, but could be as infrequent as once per week. It would last from minutes to 4 h. The attacks occurred without warning and without precipitating factors. Examination during an attack revealed rest tremor in the legs at a frequency of 4 Hz. There was no rest tremor in the hands, but they showed mild postural tremor with marked increase with action and particularly with intention on approaching a target. The voice was also tremulous, as was the handwriting. There was also mild ataxic gait and postural instability. When the episode suddenly subsided, there was no tremor of extremities or voice, and the gait and handwriting were normal. Treatment with acetazolamide, 250 mg q.i.d., was initiated, which abolished the attacks. There was some residual mild dysmetria of the arms, postural instability and inability to perform a tandem gait. But the gait was not ataxic and was narrow-based.

Intention tremor and peripheral neuropathy secondary to chronic naphthalene intoxication

Case 14

A woman first began to have pain and paraesthesia in the hands and feet in January 1968 (aged 69). Examination at another hospital revealed weakness and hypalgesia in a glove and stocking distribution, absent tendon reflexes and slowed nerve conduction velocities. A diagnosis of a peripheral neuropathy was made and she was placed on high dosages of vitamins. She showed gradual improvement.

In early 1972, she developed tremor and gait difficulty. Treatment with amantadine, phenytoin and perphenazine/amitriptyline were without benefit. She came to our neurology clinic in November 1974 complaining of tremors in the arms and legs. Examination revealed postural and intention tremors of the arms, areflexia and decreased position sense. A trial of propranolol up to 200 mg per day was without benefit, and she was referred to the movement disorder service in April 1975 when her symptoms worsened. She was admitted to the Neurological Institute in May 1975. By that time she was unable to walk because of severe proprioceptive difficulty in placing her legs and severe body tremor when standing. There was no tremor when she was sitting or lying. Tremors were present when extending her arms or legs in front of her, and they increased with action, particularly intention. They were of marked amplitude and prevented her from using the limbs for any purposeful activity. There was a mild tremor of the voice, thinness of the extremities, reduction of pain and touch sensations, marked impairment of proprioceptive sensation and absent tendon reflexes. CSF protein was 180 mg dl^{-1}; motor nerve conduction was slow; EMG revealed no acute denervation and no fasciculations; muscle and nerve biopsies revealed mild atrophy of muscle and non-specific loss of nerve fibres of moderate severity. Intravenous benztropine failed to alter the tremors. Apomorphine 2 mg s.c.

worsened the tremor, possibly because of the induction of nausea and vomiting. Ethanol 2 oz 28% p.o. failed to decrease the tremor. Haloperidol made the tremor worse and was discontinued. Carbamazepine 200 mg b.i.d. reduced the tremor. When it was discontinued, the tremor worsened. Reinstitution of carbamazepine again lessened the tremor, and she was discharged on this medication.

She has continued to be followed in our clinic. She continued to complain of some paraesthesias in the palms of her hands and the soles of her feet ('pinching of the skin'). By September 1976 there was almost no tremor, just a slight intention tremor of the hands. There was no tremor of the legs. Station and gait were normal. Sensation testing was normal. Tendon reflexes remained absent. Nerve conduction studies showed markedly reduced velocities in the left median, ulnar, peroneal and posterior tibial nerves at 18.4, 16.7, 13.8 and 11.5 m s^{-1}, respectively. Discontinuing carbamazepine failed to produce recurrence of the tremors.

In December 1976 the tremors returned. Resumption of carbamazepine provided some benefit and it has been continued ever since at a dosage of 600 mg per day. Examination in May 1977 revealed only slight intention tremor. But in October 1978 the tremors were becoming more pronounced despite carbamazepine therapy. She also had more paraesthesias. Examination revealed moderate postural, action and intention tremors of the arms and legs, and mild tremor of the voice. The tremors and paraesthesias worsened over the next five months. Her gait was also becoming unsteady and she required a walker. In March 1979 sensory examination remained normal, but her gait was wide-based and ataxic. There was no nystagmus. Over the next few months, her symptoms began to fade. By October 1979 examination revealed a remission of her problems.

We could not understand the reason for the fluctuations in her tremors, ataxia and neuropathy. Over the next two years we noticed a pattern of worsening of symptoms during the winter months. In November 1981, we obtained additional information from one of the patient's daughters. The patient had been extremely compulsive about preventing clothes damage by moths, and from autumn to spring would use mothballs excessively. She would keep the windows closed, and the entire house permeated with the aroma of the mothballs. When the patient brought me the package of mothballs that she used, I learned that it contained 100% naphthalene. She was advised to cease the habit of overusing mothballs and to keep her house aerated. The winter of 1982 passed without incident. When she was last seen in May 1982, she had only slight intention tremor of the hands, none in the legs, and a slight wide-based gait. She continues to live alone and care for herself at the age of 83.

CONCLUSIONS

From these brief case reports, I have tried to indicate that there are many types of tremors of different aetiologies that are not easily classifiable. As we learn more about them, we may be able to include them in a new classification (Capildeo and Findley, this volume, chapter 1).

REFERENCES

Bundey, S., Harrison, M. J. G. and Marsden, C. D. (1975). A genetic study of torsion dystonia. *J. Med. Genet.*, **12**, 12-19.

Campbell, J. (1979). The shortest paper. *Neurology*, **29**, 1633.

Couch, J. R. (1976). Dystonia and tremor in spasmodic torticollis, *Adv. Neurol.*, **14**, 245-58.

Fahn, S. and Singh, N. (1980). Segmental tremor vs rhythmic myoclonus: successful treatment with serotonin precursors. *Neurology*, **30**, 383-4.

Fahn, S. and Singh, N. (1981). An oscillating form of essential myoclonus. *Neurology*, **31** (no. 4, part 2), 80.

Goldsmith, J. B. (1927). The inheritance of 'facial spasm' and the effect of a modifying factor associated with high temper. *J. Hered.*, **18**, 185-7.

Klawans, H. L., Glantz, R., Tanner, C. M. and Goetz, C. G. (1982). Primary writing tremor: a selective action tremor. *Neurology*, **32**, 203-6.

Laurance, B. M., Matthews, W. B. and Diggle, J. H. (1968). Hereditary quivering of the chin. *Arch. Dis. Childh.*, **43**, 249-51.

Magnussen, I., Dupont, E., Prange-Hansen, A. and de Olivarius, F. B. (1977). Palatal myoclonus treated with 5-hydroxytryptophan and a decarboxylase inhibitor. *Acta Neurol. Scand.*, **55**, 151-253.

Rothwell, J. C., Traub, M. M. and Marsden, C. D. (1979). Primary writing tremor. *J. Neurol. Neurosurg. Psychiatr.*, **42**, 1106-14.

Tahmoush, A. J., Brooks, J. E. and Keltner, J. L. (1972). Palatal myoclonus associated with abnormal ocular and extremity movements: a polygraphic study. *Arch. Neurol.*, **27**, 431-40.

Williams, A., Goodenberger, D. and Calne, D. B. (1978). Palatal myoclonus following herpes zoster ameliorated by 5-hydroxytryptophan and carbidopa. *Neurology*, **28**, 358-9.

Yanagisawa, N. and Goto, A. (1971). Dystonia musculorum deformans: analysis with electromyography. *J. Neurol. Sci.*, **13**, 39-65.

Yanagisawa, N., Goto, A. and Narabayashi, H. (1972). Familial dystonia musculorum deformans and tremor. *J. Neurol. Sci.*, **16**, 125-36.

Zeman, W., Kaelbling, R. and Pasamanick, B. (1960). Idiopathic dystonia musculorum deformans. II. The formes frustes. *Neurology*, **10**, 1068-75.

34
Drug-induced tremor

ROGER M. PINDER

INTRODUCTION

Tremor is a relatively common feature of the pharmacological action of a wide variety of substances. The classic treatise of Pelnar, *Das Zittern*, lists a remarkable compendium of tremor-producing substances ranging from heavy metals to caffeine and opium (Pelnar, 1913). The advent of modern synthetic drugs has brought to light many more, and tremor is a frequently reported side-effect of drug treatment. Most drugs acting on the central nervous system can produce tremor as a side-effect (Findley and Gresty, 1981) to the extent that the standard psycho-pharmacological evaluation scales for side-effects in clinical trials include tremor as a major item (Guy, 1976). Unfortunately, few objective recordings have been taken of tremors produced as side-effects of drugs, and although many substances can cause tremor it may not be their principal effect and is often transient. This chapter will therefore focus on substances that consistently produce a well defined and sustained tremor in man and/or experimental animals.

Two general groups can be identified that, at least in animals, satisfy these criteria (Brimblecombe and Pinder, 1972). The first group, the members of which seem to act primarily via central cholinergic mechanisms, includes both muscarinic and nicotinic agonists as well as acetylcholine itself, anticholinesterases and a number of aminopropanols. Tremogenesis by the second group primarily involves central catecholaminergic and/or serotonergic mechanisms and is associated with neuroleptics, phenylethylamine analogues and indole derivatives. Since cholinergic, catecholaminergic and serotonergic mechanisms are intimately linked in the brain, it is doubtful whether such mechanisms can be regarded as mutually exclusive. Drug-induced tremor in animals is usually of the resting and postural types and tends to be of higher frequency than that (6–10 Hz) of physiological tremor in man (Brimblecombe and Pinder, 1972). Action and intentional tremors can be induced in animals by a number of heavy metals as well as by metal chelators such as cysteamine and penicillamine, and by carbon tetrachloride (table 34.1).

In man, drug-induced tremor is most characteristically seen in the form of postural or action tremor, causing a variable degree of disability (Findley and Gresty, 1981). However, classification of the individual tremor into the behavioural groupings of resting, postural, action and intentional tremor is difficult

445

Table 34.1 Tremogenic substances.

(1)   Drugs acting via central cholinergic systems:

acetylcholine, muscarinic and nicotinic agonists, anticholinesterases, aminopropanols

(2)   Drugs acting via central monoaminergic systems:

neuroleptics, phenylethylamines, indoles

(3)   Drugs acting via peripheral adrenergic systems:

adrenaline, β-agonists, lithium, caffeine, amphetamine, corticosteroids

(4)   Drugs producing action and/or intentional tremor:

heavy metals, metal chelators, carbon tetrachloride

because it often appears as an irregular tremulousness associated with more complex involuntary movements such as chorea and myoclonic jerking. Even drugs like the neuroleptics, which induce a parkinsonian syndrome as a side-effect, do not commonly cause a typical parkinsonian resting tremor, which is of low frequency (4–6 Hz) and is abolished by voluntary movement. Rather most tremogens produce high-frequency tremor which is aggravated by voluntary movement. Although tremogens have been widely used to select potential therapeutic agents, their relevance to the tremor of extrapyramidal or cerebellar disease is doubtful (Brimblecombe and Pinder, 1972).

A number of drugs stimulate peripheral tremogenic receptors directly, producing, an exaggerated postural physiological tremor. Physiological tremor can be increased in amplitude by, *inter alia*, endogenous catecholamines released from the adrenals, an action that is mimicked by adrenaline, β-adrenergic agonists, levodopa, amphetamine, lithium, caffeine and adrenocorticosteroids (Findley and Gresty, 1981). Such drugs are believed to act directly or indirectly through β_2-adrenoceptors located on extrafusal muscle fibre (Marsden, 1978), and although it is likely that such tremor also has a central component (Pickles *et al.*, 1981), it is essentially peripheral in nature. Drugs such as the β-blockers, which suppress forms of essential and enhanced physiological tremor, can induce heightened rebound tremor upon withdrawal. Neuroleptics and tricyclic antidepressants can exaggerate tremor in patients with essential tremor, but it is unclear whether they do so through central or peripheral mechanisms. Anticonvulsant therapy may be associated with the development of postural tremor and asterixis (Findley and Gresty, 1981).

Drugs producing action and/or intentional tremors, those acting via peripheral tremogenic receptors and those inducing an exaggeration of physiological or essential tremor will not be discussed further here. Rather an overview will be given of tremors mediated primarily through central mechanisms.

DRUGS ACTING VIA CENTRAL CHOLINERGIC MECHANISMS

Central administration

Resting tremors of high frequency have been consistently produced in conscious cats (Connor *et al.*, 1966a) and rats (Cox and Potkonjak, 1969; Matthews and Chiou, 1979) by the injection of muscarinic drugs and anticholinesterases directly into the caudate nucleus (table 34.2). Although other acetylcholine-rich areas of

Table 34.2 Characteristics of cholinergic tremor.

Drug[a]	Effective dose (µg)	Mean tremor latency (min)	Mean tremor duration (min)	Mean tremor frequency (Hz)
Acetylcholine	400	19	50	21
Carbachol	7	14	150	19
Bethanechol	31	15	120	23
Methacholine	100	19	90	19
Oxotremorine	15	29	80	22
Arecoline	100	17	95	22
Physostigmine	75	35	60	19

[a]All drugs were given by injection into the caudate nucleus of conscious cats (Connor *et al.*, 1966a).

the brain, such as the globus pallidus and the substantia nigra, do respond to some cholinergic tremogens, the primary site of action has been identified as the caudate (Connor *et al.*, 1966b). Tremors induced by muscarinic agents are inhibited by intracaudate administration of drugs that either block the postsynaptic receptor actions of acetylcholine (atropine and scopolamine) or its presynaptic synthesis (hemicholinium); they are not affected by nicotinic antagonists such as hexamethonium, even though acetylcholine, methacholine, carbachol and arecoline have substantial nicotinic properties (Connor *et al.*, 1966a,b). Such tremors are also suppressed by intracaudate injection of catecholamines, including isoprenaline, adrenaline, noradrenaline and dopamine (Connor *et al.*, 1967; Lalley *et al.*, 1970) and by monoamine oxidase inhibitors (Baker *et al.*, 1975). These findings, together with the high concentrations of acetylcholine and dopamine in the caudate, led to the idea that there is a local tremor-regulating balance between acetylcholine (excitatory) and dopamine (inhibitory) in the caudate (see Brimblecombe and Pinder, 1972). Intracaudate carbachol 1.5 µg produced a resting tremor of faster onset and shorter duration in rats than in cats, and the frequency (28 Hz) was higher (Matthews and Chiou, 1979). However, tremors induced in rats by intracaudate administration of the muscarinic agonist oxotremorine or the anticholinesterase dyflos were lower in frequency than those seen in cats (Cox and Potkonjak, 1969).

Peripheral administration

Neither pilocarpine, a muscarinic agonist, nor nicotine produced tremor in conscious cats following intracaudate administration (Connor et al., 1966b), although the peripheral nicotinic agonists tetramethylammonium and 1,1-dimethyl-4-phenylpiperazinium were effective in mice after intracerebral injection (see Brimblecombe and Pinder, 1972). Tremor can be produced in rodents by peripherally administered nicotine as well as by muscarinic agonists and anticholinesterases but not by pilocarpine (Brimblecombe and Pinder, 1972). However, the normally fleeting and high-frequency (12–20 Hz) tremor induced by parenteral nicotine in rodents is markedly sustained by previous treatment of the animals with pilocarpine (Tsujimoto and Dohi, 1976), possibly via a combination of central muscarinic activation and enhanced serotonergic function produced by pilocarpine (Dohi and Tsujimoto, 1978). Other nicotinic agonists producing tremor after peripheral administration include the desmethyl metabolite of nicotine, nornicotine, and the aminopropanol TPA (Brimblecombe and Pinder, 1972). TPA (see figure 34.2) is the most potent of a series of tremogenic aminopropanols that produce in rodents severe tremor of high frequency (12–17 Hz) and long duration (1–3 h). Their reversal by nicotinic but not by muscarinic antagonists indicates a possible mechanism of action mediated through nicotinic receptors.

Of the anticholinesterases, the reversible agents physostigmine and neostigmine have been reported to be tremogenic after peripheral administration to animals, although the irreversible organophosphorus agents such as dyflos appear to produce tremor only after central administration (Brimblecombe and Pinder, 1972; Cox and Potkonjak, 1969). Following doses of 0.25–0.8 mg kg^{-1} i.p., physostigmine produced dose-dependent tremors in rats within 5 min and lasting for about 15–20 min (Gothoni et al., 1981). The tremors were reversed by centrally active antimuscarinic agents like atropine but not by the peripheral antimuscarinic methylatropine. Physostigmine-induced tremors in rats are potentiated by drugs that reduce central catecholaminergic activity such as reserpine and chlorpromazine but inhibited by drugs like levodopa that enhance central catecholaminergic activity (Ambani and Van Woert, 1972), and are associated with a rise in brain acetylcholine levels (Sethy and Van Woert, 1973). In cats, physostigmine-induced tremors are potentiated by intracaudate serotonin (Malseed and Baker, 1973).

Muscarine itself has not been studied as a tremogen. Choline esters like carbachol, bethanechol, methacholine and acetylcholine (figure 34.1) are not active by peripheral administration because as quaternary salts they do not penetrate readily into the brain. Furthermore, methacholine and particularly acetylcholine are susceptible to hydrolysis by cholinesterases. It is interesting that the tremogenic potencies of choline esters lie in the same order as their resistance to hydrolysis, viz. carbachol > bethanechol > methacholine > acetylcholine (Brimblecombe and Pinder, 1972). However, several muscarinic agonists but not pilocarpine are active tremogens by both central and peripheral administration (figure 34.2). Arecoline, in addition to its tremogenic activity after intracaudate injection (see

Acetylcholine $(CH_3)_3\overset{+}{N}.CH_2.CH_2.O.COCH_3$ Cl^-

Methacholine $(CH_3)_3\overset{+}{N}.CH_2.CH(CH_3).O.COCH_3$ Cl^-

Carbachol $(CH_3)_3\overset{+}{N}.CH_2.CH_2.O.CONH_2$ Cl^-

Bethanechol $(CH_3)_3\overset{+}{N}.CH_2.CH(CH_3).O.CONH_2$ Cl^-

Figure 34.1 Choline esters that are tremogenic only after central administration.

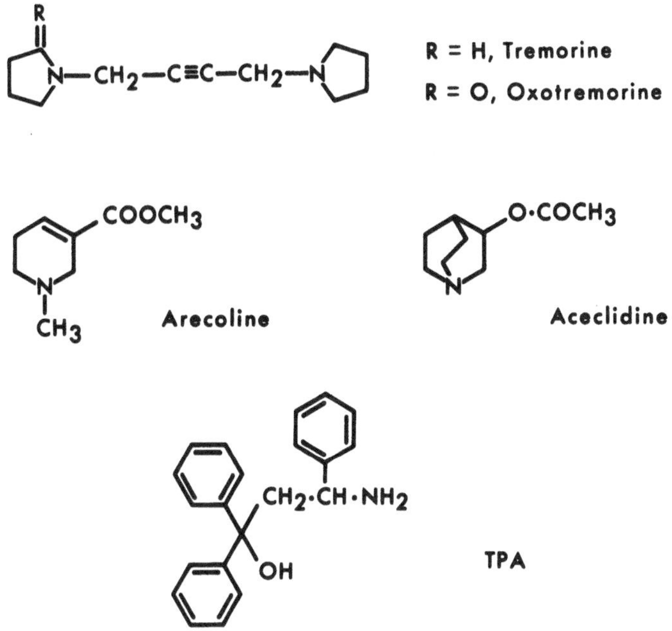

R = H, Tremorine
R = O, Oxotremorine

Arecoline

Aceclidine

TPA

Figure 34.2 Some muscarinic and nicotinic tremogens active by peripheral administration.

table 34.2), produces a well defined resting and postural tremor of high frequency (13–22 Hz) lasting about 15 min following intraperitoneal doses of 25 mg kg^{-1} in rats, while its intracerebral ED$_{50}$ in mice is about 3 μg (Brimblecombe and Pinder, 1972). Aceclidine-induced tremors have been studied only after intraperitoneal injection in mice, when dose-dependent (4–32 mg kg^{-1}) tremors of rapid onset and short duration were observed. Tremors induced by both arecoline and aceclidine are inhibited by muscarinic but not by nicotinic antagonists.

Tremorine and its pharmacologically active metabolite oxotremorine have been the most extensively studied muscarinic tremogens (Brimblecombe and Pinder, 1972). Tremorine is not active *per se* but only by virtue of biotransformation into oxotremorine (figure 34.2). Thus, tremorine has an ED_{50} of about 10-20 mg kg^{-1} after intravenous injection in mice, producing tremor after a latency of 5-10 min and lasting for 3 h, whereas oxotremorine acts immediately with an ED_{50} of only 0.05 mg kg^{-1} i.v. The frequency of tremor induced by tremorine and oxotremorine varies greatly with the species; in mice the dominant frequency is 20-24 Hz, in cats 21-23 Hz, in rats 10-15 Hz and in dogs 12-14 Hz. Although the drug has been widely used to identify potential anti-parkinsonian drugs, oxotremorine-induced tremor does not resemble the resting tremor of parkinsonism, since it occurs at a much higher frequency and is exaggerated by voluntary movement. Tremors induced by peripherally administered oxotremorine are potentiated dose-dependently by small intraventricular (i.c.v.) doses of acetylcholine (0.1-10 μg) and antagonised by even smaller doses (0.1-10 ng) of atropine (Doggett and O'Farrell, 1976). The rise in brain acetylcholine levels associated with oxotremorine-induced tremors was also inhibited by antimuscarinic drugs like atropine (Brimblecombe and Pinder, 1972; Sethy and Van Woert, 1973). Although oxotremorine releases central dopamine and noradrenaline (see Brimblecombe and Pinder, 1972), depletion of these amines by 6-hydroxydopamine i.c.v. did not modify tremor (Slater, 1974), and nor was tremor affected by intraventricular catecholamines, sympathomimetic amines or serotonin (Doggett and O'Farrell, 1976). However, oxotremorine tremor can be substantially reduced in intensity and duration by both adrenalectomy and chemical sympathectomy with intravenous 6-hydroxy-dopamine, as well as by various β-adrenergic antagonists (Barar and Madan, 1976; Weinstock *et al.*, 1978). β-Antagonists did not prevent the rise in central and plasma catecholamines induced by oxotremorine. It would appear that oxotremorine produces tremor primarily via stimulation of central muscarinic receptors and an associated increase in cholinergic influence to motor afferents, but that a secondary augmentation may occur via stimulation of β_2-adrenoceptors involved in peripheral mediation of tremor (Weinstock *et al.*, 1978).

Cholinergic tremogens in man

Although of interest in elucidating possible mechanisms of tremogenesis, cholinergic tremogens are of little therapeutic value and have not been greatly studied in man. Nicotine and arecoline are of course used very widely for social reasons, being the principal pharmacologically active ingredients of tobacco and betel nuts respectively. The doses inhaled or ingested are probably too small to produce tremor except possibly in heavy and chronic users or in cases of acute poisoning with nicotine or arecoline (Brimblecombe and Pinder, 1972). With the exceptions of bethanechol and neostigmine, which as quaternary salts fail to reach the brain readily after oral administration, cholinergic drugs are used principally in the treatment of glaucoma (table 34.3). The use of ophthalmological solutions of low

Table 34.3 Therapeutic uses of cholinergic tremogens.

Drug	Indication	Dosage/formulation
Bethanechol	gastric atonia or stasis, urinary retention	30–80 mg daily (p.o.)
Carbachol	glaucoma	3% drops
Aceclidine	glaucoma	0.5–4% drops
Physostigmine	glaucoma	0.25–0.5% drops
Neostigmine	glaucoma,	3% drops
	myasthenia gravis	15–30 mg daily (p.o.)

concentration makes it unlikely that tremor is produced as a side-effect. Oral bethanechol is still used as a stimulant of the smooth muscle of the gastrointestinal tract and the urinary bladder, while neostigmine is the standard oral anticholin-esterase for the symptomatic treatment of myasthenia gravis.

Tremor is a principal effect of poisoning not only with nicotine and arecoline but also with anticholinesterases of the organophosphorus type (Brimblecombe and Pinder, 1972). Parenterally administered physostigmine can exacerbate the tremor of Parkinson's disease, and its increasing use as an antidote to poisoning with drugs having central anticholinergic properties (e.g. atropine, tricyclic anti-depressants) may also elicit tremor as a rebound phenomenon. Physostigmine, other anticholinesterases and precursors of acetylcholine such as choline and lecithin are also being investigated as therapy for Alzheimer's disease and other dementias, on the basis that such conditions may be associated with a discrete loss of cholinergic neurones (Hier and Caplan, 1980). It is likely that with increas-ing usage or higher dosages of cholinergic agents sensitive patients, particularly the elderly, will experience tremor as a side-effect.

DRUGS ACTING VIA CENTRAL MONOAMINERGIC MECHANISMS

Catecholaminergic mechanisms

Pronounced resting tremors have been consistently produced in conscious cats (Lalley *et al.*, 1973; Baker *et al.*, 1976) and rats (Little and Dill, 1969) by local application of various phenylethylamine derivatives and related compounds to the brain. Intracaudate administration of phenylethylamines to cats gave tremors of high frequency and generally short duration, although mescaline, as well as the non-phenylethylamines tetrabenazine and bretylium, produced tremors that were sustained for more than 5 h (table 34.4). Tremogenic activity is restricted to the α-methylphenylethylamines (amphetamines) or to the ring-methoxylated deriva-tives, and is abolished by catechol or side-chain alcohol moieties. Thus, 3-methoxy-tyramine is tremogenic but not normetanephrine or dopamine, while meth-

Table 34.4 Characteristics of tremor produced in conscious cats via catecholaminergic mechanisms.

Drug[a,b]	Effective dose (μg)	Mean tremor latency (min)	Mean tremor duration (min)	Mean tremor frequency (Hz)
S(+)-Amphetamine	15	6	40	17
R(−)-Amphetamine	48	11	22	17
Methamphetamine	20	5	28	17
3-Methoxytyramine	95	8	–	17
Mescaline	65	6	> 300	21
Tetrabenazine	161	18	> 300	24
Bretylium	112	4	> 360	25

[a] All drugs were given by intracaudate injection (Lalley et al., 1973; Baker et al., 1976).
[b] Inactive drugs included dopamine (90 μg), isoprenaline (250 μg), tyramine (280 μg), normetanephrine (260 μg), ephedrine (240 μg), phenylephrine (250 μg), methylphenidate (510 μg) and 3,4-dimethoxyphenylethylamine (250 μg).

amphetamine is active but not ephedrine. A degree of stereoselectivity for tremogenic receptors is demonstrated by the greater potency of S(+)-amphetamine than its R(−)-enantiomer, which parallels the behavioural and neurochemical potencies of amphetamine derivatives.

The influence of other drugs on tremors evoked by phenylethylamine analogues and related compounds provides further evidence for a caudate tremor-regulating mechanism involving acetylcholine and dopamine. Thus, tremors induced by mescaline, tetrabenazine and bretylium were suppressed by local injections of scopolamine or hemicholinium and by dopamine or adrenaline, but were intensified by local serotonin (Lalley et al., 1973). In contrast tremors produced by S(+)-amphetamine were not influenced by pretreatment with the dopamine synthesis inhibitor α-methyl-p-tyrosine and developed independently of local acetylcholine activity since they were unaffected by cholinergic antagonists (Baker et al., 1976). Local administration of S(+)-amphetamine intensified physostigmine-induced tremor, and tremors evoked by mescaline, tetrabenazine and bretylium and abolished by hemicholinium were restored by local application of acetylcholine.

Although these results have been used to support the notion of a tremor-regulatory mechanism, the neurochemical mechanisms of action of the catecholaminergic tremogens are disparate. Amphetamine and related drugs produce a relatively rapid and transient liberation of noradrenaline and dopamine from the presynaptic neurone, leading to a sympathomimetic effect. Mescaline may block central postsynaptic noradrenergic and/or dopaminergic receptors but only at higher doses, and probably interacts more with the serotonergic system. Bretylium is an adrenergic neurone blocker preventing the release of noradrenaline, while tetrabenazine produces a slow, prolonged depletion of dopamine and noradrenaline, which are largely metabolised by monoamine oxidase (MAO) prior to release. Consequently, the major effects of bretylium and tetrabenazine are equivalent, i.e. blockade of catecholaminergic function (Goodman *et al.*, 1980). Furthermore, the application of monoamine oxidase inhibitor (MAOI) to the caudate nucleus of cats gives effects that depend upon the level of ongoing activity (Baker *et al.*, 1975). Tranylcypromine and harmaline are tremogenic whereas pargyline is not, but all three compounds suppressed ongoing cholinergic tremors induced by physostigmine. MAOIs presumably raise local levels of catecholamines, which may explain their tremolytic effects on physostigmine tremor, and they increase serotonin levels, possibly leading to a tremogenic effect. Serotonin is itself tremogenic when locally administered in the feline caudate (Malseed and Baker, 1973).

Various methoxylated phenylethylamines are also tremogenic after intrastriatal injection in conscious rats (table 34.5). The tremors are of the resting type, characterised by irregular bursts at low dosage but continuous in high dosage,

Table 34.5 Characteristics of tremor produced in conscious rats via catecholaminergic mechanisms.

Drug[a,b]	Effective dose (nmol)	Mean tremor latency (min)	Mean tremor duration (min)	Mean tremor frequency (Hz)
3-Methoxytyramine	369	14	86	6
3,4-Dimethoxy-phenylethylamine	482	16	34	6
Mescaline	242	14	109	7

[a] All drugs were given by intrastriatal injection (Little and Dill, 1969).
[b] Dopamine 395 nmol was not tremogenic.

and are of lower frequency than those seen in cats (Little and Dill, 1969). The cholinergic agonist carbachol produced tremors of the same frequency (6–8 Hz) but with a much shorter latency period. It is interesting that 3,4-dimethoxyphenyl-ethylamine is tremogenic in the rat but not in the cat. Methoxylated phenyl-ethylamines, as well as amphetamine and methamphetamine, are also tremogenic after parenteral administration in rodents, although in higher species including cats they produce only hyperkinesia (Brimblecombe and Pinder, 1972). Tetra-benazine and its close structural and pharmacological relative reserpine are tremo-genic in animals following parenteral administration, and various neuroleptics produce parkinsonian-like tremor after both acute and chronic dosage in rodents, cats, dogs and monkeys (Brimblecombe and Pinder, 1972).

Despite some difficulties in ascribing a common and precise mechanism of action to the drugs described in this section, it is clear that their tremogenic action is in some way mediated through catecholaminergic pathways. The mechanism of action of a tremogen that is only distantly related in structure to the phenylethyl-amines, LON-954 (figure 34.3), is more clearly due to a decrease in functional

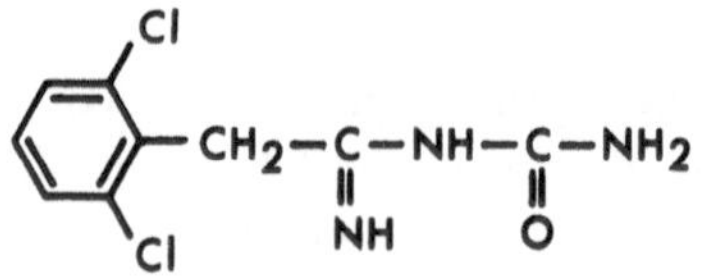

LON-954

Figure 34.3 Structure of LON-954, a tremogen acting via dopaminergic mechanisms.

dopamine levels in the brain. This acetamidine derivative produces a dose-dependent resting tremor in the mouse after oral doses of 5–100 mg kg^{-1}, which is also seen in other species including rat, cat, dog and rabbit (Coward et al., 1977a). Unlike oxotremorine, LON-954 does not produce additional parasympathomimetic effects, akinesia, rigidity or hypothermia. Smaller doses (50–100 μg) also produced tremor after intraventricular injection in mice. LON-954 tremor in the mouse is characterised by a constant frequency of about 14 Hz, beginning within 2 min of oral administration and lasting some 20–30 min. It is blocked by levodopa, apomorphine, dopamine and noradrenaline but not by anticholinergic agents, and is potentiated by neuroleptics and dopamine antagonists (Coward and Doggett, 1980; Coward et al., 1977b).

Morphine and related compounds

Pronounced resting tremors can be evoked in conscious cats by intracaudate injection of morphine (Lalley et al., 1975). Morphine-induced tremor appears about 5 min after a dose of 53 μg, having a mean frequency of about 25 Hz and lasting for just over an hour. It is antagonised by intracaudate nalorphine and also by dopamine, calcium, scopolamine and hemicholinium, but not by serotonin. Tremor inhibition by hemicholinium was reversed by local application of sub-tremogenic doses of acetylcholine. Morphine increased the intensity of physostigmine-induced tremor, and this effect was inhibited by nalorphine without influencing the underlying cholinergic tremor. Tremor production by morphine is attributed to a reduction in dopamine function, allowing cholinergic activity in the caudate to predominate.

It is possible that morphine reduces tremor via interaction with opiate receptors. Whole-body tremor or shakes can be evoked in rats by intraventricular administration of enkephalin derivatives which interact with opiate receptors (Drust et al., 1981). Furthermore, small peptides like thyrotropin-releasing hormone (TRH) can restore and potentiate oxotremorine tremor (Kruse, 1976) as well as being tremogenic per se (Bjorkman et al., 1981). However, naltrexone did not inhibit tremorine-induced tremor whereas the tremor was blocked by the tripeptide prolyl-leucyl-glycinamide (MIF-I) and related analogues (Bjorkman et al., 1979; Dickinson et al., 1981). The mechanism of action of TRH and tremolytic tripeptides does not appear to be related to opiate receptors, and morphine probably acts to produce tremor through dopaminergic mechanisms and not opiate mechanisms.

Serotonergic mechanisms

Many tremogens, including physostigmine and some of the drugs presumed to act through catecholaminergic mechanisms, are potentiated by central administration of serotonin. It is therefore not surprising that serotonin is tremogenic in both rats and cats (Brimblecombe and Pinder, 1972). In cats serotonin is more potent by intracaudate injection than intraventricularly, but both routes produce a rapid and sustained tremor of high frequency (table 34.6). Serotonin-induced tremor is abolished by local administration of the serotonin antagonist methysergide and by dopamine, and is potentiated by MAOIs. Although cholinergic antagonists did not affect serotonin-induced tremor, local application of tremogenic doses of serotonin during periods of maximal physostigmine tremor did intensify tremor activity for 30 min (Malseed and Baker, 1973).

Unlike serotonin, the precursor amino acid 5-hydroxytryptophan (5-HTP) is able to pass readily into the brain after systemic administration. Not active *per se*, 5-HTP produced fine tremors in dogs and rodents when given together with an MAOI (table 34.6). Other indole derivatives sufficiently lipophilic to reach the brain after systemic administration have also been shown to be tremogenic, including *N,N*-dimethyltryptamine and its 5-methoxy derivative as well as lysergic acid diethylamide (LSD) (table 34.6). Tremors produced by these compounds are not blocked by cholinergic antagonists but are reduced by chlorpromazine. The concept of specific central tremogenic receptors for serotonin and related compounds has been proposed, since structure–activity relationships of indole alkaloids suggest a high degree of structural specificity rather than mere dependence on lipophilicity (Singbartl *et al.*, 1973).

The most studied indole tremogens, the harmala alkaloids (figure 34.4), produce fine generalised resting tremors of consistent frequency (8–16 Hz) in a variety of species from rodent to monkey (Brimblecombe and Pinder, 1972). Harmine-induced tremor can be produced in the rat by direct injection into the caudate nucleus or substantia nigra (Cox and Potkonjak, 1971), but is more readily produced by peripheral administration. Peripherally induced harmine tremor is antagonised by dopamine, noradrenaline or apomorphine injected directly into the striatum or pallidum, and exacerbated by local serotonin (Kelly and Naylor, 1976). Its primary involvement with serotonergic pathways is established by the reduced harmine or harmaline tremor seen in rats with selective lesions of the medial or dorsal raphe nucleus and rats given intraventricular 5,6-dihydroxytryptamine, tremors that were enhanced by 5-HTP but unaffected by dopaminergic agonists (Costall *et al.*, 1976; Sjolund *et al.*, 1977). Noradrenergic mechanisms may also be involved, since harmaline tremor is reduced in rats by drugs that raise brain noradrenaline levels and is enhanced by chemical or

Table 34.6 Tremogenic indole derivatives.

Drug[a]	Species	Dose and route of administration	Mean tremor latency (min)	Mean tremor duration (min)	Mean tremor frequency (Hz)
Serotonin	cat	250–500 µg, i.c.v.	1–2	20–120	17
Serotonin[b]	cat	30 µg, intracaudate	2.5	23	15
5-Hydroxytryptophan/iproniazid	mouse	100 mg kg^{-1}, i.p.	10	60	12–16
5-Methoxy-N,N-dimethyltryptamine	rat	10 mg kg^{-1}, i.p.	immediate	10	13
Lysergic acid diethylamide (LSD)	mouse	4 mg kg^{-1}, i.p.	5–10	15–30	22–25
Harman	mouse	50 mg kg^{-1}, i.p.	3–5	30	12–14
Harmaline	mouse	10–20 mg kg^{-1}, i.p.	4–8	20–40	14–16
Harmine	mouse	10–20 mg kg^{-1}, i.p.	4–6	15–20	14–16

[a] All data from Brimblecombe and Pinder (1972), unless otherwise noted.
[b] Malseed and Baker (1973).

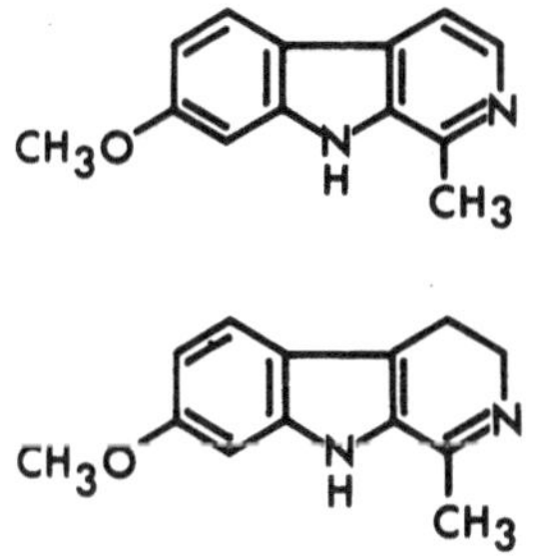

Figure 34.4 Structures of the indolic tremogens harmine and harmaline.

electrical lesions of the locus coeruleus (Yamazaki *et al.*, 1979). Electrophysiological studies in cats and dogs indicate that harmala alkaloids induce strong,
synchronous and rhythmical activity in the inferior olivary nucleus, an area of
dense serotonergic innervation (Headley *et al.*, 1976; Sjolund *et al.*, 1977). Tremors
induced by such drugs probably arise through interference with inhibitory serotonergic innervation of the inferior olive itself, presumably by modification of the
electrotonic coupling of olivary neurones to enhance their tendency to fire in
synchronous bursts at about 10 Hz. Thus, harmaline is unable to produce tremor
in infant rats until the inferior olive cells become functionally mature (Knowles
and Phillips, 1980). Harmaline tremor is therefore mediated through cerebellar
mechanisms, in contrast to cholinergic and catecholaminergic tremors which are
probably extrapyramidal in origin.

Monoaminergic tremogens in man

Tremor is an early and prominent symptom of human intoxication with hallucinogenic drugs, including those of the phenylethylamine type like mescaline as well as
indolic compounds such as LSD and 5-methoxy-*N*,*N*-dimethyltryptamine
(Brimblecombe and Pinder, 1975). These effects are undoubtedly centrally
mediated, but other phenylethylamines such as amphetamine and methamphetamine additionally produce an exaggerated postural physiological tremor by
directly or indirectly stimulating peripheral tremogenic receptors through release
of endogenous catecholamines. The harmala alkaloids also aggravate physiological
tremor in man by increasing the synchronicity of the inferior olivary neurones,
which through the cerebellum have access to descending motor pathways. The
origin of synchronicity in olivary neurones is that they are electrotonically
coupled at the dendritic level so that activity from one is propagated to the next;
the timing of periods of prolonged hyperpolarisation in the cells reflects the
dominant frequency of physiological tremor (Findley and Gresty, 1981).

Bretylium is hardly used in modern therapeutics, and tremor has not been a
consistently reported side-effect. A centrally mediated tremogenic effect is
unlikely to be seen following doses of bretylium, since it is a quaternary salt and

fails to reach the brain readily after oral administration. Furthermore, bretylium can hardly stimulate peripheral tremogenic receptors because it prevents the release of endogenous noradrenaline by the nerve impulse. 5-HTP is used only experimentally, mainly in the treatment of depression both alone and combined with MAOIs (van Praag, 1982). Tremor is the commonest side-effect of 5-HTP and of its non-hydroxylated precursor tryptophan, probably mediated through biotransformation to serotonin.

The most frequently observed tremors arising from therapeutic administration of monoaminergic tremogens are those induced by neuroleptic drugs (Simpson *et al.*, 1981). Pseudo-parkinsonism, with tremor as a major feature, appears within a few weeks of beginning neuroleptic treatment. Its incidence varies between drugs, but the butyrophenones like haloperidol as well as the older and no longer used reserpine tend to be more liable to produce pseudo-parkinsonism than the phenothiazines. A typical parkinsonian resting tremor of frequency 4–6 Hz can be seen in the upper extremities, including the classical pill-rolling movement of the fingers and hand, but more commonly neuroleptic-induced tremor appears as a postural or action tremor (Findley and Gresty, 1981). It can be treated by anti-parkinsonian agents including those of the anticholinergic type. Neuroleptics can also induce movement disorder after chronic treatment, which is termed perioral tremor or 'rabbit' syndrome, and is characterised by a frequency of about 5–7 Hz and a favourable response to anticholinergic drugs. This perioral tremor is distinguishable from the more common oral-facial tardive dyskinesia that also appears late in neuroleptic treatment.

CONCLUSIONS

Tremor can be induced in animals by a wide variety of substances and is a common side-effect of drug treatment in man. Relatively few substances, however, induce a consistent, well defined and sustained tremor. Tremogenic substances acting primarily via central cholinergic mechanisms include muscarinic drugs like oxotremorine and arecoline as well as nicotinic agents and anticholinesterases. Neuroleptics, phenylethylamine analogues and indole derivatives induce tremor primarily via central catecholaminergic and/or serotonergic mechanisms. The existence of a common neurochemical mechanism of tremogenesis is suggested by observations that both types of tremor can be inhibited by drugs that interfere with the postsynaptic actions or synthesis of acetylcholine, and by catecholamines, and may be exacerbated by acetylcholine-like compounds.

Unlike the tremor of Parkinson's disease, which has a lower frequency than that of physiological tremor and tends to disappear upon voluntary movement, many tremogenic substances induce high-frequency tremor that is aggravated by voluntary movement. Intentional tremor can itself be induced by some metals and metal chelators such as cysteamine and penicillamine. Although tremogens have been widely used to select potential therapeutic agents, their relevance to the tremor of extrapyramidal and cerebellar disease is doubtful.

REFERENCES

Ambani, L. M. and Van Woert, M. H. (1972). Modification of the tremorigenic activity of physostigmine. *Br. J. Pharmacol.*, **46**, 344–7.

Baker, W. W., Zivanovic, D. and Malseed, R. T. (1975). Contrasting local effects of MAO inhibitors on caudate tremor activities. *Eur. J. Pharmacol.*, **31**, 17–22.

Baker, W. W., Zivanovic, D. and Malseed, R. T. (1976). Tremorogenic effects of intracaudate d-amphetamine and their suppression by dopamine. *Arch. Int. Pharmacodyn. Ther.*, **223**, 271–81.

Barar, F. S. K. and Madan, B. R. (1976). Tremorine–oxotremorine induced tremor, hypothermia and analgesia, and physostigmine toxicity, in mice after pretreatment with β-adrenoceptor antagonists. *J. Pharm. Pharmacol.*, **28**, 286–9.

Bjorkman, S., Castensson, S. and Sievertsson, H. (1979). Tripeptide analogs of melanocyte stimulating hormone release-inhibiting factor (Pro-Leu-Gly-NH₂) as inhibitors of oxotremorine tremor. *J. Med. Chem.*, **22**, 931–5.

Bjorkman, S., Lewander, T., Karlsson, J. A., Korsiken, L. O. and Zetterstrom, T. (1981). Thermic and tremorogenic effects of TRH in reserpine-treated mice— the non-involvement of GABA-ergic mechanisms. *J. Pharm. Pharmacol.*, **33**, 580–5.

Brimblecombe, R. W. and Pinder, R. M. (1972). *Tremors and Tremorogenic Agents*, Scientechnica, Bristol.

Brimblecombe, R. W. and Pinder, R. M. (1975). *Hallucinogenic Agents*, Wright Scientechnica, Bristol.

Connor, J. D., Rossi, G. V. and Baker, W. W. (1966a). Analysis of tremor induced by injection of cholinergic agents into the caudate nucleus. *Int. J. Neuropharmacol.*, **5**, 207–16.

Connor, J. D., Rossi, G. V. and Baker, W. W. (1966b). Characteristics of tremor in cats following carbachol injections into the caudate nucleus. *Exp. Neurol.*, **14**, 371–82.

Connor, J. D., Rossi, G. V. and Baker, W. W. (1967). Antagonism of intracaudate carbachol tremor by local injections of catecholamines. *J. Pharmacol. Exp. Ther.*, **155**, 545–51.

Costall, B., Kelly, D. M. and Naylor, R. J. (1976). The importance of 5-hydroxytryptamine for the induction of harmine tremor and its antagonism by dopaminergic agonists. *Eur. J. Pharmacol.*, **35**, 109–19.

Coward, D. M. and Doggett, N. S. (1980). Potentiation of LON-954 tremor by typical and atypical neuroleptics—an indication of striatal dopamine antagonism. *Psychopharmacology*, **67**, 177–80.

Coward, D. M., Doggett, N. S. and Sayers, A. S. (1977a). The pharmacology of N-carbamoyl-2-(2,6-dichlorophenyl)acetamidine hydrochloride (LON-954), a new tremorigenic agent. *Arzneimittel-Forsch.*, **27**, 2326–32.

Coward, D. M., Doggett, N. S. and Thomas, J. E. (1977b). Central transmitter involvement in LON-954 induced tremorogenesis. *Neuropharmacology*, **16**, 479–84.

Cox, B. and Potkonjak, D. (1969). An investigation of the tremorgenic effects of oxotremorine and tremorine after stereotaxic injection into the rat brain. *Neuropharmacology*, **8**, 291–7.

Cox, B. and Potkonjak, D. (1971). An investigation of the tremorgenic actions of harmine in the rat. *Eur. J. Pharmacol.*, **16**, 39–45.

Dickinson, S. L., Slater, P. and Longman, D. A. (1981). Effects of naltrexone and prolyl-leucyl-glycinamide on drug-induced tremor and rigidity in the rat. *Neuropharmacol.*, **20**, 757–62.

Doggett, N. S. and O'Farrell, S. A. (1976). Modification of oxotremorine tremor and hypothermia by injections of drugs into the cerebral ventricles of the mouse. *Naunyn-Schmiedeberg Arch. Pharmacol.*, **294**, 149–55.

Dohi, T. and Tsujimoto, A. (1978). Possible mechanisms of sustained tremor induced by nicotine in pilocarpine-treated animals. *Arch. Int. Pharmacodyn. Ther.*, **235**, 62–72.

Drust, E. G., Sloviter, R. S. and Connor, J. D. (1981). Methionine enkephalin-induced shaking in rats is dissociated from brain serotonin mechanisms. *Neuropharmacology*, **20**, 473–5.

Findley, L. J. and Gresty, M. A. (1981). Tremor. *Br. J. Hosp. Med.*, **26**, 16–32.

Goodman, A. G., Goodman, L. S. and Gilman, A. (1980). *The Pharmacological Basis of Therapeutics*, 6th edn, Macmillan, New York.

Gothoni, P., Lehtinen, M. and Silen, L. (1981). Quantification of tremor in rats induced by physostigmine. *Psychopharmacology*, **74**, 275–9.

Guy, W. (1976). *ECDEU Assessment Manual for Psychopharmacology*, DHEW Publication No. (ADM) 76–33, US Government Printing Office, Washington DC.

Headley, P. M., Lodge, D. and Duggan, A. W. (1976). Drug-induced rhythmical activity in the inferior olivary complex of the rat. *Brain Res.*, **101**, 461–78.

Hier, D. B. and Caplan, L. R. (1980). Drugs for senile dementia. *Drugs*, **20**, 74–80.

Kelly, D. M. and Naylor, R. J. (1976). An intracerebral study on the role of striatal dopamine and 5-hydroxytryptamine in the production of tremor by harmine. *Neuropharmacology*, **15**, 303–8.

Knowles, W. D. and Phillips, M. I. (1980). Neurophysiological and behavioural maturation of cerebellar function studied with tremorogenic drugs. *Neuropharmacology*, **19**, 745–56.

Kruse, H. (1976). Thyrotropin-releasing hormone (TRH)–restoration of oxotremorine tremor in mice. *Naunyn-Schmiedeberg Arch. Pharmacol.*, **294**, 39–45.

Lalley, P. M., Rossi, G. V. and Baker, W. W. (1970). Analysis of local cholinergic tremor mechanisms following selective neurochemical lesions. *Exp. Neurol.*, **27**, 258–75.

Lalley, P. M., Rossi, G. V. and Baker, W. W. (1973). Tremor induction by intracaudate injections of bretylium, tetrabenazine or mescaline–functional deficits in caudate dopamine. *J. Pharmaceut. Sci.*, **62**, 1302–7.

Lalley, P. M., Rossi, G. V. and Baker, W. W. (1975). Tremor production by intracaudate injections of morphine. *Eur. J. Pharmacol.*, **32**, 45–51.

Little, M. D. and Dill, R. E. (1969). Mescaline and other O-methylated β-phenylethylamines–intrastriatal induction of tremor in rats. *Brain Res.*, **13**, 360–6.

Malseed, R. T. and Baker, W. W. (1973). Analysis of the tremorgenic effects of intracaudate serotonin. *Proc. Soc. Exp. Biol. Med.*, **143**, 1088–93.

Marsden, C. D. (1978). The mechanisms of physiological tremor and their significance for pathological tremors. In Desmedt, J. E. (ed.), *Progress in Clinical Neurophysiology*, vol. 5, Karger, Basel, pp. 1–16.

Matthews, R. T. and Chiou, C. Y. (1979). Effects of acute and chronic injections of carbachol in the rat caudate nucleus. *Neuropharmacology*, **18**, 291–4.

Pelnar, J. (1913). *Das Zittern*, Springer, Berlin.

Pickles, H., Perucca, E., Fish, A. and Richens, A. (1981). Propranolol and sotalol as antagonists of isoproterenol-enhanced physiologic tremor. *Clin. Pharmacol. Ther.*, **30**, 304–10.

Praag, H. M. van (1982). Significance of serotonin precursors as antidepressants. In Lehmann, H. (ed.), *Non-Tricyclic and Non-Monoamine Oxidase Inhibitors, Modern Problems of Pharmacopsychiatry*, vol. 18, Karger, Basel, pp. 117–38.

Sethy, V. H. and Van Woert, M. H. (1973). Antimuscarinic drugs–effect on brain acetylcholine and tremor in rats. *Biochem. Pharmacol.*, **22**, 2685–91.

Simpson, G. M., Pi, E. H. and Sramek, J. J. (1981). Adverse effects of antipsychotic drugs. *Drugs*, 21, 138–51.

Singbartl, H. G., Zetler, G. and Schlosser, L. (1973). Structure–activity relationships of intra-cerebrally injected tremorigenic indole alkaloids. *Neuropharmacology*, 12, 239–44.

Sjolund, B., Bjorklund, A. and Wiklund, L. (1977). The indoleaminergic innervation of the inferior olive. Relation to harmaline-induced tremor. *Brain Res.*, 131, 23–7.

Slater, P. (1974). Effect of 6-hydroxydopamine on some actions of tremorine and oxotremorine. *Eur. J. Pharmacol.*, 25, 130–7.

Tsujimoto, A. and Dohi, T. (1976). Characteristics of sustained tremor induced by nicotine in pilocarpine-treated animals. *Neuropharmacology*, 16, 421–6.

Weinstock, M., Zavadil, A. P., Rosin, A. J., Chieuh, C. C. and Kopin, I. J. (1978). The role of peripheral catecholamines in oxotremorine tremor in the rat and its antagonism by β-adrenoceptor blocking agents. *J. Pharmacol. Exp. Ther.*, 206, 91–6.

Yamazaki, M., Tanaka, C. and Takaori, S. (1979). Significance of central noradrenergic system on harmaline-induced tremor. *Pharmacol. Biochem. Behav.*, 10, 421–7.

35
Tremor in relation to certain other movement disorders

ROBERT R. YOUNG

INTRODUCTION

Relationships between tremor and other movement disorders are complex because, on the one hand, there are several entirely different types of tremor (Young and Shahani, 1979a) and, on the other hand, practically any one, two or even three types of tremor can and do coexist with any other movement disorder. In other words, the presence of a tremor or tremors in a patient does not confer immunity from any other movement disorder or vice versa.

There are certain exceptions to this rule that tremors and other movement disorders are not mutually exclusive. A patient with either parkinsonian or essential-familial tremor who then suffers a stroke (or other cerebral injury) that damages the corticospinal system or the ventrolateral thalamus and/or its several inputs will lose his pre-existing tremor—i.e. cerebral lesions in these particular sites produce characteristic disorders of voluntary motor control and are incompatible with those two types of tremor, observations which have been of obvious significance to neurosurgeons treating tremors. If corticospinal and other descending motor systems are so severely damaged that voluntary contraction of muscles is no longer possible, physiological or enhanced physiological tremors can also obviously not be generated in the usual way.

Another exception to the rule that any tremor can coexist with any other movement disorder concerns those tremors of the enhanced physiological variety that require, for their expression, function of the segmental stretch reflex arc. As demonstrated by Shahani (this volume, chapter 29), enhanced physiological tremors cannot be produced in patients with severe peripheral neuropathies, whether of hereditary (such as the chronic progressive type Charcot-Marie-Tooth disease), idiopathic or other varieties, providing they disrupt afferent or efferent function around the stretch reflex arc. This is another piece of evidence supporting our hypothesis that enhanced physiological tremor, which can be produced acutely by administration of beta-adrenergic agonists or eliminated acutely by adrenergic blocking agents, arises from operation of a primarily peripheral mechanism. This was first demonstrated in normal subjects by Marsden and his colleagues (Marsden *et al.*, 1967) and later confirmed and extended to patients with pre-existing tremor by Young *et al.* (1975).

However, essential–familial tremor, which has been confused with enhanced physiological tremor (Marshall, 1962), can certainly exist with all its clinical manifestations in patients whose segmental stretch reflex arcs are not functional—for example, in those patients with severe Charcot-Marie-Tooth disease who have also inherited familial tremor (Shahani, this volume, chapter 29). The tremor in these patients responds in a non-acute manner to moderate doses of oral pro-pranolol, a useful therapeutic manoeuvre for ordinary patients with essential-familial tremor first demonstrated by Winkler and Young (1971, 1974). Such observations suggest the fundamental mechanisms underlying essential-familial tremor and its therapy with propranolol involve central nervous system structures and not those in the periphery.

DEFINITIONS

Various types of tremor can and do coexist with various other movement dis-orders, but before reviewing several more important examples we must recognise a semantic problem. Such a coexistence will appear to be even more frequent if one chooses to include, under the general heading 'tremor', such disorders as clonus, nystagmus, palatal myoclonus and cerebellar ataxia or dysmetria. Most clinicians prefer to differentiate these movement disorders from tremor although physiologists may lump them together. True cerebellar tremor does exist but should be distinguished from the more common cerebellar ataxia, a disorder that is characterised by irregular errors in direction and force of voluntary movement. True cerebellar tremor is a less frequent disorder in which a rhythmic, 'static' to-and-fro tremor affects principally axial and proximal limb muscles because of certain lesions of the 'cerebellar system'. This latter term is used to emphasise the fact that motor functions subserved by the cerebellum can be adversely affected (thereby producing typical 'cerebellar symptoms') regardless of whether the causal lesion damages the cerebellum itself, its spino-cerebellar or descending inputs or its outputs.

ASTERIXIS AND MYOCLONUS

These entities are particularly telling examples of our present difficulty in defining exactly which movement disorders are tremors. The most common tremor-like movements occurring in a general hospital population arise in patients with toxic-metabolic encephalopathies and, when carefully studied, prove to be one type of myoclonus or another rather than any of the tremors usually included under that definition. Asterixis (for example, 'liver flap') is due to intermittent 50-200 ms involuntary pauses ('silent periods') in an otherwise tonically sustained EMG con-traction. These pauses produce sudden, very brief lapses of posture with a quick, jerky resumption of posture as the EMG activity switches on again following the pause. This sort of activity can appear tremulous, either because the large synchronous pauses in many muscles of one limb that produce the classical flapping lapses of posture are unusually frequent or, as first demonstrated by Leavitt and Tyler (1964), because more restricted silent periods in the EMG activity of some but not all muscles in the limb produce small, irregular tremor-like movements. Asterixis is well known to occur with various classical metabolic encephalopathies (hepatic, renal or hypercarbic) but also occurs even more frequently in patients who are febrile, toxic, drowsy, or have recently received a variety of medications including general anaesthetics. Several anticonvulsants (e.g. phenytoin and primidone), in a patient who is overmedicated with them, can also produce typical generalised asterixis.

In these settings, asterixis is only one aspect of a widespread metabolic encephalopathy in which the patient also has non-specific abnormalities of mental status, attention, etc. However, asterixis is not a generalised abnormality due to widespread cerebral dysfunction; it is an independent disorder of those motor subsystems that control tonic activation of a motoneurone pool. For example, discrete cerebral lesions such as those produced stereotactically to damage ventro-lateral thalamus (Young *et al.*, 1976) can produce unilateral asterixis of a transitory nature. The receipt of very small amounts of phenytoin, 50-100 mg i.v. for example, by patients with lesions of this sort whose asterixis has subsided can acutely reproduce unilateral asterixis for an hour or so (Shahani and Young, 1976). None of these patients has a metabolic encephalopathy—presumably those who do, and have asterixis, have a transient bilateral biochemical–neurotransmitter 'lesion' of the same system which is anatomically abnormal in patients with unilateral asterixis.

Movements produced by these brief, lightning-like, unpredictable pauses in EMG activity have many of the characteristics of myoclonus. Providing one is willing to entertain the hypothesis that myoclonic-like excessive bursts of inhibition are possible within the central nervous system and, if present, would produce involuntary EMG silence, movement disorders associated with asterixis can be grouped under the heading 'negative myoclonus'. This contrasts asterixis, in which the movement is due to an unexpected 'burst' of EMG silence, with the more well known myoclonic, excessive bursts of EMG activity, which occur in many illnesses including those such as post-hypoxic intention myoclonus where asterixis is also prominent (Young and Shahani, 1979b). Both this latter 'positive myoclonus' and asterixis or negative myoclonus produce 'jerky' (particularly in the arms) or 'bouncy' (particularly about the hip girdle and in the legs when these patients are standing) movements that look superficially like tremor. Careful surface EMG and accelerometric recordings can always demonstrate the characteristic irregularity of the movements with pauses or excessive bursts of EMG activity; clinically one often sees irregularities in these disorders separating them from true tremor. This separation is not entirely clear-cut because damped oscillations, which are self-limited but fulfil the usual definitions of tremor, occur following any sudden mechanical perturbation of a limb in which the muscles are contracting (Hagbarth and Young, 1979; Stiles, 1982) and such oscillations certainly follow each of the myoclonic bursts for a second or two.

Certain patients with cerebral lesions, particularly of progressive type such as neoplasms, develop a large-amplitude 'action tremor' of the contralateral upper limb as one of the first signs of their cerebral disorder. This 'tumour tremor', often mistaken for Parkinson's disease, has been inadequately studied and poorly described. Asterixis is produced unilaterally by certain lesions, particularly those affecting the medial cerebral hemispheres (Shahani and Young, 1976); whether this accounts for the tremors mentioned in this paragraph or whether they are due to some other disorder remains to be seen. A similar nosological situation exists for those patients with tumours (or other lesions) of the midbrain or basal ganglia in whom a tumour-induced parkinsonian syndrome is said to exist (Young, 1977). How similar are these tumour-induced movement disorders to the naturally occurring variety?

TREMORS AND NEUROPATHIC MOVEMENT DISORDERS

An important association exists between tremor and disorders of movement of peripheral origin; there are tremors that appear to be causally related to certain rare types of neuropathy. For example, Adams *et al.* (1972) reported an irregular type of action tremor that waxed and waned in amplitude and severity *pari passu* with the severity of the neuropathy in patients with steroid-sensitive, chronic-relapsing neuropathies. A similar sort of neuropathic tremor has been reported by Smith *et al.* (this volume, chapter 30). Mechanisms underlying these tremors (see Shahani, this volume, chapter 29) are not yet worked out but may involve failure of a compromised stretch reflex arc to compensate, as it normally does (Young and Hagbarth, 1980), for ubiquitous irregularities in velocity of movement due to errors in motor unit recruitment.

Most patients whose tremors are associated with a polyneuropathy have two independent disorders, neither of them terribly uncommon. It has been reported (Yudell *et al.*, 1965) that families whose members are at risk for both Charcot-Marie–Tooth disease and essential–familial tremor may have yet a third disorder, the Roussy–Levy syndrome. There is no evidence to support this hypothesis. Roussy and Levy (1926) did not describe tremor in all their patients with neuropathy. To emphasise this point, Lapresle and Salisachs (1973) reported one of Roussy and Levy's original patients who had only recently developed a senile essential–familial tremor, more than 40 years after Roussy and Levy originally studied her. This view has recently been supported by Salisachs *et al.* (1982). It is probable that certain members of the family described by Yudell *et al.* (1965) simply suffer from an association of two hereditary disorders (neuropathy and tremor) rather than yet a third new one. As will be seen, confusion has also arisen in other circumstances where a tremor is associated with another movement disorder. There are those who are prone to generate new syndromic eponyms;

such coincidences encourage them to consider the combined disorders unique, which is usually antithetical to a clear scientific approach to such illnesses and their therapies.

PARKINSON'S DISEASE

The situation with Parkinson's disease is a more frequent source of error than that generated by relationships between tremor and other movement disorders which themselves do not involve tremor. Parkinson's disease is characterised by 'tremor at rest', itself a misleading designation because this primarily distal tremor tends to be apparent in an attitude of repose where, although the patient may think his forearms are at rest, shoulder girdle and axial musculature is active in the maintenance of posture. Although every patient with Parkinson's disease need not complain of tremor at rest, it is unexpectedly difficult to determine precisely what percentage of patients with Parkinson's disease do have tremor at rest. Some patients without clinically apparent tremor at rest (at least when they are being examined by a physician) complain of tremor at other times when they are anxious, fatigued or cold. Furthermore, unpublished studies undertaken by Growdon, Shahani and myself, in which surface EMG electrodes or intramuscular needles were used to search for tremor, revealed its presence in most patients with Parkinson's disease. The abnormalities of single motor unit behaviour characteristic of parkinsonian tremor (Young and Shahani, 1979c) are (1) double discharges of single motor units at rates of 40–50 Hz during slow, non-ballistic recruitment and/or (2) synchronisation of discharge of independent motor units (figure 35.1).

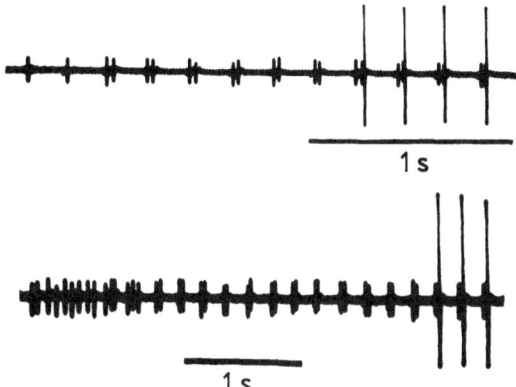

1 s

1 s

Figure 35.1 Behaviour of two single motor units in the wrist extensors of a patient with Parkinson's disease—with slowly increasing force, the smaller unit is recruited before the larger one, a unit may discharge singly or as a 'doublet' with a high instantaneous firing rate and the discharge of the larger second unit recruited is time-locked to the first. Note, at the left of the bottom trace, the smaller unit discharges normally when first recruited but then begins to discharge as a slow doublet.

In our experience, it is extremely rare to find a patient with Parkinson's disease who does not show an abnormality of one or both of these types during EMG examination even if tremor is not clinically obvious. This observation leads to the hypothesis that the pathology underlying Parkinson's disease (anatomic as well as biochemical) carries with it in every instance the pathophysiological substrate for tremor but, for reasons that remain obscure, the degree to which these tremor mechanisms are expressed is an individual affair. Apparently some patients have additional neurotransmitter or other deficits different from most patients with Parkinson's disease so their tremor is not clinically striking. There are certainly a number of as yet undiscovered neurotransmitters or modulators, of which some may also be deficient to a varying degree in patients with Parkinson's disease. Dopamine deficiency, which is now so well known, is probably not the only factor underlying Parkinson's disease, although it is perhaps the primary factor. Some other mechanism appears to determine the percentage of patients with clinically significant tremor.

Growdon *et al.* (1975), in their study of 100 consecutive unselected patients with clear-cut Parkinson's disease, found 75% had a clinically apparent tremor. In approximately 56%, this was a typical tremor at rest; in 19% the only clinically apparent tremor was an action tremor. In 10% who were assigned to the former group, their tremor at rest did not decrease in amplitude during activity and, in that sense, they might also be said to have an action tremor although we suspect they simply had a more severe tremor at rest. Altogether, action tremor, with or without tremor at rest, occurred in 55% of patients, which confirms the observation of Lance *et al.* (1963) that action tremors are rather common in patients with Parkinson's disease. Naturally, like all normal subjects, parkinsonian patients have both a minute underlying physiological tremor when they contract their muscles and an enhanced physiological tremor with anxiety, fright, fatigue, and so on. The latter is therefore one type of action tremor that can affect every patient with Parkinson's disease. Some of these patients also have a peculiar tremor during writing which does not appear under other circumstances. Finally, they may also have an essential–familial tremor. In at least 5% of patients with Parkinson's disease (Schwab and Young, 1971), a propranolol-sensitive typical essential–familial tremor is more disabling than the tremor at rest or other symptoms of Parkinson's disease. There are therefore at least four independent types of tremor that can appear in patients with Parkinson's disease and it would obviously be unwise from a scientific or therapeutic viewpoint simply to label each of them 'parkinsonian tremor'. This has been done, perhaps unwittingly, in studies of various therapies where, for example, propranolol is said to be 'effective in the treatment of parkinsonian tremor'. It is effective acutely in reducing enhanced physiological tremor in patients with Parkinson's disease who are anxious or fatigued; it is effective in the long run in patients with Parkinson's disease who also have an essential–familial tremor; but it is not effective in the therapy of the tremor at rest in these patients providing the latter has not been enhanced by various beta-adrenergic mechanisms.

TREMORS ARE ADDITIVE

When those mechanisms responsible for enhanced physiological tremor are brought into play (for discussion of the role of peripheral and stretch reflex mechanisms of this type see Young, this volume, chapter 7), the amplitude of any and all tremors already present in that subject or patient will increase. That is to say, in the case of a normal subject who has no tremor other than physiological, these mechanisms will produce an enhanced physiological tremor at a frequency that is within the range of the pre-existing physiological tremor. On the other hand, if the patient has typical parkinsonian tremor at rest, its amplitude will also be enhanced at the pre-existing frequency whenever the adrenergic mechanisms mentioned above become active. Similarly, if the patient has a pre-existing essential-familial tremor, its amplitude then also becomes enhanced without a change in frequency. A semantic problem arises: should one say that the stretch reflex mechanisms have produced a combined tremor where enhanced physiological tremor has been added to the pre-existing tremor or should one simply say that the operation of these mechanisms produces an enhanced parkinsonian tremor or enhanced essential-familial tremor, whichever the case may be? In any case, as illustrated in figure 35.2, tremors are additive so that both the tremor amplitude

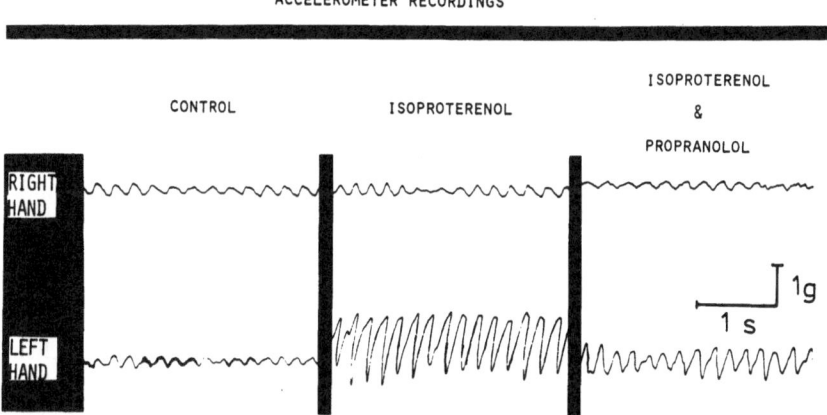

ACCELEROMETER RECORDINGS

CONTROL   ISOPROTERENOL   ISOPROTERENOL & PROPRANOLOL

RIGHT HAND

LEFT HAND

1 g
1 s

Figure 35.2 Tremors are additive. The amplitude of whichever tremor is already present (physiological, parkinsonian or, as in this patient, essential–familial) is temporarily increased by adrenergic or other mechanisms that produce enhanced physiological tremor in normal subjects. The resulting, larger, combined tremor should not be considered simply as physiological, parkinsonian or essential–familial tremor. In this experiment, beta-adrenergic agonist and antagonist were infused intra-arterially into the left forearm in minute amounts, thereby affecting tremor only in that limb. Both compounds work acutely to increase or decrease tremor amplitude – the net result, depending on the relative amounts infused, can be larger, but not smaller, than the pre-existing baseline tremor (control). However, after several days of oral propranolol therapy, this patient's essential-familial tremor virtually disappeared.

and the percentage of time during which the tremor is symptomatic become increased; the patient then complains of 'worse tremor'.

As a corollary of this enhancement hypothesis ('tremors are additive'), two independent therapeutic approaches should exist for treatment of these enhanced tremors. On the one hand, peripherally active beta-adrenergic blocking agents (or any other modality reducing the gain of the stretch reflex) should ameliorate the tremor by diminishing that fraction due to enhanced physiological tremor. On the other hand, therapies directed towards the underlying tremor—levodopa for the tremor at rest of Parkinson's disease, primidone or propranolol for the treatment of essential–familial tremor—should reduce the pre-existing tremor so that any enhancement would have a smaller baseline tremor upon which to work, so the resulting movement seen with the combined tremor would be less. Fortunately for therapists, propranolol works by both mechanisms in the treatment of patients with essential–familial tremor: (1) their pre-existing tremor can be reduced, providing propranolol is taken in large enough doses for long enough time, and (2) the anxiety- (or otherwise) enhanced component will be acutely reduced even by receipt of rather small doses of propranolol. Whereas propranolol's double mechanism of action happens to be useful from the patient's viewpoint, it confuses the nosology of these tremors, since one is tempted to attribute whatever happens following propranolol therapy to its peripheral beta-blocking action. As emphasised by Koch-Weser (1975), those central nervous system actions whereby propranolol is useful for the therapy of hypertension and angina (and perhaps tremor) are different pharmacologically and clinically from propranolol's relatively simple peripheral beta-blocking activity.

A particularly clear example of this dichotomous approach to the treatment of combined tremors may be seen in patients who have had ventrolateral thalamotomies or other surgical procedures that have eliminated their pre-existing tremor at rest or essential–familial tremor. In them, only physiological tremor remains, and they are subject to the development of enhanced physiological tremor, but no other larger tremor is possible. When they are nervous or fatigued, they still tremble a bit, but nothing like as much as occurred with anxiety before surgery. Whereas a parkinsonian patient who would previously tremble fiercely when chilled no longer does so, no-one would suggest the thalamotomy was undertaken to treat shivering nor should they suggest that lowering body temperature makes Parkinson's disease worse.

Although confusion in this area is encouraged by the fact that tremors are additive and propranolol operates by at least two different mechanisms, we are now in a position to begin to think clearly about these disorders.

CONCLUSIONS

Tremors can occur with almost any other movement disorder. 'Tremors are additive' insofar as an enhanced physiological tremor adds its excursion to an already existing tremor of the parkinsonian tremor at rest or essential–familial variety. Although this has not been an exhaustive review of tremor in all movement disorders, the principles whereby one approaches such as problem are exemplified by discussion of various tremors in Parkinson's disease. Such principles can then be applied to gain understanding of interactions between various tremors and movement disorders with either central or peripheral causes.

ACKNOWLEDGEMENT

This work was supported in part by the Parkinson's Disease Fund of the Massachusetts General Hospital.

REFERENCES

Adams, R. D., Shahani, B. T. and Young, R. R. (1972). Tremor in association with polyneuropathy. *Trans. Am. Neurol. Assoc.*, **97**, 44-8.

Growdon, J. H., Young, R. R. and Shahani, B. T. (1975). The differential diagnosis of tremor in Parkinson's disease. *Trans. Am. Neurol. Assoc.*, **100**, 197-9.

Hagbarth, K.-E. and Young, R. R. (1979). Participation of the stretch reflex in human physiological tremor. *Brain*, **102**, 509-26.

Koch-Weser, J. (1975). Non-beta blocking actions of propranolol. *New Engl. J. Med.*, **293**, 988-9.

Lance, J. W., Schwab, R. S. and Peterson, E. A. (1963). Action tremor and the cogwheel phenomenon in Parkinson's disease. *Brain*, **86**, 85-110.

Lapresle, J. and Salisachs, P. (1973). Onion bulbs in a nerve biopsy specimen from an original case of Roussy-Levy disease. *Arch. Neurol.*, **29**, 346-8.

Leavitt, S. and Tyler, H. R. (1964). Studies in asterixis. *Arch. Neurol.*, **10**, 360-8.

Marsden, C. D., Foley, T. H., Owen, D. A. L. and McAllister, R. G. (1967). Peripheral beta-adrenergic receptors concerned with tremor. *Clin. Sci.*, **33**, 53-65.

Marshall, J. (1962). Observations on essential tremor. *J. Neurol. Neurosurg. Psychiatr.*, **25**, 122-5.

Roussy, G. and Levy, G. (1926). Sept cas d'une maladie familiale particulière. *Rev. Neurol.*, **2**, 427-50.

Salisachs, P., Findley, L. J., Codina, M., LaTorre, P. and Martínez-Lage, J. M. (1982). Use and misuse of the Roussy-Levy eponym. *J. Neurol. Neurosurg. Psychiatr.*, **45**, 938-9.

Schwab, R. S. and Young, R. R. (1971). Non-resting tremor in Parkinson's disease. *Trans. Am. Neurol. Assoc.*, **96**, 305-7.

Shahani, B. T. and Young, R. R. (1976). Asterixis—a disorder of the neural mechanisms underlying sustained muscle contraction. In Shahani, M. (ed.), *The Motor System—Neurophysiology and Muscle Mechanisms*, Elsevier, Amsterdam, pp. 301-6.

Stiles, R. N. (1982). Phase lead of extensor EMG on wrist flexion during lightly-damped oscillations, postural tremor, and physiological action tremor of the hand. *Soc. Neurosci. Abstr.*, **8**, 534.

Winkler, G. F. and Young, R. R. (1971). The control of essential tremor by propranolol. *Trans. Am. Neurol. Assoc.*, **96**, 66-8.

Winkler, G. F. and Young, R. R. (1974). The efficacy of chronic propranolol therapy in action tremors of the familial, senile or essential varieties. *New Engl. J. Med.*, **290**, 984–8.

Young, R. R. (1977). The differential diagnosis of Parkinson's disease. *Int. J. Neurol.*, **12**, 219–35.

Young, R. R., Growdon, J. H. and Shahani, B. T. (1975). Beta-adrenergic mechanisms in action tremor. *New Engl. J. Med.*, **293**, 950–3.

Young, R. R. and Hagbarth, K.-E. (1980). Physiological tremor enhanced by manoeuvres affecting the segmental stretch reflex. *J. Neurol. Neurosurg. Psychiatr.*, **43**, 248–56.

Young, R. R. and Shahani, B. T. (1979a). Pharmacology of tremor. In Klawans, H. L. (ed.), *Clinical Neuropharmacology*, vol. 4, Raven Press, New York, pp. 139–56.

Young, R. R. and Shahani, B. T. (1979b). Clinical neurophysiological aspects of post-hypoxic intention myoclonus. In Fahn, S., Davis, J. N. and Rowland, L. P. (eds), *Cerebral Hypoxia and its Consequences*, Raven Press, New York, pp. 85–105.

Young, R. R. and Shahani, B. T. (1979c). Single unit behavior in human muscle afferent and efferent systems. In Poirier, L. J., Sourkes, T. L. and Bedard, P. J. (eds), *The Extrapyramidal System and its Disorders*, Raven Press, New York, pp. 175–83.

Young, R. R., Shahani, B. T. and Kjellberg, R. N. (1976). Unilateral asterixis produced by discrete central nervous system lesions. *Trans. Am. Neurol. Assoc.*, **101**, 306–7.

Yudell, A., Dyck, P. J. and Lambert, E. H. (1965). A kinship with the Roussy-Levy syndrome. *Arch. Neurol.*, **13**, 432–40.

SECTION 9
SIGNIFICANCE OF TREMOR IN THE
ONTOGENY OF THE NERVOUS SYSTEM

The phenomenon of tremor as manifest in disease is an unfortunate demonstration of the 'release' of potential nervous activity which, in the normal state, is under strict control. Previous speculation on the reasons why tremor should emerge has considered the phenomenon to be vestigial, related to rhythmical locomotor activity, or to be the consequence of necessary 'design risks' related to the inertia and viscoelastic properties of body parts. It is possible, however, that there are certain properties of tremor, or rather of the types of mechanisms that produce tremor rhythms, which may be of importance to the growth and maintenance of a self-organising intelligent network such as the nervous system. Here Professor Rodolfo Llinás speculates on how structures capable of supporting rhythmical activity may play a crucial role in determining the physical and informational growth of the nervous system.

THE EDITORS

36
Possible role of tremor in the organisation of the nervous system

R.R. LLINÁS

The essential feature of tremor is that of an activity which is sustained and regular (pathological tremors do not vary in frequency as observed over periods of several years!). Thus the mechanism responsible has the properties, essential to the workings of any organism, of a generator of motive force and of a clocking function in the sense of prediction (Pellionisz and Llinás, 1982). It is these characteristics that provoke the speculation that the existence of oscillatory rhythms, as coherent properties of CNS neurones, is of theoretical significance beyond their relationship to servo-loops (Marsden, this volume, chapter 4) or as the basis for a central motor generator in swimming and locomotion in vertebrates (Jung, 1941; Gresty and Findley, this volume, chapter 2).

It is, perhaps, the neural structures that can give rise to tremor, which in other roles are essential in the organisation of the internal coordinate reference systems in the CNS (Pellionisz and Llinás, 1979). In this respect it has long been known that during development embryos go through distinct stages of tremor and rhythmic twitching (Hamburger and Balaban, 1963; Bekoff et al., 1975). One may thus wonder if such oscillations and resonances may not be one of the key mechanisms which determine the organisation of the neuronal networks of the CNS as it relates to the external properties of the body and to the electrical properties of the neuronal elements that constitute such nets. Neuronal oscillation and resonance in fact determine much of the active movement dynamics of limbs, and thus must provide, by feedback through the afferent systems, information about the dynamics of body reference frames.

As an example, it has long been known that, in cases of Parkinson's disease, mechanical oscillatory stimulation of a finger by an external device may induce tremor that irradiates progressively upwards along the limb (Jung, 1941) in a manner similar to the Jacksonian 'march' of motor seizures following localised lesions in the motor cortex. This 'tremor march' phenomenon indicates that the different portions of the CNS which control limb movement are coupled to each other by the ability to be phase-locked and to resonate with tremors occurring in one of its portions.

Such dissipative functional structures are of the essence when considering that the limb in its totality may be utilised at a given movement as a single element and, at others, as a set of separate compartments (Kugler *et al.*, 1980). Indeed, this tremor domain expresses the degree of coupling between the different components of this limb and thus the serious possibility that the nervous system may utilise this domain to advantage in establishing an internal geometry of the co-ordination between these structures (Pellionisz and Llinás, 1980).

Tremor as establishing some aspects of the internal geometry of the central nervous system

Because tremor ultimately returns to the CNS by afferent receptor connectivity, it may be used during development to establish some of the n-dimensional vectorial transformations (in frequency hyperspace) which underlie the transformation of sensory input into coordinated motor output. Indeed the tremor and twitching of a given muscle group and the ability it has to generate sensory feedback by the production of actual movement, by the direct activation of the sensory feedback or by corollary discharge, would ultimately serve to establish the physiologically meaningful connectivity between afferent input and motor output. The importance of this interaction becomes clearer when considering that it occurs very early in development prior to the generation of truly organised movement and could thus serve as an epigenetic organising influence in determining selective stabilisation of neuronal networks (Changeux and Danchin, 1976). This mechanism of central oscillation—giving rise to tremor—in turn generating a sensory stimulus which is fed back to the central oscillator, would ultimately result in the internal moulding of the sensorimotor transformation. Since tremor is an undesirable property in the organisation of co-ordinated movement, the CNS will tend to minimise such tremor by neuronal mechanisms capable of plasticity, especially during development. In doing so, the adaptive change which ensues would tend to establish automatically the internal geometry required for transformation of sensory input (a covariant vector) into a motor output which would be in accordance with the body co-ordinate system (a contravariant transformation). In short, the tremor would serve as a mechanism to establish metric tensors (Pellionisz and Llinás, 1980; 1982).

In addition to tremor organising sensorimotor transforms, oscillatory interactions between other portions of the nervous system may be at work during development. These may coalesce, due to recurrent feedback, into the properties of matrices known as *strange attractors*, which by their self-organising properties and robustness, may serve as one of the underlying mechanisms for the establishment of network properties not immediately related to body co-ordinate systems (Hopfield, 1982). Finally, oscillation and resonance within the CNS may also serve to establish the many sets of transformations which are necessary to organise a transformation between different sensory frames of reference. Ultimately, by reconstructing external invariances, this multisensory interaction can lead to a global description of the world, i.e. an internal image of external reality.

REFERENCES

Bekoff, A., Stein, P. S. G. and Hamburger, V. (1975). Co-ordinated motor output in the hindlimb of the 7-day chick embryo. *Proc. Natl. Acad. Sci. USA*, 72, 1245–8.

Changeux, J. P. and Danchin, A. (1976). Selective stabilization of developing synapses as a mechanism for the specification of neuronal networks. *Nature (Lond.)*, 264, 705–12.

Hamburger, V. and Balaban, M. (1963). Observations and experiments on spontaneous rhythmical behaviour in the chick embryo. *Dev. Biol.*, 7, 533–45.

Hopfield, J. J. (1982). Neural networks and physical systems with emergent collective computational abilities. *Proc. Natl. Acad. Sci. USA*, 79, 2554–8.

Jung, R. (1941). Physiologische Untersuchungen uber den Parkinsontremor und andere Zitterformen beim Menschen. *Z. Neurol. Psychiatr.*, 173, 263–330.

Kugler, P. N., Scott Kelso, J. A. and Turvey, M. T. (1980). On the concept of co-ordinative structures as dissipative structures: I. Theoretical lines of convergence. In Stelmach, G. E. and Requin, J. (eds), *Tutorials in Motor Behaviour*, North-Holland, Amsterdam, pp. 3–47.

Pellionisz, A. and Llinás, R. (1979). Brain modeling by tensor network theory and computer simulation. The cerebellum: Distributed processor for predictive coordination. *Neurosci.*, 4, 323–48.

Pellionisz, A. and Llinás, R. (1980). Tensorial approach to the geometry of brain function. Cerebellar coordination via metric tensor. *Neurosci.*, 5, 1125–36.

Pellionisz, A. and Llinás, R. (1982). Space–time representation in the brain. The cerebellum as a predictive space–time metric tensor. *Neurosci.*, 7, 2949–70.

Glossary of terms

There is widespread use of certain terms to refer to the phenomenology and mechanisms of tremor. However, despite their ubiquity, there is no common agreement as to precise definition and application. The following glossary is aimed at providing a working set of definitions of terms that are commonly used in discussions on tremor of the limbs, trunk, head and eyes. An attempt to indicate major differences of opinion on terminology and suggestions for alternative terms, avoiding neologisms, has been made.

Voluntary and *involuntary* are terms widely used to describe human movements. However, as pointed out by William James and Hughlings Jackson, the distinction is not clear-cut; an infinite gradation exists between the two extremes. Hughlings Jackson, to overcome this difficulty, graded motor performance on a scale of hierarchical levels between 'less automatic' and 'more automatic'. However, whilst recognising the problem, we believe that the terms *voluntary movement* and *involuntary movement* are sufficiently ingrained in the clinical vocabulary to warrant continued use.

Asterixis

Sudden postural lapses, particularly of the outstretched hands, due to cessation of muscle contraction

[Asterixis is often called negative myoclonus]

Ataxia

Disorder of normal coordinated movement

[Aspects or subdivisions of ataxia are tremor, dysmetria and decomposition of unitary or repetitive, simple or complex movement]
[Ataxia implies disorder of movements that are normally within the subject's capability. Inappropriate movements made in extreme circumstances would not be ataxic]

Clonus

Rhythmical muscle contractions evoked by and sustained during muscle stretch

479

Co-contraction

Synchronous or near-synchronous contraction in antagonistic muscles (muscle groups)

Cogwheel phenomenon

The term *cogwheel phenomenon* should be used to refer to a rhythmical repetitive interruption of passive movement of a limb about a joint

[The term *active cogwheel phenomenon* has been used to describe repetitive interruptions to movements carried out by the patient. Some have termed active cogwheeling *action tremor*, which is an unsuitable term because all movement involves action. The correct term should be *movement tremor*]
[Some use the term *cogwheel rigidity*, assuming the phenomenon is pathognomonic of parkinsonism. It may occur in patients with a variety of other tremors]

Dysmetria

Inability to attain the target or normal performance level in a guided, goal-seeking movement

[The criteria may be a defect in the amplitude of individual movement sequences required to attain a goal or inability to match velocity and displacement of limb movement with respect to target movement]
[Dysmetria may have the appearance of tremor when the part of the body being moved has certain inertial and viscoelastic properties. Such movements have been termed *resettable tremor* because changes in the goal during the course of movement tend to arrest ongoing movement and provoke a fresh sequence of activity]

Dystonia

Sustained or intermittent muscle spasms that distort body parts into typical 'dystonic' postures

Enhanced physiological tremor

A physiological tremor of a body part that is of greater than normal amplitude but of normal frequency

[This group includes the tremor of many patients who seek aid]

Froment's sign

The *signe de Froment* is a rhythmical resistance to passive movement of a limb about a joint that can be detected specifically when there is voluntary activity of the contralateral limb

[This phenomenon may be seen in a wide variety of disorders associated with tremor]

Myoclonus

Intermittent brief muscle jerks, irregular or rhythmic, arising in the central nervous system

[Brief muscle jerks also occur in chorea and tics. These are distinguished by other features]

[Intermittent brief muscle jerks are also typical of fasciculation, which some have included as a localised form of myoclonus. However, we would prefer to restrict myoclonus to conditions in which abnormal neuronal discharge causing the muscle jerk arises in the central nervous system]

[*Rhythmic myoclonus* can be distinguished from tremor only when the driving muscle contractions are impulsive, so that there are pauses between the individual jerks. The problem of *oculo-palatal myoclonus* is discussed under *palatal myoclonus*]

[*Oscillatory myoclonus* has been used to describe a myoclonic jerk followed by exaggerated decaying oscillations]

[*Myoclonic dystonia* refers to repetitive, brief dystonic muscle spasms, which produce jerking of the body part superimposed upon a characteristic and diagnostic dystonic posture]

[Some forms of myoclonus arise spontaneously irrespective of external stimuli, and other forms may be provoked by visual, auditory, tactile or proprioceptive stimuli (*stimulus-sensitive myoclonus*)]

[Some myoclonus only appears when the patient attempts to move (*action myoclonus*)]

Nodding head tremor, head shaking

A term used especially in paediatric neuro-ophthalmology to refer to shaking movements of the head that are usually associated with abnormal eye movements; they may be in any direction and may be tremulous or non-tremulous. *Head shaking* and *head tremor* are better terms. In some instances, the head shaking develops in compensation for disordered eye movements and should be referred to as *compensatory head shaking*, if irregular, or *compensatory head tremor*, if rhythmical. These terms should be used together with an indication of direction (see below)

[The anatomical terminology available to describe the trajectory of head movement is extremely complex for the reason that there are three linear and three rotational axes of movement. We suggest the following terminology for head movements, which derives from aeronautics and has already been introduced into otological literature: *yaw, pitch, roll, surge, heave* and *bob*. Combinations of these terms will describe all possible motions of a rigid body]

Yaw

Angular motion in the horizontal plane about an axis oriented from the base to the vertex
[As in saying 'no-no']

Pitch

Angular motion in the sagittal plane about a left–right axis
[As in 'yes-yes']

Roll

Angular motion in the coronal plane about an occipito-frontal axis
[As in ear tilt down to shoulder]

Surge

Linear motion along the occipito-frontal axis
[As in the appearance of forwards and backwards movements of a pigeon's head during walking]

Heave

Linear motion along the left-to-right horizontal axis
[As in leaning sideways on skis whilst keeping the head upright]

Bob

Linear movement along the axis from the base to the vertex
[Up-and-down motion that would occur during walking]

Nystagmus

An oscillation of the eyes. Strictly speaking the term refers to an oscillation that has an asymmetrical waveform with a fast component in one direction followed by a slower component in the opposite direction

[*Congenital nystagmus* is an involuntary oscillation of the eyes, present at or shortly after birth, which is associated with no known sensory, motor or cognitive defects]

Ocular flutter

Involuntary, to-and-fro, saccadic movements of the eyes that occur without an intersaccadic interval

Ocular tremor

An oscillation of the globe

[*Physiological ocular tremor* is of minute amplitude and high frequency and cannot normally be observed]

Opsoclonus

Involuntary saccadic eye movements made in rapid succession; especially those that are multidirectional and occur without an intersaccadic interval

[*Ocular flutter* also consists of to-and-fro saccades without intersaccadic intervals and hence is the basic component of opsoclonus]

Palatal myoclonus

Palatal myoclonus is a repetitive, sustained rhythmic movement of the soft palate. The movement may be a jerk repeated about twice per second, or a slow tremor

[When there are similar movements of other structures, predominantly axial, including the eyes, the larynx, pharynx, intercostal muscles and diaphragm, the syndrome is commonly called *oculo-palatal-pharyngeal-laryngeal-(etc.) myoclonus*]

[The use of the term *myoclonus* to describe this syndrome is frequently misleading for the movements are, strictly speaking, tremulous]

[This is particularly true of *ocular myoclonus*. Most patients described with this condition have pendular eye movements although movements with an asymmetrical waveform do occur]

Pathological tremor

A tremor due to disease or disorder of the nervous system

Pendular nystagmus

A sinusoidal oscillation of the globe; strictly speaking, it should not be called nystagmus

[*Acquired pendular nystagmus* is an ocular tremor]
[*Congenital nystagmus* may have a waveform that appears to be pendular. Close inspection reveals that there are jerk-like interruptions to the waveform that do not necessarily occur in acquired pendular nystagmus]

Physiological tremor

The asymptomatic (normal) oscillation of all body parts

Reciprocal activation

Alternating activation of antagonist muscles

[The activations may overlap in time but do not start simultaneously]

Reinforced rigidity

A sustained increase in resistance throughout the range of passive movement about a joint induced by the patient voluntarily contracting muscles elsewhere

[As in the case of Froment's sign, reinforced rigidity may occur in conditions other than Parkinson's disease, even in the anxious normal subject]
[Similar reinforced rigidity can also be provoked by other stimuli such as startle or stress]

Rigidity

A sustained increase in resistance throughout the range of passive movement about a joint that is usually similar in both directions of movement

Rubral tremor

A coarse tremor, especially of the upper limbs, that is of low frequency (3-5 Hz) and is present at rest, in posture and through movement

[The term *rubral tremor* incorrectly presumes precise site of the lesion responsible; however, damage in the region of the red nucleus may interrupt cerebello-thalamic and other pathways, thereby giving rise to this form of tremor]

Spasticity

An increase in resistance to passive movement (an increase in muscle tone), more evident in one direction than another, and exhibiting a progressive exaggeration until a point is reached at which resistance collapses

Tone

The resistance encountered by the examiner when the limb or other body part is moved passively about a joint

[Types of increased tone include spasticity, rigidity, dystonia, cogwheel rigidity and reinforced rigidity]

Tremor

A rhythmic, mechanical oscillation of a body part

[By convention, tremor is identified by its appearance, irrespective of its mechanism]
[The rhythmical appearance of tremor requires that the period of the oscillation, although not necessarily its amplitude, is relatively constant]

Rest tremor

Tremor occurring when the subject is not voluntarily activating muscle(s)

[Involuntary muscle tone is often present, so strictly speaking the subject may not be at rest]
[*Static tremor* has been a term used by some for rest tremor, but has also been used for tremor provoked by maintenance of constant posture. We would not recommend its further usage]

Action tremor

Any tremor occurring on voluntary contraction of muscle

Postural tremor

Tremor provoked by the maintenance of posture

Movement tremor

Tremor provoked by any form of movement. The tremor may occur at the initiation of movement (*initial tremor*), during movement (*transition tremor*) and at the termination of movement (*terminal tremor*)

[We have chosen to introduce the term *movement tremor* because of the great confusion in terminology in this area. For instance, some have used the term *action tremor* to describe movement tremor, but posture is an action. The classical term *intention tremor* has also been used, but any form of voluntary muscular activity is intentional. Others have confined the term *intention tremor* to terminal movement tremor]

[We recognise that initial, transition and terminal tremor often occur together and may share a common mechanism. However, sometimes movement tremor may only be apparent at the beginning of, during, or at the termination of movement]

Index

ALS, *see* Amyotrophic lateral sclerosis
APT, *see* Tremor, physiological, enhanced
Acetylcholine, 313, 378
Acquired pendular nystagmus, 422–423, 484
Adrenaline (epinephrine), 49, 52, 85, 87, 89, 129, 246, 255
Alcohol, 56, 77, 85, 89–90, 230, 271
  degeneration caused by, 22, 54, 77
Alpha–gamma coactivation, 48
Alpha receptors, 86
Alzheimer's disease, 99, 105–106, 108
  liver failure in, 116
Amantadine, 86
Amyotrophic lateral sclerosis, 105
Angular transducers, 17
Animal models, of tremor
  in Parkinson's disease, 183–194
  in physiological tremor, 183–194
Anticholinergics, 85–86, 90, 331–332, 448
Antidopaminergics, 86
Antihistamines, 332
Antipsychotic agents, 89
Arecoline, 450
Asterixis, 464–466, 479
Ataxia, 71, 74–75, 479
  of cerebellum, 389
  Friedreich's, 113, 378, 383
  paroxysmal tremor and, 440–441
  sensory, 389
Atenolol, 56–57, 249, 252–253, 255
Axonal transport, 97

Baclofen, 380, 417
Ballistocardiac impulse, 41, 53, 127
Basal ganglia, 97–98, 340
Beating, 64–65
Belladonna alkaloids, 85
Benzodiazepines, 89
Beta-adrenoceptor blocking agents, 52, 54, 56–57, 71, 77, 85, 89–90, 225, 247, 265–266
  central actions of, 77

comparative effects of, 248–255
  mechanisms of, 77, 255–256
  membrane stabilising activity of, 265–266
  withdrawal syndrome of, 225, 229–230
Beta-adrenoceptors, 86, 225–244
  β_1 activity, 226–227, 232, 250
  β_2 activity, 226–227, 230, 232, 250, 256, 446
  in essential tremor, 225–260
  lymphocyte, 234, 239
  peripheral, 225
  skeletal muscle contractility in, 226
  stimulation by, 53–54, 56
Beta-blockers, *see* Beta-adrenoceptor blocking agents
Brachium conjuctivum, 71, 75
Bromocriptine, 86, 334–335
Bronchodilators, 54

Carbidopa, 89
Cardioselectivity, 248, 261
Catecholamines, 53, 129, 445, 451–454
  intracaudate, 315
Cerebello-mesencephalic-thalamic projection pathway, 22
Cerebellum, the, 22, 49, 56, 109, 413
  ataxia of, 389
  cortex of, 184–185
  cortical atrophy of, 378
  deep nuclei of, 75
  disease of, 89–90
    biofeedback in, 382
  lesions of, 71, 307–313
  output of, 71, 78
  Purkinje cells of, 167, 169, 171, 184, 191
  superior peduncle, 75, 95, 109
  toxins and, 115
  tremor in disease of, 22, 74–76, 86, 95, 115, 183–189, 353–386
Charcot, Jean Martin, 289–291, 425
Charcot-Marie-Tooth disease, 208, 392–393
  peripheral neuropathy in, 67, 133

Cholinergic agents, 378–380, 383
  central, 445
  peripheral, 447–451
  as tremogens, 449–451
  see also Acetylcholine
Chorea, 4
  Huntington's, 3, 116–117, 378
Clonidine, 231
Clonus, 5, 23, 63, 160, 301, 479
  'central generator' for, 63–65, 74
  'central pacemaker' for, 62–64
  external rythmic displacement in, 63
  'externally driven', 160, 162
  muscle spindles in, 157–164
  in Parkinson's disease, 68, 78
  rhythmic external force in, 63
  in spasticity, 60
Cogwheel phenomenon, *see* Tremor, cogwheel
Coherence analysis, 139
Coherence spectrum, 139
Congenital nystagmus, 484
Cortical infarcts, 23
Corticopontine fibres, 109
Corticospinal tract, 71
  see also Spinal cord
Corticosteroids, 129
Cumulative numbering system, 9

DBH, *see* Dopamine, beta-hydroxylase
Deafferentation, 46–47, 64, 67, 72, 76
Dementia
  in Parkinson's disease, 105, 108, 292
  senile, 106
Demyelination, 392, 400
Dentate nucleus, 75–76, 95–96, 374
Dopamine, 71, 73, 85–86, 305–306, 311,
      313–314, 332–338
  beta-hydroxylase, 97
  levels of, 96
  pathways of, 71, 73, 192
  striatal, 101
  see also Ergot alkaloids, Levodopa, Piribedil
Drug intoxication, 23
Dyschronometry, 371
Dysdiadochokinesis, 377
Dyskinesia
  diphasic, 334
  tardive, 378
Dysmetria, 22, 74, 377, 408
Dystonia
  idiopathic, 67
  myoclonic, 481
  torsion, 78, 408

EMG, *see* Electromyogram
ET, *see* Tremor, essential

Electromyogram, 59, 61–62, 65, 129–130,
      139–146, 148, 367, 373, 394
  needle, 32
  in Parkinson's disease, 299
  in physiological tremor, 389, 391
  surface, 32, 58
  tremor analysis by, 35, 59, 137–138
Electrotonic coupling, 171
Enhanced physiological tremor, *see* Tremor,
      physiological, enhanced
Ephedrine, 20, 90
Epinephrine (adrenaline), 49, 52, 85, 87, 89,
      129, 246, 255
Ergot alkaloids, 333–335
  see also Dopamine
Essential tremor, *see* Tremor, essential
Ethanol, 86, 88–89
Extrapyramidal disease, 4

Feedback, 48, 69
Festinant gate, 287
  see also Scelotyrbe festinans
Fibres
  corticopontine, 109
  GAB-ergic, 109
  serotonergic, 109
  vestibular, 109
  see also Muscle fibre
Force recordings, 29
Force tremor spectra, 31, 139–140
Forel, field of, 96, 341
Fourier transform, 18
Fourier's theorem, 18
Frequency analysis, 32, 74
Frequency domain, 18
Frequency modulation, 42
Friedreich's ataxia, 113, 378, 383
Froment's sign, 219, 222, 301, 481, 484

GABA, *see* Gamma-aminobutyric acid
GAB-ergic fibres, 109
Gamma-aminobutyric acid, 97–98, 102, 117,
      280, 361, 380, 383, 417
Gating mechanisms, inhibitory, 409–412
Globus pallidus, 96
Glutamic acid decarboxylase, 307
Golgi tendon organ, 137, 151
Goniometric transducers, 17, 127
Guillain-Barré-Strohl syndrome, 393–395,
      399
  peripheral neuropathy in, 60

HMSN, *see* Hereditary motor and sensory
      neuropathy
HRP, *see* Peroxidase, horseradish

Harmaline, 49, 71, 170, 183, 187–189, 191–192, 299, 311, 457
  tremor, 171–172, 176, 186, 455
Harmine, 457
Henneman, size principle of, 42
Hereditary motor and sensory neuropathy, 392, 400, 402–403
  Roussy–Levy syndrome in, 400
  see also Peripheral neuropathy
Hereditary system degeneration, 113
  see also Friedreich's ataxia
Herring's law, 414
Histochemistry, 97
Homovanillic acid, 306–307
Hospital Inpatient Activities Analysis, 3
Huntington's chorea, 3, 116–117, 378
4-Hydroxypropranolol, 232
5-Hydroxytryptamine, 307, 310–311, 316
5-Hydroxytryptophan, 86, 89
L-5 Hydroxytryptophan, 381
Hyoscine, 22, 426–427
Hypertension, 103
Hypoglycaemia, 54, 89
Hypokinesia, 219

ICD9, *see* Ninth International Statistical Classification of Diseases, Injuries and Causes of Death
Ibogaline, 183
Idiopathic torsion dystonia, 67
Imidazole, 380
Inferior olive, the, 25, 49, 77, 109, 167, 176, 191, 413, 423
  neurones of, 170
  synchronised rhythmic activity of, 49
Intrinsic sympathomimetic activity, 248, 251
Isoniazid, 86, 90, 380–381, 383
Isoprenaline, 49, 236
Isoproterenol, 89

Jakob–Creutzfeldt disease, 114

Kuru disease, 114

Lergotrile, 334
Lesions, cerebellar, 71, 307–313
Levodopa, 74, 85–86, 89–90, 129, 332–333
Lewy body disease, 98–99, 101, 105, 106
  see also Parkinson's disease
Lignocaine, 22–23, 426
Linear accelerometers, 17
Lipid solubility, 248, 251–252
Lisuride, 86, 334
Lithium, 77, 129

Liver failure, 116
  in Alzheimer's disease, 116
  in Parkinson's disease, 116
  in Wilson's disease, 116
Locus coeruleus, 98–100, 305, 314
Long-latency reflexes, 22, 60–61, 77
  in Parkinson's disease, 302–303
Lymphocytes, 229–230, 234, 239
  beta-adrenoceptors and, 234, 239
  in multiple sclerosis, 111

MAS, *see* Muscle activity spectrum
MSA, *see* Membrane-stabilising activity
Mechanical linear servo-systems, 45
Melanin, 99
Membrane-stabilising activity, 232, 248, 250, 261, 268
Mescaline, 451
Mesencephalic reticular formation, 410
α-Methyl-*p*-tyrosine, 71
Metoprolol, 56–57, 249, 251–253
Microneurography, 150, 157
Monoamines
  central, 451–454
  in man, 457–458
Morphine, 230, 454
Motor cortex, 69, 71, 73–74
Motor neurones, 42–45, 48, 53, 72, 129, 136–137
Motor units, 23, 27, 29–34, 42, 129, 141, 143, 467
  activity of, 32
    size principle in, 53
  dysfunction of, 35
  essential tremor, 60
  firing rates of, 30–32, 55, 197–199
  synchronisation of, 34, 43, 45, 53, 55
  twitch contractions of, 29–30, 43
Movement
  decomposition of, 377
  involuntary, 479
  tremor disorders of, 463–472, 485–486
  voluntary, 41, 479
Multiple sclerosis, 74, 90, 110–111, 348–349, 359, 381, 421, 427
  B lymphocytes in, 111
  IgG concentration in, 111
  T lymphocytes in, 111
Muscarine, 448
Muscle activity spectrum, 29–34, 136
Muscle fibre
  co-contractions of, 480
  contractions of, 28, 40
  extrafusal, 255
  intrafusal, 49, 255
  tetanic function of, 41–42, 45, 49
  unfused, 28

Muscle spindles, 45–46, 48, 53–54, 128, 133, 137, 197, 200, 227, 255, 390
  clonus of, 157–164
  discharge patterns of, 157–164
  input of, 53
  in Parkinson's disease, 203
  passive movement in, 158–160
  pathways of, 53
  primary, 55
  tremor discharge in, 157–164
  voluntary movements in, 157–158
Muscular dystrophy, 32–33
Myoclonus, 3, 16, 481
  action, 481
  asterixis and, 464–466
  dystonic, 481
  ocular, 421–428
  oculopalatal, 24
  oculopalatal-diaphragmatic, 22
  palatal, 365, 483
  palatal-diaphragmatic, 167–173
  rhythmical, 24, 433–435, 481
  startle, 15, 24
  stimulus-sensitive, 481
  see also Motor neurones
Myopathy, 32–33
Myxoedema, 40

Naphthalene, chronic intoxication by, 441–442
Neurones
  of inferior olives, 170
  noradrenergic, 256
  pause, 412
  thalamic, 74
  tonic, 411
  see also Motor neurones
Neuropathy
  in Charcot-Marie-Tooth disease, 133
  tremor in, 67, 133
  see also Peripheral neuropathy
Nicotine, 448, 450
Ninth International Statistical Classification of Diseases, Injuries and Causes of Death, 3–4, 10
Nodding, *see* Tremor, head
Noradrenaline (norepinephrine), 85, 255, 316
Norepinephrine (noradrenaline), 85, 255, 316
Nystagmus, 482–483
  congenital, 484
  pendular, 421–428, 484
    acquired, 422–423, 484
    pharmacological modification of, 425–427
    tremor in, 423–427
  periodic alternating, 416–417
  voluntary, 412

Ocular flutter, 412, 483
Ocular myoclonus, 421–428
Ocular tremor, *see* Tremor, ocular
Olivary cells, 184
  see also Inferior olive
Olivo–ponto–cerebellar atrophy, 103–104, 378
Opiate receptors, 454
Opsoclonus, 412, 483
Oscillations
  of central nervous system, 476
  saccadic, 412–414
  thalamic, 173–175
Oscillatory myoclonus, *see* Myoclonus, rhythmical
Oubaine, 426
Oxotremorine, 450

PAN, *see* Periodic alternating nystagmus
Paralysis
  by curare, 72
  by gallamine, 72
  in spasticity, 4
Paralysis agitans, 3, 4, 98, 285, 292
  see also Parkinson's disease
Paraproteinaemic neuropathy, 400–402
Paresis, 32
Parkinson, James, 285–289
Parkinsonian syndrome, *see* Parkinson's disease
Parkinsonism, *see* Parkinson's disease
Parkinson's disease, 4, 87, 98, 109, 117, 163–164, 217, 219, 221, 223, 245, 283–352, 468, 475, 484
  'arteriosclerotic parkinsonism', 103
  cerebrovascular disease in, 103
  clonus in, 68, 78
  dementia complex in, 105, 108, 292
  electromyography in, 299
  frequency spectra in, 298, 299
  general aspects of, 1–124
  idiopathic, 11–12, 98–102, 108, 285, 292
  liver failure in, 116
  long-latency reflex in, 302–303
  multiple system atrophy in, 103–104
  muscle spindles in, 203
  neurophysiology of tremors in, 125–204
  origins of tremors in, 67–74
  post-encephalitic, 98, 102, 106–108, 282
  tremor in, 22, 58, 63–64, 67–69, 72–74, 76–78, 85–90, 132, 177, 189, 192, 200, 221, 246–247, 283–352, 435–436, 467–468
    animal models of, 183–194
    essential, 60, 64, 88
    origins of, 67–74
    short-latency reflex in, 302–303
    striatonigral degeneration in, 103–104
Pathological tremor, *see* Tremor, pathological
Pause neurones, 412

Pendular nystagmus, 421-428, 484
D-Penicillamine, 90
Pergolide, 86, 334
Periodic alternating nystagmus, 416-417
Peripheral input, 62, 74
  resetting index of, 74
Peripheral neuropathy, 23, 67
  in Charcot-Marie-Tooth disease, 67
  chronic relapsing inflammation in, 399-400
  Dejerine and Sottas disease, 67
  in Guillain-Barré-Strohl syndrome, 67
  nerve entrapment syndromes in, 395-396
  stretch reflex in, 402
  tremor in, 388-406, 441-442, 466-467
Peroxidase, horseradish, 97
Phaeochromocytoma, 54
Phenobarbitone, 77, 273, 276, 279-280
Phenothiazines, 71
Phentolamine, 86
Phenylethylamines, 279, 451
Phenylethylmalonamide, 57
Phylogenesis, 24
Physiological tremor, see Tremor, physiological
Physostigmine, 378
Pick's bodies, 106
Piezoelectric accelerometer, 127
Pindolol, 249, 251
Piribedil, 335
Polyneuropathy, 46
Pontine reticular formation, 410
Postural tremor, see Tremor, postural
Power spectra, 27-28, 30, 34
Primidone, 24, 57, 77, 271-282
Progressive multifocal leucoencephalopathy, 114
Propranolol, 49, 52, 57, 60-61, 85, 88-89, 133, 227, 231, 246-253, 271, 400
  D-, 261-269
  D,L-, 261-269
  in essential tremor, 261-270
  4-hydroxy-, 232
  plasma levels of, 57, 248
  therapy by, 246-248
Purkinje cells, 167, 169, 171, 184, 191

Ramsay-Hunt syndrome, 378
Reciprocal activation, 484
Recruitment threshold, 43
Reflexes
  long-latency, 22, 60-61, 77
  in Parkinson's disease, 22, 60-61, 77, 302-303
  segmental, 135-155
    mechanisms of, 150
  short-latency, 302-303
  stretch, 19, 45-48, 77, 129-131, 133, 137 160, 162

Refsum's disease, 395
  see also Peripheral neuropathy
Relaxation time, 40
Reserpine, 71, 91
Rest tremor, see Tremor, rest
Reticular formation
  mesencephalic, 410
  pontine, 410
Rigidity, 484
  reinforced, 484
Roussy-Levy syndrome, 400
Rubral systems
  of brain, 71
  tremors of, 22-23, 75-78, 95, 359, 484
Rubro-olivo-cerebello-rubral loop, 311

Saccades, 410
  horizontal, 410
  vertical, 410
Saccadic burst cells, 410, 412
Saccadic oscillation
  macrosaccadic, 413-414
  microsaccadic, 412
Saccadic pulse generator, 410
Scelotyrbe festinans, 287,
  see also Festinant gait
Schottky barrier photodetector, 17
Sedatives, 89
Senile dementia, 106
Sensory ataxia, 389
Serotonergic fibres, 109
Serotonin, 455-457
Servo-loop mechanisms, 202
Short-latency reflexes, in Parkinson's disease, 302-303
Shy-Drager syndrome, 104-105
Sinemet, 347
Sodium valproate, 380
Sotalol, 57, 249-250, 253, 255
Spasm, 4
  see also Tremor
Spasticity, 485
  clonus in, 60
  paralysis in, 4
Spectral analysis, 18-21, 35, 138, 195
  coherence function in, 19
  total power content in, 19
  tremor and, 18-21
  velocity spectrum in, 19
Spinal cord, 69
Spinocerebellar degeneration, 381
Stereotactic surgery, 72, 75, 85, 96, 133
  in Parkinson's disease, 340, 342-346
  for tremor, 340, 342-346
Stretch reflexes, 19, 45-48, 77, 129-131, 133, 137, 160, 162
  long-latency, 60-61, 77
  peripheral neuropathy in, 402
  in physiological tremor, 45-48

Stretch reflexes (*cont'd*)
  segmental, 141, 157
  spinal, 48, 60, 77
  transcortical, 137
Stroop task, 323
Substantia nigra, 71, 76, 99–100
Sympathomimetrics, 77
Synchronisation
  central, 135–136
  input, 196, 198, 200
  long-term, 135, 141–143, 149–151, 197
  mechanisms of, 196–197
  of motor units, 34, 43, 45, 53, 55
  of physiological tremor, 128, 195
  short-term, 135–136, 196, 200

Tabes dorsalis, 46
Terbutaline, 89
Thalamotomy, 246, 348, 361
Thalamus, the, 177, 340, 345
  essential tremor in, 64, 71
  mechanism of, 189–190
  neurones of, 74
  nuclei of, 340
  oscillation of, 173–175
  rhythmic activity of, 78
  tumour of, 22
Thyrotoxicosis, 41, 54, 89, 228
Tics, *see* Tremor
Timolol, 249–250
Tocainide, 427
Tone, 485
Tonic neurones, 411
Torticollis, 208
  spasmodic, 432
Tremogens, 446, 449–450, 456–458
  cholines, 449–451
  muscarinic, 445, 448–449
  nicotinic, 445, 448–449
Tremor
  action, 23, 67–68, 78, 88, 90, 108–117, 295,
    301–302, 355–356, 358, 393, 485–486
    in Wilson's disease, 200
    in alcoholism, 54
  amplitude of, 15, 24
  analysis of, 27–35
    diagnosis by, 27–35
    by electromyogram, 35, 59, 137–138
  animal models of, 16, 183–194
  ataxic, 22, 177, 358
  atypical, 431–436
  cerebellar, 22, 74–76, 86, 95, 115, 183–189,
    353–386
    clinical aspects of, 355–363
    motor control in, 365–376
    treatment of, 377–386
  characteristics of, 15
  cholinergic, 313–315, 445, 447–451

classification of, 3–13, 37
  by appearance, 37–38
  by cause, 38
coactus, 286
cogwheel, 23, 68, 78, 219, 295
    301–302, 480
  in Parkinson's disease, 222
  rigidity, 219, 222
  definition of, 485
  drug-induced, 86–90, 247, 445–462
  dystonic, 431–435
  essential, 3–4, 24, 55–67, 88–90, 95, 118,
    191, 200, 205–283, 359, 391–392,
    400, 403, 432, 468–469
    age distribution of, 215–216
    amplitude of, 233
    animal models of, 183–194
    benign, 3–6, 10–11, 57, 65, 347–348
    beta-adrenoceptors in, 225–260
    beta-blockers in, 56
    classical, 56, 58
    diagnosis of, 219–224
    epidemiology of, 211–218
    frequency of, 60, 220, 233, 245
    in hemiplegia, 64
    mechanisms of, 58–66
    normal recruitment order in, 60
    in Parkinson's disease, 60, 64, 88
    pharmacology of, 56–57
    phase resetting index of, 246
    phenobarbitone and, 57
    prevalence of, 207, 213–216
    primidone in, 271–282
    propranolol in, 261–270
    severe, 66–67
    sex distribution of, 216
    in single motor units, 60
    symptomatic, 67
    thalamic, 67, 71
    type I, 233–235
    type II, 233–235
  in exercise, 54
  experimental resting, 69–72
  familial, 3–4
  family history of, 56
  'fatigue', 54, 132, 161
  frequency of, 15, 21–24, 47
  harmaline, 171–172, 176, 186, 455
  head, 58, 481–482
  hereditary chin, 439–440
  hyperkinetic, 365, 372
  hysterical, 437–439
  in infectious disease, 113–115
  initial, 485
  intention, 67, 75–76, 177, 200, 356,
    358–360, 399, 441–442, 445, 486
  juvenile, 56
  kinetic, 56, 67–68, 75, 358, 365, 371, 374
  measurement of, 17
  mesencephalic, 23

Tremor (*cont'd*)
movement, 463–472, 485–486
muscle spindle discharge in, 157–164
neuropathic, 67, 133
neurophysiology of, 125–204
normal, 37–84
observation of, 16
ocular, 407–428, 483
adaptive control in, 413–417
mechanisms of, 409–420
see also Nystagmus
olivo-cerebellar, 183–189
and ontogeny, 473–478
paroxysmal, 440–441
in Parkinson's disease, 22, 58, 63–64,
67–69, 72–74, 76–78, 85–90, 132,
177, 189, 192, 200, 221, 246–247,
283–352, 435–436, 467–468
animal models of, 183–194
origins of, 67–74
stereotactic surgery for, 340, 342–346
treatment of, 331–352
passive transmission in, 21
pathological, 27, 37–84, 95–123, 200–201,
247, 483
periodicity of, 15
in peripheral neuropathy, 388–406, 441–442,
466–467
pharmacological differentiation of, 85–93
physiological, 28, 37–53, 55, 77–78, 86,
90, 127–155, 160–161, 165–182,
195, 197, 200, 226, 233, 246–247,
401, 463, 469, 484
alpha rhythm and, 49
animal models of, 183–194
anxiety and, 232
causes of, 38, 53
electromyogram in, 389, 391
enhanced, 23, 27, 53–58, 68, 77, 88–89,
95, 127–134, 162, 172, 214, 225–231,
233, 301, 390, 446, 463, 468, 480
frequency of, 127
in fright, 54
mechanical factors in, 41, 135, 143–144
in peripheral neuropathy, 389–391
pharmacological influences on, 50–52
spike-triggered averaging of, 140–141
stretch reflex and, 45–48
supraspinal influences on, 49–53
synchronisation of, 128
vision and, 49–51, 77
postural, 6–7, 11, 16, 23, 55–56, 67–68,
78, 219–220, 295, 297–302, 356–357,
359–360, 365, 374, 400, 485
primary writing, 56, 58, 436–437
rare, 436–440

rate of, 195–204
rest, 6, 16, 23, 69, 74, 95–108, 183–194,
295–296, 299–300, 302, 321–329,
357, 399, 485
rubral, 22–23, 75–76, 78, 95, 359, 484
senile, 56
spectral analysis and, 18–21
static, 356, 358, 485
terminal, 358, 485
terminology of, 5, 15–16
titubation, 75, 78
transduction of, 17
transition, 485
traumatic, 103, 113, 348
undiagnosed, 440–442
in vascular disease, 112–113
voice, 88
waveform of, 15
Tremorine, 314, 450
Tricyclic antidepressants, 129
L-Tryptophan, 383
Tumours, cerebellar, 90

Vce, *see* Ventralis caudalis externus
Vci, *see* Ventralis caudalis internus
Vim, *see* Ventralis intermedius
VL, *see* Ventralis lateralis
Vop, *see* Ventralis oralis posterior
Valproic acid, 381
Ventralis caudalis externus, 341
Ventralis caudalis internus, 341
Ventralis intermedius, 340–341
nucleus of, 66, 71–73
stereotactic, 66
Ventralis lateralis, 72, 340
Ventralis oralis posterior, 340
Ventrolateral nucleus, 95
Ventrolateral thalamus, 71–73
Ventromedial tegmentum, 16, 70–71, 73,
307–313
Vestibular fibres, 109
Visualisation, fluorescent, 97
Voluntary nystagmus, 412

WHO, *see* World Health Organization
Waveform analysis, 18
Wilson's disease, 90, 359
action tremor in, 200
liver failure in, 116
World Health Organization, 3

Xanthines, 129, 228